Egan's fundamentals of
RESPIRATORY THERAPY

Egan's fundamentals of
RESPIRATORY THERAPY

Edited and revised by

CHARLES B. SPEARMAN, B.S., R.R.T.

Instructor, Department of Respiratory Therapy,
School of Allied Health Professions, Loma Linda University,
Loma Linda, California

RICHARD L. SHELDON, M.D., F.C.C.P.

Associate Professor of Medicine, School of Medicine,
Loma Linda University; Chief, Section of Pulmonary and Intensive Care Medicine,
School of Medicine, Loma Linda University and Loma Linda University
Medical Center; Medical Director, Department of Respiratory Therapy,
School of Allied Health Professions, Loma Linda University,
Loma Linda, California

Previous editions by

DONALD F. EGAN, M.D.

Chief, Pulmonary Disease Section,
Veteran's Administration Medical Center,
Asheville, North Carolina

FOURTH EDITION

with 5 contributors

with 150 illustrations

The C. V. Mosby Company

ST. LOUIS · TORONTO · LONDON   1982

MOSBY

A TRADITION OF PUBLISHING EXCELLENCE

Editor: Don Ladig
Assistant editor: Rosa Kasper
Manuscript editor: Terry Young
Book design: Jeanne Bush
Cover design: Diane Beasley
Production: Barbara Merritt

FOURTH EDITION

The C.V. Mosby Company
11830 Westline Industrial Drive, St. Louis, Missouri 63141

Library of Congress Cataloging in Publication Data

Egan, Donald F., 1916-
  Egan's Fundamentals of respiratory therapy.

  Includes bibliographical references and index.
  1. Respiratory therapy.   I. Spearman, Charles B.
II. Sheldon, Richard L.   III. Title.   IV. Title:
Fundamentals of respiratory therapy.   [DNLM:
1. Respiratory therapy.   WB 342 E28f]
RM161.E37 1982   615.8'36   82-3629
ISBN 0-8016-1504-6   AACR2

C/VH/VH 9 8 7 6 5 4 3 2 1   02/B/223

To

Dr. Donald F. Egan

for all that he has done and

to **our families**

for all they have helped us do

Contributors

DAVID H. DAIL, M.D.

Department of Pathology, The Mason Clinic,
Seattle, Washington

RICHARD D. DUNBAR, M.D.

Associate Professor of Radiology, Chief, Chest Radiology, School of Medicine,
Loma Linda University, Loma Linda, California

PATRICK M. McDONALD, R.R.T.

Technical Director, Respiratory Therapy Services,
Donald N. Sharp Memorial Community Hospital, Pulmonary Center,
San Diego, California

JAMES A. PETERS, D.H.Sc., M.P.H., R.R.T.

Chairman, Department of Respiratory Therapy; Co-Director, Human
Performance Lab, School of Allied Health Professions,
Loma Linda University, Loma Linda, California

JOHN W. YOUTSEY, Ph.D., R.R.T.

Associate Professor and Chairman, Department of Respiratory Therapy,
College of Health Science, Georgia State University, Atlanta, Georgia

Preface

In a rapidly changing world, traditions are hard to come by, especially within a new profession. This book was first written in 1969 for a new group of professionals who were then, as they are now, facing a world of rapidly changing technology and techniques. Problems regarding relationships to other professional groups within the health care delivery system arose. Dr. Donald F. Egan was the first to write a book dealing with the educational needs of allied health personnel in a new discipline, "inhalation therapy." He thereby started a tradition of educational growth within a new profession, and his success as a writer and educator did much to promote its growth. This growth continued at such a rapid rate that the name "inhalation therapy" was viewed as too restrictive, so "respiratory therapy" was substituted.

The title of this book has been changed to *Egan's Fundamentals of Respiratory Therapy* to reflect the continuation of this tradition started by Dr. Egan. It is the purpose of this new edition to reflect growth while carefully preserving fundamentals, to point out new areas of knowledge and technique and yet keep a firm hold on the basics. Tradition can serve to either facilitate or enslave a system. It is a way of allowing a new generation to stand on the shoulders of the preceding generation to see new sights and think new thoughts. A new generation of respiratory care professionals utilizing this edition will see new sights and think new thoughts and thereby stabilize a young and vigorous tradition for the next generation.

Like its predecessors, this edition is intended primarily for students of respiratory therapy and as a review source for practicing therapists and technicians. We have also tried to maintain the text's usefulness for physicians, house staff, and nursing personnel who are involved with patients requiring respiratory care. New chapters have been added to provide fundamental information about respiratory anatomy and basic pulmonary function tests and to give a systematic approach to viewing the chest x-ray. The section on pharmacology has been removed from the chapter on aerosol therapy and has been expanded into a new chapter. Four authors have joined us in these efforts, and a fifth has contributed by updating the chapter concerning the management aspects of a respiratory care department. To each of these contributors we extend our appreciation.

Much of the new information provided in this edition will be found in Chapters 3, 5, 9, and 11 and in chapters involved in the clinical application of respiratory therapy (Chapters 10 through 16).

Other chapters from the previous editions remain, with a variety of changes, from minor additions and deletions to major rewriting and updating. In all of these chapters, any changes were made in hopes of maintaining the intent that prevailed in the first three editions.

Many of the therapeutic modalities used in respiratory care continue to be questioned and a scientific basis for their use is still being sought. We have tried to reflect these controversies appropriately by discussing what is known currently, what remains to be proved, and what is reasonable clinical use of these therapies until new insights into them are gained. New references have been liberally added and, where they seemed more suitable, bibliographies have been placed at the end of each chapter to facilitate their accessibility. This text remains an introductory source and the reader is therefore encouraged to make full use of the references to further his or her knowledge.

A special thanks is in order to the following individuals for their efforts: Howard Sanders, Bob and Kris Wilkins, Gary and Cynthia Euler, Pauline Spearman, and Doreen Haberkorn for critiquing and helping during proof-reading of the text; Jo Christensen for assistance with editing; and Debbie Matook, Viki Kappel, Gay Jacobsen, Helene Crawford, and Esther Alexander for their long hours of typing and other secretarial duties.

Bud Spearman
Dick Sheldon

Contents

Egan's fundamentals of
RESPIRATORY THERAPY

Chapter 1

Gases, the atmosphere, and the gas laws

A gas, which cannot be seen or felt and has no inherent boundaries, invokes an impression of nothingness until we become aware of the tremendous activity and flexibility of its components. It can be compressed, can expand, and can produce heat. It can cool and can be liquefied. From its behavior, we can infer that a gas consists of mostly empty space, and we consider in this chapter the relationship between this space and the gas molecules.

Mobility of gases   All matter is composed of *atoms,* the characteristics of which differentiate the many different elements. In a chemical reaction these atoms can combine with identical atoms or with completely different atoms. They may separate or regroup into entirely different combinations. Compounds are made from a

1

combination of atoms, and the resulting products may possess characteristics completely different from those of the individual atoms.

The smallest particle of a substance that retains all of its properties is referred to as a *molecule*. A molecule may consist of one or more atoms. A chemical formula indicates the number of atoms in each molecule of a particular substance. For example, two hydrogen atoms and one oxygen atom make up one molecule of water (H_2O). The term *gram molecular weight* (gmw) is frequently used in chemistry and is the amount in grams equal to the molecular weight of a substance, or the sum of all the atomic weights in its molecular formula.

For example, carbon dioxide (CO_2) has one carbon and two oxygen atoms, with a total atomic weight of $12 + 16 + 16 = 44$. Therefore, the gmw of carbon dioxide is 44 g.

However, not all substances have true molecular structures, depending on the type of bonding that holds the atoms together. Those classified as *ionic compounds* are essentially mixtures of fixed proportions of minute electrically charged particles called ions, without any basic molecular structure. Atomic bonding and further details of ions are discussed in Chapter 2. Because the expression gram molecular weight is inappropriate for ionic compounds, we speak of *gram formula weight* (gfw), which has the same meaning and is calculated in the same manner as gram molecular weight. Either molecular weight or formula weight can properly be used for substances that form molecules, but only formula weight is acceptable for ionic compounds.[1]

Gases, the primary concern of this text, consist of molecules and will be discussed in terms of *molecules* and *gram molecular weights*. *Gram formula weights* are used with all other substances.

Summarizing to this point, gases consist of aggregates of small molecular particles in constant motion, and this motion is called *kinetic activity*. The density of these molecules and the amount of kinetic activity are what separate gases from solids and liquids, solids having the highest density and the least kinetic activity and liquids falling between solids and gases. However, it should not be assumed that the atoms or molecules of solids cannot move. They respond to vibration, bending, stretching, and temperature.

Gaseous molecules range in size from 10^{-8} to 10^{-7} cm in diameter, with weights varying from 10^{-23} to 10^{-20} g. Kinetic theory tells us that these particles are in *constant rapid* motion, following completely random paths and that their speed is phenomenal. Hydrogen particles move 1.84×10^5 cm/sec (greater than 1 mile/second), and oxygen 4.6×10^4 cm/sec ($^1/_3$ mile/second).[2]

During this intense activity, the particles collide with one another and with the surface of enclosing containers. The average number of collisions per second for each molecule of hydrogen is 1×10^{10}, for oxygen 4.6×10^9, and for carbon dioxide 6.2×10^9. The *mean free path* of gas molecules describes the average distance traveled by the molecules between collisions. For hydrogen, this distance is 1.66×10^{-5} cm, for oxygen 8.8×10^{-6} cm, and for carbon dioxide 5.8×10^{-6} cm.[3] Very fine particles of an insoluble substance such as carbon or metal dust, suspended in water and viewed under a microscope, can be seen to move about in an erratic random manner. This is called *brownian movement* and is produced by the kinetic activity of water molecules striking the suspended material.

To view the phenomenon of kinetic activity in familiar quantitative terms, let us imagine oxygen molecules in a pure sample of that gas to be the size of Ping-Pong balls. We can imagine large numbers bouncing off walls, the ceiling, the floor, and one another, never stopping and never settling to the floor. Considering the relative sizes of oxygen molecules to Ping-Pong balls, the mean free path, and the average number of collisions of the molecules, the Ping-Pong balls would travel an average distance of 40 feet between collisions. This gives us some concept of the great distance between molecules in relation to their size as well as the mass of "nothingness" that makes up a gas.

Pressure and temperature of gases

All gases exert pressure, whether they are free in the atmosphere, enclosed in a container, or dissolved in a liquid such as blood. In physiology, this pressure is frequently called the *tension* of a gas. Gas pressure is dependent on molecular kinetic activity and is the result of molecular bombardment on any confining surface, whether it is a steel cylinder or the earth's surface. We may consider such pressure as the striking force of molecules attempting to escape. In addition, the force of the earth's gravity, by its effect on the molecular masses of the gas, affects gas pressure. Therefore, in a container of gas, although the travel of molecules is random in all directions, pressure in the bottom of the vessel is somewhat higher because the density and frequency of collision are aided by gravity.

The amount of pressure exerted by a gas depends on the *number* of particles present and the *frequency* of their collisions. The frequency is related to the *velocity* of the gas particles since the greater the speed of travel, the greater the number of collisions per unit of time, the greater the energy of collisions, and also the greater the gas tension.

Gas particle velocity, however, is not a constant value but is directly related to gas temperature. As temperature rises, the kinetic activity increases, molecular collisions increase, and the pressure of the gas rises. Conversely, when temperatures drop, molecular activity declines, particle velocity and collision frequency drop, and pressure is lowered. An example of the relationship between gas tension and temperature is the increase in automobile tire pressure while driving on a hot pavement. This relationship between molecular activity and temperature can be more graphically illustrated by a special temperature scale, which the student will put to practical use when the gas laws are studied. But first it is important to describe the concept of *absolute temperature* and the two subscales by which it is calibrated.

The temperature at which all molecular activity ceases is a theoretic value arrived at by projection and calculation. While researchers have come close to approximating that value, it has never been achieved. If we are interested in the relative kinetic behavior of gases at various temperatures, a point of no activity produces a logical zero on which to build a scale. This is called *absolute zero* (0°_{abs}) and it is the origin of the absolute temperature scale. If it is calibrated in Celsius temperature units, it is called the *Kelvin scale* (K), and if in Fahrenheit units, the *Rankine scale* (R).

Kelvin scale

In Celsius units, molecular activity stops at about -273°C. Therefore 0°K $= -273^\circ$C, and 0°C $= 273^\circ$K, since 0°C is 273 temperature units above 0°K. When used as symbols in formulas, Celsius temperatures are often designated by a small t, and absolute temperatures by a capital T or a K. A simple equation to keep in mind is:

$$^\circ K = {^\circ}t + 273$$

Therefore, to convert Celsius degrees to Kelvin, add 273. For example:

$$25^\circ C = 25 + 273 = 298^\circ K$$
$$37^\circ C = 37 + 273 = 310^\circ K$$
$$-15^\circ C = -15 + 273 = 258^\circ K$$

Rankine scale

Used frequently in engineering but rarely in medical science, the Rankine scale is based on Fahrenheit units. Since -273°C $= -460^\circ$F (refer to formulas to convert between Celsius and Fahrenheit scales), then 0°R $= -460^\circ$F, and $^\circ$R $= {^\circ}$F $+ 460$. Fig. 1-1 is a scalar representation of the relationship between gaseous kinetic activity, or pressure, and five commonly used temperatures of the four related scales.

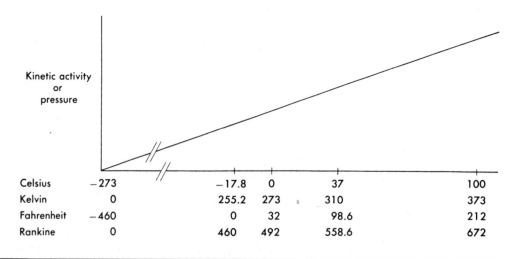

Kinetic activity or pressure

Celsius	-273	-17.8	0	37	100
Kelvin	0	255.2	273	310	373
Fahrenheit	-460	0	32	98.6	212
Rankine	0	460	492	558.6	672

Fig. 1-1   Linear relationship between gas molecular activity, or pressure, and temperature. Comparable readings of the four scales are indicated for five temperature points.

Compression   Because of the relatively great distances between molecules, gases possess the quality of *compressibility*. When pressure is exerted on a gas, the molecules are pushed closer together, and their intervening spaces are narrowed. On the other hand, if the container of a volume of gas enlarges, the gas *expands* to accommodate the new volume, and its molecules spread further apart. Fig. 1-2 illustrates the relationship between compression and expansion of a given mass of gas molecules and corresponding temperatures and pressure changes. Because the tremendous energy of molecular collision is expended as heat, compression of a gas produces *heat* as well as a buildup of pressure among the molecules. As compression brings the molecules closer together, the frequency of collisions increases, and both heat and pressure increase. Thus the heat of compression may be considered as a means of dissipating the great increase in kinetic energy that accompanies compression. Conversely, the expansion of a gas produces a drop in temperature as molecular collision frequency decreases. Cooling of expansion is used in refrigeration systems and is part of the natural phenomenon of cooling through the expansion of gases.

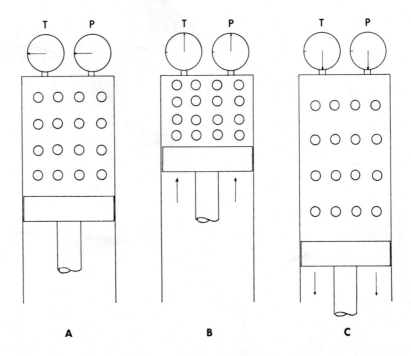

Fig. 1-2   A mass of gas in the resting state exerts a given pressure at a given temperature, in cylinder **A.** In **B,** as the piston compresses the gas, the molecules are crowded closer together, and the increased energy of molecular collisions is reflected in a rise of both temperature and pressure. Conversely, retraction of the piston in **C** allows the gas to expand, and temperature and pressure drop as molecular interaction decreases.

Molar volume of gases

One of the major principles of physics and chemistry is *Avogadro's law,* named after Italian chemist and physicist Count Amadeo Avogadro (1776-1856). This principle tells us that equal volumes of all gases at the same temperature and pressure contain the same number of molecules or, conversely, that at constant temperature and pressure, equal numbers of molecules of all gases occupy the same volume. Further, it has been established that the weights of all atoms in grams corresponding to their atomic weights, the weights of all molecules in grams corresponding to their molecular weights, and the weights of ions of all nonmolecular compounds in grams corresponding to the formula weights on the compounds always contain the same number of particles, 6.02×10^{23}. This is known as *Avogadro's number.* Although these quantities are often referred to as "gram atomic weights," "gram molecular weights," and "gram formula weights," they are each also technically known as a *mole.* A mole is any quantity of matter that contains 6.02×10^{23} atoms, molecules, or ions. Later we discuss physiologically active substances in concentrations so small that it is more convenient to refer to them in terms of *thousandths of a mole,* or *millimoles* (mM). Just as moles are the weights of substances in grams that are equal to atomic weights (gaw), molecular weights (gmw), or formula weights (gfw), millimoles are the weights of substances expressed in milligrams that are equal to atomic weights (mgaw), molecular weights (mgmw), or formula weights (mgfw).

The volume occupied by 1 mole of gas (1 gmw; 6.02×10^{23} molecules) is the *molar volume.* It allows us to calculate densities of gases and gas mixtures and to convert values for dissolved gases from volumes percent to moles per liter, a topic that is considered in detail later. It is customary, for the sake of uniformity in comparing values, to measure molar volumes under what are termed *standard conditions,* a temperature of 0°C and an ambient pressure of 1 atmosphere (atm). This is an artificial situation, however, since we do not

Table 1-1
Molar volume of selected gases under standard conditions

Gas	Symbol	Molar volume (liters)
"Ideal gas"		22.414
Ammonia	NH_3	22.094
Carbon dioxide	CO_2	22.262
Carbon monoxide	CO	22.402
Chlorine	Cl_2	22.063
Helium	He	22.426
Hydrogen	H_2	22.430
Hydrogen chloride	HCl	22.248
Nitrogen	N_2	22.402
Oxygen	O_2	22.393
Sulfur dioxide	SO_2	21.888

Modified from Pimental, G.C., editor: Chemistry, an experimental science, San Francisco, 1963, W.H. Freeman & Co., Publishers.

ordinarily handle gases in an environment of 0°C. When molar volumes are measured under common ambient conditions and then calculated to what they would be at standard conditions (a technique known as "correcting a gas volume"), we find that the natural intermolecular behavior of each gas causes its molar volume to deviate from the universal low-pressure value. Table 1-1 compares molar volumes of several gases corrected from ambient to standard or measured directly at standard conditions.

If students refer to the subject of molar gas volumes in the average chemistry textbook, they will probably find only the value 22.3 ℓ/mole given for all gases. Actually, for most purposes this is adequate, and we see in Table 1-1 that it is representative of the molar volumes of oxygen, nitrogen, and carbon monoxide, gases with which we will be concerned as we continue our study. Even carbon dioxide, a most important respiratory gas, has a value rounded off to 22.3 ℓ/mole, close to the universal normal. In summary, under standard conditions of a temperature at 0°C and a pressure of 1 atm, moles of all gases occupy 22.4 ℓ. In this test, the only exception is in a calculation involving carbon dioxide (p. 216), where the molar volume used for that gas is the more accurate one of 22.3 ℓ.

Density of gases

In considering the density of gases, certain definitions must be made clear, specifically the terms *mass, weight,* and *density.*

The term *mass* refers to the substance of an object, the quantity of matter it contains, and the number and nature of its molecules. It is characterized by inertia and is subject to the pull of gravity. *Weight* is the gravitational pull of the earth on a body. Therefore, the greater the mass, the greater the weight. Mass is proportional to weight and is measured in units against such standards as the kilogram and the pound. Weight varies with the position of mass relative to the surface of the earth, decreasing both toward the earth's center and away from its surface. The *inertia* of a body, that quality of mass that requires force to start it in motion from a resting state or to change its velocity once in motion, remains unchanged no matter where it is located.

Density may be defined as the amount of mass per unit volume of a body, the concentration of its molecules. It is usually used as *weight density.* Therefore, density is the *weight of a body per unit volume* and in our field of interest is most often described in grams per cubic centimeter (g/cc) for solids and liquids and in grams per liter (g/ℓ) for gases. Other units, such as pounds per cubic foot, can also be used. An example of figuring density would be a mass weighing 15 g and measuring 3 cc, which would have a density of 5 g/cc. A ton of feathers and a ton of bricks weigh the same, but the obvious difference is the volumes of the two because of their widely differing densities.

Specific gravity is a variation of density measurement where the density of

Table 1-2
Examples of gas
densities (D) under
standard conditions

$$D\ O_2 = \frac{gmw}{22.4} = \frac{32}{22.4} = 1.43\ g/\ell \qquad D\ He = \frac{gmw}{22.4} = \frac{4}{22.4} = 0.1785\ g/\ell$$

$$D\ N_2 = \frac{gmw}{22.4} = \frac{28}{22.4} = 1.25\ g/\ell \qquad D\ CO_2 = \frac{gmw}{22.4} = \frac{44}{22.4} = 1.965\ g/\ell$$

solids and liquids is calibrated against the density of water, and gases calibrated against oxygen or hydrogen. A liquid with the specific gravity of 1.5, for example, has a density $1\frac{1}{2}$ times that of water. Specific gravity values of gases play a negligible role in pulmonary physiology, but gas densities are of great importance.

Since density equals weight divided by volume, the density of any gas can readily be calculated by dividing its *gram molecular weight* by the universal molar volume of 22.4 ℓ. The quotient is expressed as *grams per liter*. Examples of gas densities are shown in Table 1-2.

Densities of gas mixtures are easily calculated if the percentage composition of the mixture is known. Given the following mixed gases:

$$Gas\ A = 10\%$$
$$Gas\ B = 60\%$$
$$Gas\ C = 30\%$$

$$D = \frac{(0.10 \times gmw\ A) + (0.60 \times gmw\ B) + (0.30 \times gmw\ C)}{22.4}$$

Calculate the density of a mixture of 30% hydrogen bromide (HBr) and 70% ethylene (C_2H_4):

$$D = \frac{(0.3 \times 81) + (0.7 \times 28)}{22.4} = \frac{43.9}{22.4} = 1.955\ g/\ell$$

Exercise 1-1: Calculate densities of the following, rounding off at three decimal places:
A. C_2H_2 (acetylene)
B. NH_3 (ammonia)
C. SiF_4 (silicon fluoride)
D. CO (carbon monoxide)
E. SO_2 (sulfur dioxide)
F. 5% CO_2 + 95% O_2
G. 80% He + 20% O_2
H. 70% He + 30% O_2
I. 25% CH_4 + 75% C_4H_{10}
J. 3% SO_2 + 15% N_2 + 82% O_2

Table 1-3	Element	Percent	
Approximate composition of the atmosphere	Nitrogen (N_2)	78.08	
	Oxygen (O_2)	20.95	
	Argon (Ar)	0.93	99.99%
	Carbon dioxide (CO_2)	0.03	
	Neon (Ne)	1.8×10^{-3}	
	Helium (He)	5.0×10^{-4}	
	Krypton (Kr)	1.0×10^{-4}	
	Hydrogen (H_2)	1.0×10^{-4}	0.01%
	Xenon (Xe)	1.0×10^{-5}	
	Ozone (O_3)	1.0×10^{-5}	
	Radon (Rn)	6.0×10^{-18}	

Table 1-4	Atmosphere	Strata	Approximate height (miles)
Summary of atmospheric divisions	Free space		Above 1200
	Outer	Exosphere	600-1200
		Ionosphere	50-600
		Stratosphere	8-50
	Inner	Troposphere	Up to 8

Composition of the atmosphere

The atmosphere on which we depend is a mixture of many gases plus water vapor. The elements composing the atmosphere are discussed later. Their approximate concentrations in the atmosphere are shown in Table 1-3.

The atmosphere is divided into two major segments, three subsegments, and several layers, each with specific physical and/or chemical properties,[4] as outlined in Table 1-4.

1. The first major segment is the *inner atmosphere,* extending from the earth's surface to an altitude of about 600 miles. It is composed of the following subsegments:
   a. The *troposphere* extends from the earth's surface to an outer border called the tropopause, an average distance of some 8 miles up but varying with the latitude of the earth. It is higher over the equator than over the poles. The troposphere is characterized by decreasing temperatures with altitude, reaching a low of approximately $-55°C$ ($-67°F$), and has considerable turbulence.
   b. The *stratosphere* continues from 8 to about 50 miles above the earth. The first layer of the stratosphere, from 8 to 15 miles up, is one of constant temperature around $-55°C$ ($-67°F$) and has little turbulence. The next layer, from 15 to 30 miles, shows an increase in temperature, reaching a high of $10°C$ ($50°F$). The third and last layer of the stratosphere, from 30 to 50 miles, has a sharp temperature drop to $-72°C$ ($-100°F$), and there is a return of turbulence. At approx-

imately 50 miles of altitude the stratopause separates the stratosphere from the next layer.

c. The *ionosphere* reaches from a distance of 50 miles outward to a distance of 600 miles. Here there are several layers of ions resulting from photochemical reactions between solar ultraviolet radiation and atmospheric molecules. The ionosphere is important as a reflector for the electromagnetic waves of radio communication. Temperatures in the ionosphere soar up to 2000°C (3600°F), but because the density of the air molecules is so low, such temperatures have little meaning in the usual concept of temperature. As with the other layers, a boundary called the ionopause delineates the end of the ionosphere.

2. The second major segment is the outer atmosphere, which is also called the *exosphere*. This region extends from the 600-mile limit to about 1200 miles from earth, where it blends with the vacuum of *free space*. In this marginal area, molecular collisions become progressively more rare.

The gravitational pull of the earth on atmospheric gas molecules produces the greatest density of molecules close to its surface, a density that decreases steadily outward to the vacuum of free space. It is speculated, however, that despite decreasing density, the percentage composition of the atmosphere, as described earlier, remains fairly constant to a height of about *60 miles*. Beyond this limit, with a decrease in mass air movement to keep the gases well mixed, the elements separate on the basis of their molecular weights. This phenomenon, called diffusion separation, disrupts the composition of the air as we know it on earth.

Measurement of air pressure	In the study of cardiopulmonary physiology and in therapy for cardiopulmonary diseases we are constantly dealing with the principles of gas pressure, and it is vitally important that students clearly understand this aspect of gas physics. Pressure is defined as a *force* applied to a specific *surface area*. This force is usually expressed as grams per square centimeter (g/cm^2) or pounds per square inch (lb/in^2 or psi). The force exerted by gases is a result of their kinetic molecular bombardment already discussed, and in a mixture of gases such as air, this force is the sum of molecular activity of all the constituent gases. If we visualize the atmospheric mantle surrounding the earth, we can understand that the molecular activity of atmospheric gases will exert a force against the surface of the earth. Many miles of atmosphere rest on the earth, exerting a force of pressure on the earth's surface. It is of physiologic as well as meteorologic importance to be able to measure the force exerted by the air on the earth.

Air pressure is measured indirectly by means of a barometer (*baros,* Greek for "weight"; *metron,* Greek for "measure"). Basically, a barometer consists of an evacuated glass tube approximately 37 inches tall with an inside diameter of 0.25 inches, closed at the top and with its lower end immersed in a reservoir of mercury in a flexible container. The pressure of the atmosphere on the

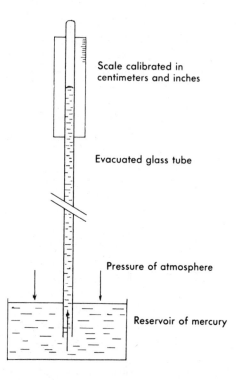

Scale calibrated in
centimeters and inches

Evacuated glass tube

Pressure of atmosphere

Reservoir of mercury

Fig. 1-3   The major components of a mercury barometer include a mercury reservoir, into which is inverted the open end of an evacuated glass tube, and a scale, by which the height of the mercury column can be read in inches and centimeters above the surface of the reservoir. The atmospheric pressure, acting on the surface of the mercury reservoir, is balanced by the weight of the column of mercury in the tube.

mercury reservoir forces the mercury up the vacuum tube, a distance above the reservoir surface relative to the atmospheric force; the height of the column of mercury in the glass tube is measured in both inches and centimeters (Fig. 1-3). This procedure balances the pressure of the atmosphere against a column of mercury in a vacuum, and if the weight per surface area of the mercury can be calculated, this value will equal the pressure of the air.

A principle of physics tells us that the *pressure* exerted by a column of fluid is equal to the height of the column times the density of the fluid. Therefore:

(1) Pressure (P) in g/cm^2 = Height in cm × Density in g/cm^3

$$P = cm \times \frac{g}{cm^3}$$

or

(2) Pressure (P) in lb/in^2 = Height in inches × Density in lb/in^3

$$P = Inches \times \frac{lb}{in^3}$$

$$= lb/in^2$$

Because of shifting air currents and the mobility of huge masses of air, atmospheric density varies over different areas of the earth's surface and is reflected in constantly changing pressures as measured at the surface. Nevertheless, it has been demonstrated that at sea level the average atmospheric pressure will support a column of mercury 76 cm (760 mm) or 29.9 inches high. If we also know that mercury has a density of 13.6 g/cm^3 (i.e., is 13.6 times as heavy as water) or 0.491 lb/in^3, then we can calculate the *atmospheric pressure* (P_B) by the formulas just given:

(1) P in g/cm^2 = 76 × 13.6 = 1034 g/cm^2

(2) P in lb/in^2 = 29.9 × 0.491 = 14.7 lb/in^2

These two values, 1034 g/cm^2 and 14.7 lb/in^2, are used as standards and are called *1 atmosphere of pressure* (1 atm). It is not necessary, however, in recording air pressure to calculate the actual g/cm^2 or lb/in^2 but only to record the height of the mercury column. Pressure might be reported as 77.2 cm (772 mm) or 30.4 inches of mercury (Hg). This means that the atmospheric pressure is of such a magnitude that it is able to hold up a column of mercury 772 mm or 30.4 inches high. This translates to actual force per surface area values of 1050 g/cm^2 and 14.9 lb/in^2.

Mercury is used as the agent for measuring the air pressure because its density is such that at ordinary pressures it assumes a height that is easy and convenient to read. It would be possible, although not practical, to construct a barometer of water. At 1 atm (76 cm Hg or 29.9 inches Hg), water, which is 13.6 times lighter than mercury, would rise to a height of *33.9 feet*. However, when very small pressures are being measured, expressing the pressure in terms of *centimeters of water* may be more convenient than in centimeters or millimeters of mercury. For example, a pressure of 2 cm Hg (20 mm Hg) is the same as 27.2 cm H_2O (2 × 13.6). A pressure gauge calibrated in centimeters of water would be easier to read than one calibrated in centimeters or millimeters of mercury. In physiologic work the student becomes accustomed to thinking and speaking in terms of both millimeters of mercury and centimeters of water. Inches of mercury or water are rarely used.

A device called an *aneroid barometer* is frequently used because of its convenient small size. It consists of a sealed evacuated metal box with a flexible, spring-supported top that responds to changes in atmospheric pressure (Fig. 1-4). Motion of its top is magnified by levers to activate a geared pointer, which indicates the pressure on a scale calibrated against a mercury barometer. Less precise than a mercury instrument, the aneroid barometer is practical for nonscientific or domestic use.

To complete the study, we should consider that method of measuring pressure that uses the *dyne*, frequently used in meterology and physics. A dyne is defined as a unit of force that, when acting on 1 g of mass, gives to the mass an *acceleration of 1 cm/sec/sec*, or 1 cm/sec^2. A freely falling 1-g mass (under the influence of gravity) will accelerate at the rate of 980.7 cm/sec for every second it falls. It therefore accelerates 980.7 cm/sec/sec, or 980.7 cm/sec^2. This can be thought of as a force of 1 g acting on itself (1 g force action on 1 g mass),

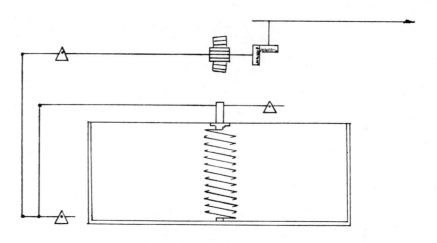

Fig. 1-4   Aneroid barometer. (See text for description.)

producing an acceleration of 980.7 cm/sec^2. Therefore an acceleration of 1 cm/sec^2 on a 1-g mass would be produced by a force of 1/980.7 g, or 1.02×10^{-3} g, and this is practically the equivalent of a milligram. For easy visualization, then, a dyne can be considered as the amount of force that would be exerted by a *milligram weight*.

Meteorologists often express air pressure in dynes, using their own terms of *barye, bar,* and *millibar* (mb). To understand this system, note the following relationships:

$$1\ atm\ =\ Height\ of\ Hg \times Density\ of\ Hg\ =\ 76 \times 13.6\ =\ 1034\ g/cm^2$$

or

$$1\ atm\ =\ 1034\ g/cm^2 \div 1.02 \times 10^{-3}\ (or\ 1034 \times 980.7)\ =\ 1.014 \times 10^6\ dynes/cm^2$$

The meteorologic units of pressure are defined as follows:

$$1\ barye\ =\ 1\ dyne/cm^2$$
$$1\ bar\ =\ 10^6\ dynes/cm^2\ =\ 10^6\ baryes$$
$$1\ mb\ =\ 10^3\ dynes/cm^2\ =\ 10^{-3}\ bar\ =\ 10^3\ baryes$$

Thus 1 standard atmosphere of pressure (1 atm) $=\ 1034\ g/cm^2\ =\ 1.014 \times 10^6\ dynes/cm^2\ =\ 1.014\ bars\ =\ 1014\ mb$. In meteorology, atmospheric pressure is most frequently expressed as *millibars*. Millibars can be approximately converted to g/cm^2 by multiplying by 1.02. In summary, then, the pressure of 1 atm can be expressed as follows:

760 mm (76 cm) Hg
29.9 inches Hg
33.9 feet H$_2$O
1034 g/cm^2
14.7 lb/in^2
1.014×10^6 dynes/cm^2
1014 mb

Exercise 1-2: Calculate the following pressures to the nearest tenth:
A. 752 mm Hg, in g/cm^2
B. 31.4 inches Hg, in lb/in^2
C. 766 mm Hg, in lb/in^2
D. 28.4 inches Hg, in g/cm^2
E. 30.7 inches Hg, in feet H_2O
F. 1022 g/cm^2, in mm Hg
G. 15.2 lb/in^2, in inches Hg
H. 15 cm H_2O, in mm Hg
I. 1018 mb, in mm Hg
J. 766 mm Hg, in mb

In cardiopulmonary physiology, the effect of gases is frequently considered in terms of their partial pressures. *Dalton's law of partial pressures* tells us that the total pressure of a gaseous mixture is equal to the sum of the partial pressure of the constituent gases and that the partial pressure of each gas in the mixture is the pressure it would exert if it occupied the entire volume alone. Therefore, each gas contributes its share of the total pressure of a mixture in proportion to its percentage of the mixture. A gas that is composed of 25% of a mixture of gases would exert a partial pressure of 25% of the total pressure.

As an example, *dry* air may be considered to consist of only two major gases, O_2 at 21% and N_2 at 79%. Assuming a normal atmospheric pressure of 760 mm Hg, we can show individual partial pressures as follows:

$$P_B \text{ (dry)} = 760 \text{ mm Hg}$$
$$P_{O_2} = 760 \times 0.21 = 160 \text{ mm Hg}$$
$$P_{N_2} = 760 \times 0.79 = \underline{600 \text{ mm Hg}}$$
$$760 \text{ mm Hg}$$

Hypobarism and hyperbarism

Hypobarism and *hyperbarism* refer to air pressures significantly below and above, respectively, the sea level normal of 760 mm Hg, or 1034 g/cm^2. They are of great importance in the exploration of the oceans and outer space. One aspect of medicine under current investigation is that of hyperbaric medicine, in which the patient is subjected to the effects of several atmospheres of pressure.

The amount of atmospheric pressure individuals are exposed to depends on their location. Atmospheric pressure decreases with an increase in altitude. At any point above the earth there is less air beyond it to exert pressure than there is on the earth's surface. The opposite must also be true. As an individual descends into the earth, more atmosphere exerts pressure on every square centimeter of surface area.

Increasing pressure is most dramatically exemplified by descent into the sea. Since water is heavy and not compressible, an individual making a deep dive for a prolonged time must surround him- or herself with a layer of air that compensates for the tremendous pressure of the water. A state of hyperbarism is reached much more quickly since each 33 feet of depth in sea water represents an increase of 1 atm.

Since we are ultimately interested in the amount of oxygen available to the body cells and will soon study the relationship between this availability and the pressure of oxygen partial pressure, let us consider the effect of changing atmospheric pressure on oxygen partial pressure. We assume a concentration of oxygen in dry air of 20.95% (this is expressed as the F_{O_2}, or fractional concentration of O_2). At a P_B of 760 mm Hg, the $P_{O_2} = 760 \times 0.2095 = 159$ mm Hg. Although the F_{O_2} of air at 25,000 feet is still 0.2095, the P_B is only 282 mm Hg and the P_{O_2} is thus 59 mm Hg. Although the F_{O_2} at sea level and at 25,000 feet is the same, the kinetic activity of oxygen at the high altitude is equal to that of a mixture containing only 7.8% oxygen on the ground. In contrast, at a depth of 66 feet into the sea, the weight of water exerts a pressure equal to that of 3 atm, or 2280 mm Hg. Air breathed by a diver at this depth would also be subjected to this same pressure, and its P_{O_2} would be 20.95% of 2280, or 477 mm Hg.

In Appendix 3 some characteristics of dry air are compared (such as pressure, oxygen levels, and density) when the air is at various altitudes from 300,000 feet above and 297 feet below sea level. Sea level values are outlined at *0*, with altitudes above and sea depths below. The air density values (g/ℓ) assume a sea level temperature of 15°C, at which temperature air has a density of 1.250 g/ℓ. The relationship between gas density and temperature is described in detail later. The column *Atm* indicates the fraction or multiple of 1 atm pressure found at the various levels of altitude and depth; *%O_2 Equiv* refers to percentages of oxygen in breathing mixtures at sea level that would have oxygen partial pressures equal to those recorded in the *P_{O_2}* column. Students are not expected to memorize this table but to study it to understand the wide environmental variation to which a body may be subjected when it ventures from the surface of the earth. Some of the principles illustrated in the table will have important clinical meaning later.

Exercise 1-3: Assuming an F_{O_2} of 0.2095, calculate the following to the nearest tenth:
A. The P_{O_2} of dry air at a P_B of 752 mm Hg
B. The P_{O_2} of dry air at 1068 mb, in mm Hg
C. The P_B in mm Hg with a P_{O_2} of 140 mm Hg
D. The P_{O_2} of dry air at 50 feet of seawater
E. The seawater depth with an O_2 equivalent of 100%

The discussions so far have concerned only dry gases, but it is important to consider the role played by water in gas physics. Invisible moisture is present in the atmosphere in the form of vapor, which assumes the state and characteristics of a gas and is sometimes refered to as "molecular water" to distinguish it from visible gross "particulate water," such as mist. Molecular water is subjected to the same kinetic activity as other gases and, like them, exerts its own partial pressure, called *vapor pressure*. Atmospheric conditions vary the amount of water vapor in the air, but molecular water is constantly entering the air whenever air is exposed to a water surface.

Water enters the atmosphere by vaporization. A volume of water, like a gas, is in constant molecular activity. The energy of some molecules near the surface causes them to escape into the surrounding air, just as long as there is room for them in the air mixture. Thus a steady flow of air across the water surface accommodates a continuing flow of escaping water molecules, and *evaporation* progressively reduces the volume of water (Fig. 1-5, *A*). Another principle of physics provides that heat is required to produce the change in state from liquid to gas that occurs in vaporization. This heat is taken from the air immediately adjacent to the water supply, thereby cooling the air. This cooling from vaporization is responsible for the cooling effects during the summer of large bodies of water. However, if a cover is placed over a volume of water, air trapped over the surface and below the cover will be filled with all the water vapor molecules it can hold and will be *saturated with water vapor*. At this point, vaporization does not stop, but a state of equilibrium is established. For every molecule escaping from the water, another molecule returns to the reservoir from the overlying saturated air (Fig. 1-5, *B*).

Two factors that influence vaporization are temperature and pressure. Vaporization is directly related to temperature, and this relationship can be looked at from two directions. First, the warmer the air, the more vapor it can

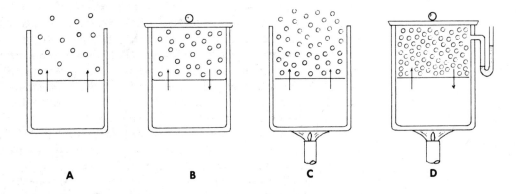

A **B** **C** **D**

Fig. 1-5 The factors influencing vaporization of water are shown in these four sketches. **A,** The kinetic activity of molecules at the surface carries the molecules into the surrounding air, and evaporation gradually reduces the reservoir. **B,** If the container is covered, vaporization does not stop, but a state of equilibrium is reached when the air trapped in the container becomes saturated. At this point, water molecules leave and return to the reservoir in equal numbers. **C,** If the open container is heated, the increased molecular activity speeds the rate of vaporization. **D,** When the container is both covered and heated, more vapor will crowd into the trapped air, raising the vapor pressure as indicated by the attached manometer.

hold. In other words, the *capacity* of air for water vapor increases with temperature. Therefore, if warm air passes over a water surface, the air's greater capacity will permit an increased escape of molecules from the water per unit of time, and evaporation will be faster. Second, if heat is applied to the water, the increased kinetic energy of the escaping molecules will allow more molecules to escape the surface per unit of time (Fig. 1-5, *C*). If a cover is placed over a surface of heated water, the increased kinetic energy of the escaping molecules will force more of them into the trapped air, increasing the saturation of the air and increasing the vapor pressure (Fig. 1-5, *D*). Therefore, the water content and the degree of saturation of air or any gas are a function of temperature.

The effect of pressure on vaporization is the opposite. It is convenient to visualize vaporization as the escape of water molecules from the surface against the opposition of adjacent air molecules. As the surrounding air pressure increases or decreases, vaporization will be correspondingly decreased or increased.

The amount of water in a given mass of air (or any gas) can be recorded in one of three ways.

Absolute humidity. This is a measurement of the content or actual weight of water present in a given volume of air expressed in grams per cubic meter (or pounds per cubic foot or yard). Water may be physically extracted from a known air volume by an absorbing agent and weighed, or it may be computed by meteorologic data according to the techniques of the U.S. Weather Bureau.[5]

Relative humidity. This is the percentage of water in the air *(content)* as compared to the amount of water the air could hold if saturated *(capacity)*, which is taken as 100. *Content divided by capacity* equals a value called relative humidity (RH). If air contains half the water at a given temperature that it has the capacity to contain, the RH equals 50%. At room temperature, air has the capacity of approximately 18 g/m^3. If the water content is measured as 12 g/m^3, the air is 67% saturated, and the RH is 67%. Instruments called *hygrometers* allow direct and simple measurement of RH without the necessity of extracting and weighing water content of air samples.

Water vapor pressure. In contrast to other gases in a mixture, partial pressure of water vapor does not depend on its fractional concentration in the mixture but entirely on temperature and relative humidity. Actual measurements of water vapor pressure in saturated air have been made over a wide range of temperatures, and their values are available in handbooks of chemical data. The vapor pressure in any gas that is less than saturated is found by multiplying its capacity (saturated tension) at a given temperature by the RH. Therefore, at a stated temperature, vapor tension of a gas with a 50% RH is one half that of the saturated gas. *For specific conditions of humidity and temperature, water vapor pressure is an absolute value, regardless of the concentrations of other gases present.* So the partial pressure of other gases is calculated as the product of their fractional concentration times the total atmospheric pressure minus the water vapor pressure (which must be computed first). In pulmonary physiology, gases are considered either to be dry, with no water vapor, or to be saturated. Appendix 4 lists the water vapor tensions of saturated gas within the usual physiologic range of interest. The column to the right represents that portion of any atmospheric pressure at given temperatures resulting solely from water vapor. Therefore, at 25°C, in a gas saturated with water and regardless of other gas concentrations, 23.8 mm Hg of the total P_B is a result of the action of water molecules. If the gas were a mixture under an atmospheric pressure of 760 mm Hg, and the fractional concentration of oxygen were 0.21, the oxygen partial pressure would be 0.21 (760 − 23.8) = 154.6 mm Hg. This principle is used extensively in the next section.

The *dew point* of air is that temperature at which the air becomes saturated with water vapor. Imagine a water content of air sufficient to comprise an RH of 90%. Should the air temperature drop, the water *capacity* of the air lessens. A temperature can be reached at which the water content now fully saturates the air, and the RH is 100%. At this point, excess water vapor begins to condense as visible droplets on small objects, such as blades of grass. This temperature is the dew point. This phenomenon is frequently observed on cooling iced beverage glasses in warm humid weather. As the temperature of the glass drops, the air adjacent to the glass also cools, and finally at the dew point, water in the air begins to condense on the glass surface.

When an air mass near the earth's surface reaches its dew point, excess water often precipitates as very fine but visible water particles, so light that they remain suspended in air as mist or fog. When larger air masses at higher altitudes are chilled by cold air currents, excess water usually falls out as rain or snow. Urban and industrial contamination of air has produced a mixture of fog and smoke or other vapors called *smog,* which has important public health significance. Smog may be held close to the ground by a *temperature inversion.* This occurs when the air, instead of showing a progressive cooling from the ground up, contains a layer of warm air at heights from 300 to 3000 feet. In such a state the air is very quiet, with little or no current to carry away contaminants.

To prepare for the use in physiologic calculations of the characteristics of pressure and humidity, students should understand certain conventions adopted in the interest of uniformity. The following definitions should be learned:

1. Standard temperature and pressure (STP) means 0°C and 760 mm Hg.
2. Body temperature (BT) means 37°C.
3. Ambient temperature (AT) or pressure (AP) means the existing environmental temperature or pressure (as opposed to standard).
4. Saturated gas (S) means a volume of gas with a relative humidity of 100% at any given temperature.
5. Dry gas (D) means a volume of gas with *no* vapor in it.

These abbreviations are usually used in combination. For example:

1. STPD means a volume of dry gas at a temperature of 0°C and atmospheric pressure of 760 mm Hg.

2. BTPS means a volume of gas saturated with water vapor at 37°C and the ambient environmental pressure.
3. ATPS means a volume of gas saturated with water vapor at ambient temperature (room temperature) and pressure.

When reporting data on gases for physiologic evaluation the following rules are generally used:

1. Volumes of gases in the lungs are recorded as BTPS.
2. Gases that undergo chemical reaction in the body, such as blood gases, are recorded as STPD.
3. If saturated gas volumes are to be used in physiologic calculations, they are first corrected to their dry volume, then calculated back to the saturated value. How this is done is discussed later.

Gas laws

Our prime concern with the laws governing gas behavior is the consideration of the relationships among the interdependent variables of temperature, pressure, volume, and mass. These relationships are often studied under ideal conditions based on theoretic principles that are true under certain limited conditions. Fortunately, these limitations apply to the usual physiologic ranges usually dealt with. The *real behavior* of gases deals with actual deviations from *ideal behavior*.

The *ideal* gas laws are widely used in chemistry, physics, and pulmonary physiology. The last is most frequently concerned with changes in gas volumes brought about by changes in temperature and pressure. The role of humidity is mediated through its effect on pressure. Clinical pulmonary physiology is vitally concerned with these measurements as they relate to lung volume and what happens to these volumes with environmental or pathologic changes. An effective technologist, whether working in a laboratory or in clinical medicine, must understand the fundamentals of the gas laws described. (In the following definitions and applications of the gas laws, "temperature" always means absolute temperature.)

The four properties of gases (pressure, volume, temperature, and mass) are considered to be variables. The relationships among them can be expressed as:

$$PV/Tn = k$$

All gases consist of all these parameters, and although the proportionality constant *(k)* does not change with any specific sample, the component properties (such as pressure and temperature) can vary among themselves.

There are a number of gas laws named after the person who first described the law. Following are three of the most important:

Boyle's* law. If temperature (T) and mass (n) remain unchanged, volume (V) varies *inversely* with the pressure (P). This means that at a constant temperature and mass, as increasing pressure is applied to a given volume of gas,

*Robert Boyle, British physicist and chemist, 1627-1691.

the volume decreases. However, there must be a limit to the shrinkage of the gas volume because the mass of gas cannot simply disappear as the pressure increases. The increments in volume reduction become smaller as the units of pressure increase, until a point is reached at which this relationship between pressure and volume no longer exists. At this point the ideal behavior of the gas ceases, and physical changes in the characteristics of the gas occur. These inverse relationships can be expressed as PV = k, eliminating T and n since they do not vary in this instance and do not influence the relationship.

Charles'* law. If pressure and mass are kept unchanged, volume varies *directly* with changes in absolute temperature. This means that if a mass of gas is kept under a constant pressure, as the absolute temperature of the gas is increased or decreased, the volume will increase or decrease accordingly. As in Boyle's law, the mass of gas cannot be cooled into nothingness, and at a certain point the ideal behavior ceases, and other factors come into play. This direct relationship between temperature and volume can be expressed as V/T = k, since for the quotient to remain stable, the other must change proportionately in the same direction.

Gay-Lussac's† law. If volume and mass remain fixed, the pressure exerted by a gas varies *directly* with the absolute temperature of the gas. If the volume of mass of gas is kept unchanged (e.g., in a rigid cylinder), as the absolute temperature of the gas is increased or decreased, its pressure will increase or decrease accordingly. The linear relationship is shown in Fig. 1-1, which demonstrates that, theoretically, with no pressure exerted by a gas at $0°K$, changes in pressure are proportional to changes in absolute temperature values and are expressed as P/T = k.

When the gas laws are put to practical use we will be concerned with changes in volume, pressure, and temperature in a given gas sample with a fixed number of molecules. Therefore, since mass will not be a variable in these circumstances, it can be disregarded, and the three gas laws just defined can be combined into the single simplified expression:

$$PV/T = k$$

Combined gas laws

When gas is subjected to changes in pressure, volume, temperature, and mass, individually or in combination, the total product divided by the quotient of PV/Tn remains unchanged. In effect, these variables represent the *matter* of the gas, which is neither increased nor decreased but is "redistributed" among the variables. This can be stated as follows:

$$\frac{P_1 V_1}{T_1 n_1} = \frac{P_2 V_2}{T_2 n_2}$$

---

*Jacques Alexandre César Charles, French physicist and chemist, 1746-1823.
†Joseph Louis Gay-Lussac, French chemist and physicist, 1778-1850.

The subscript *1* indicates a *before* value, and *2* an *after* value. So the products and quotients of the gas variables before a change must be the same after.

In pulmonary physiology it is important to know how much change there will be in a gas volume if it is subjected to changes in pressure and/or temperature. Since the total mass of a gas will not be affected, the quantity *n* can be eliminated from the equation, but careful analysis of gas problems is necessary to determine whether such a shortened version of the equation can be used. With the equation now written as

$$\frac{P_1 V_1}{T_1} = \frac{P_2 V_2}{T_2}$$

it is apparent that knowing five of the six factors, it is possible to calculate the sixth. If we know the original volume (V_1), the original temperature (T_1), and the original pressure (P_1), plus the new pressure (P_2) and temperature (T_2), it is possible to calculate the new volume using the following equation:

$$V_2 = \frac{V_1 \times P_1 \times T_2}{P_2 \times T_1}$$

By substituting specific values in the equation we can correct a gas volume for changes in pressure and temperature.

This is a form of the *combined gas laws* that make up the basis for most of the gas volume calculations. In examining the equation, it can be seen that the new corrected gas volume (V_2) is a proportion of the original volume (V_1) according to the changes in pressure and temperature. If the equations are written to demonstrate the laws described, they appear as follows:

$$\text{Boyle's law: } V_2 = V_1 \times \frac{P_1}{P_2}$$

$$\text{Charles' law: } V_2 = V_1 \times \frac{T_2}{T_1}$$

In summary, Boyle's law states that if the pressure of a gas is increased, the volume will decrease. In this case, P_2 will be greater than P_1, and in the above equation, since V_1 will be multiplied by a fraction less than 1, V_2 will be reduced. The opposite relationship exists in regard to temperature and Charles' Law. As temperature increases, the volume increases.

Exercise 1-4: Set up the combined gas laws to solve for the following:
A. P_2
B. T_1
C. V_1
D. T_2

Correction of dry gas volumes

The following technique is suggested for the student to use in all gas volume calculations to avoid mistakes of omission. When proficiency has been reached, shortcuts to suit individual needs can be employed.

Problem 1: Given 100 ml of dry gas measured at 37°C and 760 mm Hg P_B, what would be its volume at 60°C?

Solution: $V_1 = 100$ $V_2 = ?$
$P_1 = 760$ $P_2 = 760$
$t_1 = 37$ $t_2 = 60$
$T_1 = 37 + 273 = 310$ $T_2 = 60 + 273 = 333$

$$V_2 = \frac{V_1 P_1 T_2}{P_2 T_1} = \frac{100 \times 760 \times 333}{760 \times 310} = 107.4 \text{ ml}$$

(*Note:* Since $P_1 = P_2$, both *could* have been eliminated from the equation, but it is better for the beginner to include all data.)

Problem 2: Given 100 ml of dry gas measured at 37°C and 760 mm Hg P_B, what would be its volume at 800 mm Hg?

Solution: $V_1 = 100$ $V_2 = ?$
$P_1 = 760$ $P_2 = 800$
$t_1 = 37$ $t_2 = 37$
$T_1 = 37 + 273 = 310$ $T_2 = 37 + 273 = 310$

$$V_2 = \frac{V_1 P_1 T_2}{P_2 T_1} = \frac{100 \times 760 \times 310}{800 \times 310} = 95 \text{ ml}$$

Problem 3: Given 100 ml of dry gas at 37°C and 760 mm Hg, what would be its volume at 60°C and 800 mm Hg?

Solution: $V_1 = 100$ $V_2 = ?$
$P_1 = 760$ $P_2 = 800$
$t_1 = 37$ $t_2 = 60$
$T_1 = 310$ $T_2 = 333$

$$V_2 = \frac{V_1 P_1 T_2}{P_2 T_1} = \frac{100 \times 760 \times 333}{800 \times 310} = 102 \text{ ml}$$

Exercise 1-5: Convert the following dry gas volumes, as indicated (to three digits):
A. 150 ml at 25°C and 752 mm Hg, to 0°C
B. 2.5 ℓ at 18°C and 762 mm Hg, to 748 mm Hg
C. 325 ml at 20°C and 770 mm Hg, to 37°C and 760 mm Hg
D. 22.4 ℓ at 15°C and 730 mm Hg, to 5°C and 755 mm Hg
E. 95 ml at 28°C and 784 mm Hg, to 20°C and 768 mm Hg

Correction of gas volumes containing water vapor

Most physiologic gas volume calculations involve gases saturated with water vapor and require correction of volumes from the saturated to the dry state or the reverse. Since water vapor is, in essence, a space-occupying gas in a mixture of gases, its removal from a gas volume will shrink the volume, and its addition will increase the volume. Therefore, in the examples and exercises that follow, whenever a volume of gas saturated with water vapor is calculated to what it would be in the dry state (corrected from saturated to dry), the dry volume will be smaller unless other conditions of pressure and temperature counteract the shrinkage. The opposite must also be true. Correcting from dry to saturated will give a larger volume.

At a fixed temperature, if a gas sample is in a container permitting it to respond to ambient pressure, it reaches a static volume where the pressure it exerts exactly balances ambient pressure. Water vapor, if added to dry gas at ambient pressure, will have two effects. First, the increased number of molecules will obviously enlarge the volume until the total molecular kinetic activity again equilibrates with ambient. Second, because water vapor exerts a pressure that is dependent only on temperature and RH and is independent of other gases with which it mixes, the partial pressures of the other gases will be accordingly reduced to maintain parity with ambient pressure.

The effect of moisture in gas volume calculations is mediated through the partial pressure it exerts at a given temperature and saturation, and it slightly modifies the application of Boyle's law. The relevance of Boyle's law to this situation can be understood if we view it as follows. The law tells us that gas volume varies inversely with the ambient pressure. Let us imagine some water vapor being instantaneously added to a sample of dry gas, with the temperature remaining constant. Because of the added water molecules, the kinetic activity and the pressure of the now wet gas will momentarily exceed the ambient pressure that is applied to it. The volume will expand until molecular activity and pressure of the larger number of molecules finally decrease to equilibrate with ambient. Just before the addition of the vapor molecule the gas was in equilibrium with ambient pressure, and therefore, in volume correction data, the initial pressure to be used is ambient. As soon as vapor molecules are added, the pressure of the gas goes up. This has the same effect on gas volume as if the ambient pressure went down a like amount. Therefore, the final pressure affecting gas volume is the ambient minus the vapor pressure, and in conformity with Boyle's law, the volume increases.

This final pressure can be calculated through a formula and is designated as P_C. P_C therefore equals $P - P_{H_2O}$ at t, where P is the total effective pressure, t is the temperature of the gas, and P_{H_2O} is the vapor pressure at t as listed in the right column of the table in Appendix 4, if we are dealing with gas saturated with water vapor. Boyle's Law can now be expressed as follows:

$$V_2 = \frac{V_1 \times (P_1 - P_{1H_2O} \text{ at } t_1)}{(P_2 - P_{2H_2O} \text{ at } t_2)} = \frac{V_1 \times P_{1C}}{P_{2C}}$$

Let us assume that V_1 is dry gas, V_2 is water-saturated gas, and pressure and temperature remain unchanged. Because V_1 is dry there will be no P_{H_2O} to subtract from P_1. Therefore P_{1C} will be unchanged from P_1 and will be larger than P_{2C}, making V_2 larger than V_1. This is expected since it is the same as adding moisture to a volume of gas and then calculating the new volume. Use of the *corrected pressure* in Boyle's law simultaneously adjusts for changes in both pressure and humidity. The format for arranging data as demonstrated above will be modified a bit to accomodate water vapor effect:

V_1	= Initial volume	V_2	= Final volume
P_1	= Initial pressure	P_2	= Final pressure
t	= Initial temperature	t_2	= Final temperature
P_{1H_2O}	= Partial pressure of water vapor at t_1	P_{2H_2O}	= Partial pressure of water vapor at t_2
P_{1C}	= Corrected initial pressure = $P_1 - P_{1H_2O}$	P_{2C}	= Corrected final pressure = $P_2 - P_{2H_2O}$
T_1	= $t_1 + 273$	T_2	= $t_2 + 273$

$$V_2 = \frac{V_1 \times P_{1C} \times T_2}{P_{2C} \times T_1}$$

The following examples illustrate how the combined gas laws can make corrections for changes in any or all of the variables of pressure, temperature, and water vapor.

Problem 1: Given 100 ml of saturated gas at 760 mm Hg and 25° C, what would be its volume if dry at the same pressure and temperature?

Solution:

V_1	= 100	V_2	= ?
P_1	= 760	P_2	= 760
t_1	= 25	t_2	= 25
P_{1H_2O}	= 23.8	P_{2H_2O}	= 0
P_{1C}	= 736.2	P_{2C}	= 760
T_1	= 298	T_2	= 298

$$V_2 = \frac{V_1 P_{1C} T_2}{P_{2C} T_1} = \frac{100 \times 736.2 \times 298}{760 \times 298} = 96.8 \text{ ml}$$

Problem 2: Given 100 ml of saturated gas at 760 mm Hg and 25° C, what would be its volume saturated at the same pressure and 37° C?

Solution:

V_1	= 100	V_2	= ?
P_1	= 760	P_2	= 760
t_1	= 25	t_2	= 37
P_{1H_2O}	= 23.8	P_{2H_2O}	= 47
P_{1C}	= 736.2	P_{2C}	= 713
T_1	= 298	T_2	= 310

$$V_2 = \frac{V_1 P_{1C} T_2}{P_{2C} T_1} = \frac{100 \times 736.2 \times 310}{713 \times 298} = 107.5 \text{ ml}$$

Problem 3: Given 100 ml of saturated gas at 754 mm Hg and 20° C, what would be its volume as dry gas at 764 mm Hg and 37° C?

Solution:

V_1	= 100	V_2	= ?
P_1	= 754	P_2	= 764
t_1	= 20	t_2	= 37
P_{1H_2O}	= 17.5	P_{2H_2O}	= 0
P_{1C}	= 736.5	P_{2C}	= 764
T_1	= 293	T_2	= 310

$$V_2 = \frac{V_1 P_{1C} T_2}{P_{2C} T_1} = \frac{100 \times 736.5 \times 310}{764 \times 293} = 102.1 \text{ ml}$$

Problem 4: Given 100 ml of saturated gas at 754 mm Hg and 20° C, what would be its volume saturated at 764 mm Hg and 37° C?

Solution:

$$V_1 = 100 \qquad V_2 = ?$$
$$P_1 = 754 \qquad P_2 = 764$$
$$t_1 = 20 \qquad t_2 = 37$$
$$P_{1H_2O} = 17.5 \qquad P_{2H_2O} = 47$$
$$P_{1C} = 736.5 \qquad P_{2C} = 717$$
$$T_1 = 293 \qquad T_2 = 310$$

$$V_2 = \frac{V_1 P_{1C} T_2}{P_{2C} T_1} = \frac{100 \times 736.5 \times 310}{717 \times 293} = 108.5 \text{ ml}$$

Exercise 1-6: Correct the following gas volumes to four digits:

A. 250 ml, saturated at 750 mm Hg and 20° C, to saturated at 764 mm Hg and 25° C

B. 1.75 ℓ, dry at 752 mm Hg and 26° C, to saturated at 770 mm Hg and 33° C

C. 58 ml, saturated at 748 mm Hg and 21° C, to dry at 730 mm Hg and 30° C

D. 430 ml BTPS at 766 mm Hg, to STPD

E. 2.28 ℓ, saturated at 1006 mb and 72° F, to saturated at 1022 mb and 90° F

Correction of barometric reading

    Because the aneroid barometer is composed of brass, it reacts by expansion and contraction to ambient temperature changes. Even more important, the column of mercury found on the barometer not only responds to atmospheric pressure changes but, like a large thermometer, is significantly affected by temperature. Therefore, when we read the mercury level of a barometer, we see the effects of both pressure and temperature. For accuracy we must correct our *observed* reading for changes in the mercury column caused by temperature. A formula based on expansion coefficients of brass and mercury at any given temperature is the basis for a table of correction factors prepared by the U.S. Weather Bureau, and reproduced in part in Appendix 5, for the pressures and temperatures most frequently encountered. The values in the table are *subtracted* from the observed reading. At 30°C an observed barometric reading of 750 mm Hg would be corrected for temperature by subtracting 3.66 from 750 for a corrected reading of 746.34 (usually rounded off to 746.3 or just 746). For P_{BS} between those listed in the table, interpolation is used. For an example, the correction factor for 764 mm Hg at 25°C is 3.09 (factor for 760 mm Hg) + 0.4 of the difference between 3.09 and 3.13 (factor for 770 mm Hg). Since 0.4(3.13 − 3.09) = 0.4 × 0.04, or 0.016, the final factor is 3.09 + 0.016, or 3.106, rounded off to 3.11. From a practical point of view, the only temperature variations affecting barometric readings are those of the room housing the barometer. Since it is unlikely that the temperature of the average laboratory would exceed seasonal changes of 16° to 27°C (60° to 80° F), or the P_B range of 740 to 780 mm Hg, the correction factors would usually be between 1.9 and 3.4.

When given a problem in gas volume correction, the student can assume that the barometric value is already corrected unless the data specifies an *observed* reading. Normally, however, when the P_B is not specified it is assumed to be 760 mm Hg.

If a student were asked to correct a volume of a patient's exhaled air at an *observed* P_B of 753 mm Hg, with a room temperature of 21°C, to STPD, the first step would be to correct the observed pressure for room temperature effect and to record the corrected pressure as P_1. The 760 mm Hg of the STPD needs no correction because it is a *stated* value, not observed. Therefore, the data would read:

$$
\begin{array}{llll}
V_1 & = ? & V_2 & = ? \\
P_1 & = 750.4 & P_2 & = 760 \\
t_1 & = 21 & t_2 & = 0 \\
P_{1H_2O} & = 18.7 & P_{2H_2O} & = 0 \\
P_{1C} & = 731.7 & P_{2C} & = 760 \\
T_1 & = 294 & T_2 & = 273
\end{array}
$$

Using the principles discussed for correction of gas volumes, any gas volume can be determined, no matter how bizarre.

Exercise 1-7: Set up the final formula to correct V_1 to V_2 according to the following conditions of observed pressures (correct P_B to one decimal place):
A. Dry, 730 mm Hg, 30°C to saturated, 730 mm Hg, 30°C
B. Saturated, 750 mm Hg, 24°C to saturated, 760 mm Hg, 24°C
C. Saturated, 744 mm Hg, 20°C to dry, 744 mm Hg, 25°C
D. Dry, 756 mm Hg, 15°C to saturated, 738 mm Hg, 22°C
E. Dry, 766 mm Hg, 24°C to dry, 738 mm Hg, 30°C

Use of factors in gas volume calculations

Factors are constant values. Instead of doing the individual arithmetic for each calculation, prepared factors are used. In gas volume determinations, three frequently encountered computations are (1) correction from ATPS to BTPS, (2) correction from ATPS to STPD, and (3) correction from STPD to BTPS. For each of these there are factors that reduce the amount of arithmetic needed. The student needs to understand the derivation of these factors.

Factors to correct volumes from ATPS to BTPS. The values in the first column of Appendix 4, when multiplied by V_1, will correct a gas volume from ATPS to BTPS. The factors listed give a close approximation because, as the footnote to the table explains, all the factors are based on a P_B of 760 mm Hg. The answer obtained using a factor might differ from one derived from detailed calculations, but the discrepancy is usually small. Derivation of the factors can be illustrated by an example. Let us correct a volume of gas (V_1) saturated at 760 mm Hg and 25°C to a gas saturated at 760 mm Hg at 37°C (ATPS to BTPS):

$$
\begin{array}{ll}
V_1 = ? & V_2 = ? \\
P_1 = 760 & P_2 = 760 \\
t_1 = 25 & t_2 = 37 \\
P_{1H_2O} = 23.8 & P_{2H_2O} = 47 \\
P_{1C} = 736.2 & P_{2C} = 713 \\
T_1 = 298 & T_2 = 310
\end{array}
$$

$$
V_2 = \frac{V_1 P_{1C} T_2}{P_{2C} T_1} = \frac{V_1 \times 736.2 \times 310}{713 \times 298} = V_1 \times 1.075
$$

Note that the product or quotient for the pressure, temperature, and humidity corrections equals 1.075, the same value found in Appendix 4 corresponding to a gas temperature of 25° C. If, in the example above, P_1 were 752 mm Hg and P_2 were 758 mm Hg and the calculation were done by the detailed method, the value by which V_1 would be multiplied would be 1.066.

Factors to correct volumes from ATPS to STPD. Factors in Appendix 6, when multiplied by V_1, will correct V_1 from ATPS to STPD. The barometric readings of the left column are *observed* values, *not* corrected for temperature. To use the table, a direct reading from the barometer must be used since the factors include temperature adjustment. As an example, let us corect a saturated gas volume at an observed P_B of 770 mm Hg and a room temperature of 20° C to dry gas at 760 mm Hg and 0°C. The first step would be to correct 770 mm Hg for 20°C to 767.5 mm Hg. The data, therefore, would be as follows:

$$
\begin{array}{ll}
V_1 = ? & V_2 = ? \\
P_1 = 767.5 & P_2 = 760 \\
t_1 = 20 & t_2 = 0 \\
P_{1H_2O} = 17.5 & P_{2H_2O} = 0 \\
P_{1C} = 750 & P_{2C} = 760 \\
T_1 = 293 & T_1 = 273
\end{array}
$$

$$
V_2 = \frac{V_1 P_{1C} T_2}{P_{2C} T_1} = \frac{V_1 \times 750 \times 273}{760 \times 293} = V_1 \times 0.919
$$

The listed factor for 770 mm Hg and 20°C is also 0.919.

Factors to correct volumes from STPD to BTPS. Factors for this conversion are given in Appendix 7. With ambient pressure as the only variable, the factor for correction to an ambient pressure of 750 mm Hg is derived as follows:

$$
\begin{array}{ll}
V_1 = ? & V_2 = ? \\
P_1 = 760 & P_2 = 750 \\
t_1 = 0 & t_2 = 37 \\
P_{1H_2O} = 0 & P_{2H_2O} = 47 \\
P_{1C} = 760 & P_{2C} = 703 \\
T_1 = 273 & T_2 = 310
\end{array}
$$

$$
V_2 = \frac{V_1 P_{1C} T_2}{P_{2C} T_1} = \frac{V_2 \times 760 \times 310}{703 \times 273} = V_1 \times 1.227
$$

The listed factor for 750 mm Hg is also 1.227.

Calculations involving weight and density of gas

Gas problems that depend on variations in weight and density of gases are frequently encountered in chemistry and physics, although rarely in pulmonary physiology. Nevertheless, the student should learn how to use the general gas laws equation to solve problems. It was indicated earlier that the n in the gas laws equation refers to the number of gas molecules representing gas weight or density. When analyzing a problem involving weight or density, the student will find it helpful to remember that at P_B of 760 mm Hg and 273°K, 1 gmw of a gas occupies 22.4 ℓ. Following are typical problems:

Problem 1: If the density of oxygen is 1.43 g/ℓ at 0°C and 1 atm, what is its density at 20°C and 720 mm Hg? (*Note:* Although volume is not mentioned, it is implied in the use of the term *density*, g/ℓ. Thus V_1 equals V_2 and need not be considered.)

Solution:
$V_1 = ?$ $\qquad$ $V_2 = ?$
$P_1 = 760$ $\qquad$ $P_2 = 720$
$T_1 = 273$ $\qquad$ $T_2 = 293$
$n_1 = 1.43$ g/ℓ $\qquad$ $n_2 = ?$ g/ℓ

$$n_2 = \frac{n_1 \times P_2 \times T_1}{P_1 \times T_2} = \frac{1.43 \times 720 \times 273}{760 \times 293} = 1.26 \text{ g/}\ell$$

Problem 2: What volume will be occupied by 2.35 g of SO_2 at 25°C and 750 mm Hg? (*Note:* The *before* values will be the volume occupied by 1 gmw at STP to permit the setting of a ratio.)

Solution:
$V_1 = 22.4$ ℓ $\qquad$ $V_2 = ?$ ℓ
$P_1 = 760$ $\qquad$ $P_2 = 750$
$T_1 = 273$ $\qquad$ $T_2 = 298$
$n_1 = 64$ g $\qquad$ $n_2 = 2.35$ g

$$V_2 = \frac{V_1 \times P_1 \times T_2 \times n_2}{P_2 \times T_1 \times n_1} = \frac{22.4 \times 760 \times 298 \times 2.35}{750 \times 273 \times 64} = 0.910 \text{ } \ell$$

Problem 3: How many grams of air will a 500-ℓ tank hold if it is filled to 3 atm at 15°C? Assume the gram molecular weight of air to be 29. (*Note:* $n_1 = $ Density $\times 500 = [29/22.4] \times 500 = 647$ g)

Solution:
$V_1 = 500$ ℓ $\qquad$ $V_2 = 500$ ℓ
$P_1 = 1$ $\qquad$ $P_2 = 3$
$T_1 = 273$ $\qquad$ $T_2 = 288$
$n_1 = 647$ g $\qquad$ $n_2 = ?$ g

$$n_2 = \frac{n_1 \times P_2 \times T_1}{P_1 \times T_2} = \frac{647 \times 3 \times 273}{1 \times 288} = 1840 \text{ g}$$

Another factor the student should be aware of is the *molar gas constant*. It is a numeric value of the constant of the ratio $PV/nT = k$, where n is the number of moles of gas and V is 22.4 ℓ at 1 atm and 273°K. For respiratory physiologic use of the gas laws, the molar gas constant is not as helpful as the tabular system explained on the preceding pages.

Properties of gases at extreme temperatures and pressures

The *theoretic* responses of gases to changes in pressure, volume, temperature, and density have not been discussed. Now it is important to consider variations from theory when gases are subjected to both low temperatures and high pressures, revealing their *real* characteristics. This will help prepare the student in dealing with the commercially prepared gases used in treating patients.

A term that needs to be considered at this point is *van der Waals forces*. According to Webster's New Collegiate Dictionary, these are the "relatively weak attractive forces between neutral atoms and molecules." These weak forces oppose the kinetic activity of the molecules. Although it is independent of temperature, the effectiveness of van der Waals forces is related to both temperature and pressure. For example, at a high temperature the increased kinetic molecular activity far overshadows the van der Waals energy, rendering the latter relatively unimportant, whereas at very low temperatures the resulting decrease in kinetic action makes the molecules much more responsive to mutual attraction. At the same time, low pressures exerted on a gas permit the molecules to move freely with little influence from other molecules, in contrast to the molecular crowding of high pressures, which permits greater increase in the van der Waals effect. In addition to the attractive force between gas molecules, another factor that influences the relationship between pressure and volume is attributed to the space occupied by the molecules themselves. When moderate to low pressures are exerted on a given container full of gas, the total mass of matter is a negligible fraction of the total volume of the gas. As the volume is reduced by increasing pressure, however, the resulting molecular density, which is not compressible, comprises a proportionately larger portion of the overall gas volume, disturbing the volume response to pressure predicted by the ideal gas laws.

These observations can be summarized by generalizing that at very low temperatures or very high pressures, gases deviate in their behavioral patterns as predicted by the classic gas laws because of the influence of the van der Waals intermolecular attractive forces and the volume of compressed gas molecules. For those scientists and technicians whose work requires maximum precision, a modification of Boyle's law is available that includes correction for the van der Waals effect and density of molecules; also handbooks of chemistry and physics have prepared tables of constants to facilitate such calculations for a wide variety of gases. The interest here, however, is in the effects of excessive temperatures and pressures on the *state* of gases, since those we use may be in liquid or solid as well as gaseous forms. The most familiar example of the three states of matter is that of water, which we know as a solid (ice), gas (vapor), and liquid. Before discussing the state of matter in relation to therapeutic gases, it is important to describe and define some physical terms that make it easier to understand the characteristics of prepared gases.

Units of heat

Calorie. The quantity of heat required to raise the temperature of 1 g of water from 14.5° to 15.5°C is used as the standard and is called a *calorie* (cal). In general use, the definition simply describes the amount of heat necessary to raise the temperature of 1 g of water 1°C. In dealing with large quantities, the term *large calorie* (Cal) is sometimes used and is equal to 1000 cal. If it is desired to calculate the heat produced by a chemical reaction, the ingredients are placed in the reaction chamber of an instrument called a calorimeter. The heat of the chemical reaction is absorbed by a carefully weighed mass of water surrounding the reaction chamber, and the temperature change in the water is measured. The weight of water in grams multiplied by the Celsius rise in temperature calculates the total calories produced, which can then be expressed as calories per unit of weight of the reacting substances.

British thermal unit. The Btu is the English measurement system counterpart of the calorie and is the amount of heat required to raise the temperature of 1 pound of water 1°F. One British thermal unit is equal to 252 cal. Scientists generally use the calorie, but persons in engineering and commerce usually employ the Btu along with other elements of the English system. This dichotomy of standards places a burden on the respiratory therapist, who must be familiar with both systems. Respiratory therapy involves contact with scientific data and the metric system as well as commercial gases and other equipment standardized in the English system.

Heat capacity. This refers to the number of calories required to raise the temperature of 1 g of a substance 1°C or 1 pound of a substance 1°F. By definition, the heat capacity of water is 1 cal in the metric system and 1 Btu in the English system.

Specific heat. This value is a ratio between the amount of heat required to raise the temperature of 1 g of a substance 1°C or 1 pound of a substance 1°F at a specific temperature, and the amount of heat required to raise the temperature of 1 g of water 1°C or 1 pound of water 1°F at the specified temperature. Numerically, specific heat is equal to heat capacity in either of the systems, but because it is a ratio, it is a pure number with no inherent dimensions and has the same meaning in any system of units. For example, the specific heat of hydrogen, measured at 1 atm and 21°C (70°F) is 3.41. This means that:

$$\frac{\text{Heat required to raise 1 g } H_2 \text{ 1°C, or 1 lb } H_2 \text{ 1°F}}{\text{Heat required to raise 1 g } H_2O \text{ 1°C, or 1 lb } H_2O \text{ 1°F}} = 3.41$$

Therefore, it takes 3.41 times as much heat to raise the gas temperature of hydrogen as that of water—3.41 calories for 1 g of gas as against 1 calorie for 1 g of water, or 3.41 Btu per pound of gas as against 1 Btu for 1 pound of water.

Because specific heat is among the data frequently provided for medical and commercial gases, special mention should be made of the two ways in which it can be measured. First, the specific heat can be calculated by heating a *constant volume* of a gas, in which case the heat energy applied is transformed into increasing molecular energy. Second, the heated gas may be kept at a *constant pressure,* as in a flexible container; in this instance because the expanding gas performs work (uses up heat) in displacing the surrounding atmosphere, more energy is required to bring the gas to the specific temperature. Therefore, a gas has two specific heats, that of constant volume (C_V) and that of constant pressure (C_P), which is larger. In the previous example of hydrogen, 3.41 is the C_P value, whereas the C_V is 2.40.

Among the specifications of a given gas, the specific heat can be listed as *Btu/(lb-mole) (°F)*, or less frequently as *cal/(g-mole) (°C)*. This gives the heat value for a pound molecular weight, or a gram molecular weight. If we wish to convert the figure to a simpler pound or gram relation, it is only necessary to divide the number by the molecular weight of the gas. Expressed as pound mole or gram mole specific heat, hydrogen is 6.89, or 3.41 times 2.02 (the molecular weight of hydrogen).

Change of state

All matter can change from a solid to a liquid to a gas. This is called a change of state. In respiratory therapy we deal with the so-called *permanent gases* because, in our study, they are in the gaseous state. Still, these same gases can also be liquids or solids, depending on the pressures or temperatures to which they are exposed. In the interest of economy and for ease of transportation and storage, it is often convenient to transform permanent gases into a liquid or solid state. Therapists should understand the basic thermodynamics of changes of state for those substances they use as therapeutic gases, as well as the function and performance of their mechanical equipment. It is important to understand the terms and expressions used to describe the specifications of commercially prepared gases.

We should mention here that while all materials can exist in all three states, it is possible to have a material that goes from a solid to a gas without being a liquid. This is called *sublimation*.

If the three states of a given substance were drawn on a graph that included combinations of temperature, in O°C, and pressure, in atmospheres, three lines could be used. If a line were drawn indicating the temperatures and pressures when a liquid becomes a vapor, when a solid becomes a liquid, and when a solid sublimates to become a vapor, these three lines would intersect at one point called the *triple point*. The significance of this point is that it is the only combination of temperature and pressure that allows the solid, liquid, and vapor forms of a given substance to exist in equilibrium with one another. Every substance has its own triple point. Fig. 1-6 diagrammatically shows the triple point of water. Line *AB* plots the boiling points of water at various pressures and also indicates the saturated vapor pressure at different temperatures. This emphasizes the relationship between increasing pressure and increasing boiling points of water. Line *AB* terminates at the so-called *critical point* (described later). Line *AD* represents conditions for water to sublimate, which is to move directly from ice to a vapor, or back. *AC* indicates the transition points between ice and liquid water (the melting or freezing point). The steepness of *AC* indicates the relatively small effect exerted by pressure on melting or freezing points. At any plot of pressure and temperature that falls within the confines of the points *CAB*, water can exist *only* as a liquid. At points below *DAB*, pressures are too low for water to be anything other than gaseous. However, if the temperature is above the triple point, an elevation of pressure would transform the vapor into a liquid, and if below this point, directly into ice. The points *DAC* delineate the pressure-temperature condi-

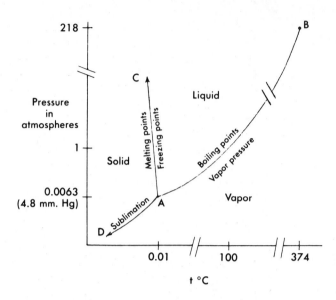

Fig. 1-6   The intersection of the three lines at *A* represents the *triple point* of water. Thus, at a temperature of 0.01°C and a pressure of 4.8 mm Hg, the three states of water (solid, liquid, and vapor) exist in equilibrium. The graphs show the pressure-temperature relationships of boiling, freezing, and sublimation of water.

tions necessary for the formation of ice. Therefore, at all points along each line, two phases of matter exist in complete equilibrium, but only at the triple point do all three equilibrate simultaneously.

It is interesting to note that if the pressure on a volume of water is reduced from 1 atm (760 mm Hg) to 0.0063 atm (4.8 mm Hg), the boiling point of water will drop from 100°C to almost 0°C. However, because the reduced pressure slightly alters the melting point of ice, the lines intersect at 0.01°C. Therefore, at a pressure of 4.8 mm Hg and a temperature of 0.01°C, ice, water, and water vapor coexist in equilibrium, not in a static state but actively, as molecules of the substance transform themselves from one form to the other forms. To appreciate the wide variation in range of triple points, note that the value for Freon-14 is −184°C and 0.88 mm Hg, whereas that of krypton is −157°C and 548 mm Hg.

The student should keep in mind that changes in state are always made at the expense of energy. This energy is supplied by heat that is either given or taken by the matter undergoing change.

Liquid to solid and solid to liquid. A solid will convert to its liquid form at a given temperature known as its *melting point.* The range of melting points is considerable. For example, carbon has a melting point in excess of 3500°C, and helium, less than −272.2°C. Melting is little affected by pressure, as noted earlier. In order to excite molecules from a fixed state to a fluid state, heat is

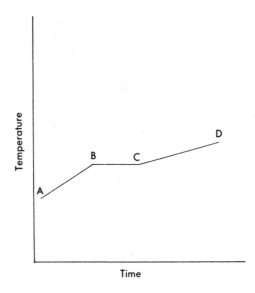

Fig. 1-7   *Heat of fusion* is illustrated by the temperature-time graph. Heat applied to a solid raises its temperature from *A* to *B;* at *B,* the solid begins to liquefy (melt). From *B* to *C,* the applied heat is utilized to accomplish the change in state, and the temperature of the substance does not rise further until liquefaction is complete, *C* to *D.*

required, which may be applied to the substance or may be extracted by the substance from its surroundings.

The heat needed to melt a substance is referred to as the *heat of fusion* (sometimes called the latent heat of fusion) and is defined as the calories required to change 1 g of the substance, or the Btu to change 1 pound of the substance, from the solid to the liquid state without changing its temperature. It is called *latent* because at a specific temperature (the melting point), the energy of the applied heat is used to effect the molecular change from solid to fluid and does not change the temperature of the mass. Only after the change of state has taken place does continued heat elevate the temperature of the newly formed liquid. Fig. 1-7 depicts the melting point of a solid mass to which heat has been applied. The solid is heated from *A* to *B,* with a simultaneous rise in temperature, but at *B,* liquefaction begins, and from *B* to *C* the temperature of the matter does not vary as the heat energy is used in the physical change. After melting is complete, at *C,* continued heat raises the temperature of the liquid from *C* to *D.* The temperature at *BC* is the melting point of the substance. Although pressure has little influence on melting, for the sake of uniformity, scientific tables often report heats of fusion at the triple points. Thus the latent heat of fusion of ice is 80 cal/g, calium chloride is 54 cal/g, oxygen is 3.3 cal/g, and argon is 6.7 cal/g, to give some idea of the diversity of energy needed for this change in state.

Freezing is the reverse of melting. Because considerable energy is utilized in transforming a solid into a liquid, this "stored" energy is released during the process of freezing; thus, in a sense, freezing is a heating process in that the freezing liquid must give up heat (by being exposed to cold) as its molecules assume the stable configuration of a solid mass. Therefore, for pure substances, freezing and melting points are the same.

Liquid to vapor and vapor to liquid. These changes of physical states are the most relevant to therapeutic gases, and we have already considered the mechanism of evaporation as the escape of molecules from a liquid surface to mix with the ambient gases adjacent to the surface. Maximum change of state from liquid to vapor (vaporization), however, occurs through the phenomenon of boiling, which differs significantly from evaporation. In evaporation, water molecules diffuse into ambient gases, whereas the vapor released by boiling escapes with sufficient force to displace surrounding gas. Also, where simple evaporation is purely a surface activity, boiling produces large bubbles of vapor throughout the depth of the liquid, which rise to the surface to escape. Boiling occurs at the *boiling point,* a temperature at which the vapor pressure of a liquid equals the pressure exerted on the liquid by the weight of the atmosphere and is influenced by two important factors. First, the boiling point is directly related to the atmospheric pressures on the liquid surface since the weight of the air molecules retards the escape of vapor molecules. The greater the pressure applied, the greater must be the kinetic energy of the fluid molecules to escape against the pressure. Energy than can only come from increasing heat. On the other hand, lower ambient pressures allow the easier escape of molecules, and boiling can occur at much lower temperatures. Second, dissolved substances exert a cohesive force that increases the bonding among the molecules so that greater heat energy is required to free them into the vapor state, elevating the boiling point. Although we are accustomed to associate the phenomenon of boiling with high temperatures, such as water at 100°C (212°F), the boiling points of the liquid state of substances we call gases have exceedingly low values. For example, tungsten boils at 5900°C, neon boils at -246°C, ozone at -112°C, and oxygen at -183°C.

Just as energy is needed to liquefy a solid, energy is also required to vaporize a liquid, and this energy is called the *heat of vaporization* (sometimes referred to as the "latent heat of vaporization," or simply "latent heat"). It is defined as the calories required to vaporize 1 g of a liquid, or the British thermal units to vaporize 1 pound of a liquid at its normal boiling point. When water is put on a stove to boil, its temperature rises steadily until the boiling point is reached, and then it maintains a constant temperature even though heat continues. This latent heat reflects the energy necessary to release the energy holding together the water molecules, freeing them to become vapor. It is interesting to note that the heat of vaporization for water is 540 cal/g, at 100°C, which is considerably higher than the heat of fusion of ice. This demonstrates that more energy is required to free water molecules into the vapor state than to rearrange them from the solid to the liquid state.

The therapist will often see the latent heat of vaporization listed in the specifications of commercial gases as Btu/lb-mole. For example, the latent heat of methane (CH_4, molecular weight 16.04) is given as 3519 Btu/lb-mole at its normal boiling point of $-126°C$ ($-258.6°F$). This means that to convert 16.04 pounds of methane (1 lb-mole) from a liquid to a gas, 3519 Btu of heat must be supplied. Since *latent heat* refers to the heat required to change 1 pound or 1 g of a substance, the above value can be reduced to the basic units of both the English and metric systems as follows:

(1) $\dfrac{Btu/lb\text{-}mole}{gmw} = Btu/lb$ $\dfrac{3519}{16.04} = 219\ Btu/lb$

(2) Because 1 Btu = 252 cal and 1 lb = 454 g

$\dfrac{Btu/lb\text{-}mole \times 252}{454} = Btu/lb\text{-}mole \times 0.554$

$= cal/g\text{-}mole$ $3519 \times 0.554 = 1950\ cal/g\text{-}mole$

(3) $\dfrac{Btu/lb\text{-}mole \times 0.554}{gmw} = cal/g$ $\dfrac{3519 \times 0.554}{16.04} = 122\ cal/g$

For every liquid there is a temperature above which the kinetic energy of the molecules is so great that the attractive forces cannot maintain them in a liquid state. This temperature is called the *critical temperature*. Because there is no pressure able to maintain the molecules of the matter in a liquid state above this temperature, the critical temperature is the highest temperature at which a substance can exist as a liquid. If an evacuated sealed tube partially filled with liquid is heated, vapor will escape into the vacuum. The density of the vapor will steadily increase as that of the liquid substance decreases, and when the critical temperature of the liquid is reached, the densities of both vapor and the remaining liquid will be equal, and the two phases of matter will become identical without a line of demarcation between them. Further elevation of the temperature will transform the entire mass into vapor. The pressure exerted by the vapor within the evacuated tube at the critical temperature is the *critical pressure,* and on a plotted vapor pressure-temperature curve, the two values identify what is known as the *critical point*. Each substance has its own critical point at which the gas phase is in equilibrium with the liquid phase, and the two are not visibly separated. Point *B* in Fig. 1-6 represents the critical point of water at a pressure of 218 atm and a temperature of 374°C. Here the densities of the liquid and vapor phases are not distinguishable, the two are in equilibrium, and beyond this temperature no pressure can revert the mass to liquid. Compare the high values for water with the critical values of the gases in Table 1-5.

Table 1-5 Critical points of three gases		°C	°F	atm
	Helium	−267.9	−450.2	2.3
	Oxygen	−118.8	−181.1	49.7
	Carbon dioxide	31.1	87.9	73

The terms *gas* and *vapor* are often erroneously used interchangeably, but the concept of critical temperature will help to differentiate them. Gas is a substance with a critical temperature so low that at usual ambient conditions of temperature and pressure, it cannot exist as a liquid with a surface exposed to the atmosphere. If the temperature of a gas is above its critical value, it cannot be compressed into a liquid by a pressure of any magnitude. Such substances are referred to as *permanent gases*. On the other hand, vapor is the gaseous state of a substance that also exists simultaneously in a liquid or solid state. Oxygen therefore is a permanent gas, since it has no solid or liquid phase under ambient conditions. Water is both a liquid and a gas at room temperature and 1 atm of pressure, and therefore its gaseous phase is a vapor. Appendix 8 lists the critical temperatures of several gaseous and vaporous substances.

Although we have described the critical points of matter in terms of the stability of liquids, they apply as readily to the transition of gas to liquid. To effect a change of state from gas to liquid we must cool the gas below its critical temperature and then compress it. Theoretically, it is possible to liquefy a gas by cooling alone, dropping its temperature below the substance's boiling point, but under no circumstances is it possible to liquefy it by pressure alone if its temperature is above its critical point. The further below its critical temperature a gas can be cooled, the less pressure is needed to liquefy it. Therefore, any gas whose critical temperature is above ambient can be liquefied by pressure alone because allowing the gas to equilibrate with ambient temperature actually keeps it below its critical temperature. Carbon dioxide has a critical temperature slightly above normal room temperature (31°C), with a corresponding critical pressure of 73 atm, but at room temperature of 21.5°C, less than 60 atm of pressure is needed to convert the gas to liquid.

Only those gases whose critical temperatures are above ambient can be kept in the liquid state for everyday use at room temperature, and they must be under pressure in strong storage cylinders. The anesthetic gases cyclopropane and nitrous oxide, along with carbon dioxide, are commercially supplied as tanked liquids, and Table 1-6 compares their critical points with the approximate pressures at which they are kept at room temperature to maintain their

Table 1-6 Pressures needed to maintain liquid state of gases at room temperature		Critical temperature		Critical pressure		Approximate pressure in commerical cylinder at room temperature	
Gas	°C	°F	atm	psi	atm	psi
Cyclopropane	125	257	54.2	797	5.4	79
Nitrous oxide	36.5	97.7	71.8	1054	50.6	745
Carbon dioxide	31.1	87.9	73.0	1071	57.0	838

liquid state. There are many industrial gases that are converted to the liquid state for ease of mass transportation, and with critical temperatures above ambient, they need only to be kept under sufficient pressure to ensure their liquid form. With release of pressure the liquid reverts immediately to gas.

Oxygen presents a more complicated problem, but because of its widespread medical and industrial use, moving and storage are made easier by keeping it in the liquid state. In contrast to the three gases illustrated above, oxygen has a low critical temperature of $-118.8°C$ ($-181.1°F$), and we know that no pressure will be able to keep it in liquid form above that value. In the manufacture of oxygen, large quantities of filtered air are subjected to tremendous pressures of up to 200 atm. This produces a great deal of heat, and the compressed gas is passed through heat exchangers and then subjected to a pressure drop of 5 atm. The rapid cooling brings the oxygen in the air below its boiling point of $-183°C$ ($-297°F$), and it liquefies. If oxygen can be kept in an insulated container so that its temperature does not exceed its boiling point, it will remain liquid at atmospheric pressure. Should higher temperatures be necessary, higher pressures must be used, but at no time can oxygen be allowed to exceed the critical temperature of $-118.8°C$ because it then converts immediately to gas.

Solid to vapor and vapor to solid. Solid matter, as well as liquid, can vaporize, and at any given temperature, solids have definite vapor pressures. The strong odor given off by napthalene (mothballs) is evidence of the escape of vapor from a solid. The direct transition from the solid to the gaseous state is called *sublimation,* and because a change of state is involved, energy is transferred. The heat, in calories per gram or British thermal units per pound, required to convert 1 g or 1 pound of a solid into a vapor is called the *heat of sublimation.* Sublimation resembles boiling because it occurs when the vapor pressure of the solid equals that of the opposing ambient pressure and because increasing and lowering of the ambient pressure directly displaces the subliming point. If temperature is below the melting point, a pressure drop produces boiling. At exactly 0°C, the vapor pressure over ice is 4.6 mm Hg, and if a vacuum less than this pressure is applied to the ice, the ice will sublime directly into water vapor.

Carbon dioxide is an interesting example of sublimation. If the gas is cooled to its critical point of $-57°C$, it will freeze, and the vapor will equilibrate with the solid at a pressure of 5.1 atm. When solid carbon dioxide is exposed to the atmosphere, the drop in pressure from 5.1 to 1 atm causes the solid state to sublime directly into vapor. Most people are familiar with the behavior of commercially prepared solid carbon dioxide, called "dry ice," as it gradually disappears when exposed to ambient conditions, leaving no trace of moisture. On the other hand, if solid carbon dioxide is subjected to pressures in excess of 5.1 atm and allowed to warm above $-57°C$, it will melt into a liquid without boiling.

It is possible to produce carbon dioxide snow by suddenly releasing the compressed liquid from a commercial tank. A rush of very cold vapor will emerge, carrying with it fine snowlike particles of solidified carbon dioxide. The rapid vaporization of the liquid in the tank requires heat, and the liquid removes this heat from itself, freezing part of the material so that the remainder may vaporize.

Consider that a given mass of matter is progressing through changes of state from solid to liquid to vapor. The step from solid to liquid uses energy that is called heat of fusion. The conversion of liquid to vapor requires heat of vaporization. Even though the direct transformation from solid to vapor eliminates the liquid phase, the same total energy is required, and the heat of sublimation is therefore equal to the sum of the heats of fusion and vaporization.

In summary, all matter can theoretically exist in three physical states, depending on specific conditions of pressure and temperature. Those substances that we commonly refer to as gases are in the vaporous state because ambient pressure and temperature cannot maintain them as liquids or solids.

The ideal gas laws are not applicable to conditions of extreme pressure and temperature because the relationships between pressure, temperature, and volume described by the laws break down as the factors of intermolecular force, molecular mass, and change of state influence the behavior of gases subjected to these extremes. This does not decrease the practical clinical value of the gas laws, but understanding the deviations from the laws permits us to see how matter can be manipulated and modified to serve specific purposes. In Appendix 8, some of the pressure-temperature characteristics of a few selected gases and water are compared so that the student can see the tremendous range of values that distinguish one type of matter from another.

References

1. Williams, A.L., et al: Introduction to chemistry, Reading, Mass., 1973, Addison-Wesley Publishing Co., Inc.
2. Saunders, F.A.: A survey of physics for college students, New York, 1936, Henry Holt and Co.
3. Quagliano, J.V.: Chemistry, Englewood Cliffs, N.J., 1964, Prentice-Hall, Inc.
4. Armstrong H.G.: Aerospace medicine, Baltimore, 1961, The Williams & Wilkins Co.
5. List, R.J., editor: Smithsonian meteorological tables, Washington D.C., 1958, The Smithsonian Institute.

Chapter 2 Solutions and ions

An understanding of some of the characteristics of solutions and ions is necessary to the study of the chemical characteristics of physiology. This is especially true of respiratory gas transport and acid-base balance. In this chapter, these characteristics are reviewed, as well as the structure of atoms, atomic stability, atomic bonding, and ionic and covalent compounds.

Atomic structure

One definition of an atom describes it as the smallest particle of an element that can take part in a chemical change. It can be thought of as the ultimate in the breakdown or degradation of matter, the final indivisible particle. Modern physics, however, has shown that this is not true because atoms can be fragmented, but extraordinary effort is required and it does not occur in usual chemical reactions. An element is a substance composed of one kind of atom, and a compound is a substance consisting of two or more different kinds of atoms. It is the constituent atoms that impart to matter its great variety of characteristics, through a myriad of combinations of the 105 different atoms currently identified.

Components of an atom. An atom can be imagined as a miniature orbital system, much like a sun and planets, with a *nucleus* surrounded by smaller particles called *electrons,* circling it mostly in pairs but with a few singles. The composition of the nucleus and the number of orbiting electrons are different and unique for each of the different kinds of atoms. It is estimated that the diameters of atoms range from 1×10^{-8} cm to 5×10^{-8} cm. The nucleus is the largest part of an atom, with a diameter of approximately 10^{-13} cm, and while it may contain many kinds of matter referred to as "particles," two particles comprise virtually all of its mass. *Protons* are particles with a positive electrical charge. They give to the nucleus an overall positive electrical charge, while *neutrons* have no electrical charge. Protons and neutrons have about the same mass (1.67×10^{-24} g) and constitute most of the weight of the atom. Other unstable nuclear components such as positrons, mesons, hyperons, and neutrinos do not contribute to the mass or chemical characteristics of atoms. For students' purposes, atomic nuclei can be considered as consisting solely of protons and neutrons, although there is one atom that has no neutrons. *Electrons* are particles of matter with a mass of some 9.1×10^{-28} g and are negatively charged, as opposed to protons.

Fig. 2-1 illustrates the structure of the two simplest and lightest atoms, hydrogen and helium. Note that hydrogen is the atom referred to previously with no neutrons in its nucleus; essentially, hydrogen consists only of one proton and one electron, the latter represented by an orbiting dot in the sketch. Helium has double the number of electrons and protons of hydrogen and includes two neutrons in its nucleus.

More typical of an "average" atom is the metal potassium (Fig. 2-2). Its mass is composed of 19 protons and 20 neutrons, with its electrons arranged in pairs with one single electron around the nucleus. In the resting or inactive ground state, the atom is electrically neutral. Since the nucleus of an atom of a given element has its own characteristic number of protons, it must have the same number of orbiting electrons to maintain electrical neutrality. The potassium atom therefore has 19 electrons distributed among four orbits.

Electron orbits. The orbits are known as *electron shells,* or *principal energy levels.* The simplest of the atoms—hydrogen and helium—have but one electron shell each, while the 19 most complex atoms have seven. The principal energy levels are designated both by numbers 1 through 7 and by capital letters K through Q. To help specifically designate increasing numbers of electrons among the more complex atoms, the principal energy shells may have one to four *subshells* identified by lowercase letters s, p, d, and f. Fig. 2-3 diagrams one half of one of the large atoms, demonstrating all seven electron shells and the number of subshells in each. Principal levels *1(K)* and *7(Q)* have only one orbit each for their electrons, while levels *4(N)* and *5(O)* have four sublevels. Level *2(L)* has two subshells, and levels *3(M)* and *6(P)* each has three subshells.

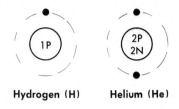

Hydrogen (H)   Helium (He)

Fig. 2-1   Atomic structure of hydrogen and helium. Hydrogen has no neutrons and only one orbiting electron and one proton. Helium is heavier, with two protons and two neutrons.

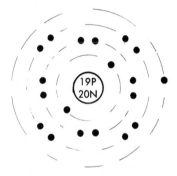

Fig. 2-2   Atomic structure of potassium. The significance of the single outer orbiting electron is clarified later.

Space limitations prevent discussion of other atomic details, but even the subshells as represented in Fig. 2-3 show how subordinate orbits or electron pathways known as *orbitals,* each limited to a maximum of one pair of electrons, help make up the structure of the atom. Single electrons may occupy an orbital of incompletely filled subshells. Subshell *s* has only one orbital, *p* has three, *d* has five, and *f* has seven orbitals. These illustrations oversimplify reality for the sake of explaining general principles. Actually, the electron shells are not all spherical, and there are overlaps among principal levels 3 through 7. For example, subshell *3d* falls between subshells *4s* and *4p,* and subshell *4d* is found between *5s* and *5p.* These spatial arrangements of the electrons relate to internal energies of the atoms and help to explain the progressive sequence of increasing atomic complexity.

The pattern of electron spacing among all the different kinds of atoms is summarized in Table 2-1. The maximum number of electrons that can be accommodated in each subshell and orbital is shown on the left, while the total for each principal level is shown in the center, and the cumulative totals are

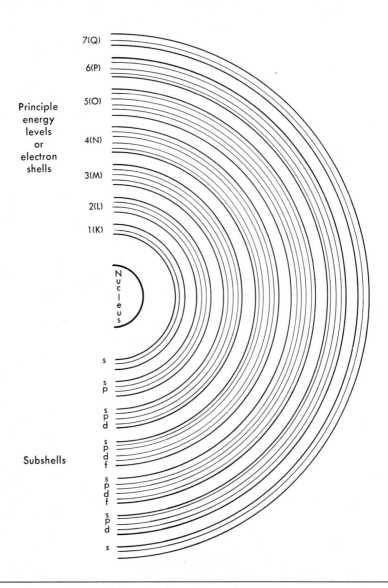

Principle
energy
levels
or
electron
shells

Subshells

Fig. 2-3   Imaginary section through one of the large atoms showing the maximum number of available shells and subshells for orbiting electrons. Placing all orbits on the same plane is an inaccurate simplification for the sake of illustration, as is the deliberate omission of overlapping of shells 3 through 7.

Table 2-1	Maximum number electrons per subshells			Maximum number electrons per principal shell			
Electron distribution among subshells and principal shell	Subshell	Orbitals	Electrons	Shell	Subshells	Electrons	Total electrons
	s	1	2	1(K)	s	2	2
	p	3	6	2(L)	sp	8	10
	d	5	10	3(M)	spd	18	28
	f	7	14	4(N)	spdf	32	60
				5(O)	spdf	32	92
				6(P)	spd	18 (11)*	110 (103)
				7(Q)	s	2	112 (105)

*Maximum number of electrons actually in level 6(P) of the known elements is 11 (2-6-3). Other numbers in parentheses are based on this figure.

shown on the right. These figures are *possible* maximum numbers of electrons, but all shells and subshells that contain electrons are not necessarily filled. Another view of electron distribution is given in Table 2-2, which is a section from a larger table of all 105 elements showing the location of electrons in their principal levels and sublevels. For the sake of space economy this segment includes only the first 36 elements and the last and most complex element for comparison. Designations of principal energy levels, subshells, and maximum numbers of electrons per subshell are given at the top of the table. The *atomic numbers* (Z) refer to the numbers of both nuclear protons and orbiting electrons of each element and provide a practical method listing the elements.

For this study, the main interest is with the outermost orbiting electrons. These are known as *valence electrons* and are responsible for the bonding of atoms into crystals, molecules, and compounds. This concept of "valence electrons" is vital to developing a working concept of molecular design and must be well understood by the student.

Atomic stability. Atomic stability exists when the *outermost energy level* of an atom contains just eight electrons. However, this description cannot be dogmatically applied to all elements since many of the more complex atoms have electron distributions that do not follow such simple scheme. Nevertheless, the outer orbit octet principle applies to many of those that are of interest in the study of physiology and are found among the 36 elements listed in Table 2-2.

Table 2-2 shows that subshells s and p, in any principal level but K, must be filled with their allocated electrons to be stable and that until stability is reached, no electrons may occupy a higher subshell. A major exception to this rule involves energy level K, which has only one subshell. Stability in this example is reached with only two electrons filling subshell s. Therefore, an atom with two electrons in its one and only energy level (K), or eight electrons in the highest of any of the other six levels, is a stable atom. There are only six elements whose atoms are naturally stable, rendering them chemically inert. They are the *inert gases,* helium (two electrons), neon, argon, krypton, xenon,

Table 2-2
Electronic configurations of the atoms

Atomic number (Z)	Element	(K) s	(L) s	(L) p	(M) s	(M) p	(M) d	(N) s	(N) p	(N) d	(N) f	(O) s	(O) p	(O) d	(O) f	(P) s	(P) p	(P) d	(Q) s
1	H	1																	
2	He	2																	
3	Li	2	1																
4	Be	2	2																
5	B	2	2	1															
6	C	2	2	2															
7	N	2	2	3															
8	O	2	2	4															
9	F	2	2	5															
10	Ne	2	2	6															
11	Na	2	2	6	1														
12	Mg	2	2	6	2														
13	Al	2	2	6	2	1													
14	Si	2	2	6	2	2													
15	P	2	2	6	2	3													
16	S	2	2	6	2	4													
17	Cl	2	2	6	2	5													
18	Ar	2	2	6	2	6													
19	K	2	2	6	2	6		1											
20	Ca	2	2	6	2	6		2											
21	Sc	2	2	6	2	6	1	2											
22	Ti	2	2	6	2	6	2	2											
23	V	2	2	6	2	6	3	2											
24	Cr	2	2	6	2	6	5	1											
25	Mn	2	2	6	2	6	5	2											
26	Fe	2	2	6	2	6	6	2											
27	Co	2	2	6	2	6	7	2											
28	Ni	2	2	6	2	6	8	2											
29	Cu	2	2	6	2	6	10	1											
30	Zn	2	2	6	2	6	10	2											
31	Ga	2	2	6	2	6	10	2	1										
32	Ge	2	2	6	2	6	10	2	2										
33	As	2	2	6	2	6	10	2	3										
34	Se	2	2	6	2	6	10	2	4										
35	Br	2	2	6	2	6	10	2	5										
36	Kr	2	2	6	2	6	10	2	6										
105	Ha	2	2	6	2	6	10	2	6	10	14	2	6	10	14	2	6	3	2

and radon. The first four are in Table 2-2 as Z-2, Z-10, Z-18, and Z-36, while the remaining two are larger atoms, Z-54 and Z-86.

All atoms other than those of the inert gases have varying degrees of chemical activity, which is a reflection of an attempt to reach stability by giving electrons to, by accepting electrons from, or by sharing electrons with other atoms. For example, atoms with one, two, or three valence electrons (such as Z-11, sodium; Z-12, magnesium; and Z-13, aluminum) tend to release them, emptying the outer orbits and letting the next lower shells satisfy electronic stability. In contrast, those with five, six, or seven valence electrons (such as Z-15, phosphorus; Z-16, sulfur; and Z-17, chlorine) tend to accept three, two, or one electron to reach stable octets. Atoms with four valence electrons (such as Z-6, carbon; and Z-14, silicon) can either release or accept four electrons. Some atoms neither donate nor accept electrons but reach stability by sharing them with other atoms. Finally, because the outer subshells of the inert gases are filled, there are no valence electrons available for either exchange or sharing.

Valence. The term *valence* is an expression of atomic combining capacity and refers to the number of electrons able to participate during chemical reactions. In current textbooks there is an increasing use of the term *oxidation number,* which, although not a true synonym of valence, has the same implication as valence in atomic bonding and the same numeric value. Valence is designated by positive and negative superscripts following elemental symbols such as Na^+ and $S^=$. It has already been mentioned that atoms at rest are electrically neutral, with equal numbers of protons and electrons. In a chemical reaction, if one atom releases electrons to another to reach stability, the first atom will be left with more positive protons than negative electrons and will therefore have a net positive charge. Electron donors such as potassium (K^+) and calcium (Ca^{++}) are said to have positive valences (or oxidation numbers) equal to the number of electrons received, such as chlorine (Cl^-), and oxygen $(O^=)$. Elements that donate electrons are said to be *oxidized,* or to undergo *oxidation,* while those that are electron acceptors are *reduced,* or undergo *reduction.* An element that is itself oxidized reduces another and is called a *reducing agent.* The opposite is an *oxidizing agent.* If this seems backward, remember that an electron is negatively charged and by accepting an electron (e^-), the accepting atom's total charge becomes reduced.

While most of the elements Z-1 through Z-20 are common and familiar and their usual valences are well known, these are valences unexpected from the electron configuration. For example, nitrogen not only has multiple valence values but also multiple valence signs such as $+5$, $+3$, and -3. These apparent inconsistencies arise from the orientation of electrons within subshell orbitals, rendering their exchange susceptible to various chemical, thermal, and pressure influences. On the other hand, manganese (Z-25) has possible valences of $+2$, $+3$, $+4$, $+6$, and $+7$. Here, as many of the larger atoms, there are unfilled subshells (i.e., 3d) proximal to the outermost s and p orbits. Chemical reactions of these atoms may involve electrons in the *next* to outermost shell as well as the valence electrons. At no time, however, can the valence number exceed seven. In general, the most common valence number will be the first number given for the elements listed in Appendix 9.

Atomic bonding

A chemical bond is a force that holds atoms together in crystals or molecules. Following are two descriptions of the two major kinds of atomic bonding, *ionic* and *covalent*.

Ionic (electrovalent) bonding. It is in this type of bonding between atoms that the electron exchange just described takes place. When electrons are gained or lost, the atoms are left with either increased positive or negative charges. These charged atoms are called *ions*. Those with positive charges (e.g., Na^+) are *cations,* and those with negative charges (e.g., F^-) are *anions*. The symbols for ions and the valence designation of elements are the same.

Fig. 2-4 illustrates the electron exchange between potassium and chlorine to form the salt potassium chloride (KCl). Only the valence electrons in the outermost shells are shown since they are the only electrons participating in any bonding examples used. Although potassium has one more energy level than does chlorine, the major difference in electron distribution lies in the outermost shells. Here, potassium has one electron, and chlorine has seven. If potassium donates its electron to chlorine (is oxidized and reduces chlorine), potassium's M shell, with eight electrons, becomes its outermost, and the atom achieves stability. The loss of an electron converts the potassium atom into an ion, leaving it with 19 protons compared to 18 electrons, giving it a net ionic charge, valence, and oxidation number of +1. When the chlorine accepts the electron from potassium (is reduced and oxidizes potassium), the electron octet of chlorine's M shell is completed and is stabilized. Chlorine is now an ion

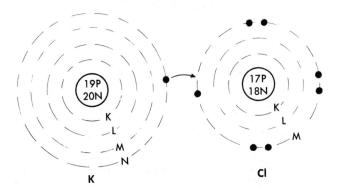

Fig. 2-4   Ionic bonding of potassium to chloride by the transfer of a single electron from potassium to chloride. (See text for details.)

with 18 electrons and 17 protons and a -1 electrical charge, valence, and oxidation number.

Electrovalent bonding is characteristic of the highly reactive elements with strong electropositivity and negativity that need to lose or gain one to three electrons to reach stability. Metals are in this group, as are such negative valence elements as fluorine, chlorine, oxygen, and sulfur. Some elements such as fluorine, chlorine, and oxygen can be part of both ionic and covalent bonding, depending on the nature of the specific reaction.

Ionic compounds do not form true molecules. Instead, cations and anions are held together in aggregates called crystals and referred to as giant molecules, or macromolecules. In aqueous solution, crystals break down into their constituent ions, a process called *dissociation*.

Covalent bonding. Electrons are shared in pairs rather than exchanged in covalent bonding. This type of union is formed between elements with less contrasting properties than those of ionic compounds. It is formed between two atoms of the same element and between hydrogen and carbon in the numerous organic compounds of which they are major ingredients. The elementary gases such as H_2, N_2, O_2, Cl_2, Br_2, and I_2 are covalent compounds, as are HCl, H_2O, NH_3, SO_2, SO_3, and CH_4, to cite a few common substances.

In contrast to the crystalline structure of ionic compounds, atoms covalently bonded form molecules, the smallest intact units of matter capable of independent existence. Their formulas are molecular formulas that can be used to calculate true *gram molecular weight*. Because ionic compounds have no molecular form and dissociate into their ultimate particles, ions, they have only empiric formulas, which express the ratios of their combined elements and from which gram formula weights can be derived.

There are two varieties of covalent bonds, *nonpolar* and *polar*. The term *polar,* as used here, refers to the distribution of electrical charges throughout the covalent molecule. If positive and negative charges are evenly spread about a particle so that neither dominates any area, the particle is said to be nonpolarized, or nonpolar. In contrast, a particle on which positive charges gather predominately in one region and negative charges in another is considered polarized (possessing positive and negative poles) and is *polar* in nature. The net electrical activity of both particles may actually be neutral, but because of concentrations of opposing charges, the polarized particle is more responsive to electrical influences surrounding it than is the relatively inert nonpolar particle.

Polarization of covalent molecules is dependent on three factors. First, molecules that are symmetrically constructed with spatially balanced atoms tend to have a uniform spread of electrical charges without polarization, while those with less symmetry are apt to concentrate their charges into poles. Second, the nuclei of some atoms have a greater attraction for electrons than do the nuclei of others and gather most of the electrons in their vicinity. This creates an area, or pole, of negativity that must be countered by an opposing positive pole. Third, when one atom has a larger number of electrons than its partner, the following imbalance generates molecular polarity.

Nonpolar covalent bonding. Fig. 2-5 illustrates the covalent bond of two atoms of fluorine in a molecule of fluorine gas with the formula F_2. Each atom needs one electron to build a stable octet in its outer shell. The atoms combine their single electrons into a pair shared by both, creating a diatomic molecule. This is an example of a single bond, single element, symmetric, nonpolar covalent compound. Fig. 2-6, on the other hand, demonstrates the structure of

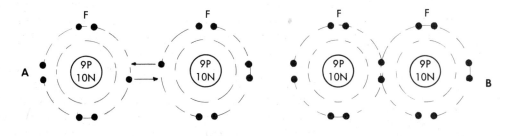

Fig. 2-5   Single bond, single element, symmetrical, nonpolar covalent bonding joins two atoms of elemental fluorine (**A**) into a molecule of fluorine gas (**B**), each atom sharing an electron from the other.

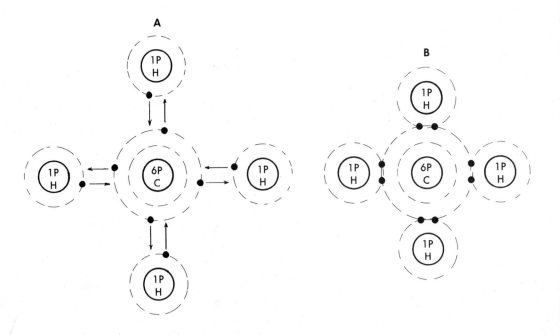

Fig. 2-6   Multiple bond, dissimilar element, symmetrical, nonpolar covalent bonding joins one atom of carbon with four atoms of hydrogen (**A**), to make the organic compound, methane, CH_4 (**B**).

methane (CH₄), a multiple bond, dissimilar element, symmetric, nonpolar covalent compound.

In contrast to ionic compounds, nonpolar covalent substances have no ions into which they can dissociate in water, nor do they form ions easily in solution because of their electrically neutral status.

Polar covalent bonding. By definition, polar covalency implies opposing molecular regions of electrical charges. Molecules so unbalanced are referred to as *dipoles* (possessing two poles). Fig. 2-7 shows that hydrogen chloride (HCl) is such a dipole (also called a polar covalent compound). The predominance of electrons about the chloride atom compared with the hydrogen atom gives a negativity to the chloride portion of the molecule, leaving the hydrogen end positive. The polarity is indicated in the sketch by the charge signs at each pole of the molecule.

One atom of oxygen holds two atoms of hydrogen in double, polar, covalent bonding to make a molecule of water. Fig. 2-8 illustrates the characteristic structure of a water molecule where the hydrogen atoms diverge from one another at an angle of 105 degrees. This gives polarity to the molecule, with negativity at the oxygen end and positivity around the hydrogens.

Generally speaking, and in contrast to nonpolar substances, polar molecules *ionize* in aqueous solution. This means that the molecules break into ions that are formed when the molecules dissolve, as opposed to the dissociation into

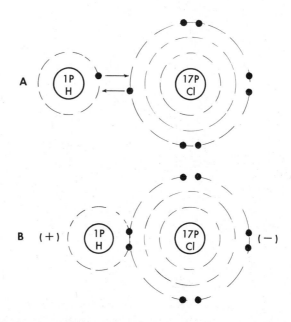

Fig. 2-7   **A,** Hydrogen chloride is a single bond, dissimilar element, asymmetrical, covalent bonded compound. **B,** It forms dipoles, with areas of opposing electrical charges. (See text for explanation).

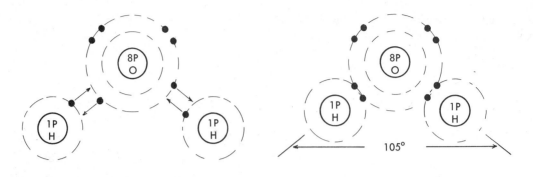

Fig. 2-8 The water molecule is a double covalent, polar compound, with two atoms of hydrogen attached to one atom of oxygen at an angle of 105 degrees to one another.

ions already present in ionic compounds. In terms of ion formation, polar covalent compounds are intermediate between the strong ion production of electrovalent substances and the negligible activity of those with nonpolar covalent bonds. Even within the polar group there is considerable variation. Hydrochloric acid readily forms many ions in a water solution, while water generates very few.

Equivalent weights

Weights of reacting substances that have equal chemical power are referred to as *equivalents, equivalent weights,* or *chemical equivalents.* Therefore, when A reacts chemically with B, one equivalent of A will react exactly with one equivalent of B, and there will be no excess of reactants remaining.

There are two magnitudes of equivalent weight measurements related to one another in the ratio of 1:1000. Therefore, the term *equivalent* is a general one, and in specific uses the proper unit must be stated. The two levels of equivalents are the *gram equivalent weight* (gEq) and the *milligram equivalent weight,* or *milliequivalent* (mEq). A gram equivalent weight is related to a milligram equivalent weight as a gram is related to a milligram. One gram equivalent equals 1000 mEq. To avoid confusion, this text follows the usual format of defining and describing chemical equivalents in terms of the gram equivalent weight. This concept of gram molecular weight must be mastered by the student.

Gram equivalent weight

The gram equivalent weight of a substance is its quantitative chemical reacting unit and is defined as the *gram mass that contains, replaces, or reacts with (directly or indirectly) the Avogadro number (1 mole) of hydrogen atoms.*

Equivalent weight of an element or radical. The equivalent weight of an element or radical is the weight in grams that combine with or replace in a chemical reaction 1 gram atomic weight (1 mole) of hydrogen or other mono-valent elements. For example:

1. In hydrochloric acid (HCl), one atom of chlorine combines with one atom of hydrogen. In terms of moles or gram atomic weights, this means that 35.5 g of chlorine (gram atomic weight of chlorine) combines with 1 g of hydrogen (gram atomic weight of hydrogen). Therefore the equivalent weight of chlorine is the same as its gram atomic weight, 35.5 g.

2. One atom of sulfur (S) combines with two atoms of hydrogen (H) in hydrogen sulfide (H_2S), which means that 32 g of sulfur (1 mole) combines with 2 g of hydrogen (2 moles). Therefore, 0.5 gram atomic weight of sulfur combines with, or is equivalent to, 1 atomic weight of hydrogen. The gram equivalent weight of sulfur is therefore 0.5 its gram atomic weight, or 16 g.

3. The formula of sulfuric acid (H_2SO_4) shows us that one sulfate group (SO_4) combines with two atoms of hydrogen. Therefore, 0.5 gram formula weight, or 0.5 mole of sulfate, is the equivalent of 1 mole of hydrogen atoms. The equivalent weight of SO_4 is 0.5 its gram formula weight, or 48 g.

These samples demonstrate that the numeric value of the gram equivalent weight of an element or radical is simply its gram atomic, or gram formula, weight divided by its valence, with no regard for the valence sign. If an element has more than one valence, the valence must either be specified or apparent from the element's observed chemical combining properties. Therefore, with a valence of $+1$, the gEq of Na is its gram atomic weight of 23 g; the gEq of Cu^{++} is its atomic weight divided by 2, or 31.7 g; the gEq of $Br^{=}$ is its atomic weight divided by 3, or 26.6 g.

Equivalent weight of an acid. This is the weight in grams of the acid that contains 1 gram atomic weight (1 mole) of *replaceable* hydrogen. Following are a few examples.

1. In the reaction $HCl + Na^+ \rightarrow NaCl + H^+$, the single hydrogen atom of hydrochloric acid is replaced by sodium. It can therefore be concluded that 1 mole of hydrochloric acid has 1 mole of replaceable hydrogen and by definition, the gram equivalent weight of hydrochloric acid is the same as its gram formula weight, or 36.5 g.

2. The two hydrogen atoms of sulfuric acid (H_2SO_4) are both considered replaceable. Therefore, 1 mole of the acid contains 2 moles of replaceable hydrogen. For the ratio to conform to the definition given above, 0.5 mole of acid must contain 1 mole of replaceable hydrogen. The gram equivalent weight of sulfuric acid is therefore 0.5 its gram formula weight, or 49 g.

3. Carbonic acid (H_2CO_3) has two hydrogen atoms, but in reactions under physiologic conditions, only one is considered replaceable. This is illustrated in the reaction $H_2CO_3 + Na^+ \rightarrow NaHCO_3 + H^+$. Only one

hydrogen atom is released, the other remaining bound. Despite the presence of two hydrogen atoms, 1 mole of acid contains only 1 mole of replaceable hydrogen, and the gram equivalent weight of carbonic acid is its gram formula weight, or 62 g.

4. As a general rule, the gram equivalent weight of an acid can be calculated by *dividing its gram formula weight by the number of atoms of hydrogen atoms in its formula*. Exceptions to this rule are those acids whose hydrogen atoms are not completely replaceable or are variably replaceable according to specific reactions. The major exceptions in the area of interest are carbonic acid, illustrated above, and phosphoric acid (H_3PO_4), an important physiologic buffer. Equivalent weights of both are determined by the conditions of their chemical reactions.

Equivalent weight of a base. The equivalent weight of a base is the weight of the base in grams that contains 1 gfw (1 mole) of *replaceable* hydroxyl (OH^-) radicals. Like the acids just described, the gram equivalent weight of a base is calculated by *dividing its gram formula weight by the number of OH groups in its formula*.

Equivalent weight of a salt. The equivalent weight of a *normal* salt (i.e., a salt molecule that does not contain replaceable hydroxyl groups or hydrogen) is the gram weight that contains 1 gEq of either of its components. Only one needs to be analyzed since, of necessity, the other will have the same chemical equivalency.

1. For example, the gram equivalent weight of chlorine (Cl) is 1 gram atomic weight, or 35.5 g. Since a mole of sodium chloride (NaCl) contains 1 gram atomic weight, or 1 gEq of chlorine, the equivalent weight of sodium chloride is its gram formula weight, 58.5 g.

2. Because sodium is a monovalent element, we know that its gram equivalent weight is 1 gram atomic weight. In the formula for the salt sodium sulfate (Na_2SO_4), the subscript 2 indicates that there are 2 gram atomic weights of sodium per mole of the salt. If 1 mole of sodium sulfate has 2 gEq of sodium, then 0.5 moles would contain 1 gEq. The gram equivalent weight of sodium sulfate, therefore, is 0.5 its formula weight, or 71 g.

3. The gram equivalent weight of a normal salt can easily be calculated by *dividing its gram formula weight by the total of either positive or negative valence*. The total valence is the valence of a given element multiplied by the subscript of that element or radical as it appears in the formula of the salt. Thus the gram equivalent weight of ferric oxide (Fe_2O_3) is $159.8 \div 6$, or 26.6 g (using Fe $+3$ valence times the 2 Fe, or if one chooses using the two negative charges on the three oxygens; the product of either method is 6, used as the denominator above).

4. For a *complex* salt such as an acid, basic, or double salt, the gram equivalent weight of the components of sodium dihydrogen phosphate (NaH_2PO_4) are:

$$
\begin{array}{lll}
\text{for Na}^+ & \text{gfw of salt} \div & 1 \\
\text{H}^+ & & 2 \\
\text{PO}_4^= & & 3
\end{array}
$$

Exercise 2-1: Assuming complete replaceability of H and OH, calculate the equivalent weights of the following:

A. HBr
B. H_3PO_4
C. HNO_2
D. H_3AsO_4
E. H_2S
F. KOH
G. $Zn(OH)_2$
H. $Al(OH)_3$
I. NH_4OH
J. $Mg(OH)_2$

Exercise 2-2: Calculate the gram equivalent weights of the following:

A. MgF_2
B. $CaCl_2$
C. Na_3PO_4
D. $Ca_3(PO_4)_2$
E. $Al(OH)_2Cl$

Converting gram weight to equivalent weight. To determine the number (or fraction) of gram equivalent weights in a given substance, *the gram weight of the substance is divided by its calculated equivalent weight.* Therefore, 58.5 g of NaCl divided by its gram equivalent weight of 58.5 g equals 1 gEq, whereas 29.25 g of NaCl divided by 58.5 g equals 0.5 gEq. Or, 407.8 g of $AgNO_3$ divided by 169.9 g equals 2.4 gEq.

Finally it should be pointed out that an equivalent of a compound or a fraction or multiple of a compound contains the same degree of equivalency of each of its components. For example:

$$
(1)\ \ 1\text{ gEq NaCl} \ \ = \frac{23 + 35.5}{1} \ \ = 58.5\text{ g}
$$

$$
1\text{ gEq Na} \ \ = \frac{23}{1} \ \ = 23\text{ g}
$$

$$
1\text{ gEq Cl} \ \ = \frac{35.5}{1} \ \ = \frac{35.5\text{ g}}{58.5\text{ g}}
$$

$$
(2)\ \ 2\text{ gEq Na}_2\text{CO}_3 = \frac{2[23(2) + 60]}{2} = 106\text{ g}
$$

$$
2\text{ gEq Na} \ \ = \frac{2(23)}{1} \ \ = 46\text{ g}
$$

$$
2\text{ gEq CO}_3 \ \ = \frac{2(12 + 48)}{2} \ \ = \frac{60\text{ g}}{106\text{ g}}
$$

Therefore, if 2 gEq of sodium is required, the other ingredients could be disregarded, and 117.0 g of NaCl, 106 g of Na_2CO_3, or 109.3 g of Na_2PO_4 would be measured out.

Exercise 2-3: Calculate the number of gram equivalent weights in the stated quantities of the following compounds:
A. 62 g MgF_2
B. 50 g $CaCl_2$
C. 120 g $Na_3(PO_4)$
D. 10 g $Ca_3(PO_4)_2$
E. 1.5 kg $CuCl_2$

Milligram equivalent weight   When referring to small amounts of chemically reactive substances, especially as found in physiologic chemistry, the term *milligram equivalent,* or *milliequivalent weight (mEq),* is often used. A milliequivalent is 0.001 of a gram equivalent weight and is expressed in milligrams instead of grams. Just as a gram consists of 1000 mg, 1 gEq is equal to 1000 mEq. It should be restated here that the terms *equivalent* or *equivalent weight* are general ones, without specification of units of measurement. They apply equally to scales of grams and milligrams. For examples, the *gram* equivalent weight of sodium chloride is 58.5 *g,* but it can also be said that its *milliequivalent* weight is 58.5 *mg.* In other words, the equivalent weight of sodium chloride is 58.5, and it is up to the respiratory therapist to apply gram or milligram units as the occasion requires. Therefore, because 58.5 g of sodium chloride is 1 gEq, 58.5 mg is actually 0.001 gEq; but to minimize the transition in translating decimals back and forth, it is easier to call the smaller amount 1 mEq. Again, 0.5 gEq can also be called 500 mEq, and 1340 mEq can be called 1.34 gEq.

When calculating equivalents, if weights of substances are given in grams, equivalents are probably better expressed in gram equivalent weights, and if weights of the substance are given in milligrams then it is better to express them in milliequivalent weights. Also, if specified weights of substances, when given in or converted to grams are numerically greater than their equivalent weights, the results should be given in gram equivalents; if they are less, they should be given in milliequivalents. Note that in dealing with medical problems of patients, the term *milliequivalents* is exclusively used since the concentrations of compounds in the blood such as Na^+, Cl^-, K^+, HCO_3^-, and others are very small. For example:

(1) Convert 150 mg of $CaCl_2$ to equivalents:

(a) 1 gEq = gfw ÷ 2 = 55.5 g *or*
1 mEq = mgfw ÷ 2 = 55.5 mg

(b) 150 mg = 0.150 g

therefore

(c) 0.150 g ÷ 55.5 g = 0.0027 gEq (awkward) *or*
150 mg ÷ 55.5 mg = 2.7 mEq (better)

(2) Convert 45 g MgO to equivalents:

(a) 1 gEq = gfw ÷ 2 = 20.2 g *or*
1 mEq = mgfw ÷ 2 = 20.2 mg

(b) 45 g = 45,000 mg

therefore

(c) 45,000 mg ÷ 20.2 mg = 2,228 mEq (awkward) *or*
45 g ÷ 20.2 g = 2.23 gEq (better)

Exercise 2-4: Convert the following to the proper corresponding weights or equivalents:
A. 5.3 g Na_2CO_3
B. 6.8 mg $CaSO_4$
C. 1.2 g $CuCl_2$
D. 2.3 mEq $AlBr_3$
E. 9.5 mEq $AgNO_3$

Use of equivalent weight

The importance of the equivalent weight as a chemical unit of measurement is its use in calculating quantities of substances reacting with one another and the products of such reactions. Consider the following (note that it is more meaningful to depict water as a 1:1 compound of a hydrogen atom and a hydroxyl group, HOH, than a 2:1 of hydrogen and oxygen as in H_2O):

$$Ca(OH)_2 + 2HNO_3 \rightarrow Ca(NO_3)_2 + 2HOH$$

Number of moles	1	2	1	2
Gram formula weight	74	2×63	164	2×18
	74	126	164	36
		(200)		(200)

This equation, with equal weights of substances on both sides, shows the quantities and proportions of both reactants and products involved in the reaction. It can be simplified, however, by deleting the coefficients and still show the proportion of ingredients that will exactly react. If the equation is rewritten entering only one equivalent for each substance and the corresponding gram equivalent weights, the formula would be written:

$$Ca(OH)_2 + HNO_3 \rightarrow Ca(NO_3)_2 + HOH$$

Number of equivalents	1	1	1	1
Gram equivalent weights	37	63	82	18
		(100)		(100)

By writing the equation in terms of equivalent weights, balancing it is unnecessary, and the proportions of reactants and products are the same as above.

In medicine, it has become customary to refer quantitatively to certain essential substances that are highly reactive in the body in terms of their equivalent weights. This is especially true of such elements as sodium, potassium, and chlorine and the bicarbonate radical HCO_3^-, which are in small enough quantities to be measured in milliequivalents. To the physiologist the number of chemically reactive units (mEq) present in the blood is more meaningful than bulk weight in milligrams. The therapist should be aware of the method the laboratory uses in reporting these elements.

In the hospital clinical laboratory these blood chemicals (also known as *electrolytes*) are quantitatively measured in milligrams per 100 ml of blood, customarily referred to as *mg%* or *mg/dl*. This text uses the modern designation of mg/dl, *dl* being the abbreviation of deciliter, one tenth of a liter, or 100 ml. These values are then converted by the technologist into the corresponding equivalent weights and reported as milliequivalents per liter of blood, or mEq/ℓ. Transposition between mEq/ℓ and mg/dl is performed as follows:

(1) $mEq = \dfrac{mg}{equiv\ wt}$

$mEq/\ell = \dfrac{mg/dl \times 10}{equiv\ wt}$

(2) $mg = mEq \times equiv\ wt$

$mg/dl = \dfrac{mEq/\ell \times equiv\ wt}{10}$

Therefore, if a blood sample contains 322 mg/dl of sodium, it would be reported as

$$\frac{322 \times 10}{23} = 140\ mEq/\ell$$

As a check, $140\ mEq/\ell = \dfrac{140 \times 23}{10}$ or 322 mg/dl.

Table 2-3 Concentrations of ingredients listed on label of Ringer's solution container		mg/dl		Approximate mEq/ℓ
	NaCl	600	Na	130
	$NaC_3H_5O_3$(Na lactate)	310	Cl	109
	KCl	30	$C_3H_5O_3$	28
	$CaCl_2$	20	K	4
			Ca	3

Table 2-4 Calculated milliequivalents (mEq) of ingredients of lactated Ringer's solution		Na	Cl	Lactate	K	Ca
	NaCl	102.6	102.6			
	NaLac	27.7		27.7		
	KCl		4.0		4.0	
	$CaCl_2$	____	3.6	____	____	3.6
	TOTAL MEQ/ℓ	130.3	110.2	27.7	4.0	3.6

In hospital practice, electrolyte replacement is commonplace therapy. This is accomplished by the intravenous infusion of solutions in which the electrolyte content is stated in milligrams per 100 ml of solution and as milliequivalents per liter. A typical example is a solution known as lactated Ringer's injection, the label of which lists its ingredients as show in Table 2-3.

Table 2-4 lists the equivalents of electrolytes more accurately, as calculated from milligram percentage, using the formula above for converting to mEq/ℓ.

Equivalents can be calculated for any volume of solution. As an example, one oral preparation lists the potassium chloride content as 3 g for each 15-ml (tablespoonful, approximately) dose. Each dose therefore provides 40.2 mEq of both potassium and chloride.

Exercise 2-5: Convert the following to the corresponding mEq/ℓ or mg/dl:
A. 296 mg/dl Na
B. 82 mm Eq/ℓ Cl
C. 23 mg/dl K
D. 9 mg/dl Ca
E. 26 mEq/ℓ HCO_3

Definition of a solution

A solution is a mixture of two substances with one evenly dispersed throughout the other. The substance dissolved, or going into solution, is called the *solute,* and the medium in which it is dissolved is called the *solvent.* The ease with which a solute mixes with a solvent is a measure of its solubility. The four factors influencing solubility are:

1. *Nature of the solute.* The degree to which all substances go into solution in a given solvent is a physical characteristic of matter, with wide variability.
2. *Nature of the solvent.* As with solutes, solvents vary widely in their ability to incorporate substances into solutions.
3. *Temperature.* In general, the solubility of most solid solutes increases with temperature; the solubility of gases, however, varies inversely with temperature.
4. *Pressure.* Solubility varies directly with pressure.

A solution is described as *dilute* if it has a relatively small amount of solute in proportion to solvent. Fig 2-9 shows three different states of a solution. In Fig. 2-9, *A,* the solution is considered dilute because it has relatively few solute particles. A saturated solution is one with the maximum amount of solute that can be held by a given volume of a solvent at a constant temperature, in the presence of an excess of solute. In such a mixture the dissolved solute is in equilibrium with the undissolved solute. Saturated solutions are usually prepared by adding a known excess of solute to the solvent, allowing the excess to remain in contact with the solution. Fig. 2-9, *B,* is a saturated solution, and

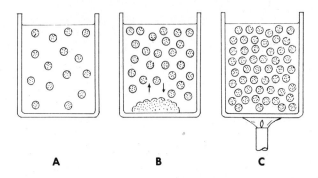

Fig. 2-9   In the dilute solution, **A,** the solute particles are relatively few in number, whereas in the saturated solution, **B,** the solvent contains all the solute it can hold in the presence of an excess of solute. Heating the solution, **C,** dissolves more solute particles, which may remain in solution if gently cooled, creating a state of supersaturation.

the excess solute is depicted as an undissolved mass at the bottom of the container. Although there is more solute in contact with solvent than the latter can accommodate at a fixed temperature, the excess must not be thought of as completely inert. Particles of solute precipitate into the solid state at the same rate that new molecules leave the supply of solute and go into solution. This is the state of equilibrium that characterizes a saturated solution. A solution is said to be *supersaturated* when it contains more solute in solution than does a saturated solution at the same temperature and pressure. If a saturated solution is heated, upsetting the solute equilibrium and allowing more solute to go into solution, and the remaining undissolved solute is filtered and the solution allowed to cool gently, then the solution will contain an excess of dissolved solute. Solution *C* in Fig. 2-9 can be considered the result of applying heat to the solution *B,* driving the remainder of the excess solute into solution. The additional dissolved particles may remain in solution, even after cooling to the temperature of the original saturated state, if extreme care is taken. Such a supersaturated solution is unstable, and the excess of dissolved solute may be precipitated out of solution by such physical stimuli as shaking or vibrating, or by adding to the solution a small amount of the solid solute.

Most of the solutions of physiologic importance in the body are *dilute,* and solutes in dilute solution demonstrate many of the properties of gases. This behavior is a result of the relatively large distances between the molecules of solute in dilute concentrations. Following are brief descriptions of four of the major characteristics of solutions:

1. *Vapor pressure depression.* The vapor pressure of a solution is less than that of the pure solvent. This is attributed to interference with the escape of solvent molecules by solute molecules at the liquid surface.
2. *Boiling point elevation.* The boiling point of a solution is higher than that

of the pure solvent, and its elevation is directly proportional to the number of solute particles in a given weight of solvent.

3. *Freezing point depression*. The freezing point of a solution is lower than that of a pure solvent, and its depression is directly proportional to the number of solute particles in a given weight of solvent.

4. *Osmotic pressure*. This is discussed separately later.

Quantitative classification of solutions	1. *Ratio solution*. The relationship of the solute to the solvent is expressed as a proportion (e.g., 1:100, parts per thousand, etc.). This is used frequently in describing concentrations of pharmaceuticals.

2. *Weight per volume (W/V) solution*. Often erroneously referred to as a "percent solution," the W/V solution is the one most commonly used in pharmacy and medicine for solids dissolved in liquids. It is calibrated in *weight of solute per volume of solution as grams of solute per 100 ml of solution*. Therefore, although 50 g of glucose in 1 L of solution is not a true percent relationship, it is customarily called a 5% (W/V) solution. In contrast, a liquid dissolved in a liquid is measured as volumes of solute to volumes of solution.

3. *Percent solution (%)*. Used in chemistry, a percent solution is calibrated as *weight of solute per weight of solution*. Five grams of glucose dissolved in 95 g of water is a true percent solution since the glucose is 5% of the total solution weight of 100 g.

4. *Molal solution (m)*. Less frequently used in physiologic chemistry than are the molar solution and the normal solution, a molal solution contains *1 mole of solute per kilogram of solvent (or 1 millimole per gram of solvent)*. A 1-m solution of sodium chloride contains 58.5 g (1 gfw) dissolved in 1000 g of solvent. This designation is of value when stability of precise concentrations of moles are desired over a wide temperature range. Volumes of liquid vary with temperature changes as do gases, although to only a fraction of the magnitude of gas volume changes. With its solvent measured in weight, the concentration of a molal solution is independent of temperature. For a specific solution at all temperatures a given *weight* of the solvent, regardless of its *volume,* will contain the same number of moles. |

    a. What is the molality of a solution with 162.4 g of $FeCl_3$ dissolved in 500 g of water?

        (1) 1 m solution = 162.4 g (1 gfw)/1000 g H_2O
        (2) 162.4 g/500 g = 324.8 g/1000 g
        (3) 324.8 g ÷ 162.4 g = 2 gfw/1000 g
        (4) Solution = *2 molal (2 m)*

    b. How much K_2SO_4 must be dissolved in 250 g water to make a 0.75-m solution?

        (1) 1 m solution = 174.2 g (1 gfw)/1000 g H_2O
        (2) 0.75 m solution = 174.2 × 0.75 = 130.65 g/1000 g

    (3) 130.65 g/1000 g = 32.66 g/250 g
    (4) *32.66 g/250 g* H_2O = 0.75 m

    5. *Molar solution (M)*. Chemically and physiologically the molar solution and the normal solution are the most important of all solutions. A molar solution has *1 mole of solute per liter of solution (or 1 millimole per milliliter of solution)*. A 1-M solution of sodium chloride contains 58.5 g (1 gfw) per liter of solution; a 0.5-M solution has 29.25 g/ℓ of solution; a 2-M solution has 117 g/ℓ of solution, etc. The solute is measured into a container, and the solvent is added to the total solution volume desired. The molar solution is chemically important because equal volumes of solutions of equal molarity contain the same number or fractions of solute moles.

    a. What is the molarity of a solution with 1.07 g NH_4Cl dissolved in 100 ml of solution?

        (1) 1 M solution = 53.5 g (1 gfw)/1000 ml solution
        (2) 1.07 g/dl = 10.7 g/1000 ml
        (3) 10.7 g ÷ 53.5 g = 0.2 gfw/1000 ml
        (4) Solution = *0.2 molar (0.2 M)*

    b. In what volume of solution must 41 g $Ca(NO_3)_2$ be dissolved to make a 3 M solution?

        (1) 1 M solution = 164 g (1 gfw)/1000 ml solution
        (2) 3 M solution = 164 g × 3 = 492 g/1000 ml
        (3) 492 g/1000 ml = 41 g/83.3 ml
        (4) 41 g dissolved in *83.3 ml* solution = 3 M solution

    6. *Normal solution (N)*. Widely used in chemistry and biochemistry, the normal solution has *1 gEq of solute per liter of solution (or 1 mEq per milliliter of solution)*. Accordingly, 1 gfw of HCl, $^1/_2$ gfw of H_2SO_4, $^1/_3$ gfw of AlF_3, and $^1/_6$ gfw of $Al_2(SO_4)_3$, each dissolved in 1 ℓ of solution, make 1-N solutions of the respective solutes. For all *monovalent* solutes, normal and molar solutions are the same because the equivalent weights of such solutes equal their gram formula weights. Equal volumes of solutions of the same normality contain chemically equivalent amounts of their solutes. If the solutes react chemically with one another, then equal volumes of the solutions will react completely, and neither substance will remain in excess. Solutions of known normality are often used as *standard solutions* in an analytic process known as titration for determining the concentrations of other solutions.

    a. What is the normality of a solution with 39.75 g of Na_2CO_3 dissolved in 250 ml of solution?

        (1) 1 N solution = 53 g (1 gEq = 1 gfw ÷ 2)/1000 ml solution
        (2) 39.75 g/250 ml = 159 g/1000 ml
        (3) 159 g ÷ 53 g = 3 gEq/1000 ml
        (4) Solution = *3 normal (3 N)*

    b. What weight of K_3PO_4 must be dissolved in 5 ml of solution to make a 1.5-N solution?

(1)1 N solution = 70.8 g (1 gEq = 1 gfw ÷ 3)/1000 ml solution   *or*
70.8 mg (1 mEq = 1 gEq ÷ 1000)/ml solution
(2) 1.5 N solution = 70.8 × 1.5 = 106.2 g/1000 ml   *or*
70.8 × 1.5 = 106.2 mg/ml

Exercise 2-6: Calculate the following:
A. How many grams of solute are there in 300 ml of a 3% (W/V) solution?
B. What volume will contain 70 mg of solute of a 7% (W/V) solution?
C. How many grams of solute and solvent are needed for 250 g of a 10% solution?
D. What weight of water is needed to dissolve 13 g of $BaCl_2$ to make a 0.25 m solution?
E. What is the molarity of a solution with 16 g of CH_3OH (methyl alcohol) in 200 ml of solution?
F. How many milliliters of 0.1-M $AgNO_3$ solution contain 8.5 g of solute?
G. How many grams of $C_{12}H_{22}O_{11}$ (cane sugar) are there in 50 ml of a 3-M solution?
H. What is the normality of a solution with 13.25 g of Na_2CO_3 in 500 ml of solution?
I.   How many milliliters of 2-N solution of $AlCl_3$ contain 8.9 g?
J.   How many milligrams of $Al_2(SO_4)_3$ are there in 10 ml of 0.2-N solution?

Osmotic pressure   One of the physical characteristics of solutions that has great physiologic significance is *osmotic pressure*. This is a measureable force produced by mobility of the solvent particles under certain conditions. Imagine a thin porous sheet constructed so as to permit the passage through it of molecules of solvent but not solute. Such a structure is called a *semipermeable membrane*. Should such a membrane be placed so as to divide a solution into two compartments, molecules of solvent would pass freely through it from one side to the other (Fig. 2-10, *A*). However, the number of molecules that pass (or diffuse) in one direction must be equaled by the number passing in the opposite direction to maintain an equal ratio between solute and solvent particles (which determines the concentration of the solution) on both sides of the membrane.

If a solution is put on one side of the semipermeable membrance and pure solvent on the other, solvent molecules will move through the membrane, but only in one directron, from the pure solvent to the solution, continuing to move until the supply of solvent is exhausted. The force driving the solvent molecules through the membrane is termed *osmotic pressure* and can be measured by connecting the expanding column of the solution to a manometer (Fig. 2-10, *B* and *C*). This pressure can be considered as a force that tries to distribute solvent molecules so there will be the same ratio between solute and solvent particles and thus the same concentration on both sides of the membrane. Osmotic pressure can also be visualized as the attractive force of solute

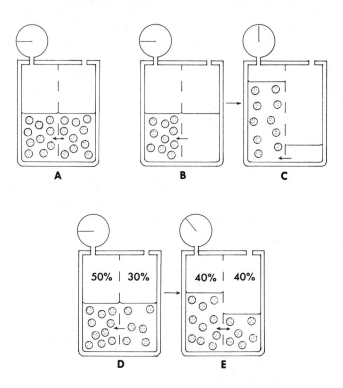

Fig. 2-10   Osmotic pressure is illustrated by the solutions in the above five containers. The containers are divided into two compartments by semipermeable membranes that permit the passage through them of solvent molecules but not solute *(dotted circles)*. The numbers of solute particles represent relative concentrations of the solutions, and since they are fixed in number and are confined by the membranes, volume changes are a function of the diffusible solvent, movements of which are indicated by the arrows through the membranes. The arrows between containers **B** and **C**, and **D** and **E**, indicate progressive sequences of osmotic pressure. (See text for further description.)

particles in a concentrated solution. If the conditions include placing a 50% solution on one side of the membrane and a 30% solution on the other, again the solvent molecules will penetrate the barrier from the dilute side to the concentrated side (Fig. 2-10, *D* and *E*). The greater number of solute particles per solvent molecules in the concentrated solution attract solvent molecules away from the smaller concentration of solute particles in the dilute solution. Migration of solvent molecules will continue until the attractive force (osmotic pressure) of solute is equal on both sides of the membrane. Such an equilibrium implies an equal ratio of solute/solvent particles in both compartments, or an equal concentration of 40%. At this point, solvent particles move equally in both directions.

Osmotic pressure is directly proportional to the concentration of solute and will be twice as strong in a 2% solution as in a 1% solution. For a given amount of solute, the osmotic pressure is inversely proportional to the volume, an application of Boyle's law to liquids. Also, osmotic pressure varies directly with temperature, increasing $1/273$ for each Celsius degree.

Body cell walls are semipermeable membranes, and through the action of osmotic pressure, the distribution of water throughout the body is kept within physiologic ranges. The term *tonicity* refers to the relative degree of osmotic pressure exerted by a solution. In a general way, the average body cellular fluid has a tonicity equal to that of a 0.9% NaCl solution, often referred to as physiologic saline. For comparative purposes any other solution with similar tonicity is called *isotonic,* one with greater tonicity is called *hypertonic,* and one with less *hypotonic.* Some cell walls possess *selective permeability,* allowing the passage not only of water but of specific solutes, and through this mechanism nutrients and physiologically active substances are distributed throughout the body.

Dilution calculations

It is often necessary to make a dilute solution from a stock preparation, and this can be done accurately if the concepts of solution concentrations are understood. Such dilution problems usually involve medications and are based on the pharmacologic weight/volume percent principle defined earlier. Diluting a solution increases its volume without changing the amount of solute it contains but reduces its concentration. Therefore the amount of solute in a given sample after dilution is the same as was present in the smaller original volume. The amount of solute present in a sample of a solution can be expressed as *volume* times *concentration.* For example, the amount of solute in 50 ml of a 10% solution (10 g/dl) is $50 \times 0.1 = 5$ g. In diluting a solution, then, the initial volume times the initial concentration equals the final volume times the final concentration. This can be simplified with the formula

$$V_1 C_1 = V_2 C_2$$

and when three of the data are known, the fourth can be calculated.

1. Given 10 ml of a 2% solution, dilute to a concentration of 0.5%. This requires finding the new volume.

$$V_1 C_1 = V_2 C_2$$
$$V_2 = \frac{V_1 C_1}{C_2} = \frac{10 \times 2}{0.5} = 40 \text{ ml}$$

Thus 30 ml added to 10 ml of 2% solution make 40 ml of 0.5% solution.

2. If 50 ml of water are added to 150 ml of a 3% solution, calculate the new concentration.

$$V_1 C_1 = V_2 C_2$$
$$C_2 = \frac{V_1 C_1}{V_2} = \frac{150 \times 3}{200} = 2.25\%$$

3. Given 50 ml of solution, dilute it to concentration. Here, concentration is given as normality, but it can be used as well as percent.

$$V_1 C_1 = V_2 C_2$$

$$V_2 = \frac{V_1 C_1}{C_2} = \frac{50 \times 0.333}{0.1} = 167 \text{ ml}$$

Exercise 2-7: Calculate the following:
A. To what volume would 15 ml of a 6% solution be diluted to make a 4% solution?
B. How much water would be added to 65 ml of a 3% solution to make 2.5%?
C. What was the concentration of 25 ml of solution, if the addition of 14 ml of water produced a 6.5% solution?
D. How much 3-M solution is needed to make 12 ml of 0.2-M solution?
E. If 92.75 mg of Na_2CO_3 is dissolved in 0.5 ml of water, what would be the normality of the solution after the addition of 0.67 ml of water?

Other solutions

Two types of liquid mixtures that are considered with solutions but that do not have specific characteristics of solutions are *collids* and *suspensions*. Collids (sometimes called *dispersions* or *gels*) consist of large molecules, or clumps of molecules, that are able to attract and hold large numbers of water molecules. Egg white, glue, soap, and gelatin are common examples. Colloid solutions are cloudy or opalescent, exert only slight osmotic pressure, and have little effect on boiling or freezing points. *Suspensions,* of which clay in water is a typical example, consist of large particles that are merely suspended in a liquid vehicle without the normal relationship between solvent and solute found in solutions. Dispersion of the suspended particles depends on physical agitation, and when the mixture is allowed to stand, the particles settle out.

Electrolytes and ions

One of the most important cardiopulmonary functions is the stability of acid-base balance. To understand its fundamentals, the student must first understand the principles of electrolytes and ions. The mechanism for regulation of acidity and alkalinity of the body and the transportation of respiratory gases, to and from the tissues, are interrelated. Neither can be completely understood without knowledge of the other.

Any substance in aqueous solution capable of carrying an electric current is called an *electrolyte;* nonconductors are called *nonelectrolytes.* In general, solutions of ionic or electrovalent compounds are good conductors of electricity. Nonpolar covalent compounds, however, have a wide range of conductivity, from the highly conductive hydrogen chloride to the barely conductive carbonic acid.

Nonelectrolytes and electrolytes differ also in their effects on the freezing and boiling points of water. Any substance dissolved in water will lower the freezing point and raise the boiling point. If the solute is a true nonelectrolyte, a 1-m solution will depress the water's freezing point 1.86° C and elevate its boiling point 0.52° C. In contrast, a 1-m solution of an electrolyte alters these points two to four times more than does the nonelectrolyte. The effect of solute on solvent freezing and boiling is a function of the concentration of solute particles. The more particles of solute per weight of solvent, the greater the displacement of freezing and boiling temperatures. Therefore, there must be more particles of solute per weight of solvent in an electrolyte solution than in a nonelectrolyte solution of equal molality.

Solutions of the same molality have the same number of moles (gram molecular or gram formula weights) of solute in the same weight of solvent. For example, a 1-m solution of simple glucose ($C_6H_{12}O_6$), a nonpolar covalent substance, will contain 1 gmw of sugar, or 6.02×10^{23} molecules per kilogram of water. This concentration of molecular particles lowers the freezing point of water 1.86° C and elevates its boiling point 0.52° C. A 1-m solution of sodium chloride, on the other hand, depresses the freezing point and elevates the boiling almost twice as much as does sugar. This means that the salt solution must have a larger number of particles in solution that does the sugar, or more than 6.02×10^{23} particles per kilogram of water. Because sodium chloride is an electrovalent compound, in solution 1 mole does not form 6.02×10^{23} molecules of sodium chloride but breaks down into a larger number of the smaller sodium and chloride ions. It is the larger number of these small ions that exerts a greater influence on the freezing and boiling of water than does the smaller number of larger sugar molecules. This is called the "colligative" property of the solute.

Ion formation

Ion formation includes the following three principles: (1) electrolytes in solution exist as ions, (2) ions are atoms or groups of atoms that carry electric charges, and (3) water solutions of electrolytes contain equal numbers of positive ions (cations) and negative ions (anions).

Ionic (electrovalent) solutions. Lacking molecular structure, ionic compounds exist as an orderly arrangement of ions in masses called crystals. Ions are present in such compounds even in the dry undissolved state. The process of dissolving consists of separating crystals into individual ions. The ions are freed from their mutual bonds and immediately distribute themselves uniformly throughout the solvent. This phenomenon is referred to as *ionic dissociation,* or just dissociation, since the ions released are ions already present in the solute rather than newly formed.

A common example of ionic or electrovalent dissociation in aqueous solution is that of sodium chloride, shown as follows:

$$Na^+Cl^- \text{ (s)} \rightarrow Na^+ \text{ (aq)} + Cl^- \text{ (aq)}$$

where *s* is solid state (g is gas; l is liquid), and *aq* is "in water." Charge signs in the compound formula indicate ions existing in the solid crystalline state before dissolving. The arrow indicates complete dissociation into ions. For the sake of simplicity this equation could be written:

$$NaCl \rightarrow Na^+ + Cl^-$$

Solutions of sodium chloride contain equal numbers of sodium and chloride ions to maintain electrical equilibrium. Calcium chloride ($CaCl_2$), in contrast, produces twice as many anions as cations, but the total charges remain equal:

$$Ca^{++}Cl_2^- \rightarrow Ca^{++} + Cl^- + Cl^-$$

It was originally thought that the role of water as a solvent was purely passive, providing a uniform medium in which electrolytic dissociation could spontaneously occur. The dipole water molecule is now recognized as being critically important in this phenomenon, participating in solute dissociation and regulating the degree to which ions are produced.

Fig. 2-11 represents the dissociation of sodium chloride. A crystalline mass of sodium and chloride ions rests on the bottom of the container. Water molecular dipoles are separating the crystalline ions through the electrical attraction of their polar charges. Negative oxygen poles of water molecules draw away from the crystal the positive sodium ions, while positive hydrogen poles relate similarly to chloride ions. As the ions diffuse throughout the solvent, each is loosely held by several water molecules surrounding it and facing it with oppositely charged poles. The number of water dipoles associated with a particular ion depends on the size and charge of the ion, and Fig. 2-11 is not intended to be quantitatively accurate. An ion associated with water dipoles is

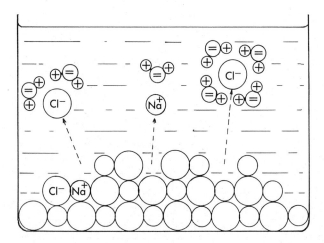

Fig. 2-11   Sodium chloride is shown as a crystalline mass of ions being dissociated by the attraction of water dipoles. (See text for a more detailed description.)

said to be *hydrated*. Hydration is a kinetic state, as water molecules continually interchange from ion to ion and between ions and the solvent mass.

Generally, ionic compounds are strong electrolytes, strength being a function of the degree of electrical conductivity. Conductivity, in turn, depends on the number of ions formed; the larger the concentration of ions made available by a solute, the stronger the electrolyte is.

Polar covalent solutions. Molecular covalent compounds have no ions of their own. In solution, however, through action similar to that described for the dissociation of sodium chloride, water dipoles can break the covalent bonds of polarized molecules and produce ions. In this circumstance ions are made from molecules in water where none existed before, and such a phenomenon is called *ionization,* as differentiated from ionic dissociation.

Ionization of a strong polar covalent electrolyte. Hydrogen chloride is a good example of a strong covalent electrolyte. In the pure liquid state from compression and cooling of the gas, or when dissolved in an organic nonpolar covalent solvent such as benzene, hydrogen chloride does not conduct electricity, demonstrating a lack of ions of its own; but when dissolved in water, it becomes an active electrolyte. The dramatic change in properties after hydrogen chloride dissolves is attributed to a function of the water solvent molecules. Fig. 2-12 illustrates the fundamental reaction between hydrogen chlo-

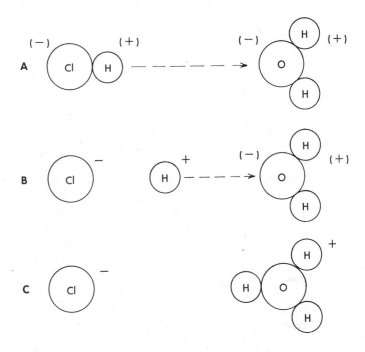

Fig. 2-12   Ionization of hydrogen chloride molecule by a water dipole. The hydrogen atom is separated from the chloride by the negative pole of a water molecule. (See text for details.)

ride molecules and water dipoles. Fig. 2-12, *A*, shows the negative pole of a water molecule reacting with the positive pole of a hydrogen chloride molecule. The effect is seen in Fig. 2-12, *B*, where the water dipole, through electrical attraction, has pulled the hydrogen from the chloride atom, leaving the chloride with the shared electrons, creating a chloride anion and a hydrogen cation. Ionization has been accomplished. Hydrogen ions, however, cannot exist alone in solution but only in combination with a dipole water molecule as shown in Fig. 2-12, *C*. The hydrated hydrogen ion becomes a group of three atoms with an overall net electrical charge of $+1$. It is called a *hydronium ion*. In terms of chemical action the hydronium ion is the hydrogen ion with the same meaning as the notation H^+. For convenience, the latter is more commonly used in chemical equations involving hydrogen ions, and it is used almost exclusively in the remainder of this text. Note that the simple hydrogen ion, H^+, is actually a proton. From Fig. 2-1 it can be seen that when a hydrogen atom loses its electron to become an ion, the only electrical charge left is the single nuclear proton. The hydronium ion therefore is actually a hydrated proton.

The ionization of hydrogen chloride depicted in Fig. 2-12 can be expressed chemically as follows:

$$HCl(g) + H_2O(\ell) \rightarrow H_3O^+ (aq) + Cl^- (aq)$$

or

$$HCl \rightarrow H^+ (aq) + Cl^- (aq)$$

or simply

$$HCl \rightarrow H^+ + Cl^-$$

Notice that the formula for HCl is written without charge signs, as opposed to Na^+Cl^-, to demonstrate its molecular (rather than ionic) structure. The student should understand that the process of ionization changes the nature of the substance ionized. Hydrogen chloride, as a gas or a solute in a nonpolar solvent, is transformed into hydrochloric acid when ionized in an aqueous solution. It then acquires properties characteristic of acids.

Ionization of a weak polar covalent electrolyte. Many of the organic compounds of the body are weak electrolytes and play importan roles in maintaining homeostasis. The mechanism of acid-base balance, an understanding of which is important in the management of pulmonary disease patients, is dependent on the principles of low-level ionization.

Acetic acid is an example of a weak electrolyte, an organic acid (the major ingredient of vinegar), with a formula that can be written two ways. It can be represented as $C_2H_4O_2$ or written as CH_3COOH, which is consistent with the custom of recording organic acids with the anion first and the hydrogen cation last. Acetic acid therefore consists of the *acetate ion,* CH_3COO^-, with a single negative oxidation number and a hydrogen ion, H^+. When acetic acid is characterized as a weak electrolyte it is implied that it has some, but not much, molecular polarity and a strong covalent bond that is difficult for the water dipole to break. Its ionizing equation is:

$$CH_3COOH + H_2O \rightleftharpoons H_3O^+ + CH_3COO^-$$

or

$$CH_3COOH \rightleftharpoons H^+ + CH_3COO^-$$

The use of the double arrows in this equation is an indication that the reaction can go in both direction simultaneously and is a reversible reaction. While molecules of acetic acid are breaking down into ions (movement to the right), some of the ions are recombining into molecules (movement to the left). The arrows represent a state of equilibrium where the number of molecules ionizing are equaled by the number reformed from ions. Some degree of quantitation can be expressed by the equation's arrows. A single arrow to the right shows a complete reaction in that direction with no equilibrium established between molecules and ions, but a conversion of all molecules to ions, leaving only ions to remain in solution. Therefore, $HCl \rightarrow H^+ + Cl^-$ means full ionization of hydrogen chloride, the sign of a strong electrolyte. The reaction $Na^+Cl^- \rightarrow Na^+ + Cl^-$ similarly shows complete dissociation of the electrovalent salt into its component ions, also indicating a strong electrolyte. In general, less than complete ionization is often shown by two arrows of equal length, but a known very weak electrolyte can be clearly identified by unequal arrows as used above for acetic acid. This means the compound has a stronger tendency to remain molecularly bound than to ionize.

Weak electrolytes exist in aqueous solution mostly as molecules with only a few ions. Fig. 2-13 illustrates the degree of ionization of acetic acid compared

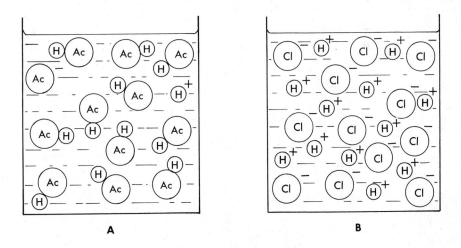

A   **B**

Fig. 2-13   **A,** The weak electrolyte, acetic acid (CH_3COOH), exists almost entirely as intact molecules, with only one cation and one anion each illustrated. **B,** In contrast, the strong electrolyte, hydrogen chloride, is completely ionized.

with hydrochloric acid and emphasizes the larger number of ions in a strong electrolyte rather than in a weak electrolyte.

Ionization of water. Water is one of the weakest electrolytes, yet on its seemingly negligible amount of ionization depend physiologic acid-base balance and our system of recording it. Attraction between a pair of water dipoles can develop a bond uniting the oxygen of one and a hydrogen of the other that is stronger than the internal covalent bond of the second molecule. Fig. 2-14 illustrates the union of two water molecules and then their separation into hydronium and hydroxide (OH^-) ions according to the reaction:

$$H_2O + H_2O \rightleftharpoons H_3O^+ + OH^-$$

or

$$H(OH) + H(OH) \rightleftharpoons HH(OH)^+ + OH^-$$

or more simply

$$HOH \rightleftharpoons H^+ + OH^-$$

The hydronium ion formed is exactly like that generated in the ionization of hydrogen chloride. The formula H_2O indicates that a molecule consists of two hydrogen atoms linked to one oxygen atom; HOH indicates the same thing but in addition emphasizes the two ions that derive from a very few of the molecules. The latter is the preferred notation, especially in an ionization

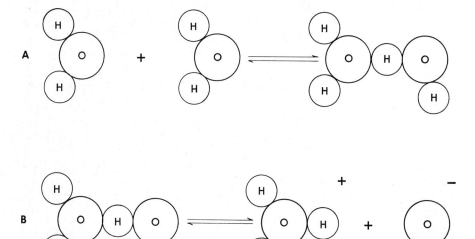

Fig. 2-14   Ionization of water. **A,** A rare union of the oxygen of one water dipole with a hydrogen atom of another. **B,** The two dipoles separate into hydronium and hydroxide ions. (See text for description of ion formation.)

equation, while the more common H_2O is normally used in other circumstances.

The hydronium ion in the second equation is written $HH(OH)^+$ to be consistent with the HOH of water and to underscore its ionic structure. This is not an official notation and is used here for emphasis. In general, however, the hydrogen ion will be designated in this text as H^+.

The ionization equation, with its unequal arrows, indicates the weakness of water as an electrolyte. Nonetheless, because some ionization does occur, water may be thought of as a very dilute aqueous solution of hydrogen and hydroxide ions or a solution of these two ions in molecular water.

Nonpolar covalent solutions. An even distribution of charges gives to nonpolar covalent compounds an electrical symmetry that prevents polarity. It creates strong internal molecular bonding that resists the attraction of water solvent dipoles. A nonpolarized molecule may be imagined as presenting a defensive perimeter on which any given point is electrically neutral because of surrounding balanced charges. Methane, diagrammed in Fig. 2-6, is a good example of a nonpolar covalent substance. Solutions of these compounds produce no ions, conduct no electrical current, and are nonelectrolytes.

Ionic charac-teristics of acids, bases, and salts **Acids**	There are two definitions of an acid. The older description states that an acid is a compound whose aqueous solution contains hydrogen ions. Such substances consist of a hydrogen atom or atoms covalently bonded to a negative valence nonmetal or radical, which gives the acid its name. By definition, an acid must be an electrolyte that produces hydrogen ions and anions. More consistent with modern chemical views is the Brønsted-Lowry definition, which simply calls an acid any compound that is a *proton donor*. This includes substances other than those we recognize as traditional acids. For example, the ammonium ion (NH_4^+) qualifies as an acid since it can release a proton (H^+) in the following reaction, which produces ammonia gas (NH_3):

$$NH_4Cl + NaOH \rightarrow NH_3 + NaCl + HOH$$

The sodium and chloride ions are called *spectator ions* because they are not involved in the proton transfer, the important event of this reaction. By eliminating the spectator ions, we can write the equation ionically and demonstrate the acidity of the ammonium ion:

$$NH_4^+ + OH^- \rightarrow NH_3 \text{ (g)} + HOH$$

The ammonium ion donated a hydrogen ion (proton) to the reaction, and it was accepted by the hydroxide ion (OH^-), converting the former into ammonia gas and the latter into water. There is little difference between the two acid definitions, and the use of the term *acid* in this text generally refers to compounds that are readily seen to be sources of hydrogen ions in solution.

In Chapter 1, under the discussion of equivalent weight, the term *replace-*

able hydrogen was used in relation to acids. The term *ionizable hydrogen* can now be used for a synonym with the former, but it is a little more specific for use here. The following demonstrates two levels of acid complexity.

Acids with single ionizable hydrogen. Simple compounds such as the following ionize into one cation and anion each:

$$HCl \rightarrow H^+ + Cl^-$$
$$HBr \rightarrow H^+ + Br^-$$
$$HNO_3 \rightarrow H^+ + NO_3^-$$

Acids with multiple ionizable hydrogens. All of the potential hydrogen ions in an acid may not be made available at once but in stages. The degree of ionization tends to increase as an electrolyte solution becomes more dilute. Concentrated sulfuric acid ionizes only one of its two hydrogen atoms per molecule:

$$H_2SO_4 \rightarrow H^+ + HSO_4^-$$

With further dilution, second stage ionization occurs:

$$H_2SO_4 \rightarrow H^+ + H^+ + SO_4^=$$

Similarly, three stages of phosphoric acid ionization can be summarized as follows:

$$H_3PO_4 \rightarrow H^+ + H_3PO_4^-$$
$$H^+ + H^+ + HPO_4^=$$
$$H^+ + H^+ + H^+ + PO_4^=$$

The greater the concentration of hydrogen ions, the more acid or the stronger acid is the solution. Acids characteristically have a sour taste. They react with metals to produce hydrogen gas and with bases to form salts and water.

Bases

The older definition of a base describes it as a compound whose aqueous solution contains hydroxyl groups and that destroys the properties of dissolved acids when mixed. These compounds are called *hydroxides* and consist of metals, or the metal equivalent ammonium cation (NH_4^-), ionically bound to a hydroxide ion or ions. A Brønsted-Lowry base is any compound that *accepts a proton,* including many substances other than hydroxides. Bases are negatively charged.

Hydroxide bases. In aqueous solution the following are typical dissociations of hydroxide bases:

$$Na^+OH^- \rightarrow Na^+ + OH^-$$
$$K^+OH^- \rightarrow K^+ + OH^-$$
$$Ca^{++}(OH^-)_2 \rightarrow Ca^{++} + 20H^-$$

Inactivation of an acid, as part of the definition of a base, is accomplished by OH^- reacting with H^+ (proton acceptance by the base), forming water:

$$NaOH + HCl \rightarrow NaCl + HOH$$

Nonhydroxide bases. Two examples follow:

Ammonia. In the description of acids it was demonstrated how an ammonium ion can be called an acid by donating a proton and becoming ammonia. Ammonia also qualifies as a base by reacting with water to produce OH^-:

$$NH_3 + HOH \rightleftharpoons NH_4^+ + OH^-$$

and by neutralizing H^+ directly

$$NH_3 + H^+ \rightleftharpoons NH_4^+$$

In both instances NH_3 accepted a proton to become NH_4^+.

Carbonates. The reactions of this group, of which sodium carbonate is an example, are very relevant to pulmonary physiology. The carbonate ion, $CO_3^=$, can react with water to produce OH^-. First,

$$Na_2CO_3^= \rightleftharpoons 2Na^+ + CO_3^=$$

then

$$CO_3^= + HOH \rightleftharpoons HCO_3^- + OH^-$$

The carbonate ion accepted a proton from water, became the bicarbonate ion, and produced a hydroxide ion. The carbonate ion can also directly react with H^+ to inactivate it as follows:

$$CO_3^= + H^+ \rightleftharpoons HCO_3^-$$

Bases have a bitter taste and most feel slippery or soapy. The soluble hydroxides or carbonates of sodium and potassium are sometimes referred to as *alkalis*. Finally, bases react with acids to form salts and water.

Salts

The most common of compounds, salts are composed of metal or ammonium ions electrovalently joined to anions other than the hydroxyl. There are many ways of producing salts, but the simplest is by the reaction between an acid and a base, as noted in the descriptions of these last two compounds:

$$HCl + NaOH \rightarrow NaCl + HOH$$

There are three classifications of salts, which depend on the degree of hydrogen and hydroxyl replacement from the parent acids and bases.

Normal salt. A normal salt is a compound formed by the complete replacement of hydrogen ions from its acid as follows:

$$H^+Cl^- + Na^+OH^- \rightarrow Na^+Cl^- + H^+OH^-$$
$$H^+NO_3^- + K^+OH^- \rightarrow K^+NO_3^- + H^+OH^-$$

Acid salt. An acid salt results from only partial replacement of hydrogen ions from the related acid, leaving some "acidity" (hydrogen ion or ions) in the salt:

$$H_2^+CO_3^= + Na^+OH^- \rightarrow Na^+HCO_3^= + H^+OH^-$$

Sodium bicarbonate can also be called sodium acid carbonate because of its hydrogen atom. Both hydrogen atoms in H_2CO_3 may ionize under proper conditions, but in the physiologic environment of the human body, the single hydrogen ionization is the only reaction possible. To underscore the ions involved, carbonic acid can be rewritten to show it composed of only one hydrogen ion and the univalent bicarbonate ion, HCO_3^-. The reaction would look like this:

$$H^+ + HCO_3^- + Na^+OH^- \rightarrow Na^+HCO_3^- + H^+OH^-$$

Basic salt. A basic salt contains an unreplaced hydroxide ion from the base generating it, such as:

$$Ca^{++}(OH^-)_2 + H^+Cl^- \rightarrow Ca^{++}(OH^-)CL^- + H^+OH^-$$

There are no basic salts that are relevant to pulmonary physiology.

Measurement of electrolytic activity

Electrolytic equilibrium

The physiologically active chemical compounds of the body are, for the most part, weak electrolytic covalent substances, and their ionic behavior can be stated as follows:

1. A proportion of the molecules in an aqueous solution of a weak covalent electrolyte ionize, and the remainder of the molecules persist intact. At a given temperature and concentration, equilibrium is maintained between the ions and the unionized molecules.
2. After the establishment of ionic equilibrium, the product of the molar concentration (moles per liter) of the ions divided by the molar concentration of the unionized molecules is a constant value at a given concentration of solution and temperature. This is a special type of equilibrium constant called an *ionization constant,* or K. It cannot be emphasized too strongly that such a relationship exists *only* with aqueous solutions of *weak* electrolytes.

Degree of dissociation or ionization

As pointed out earlier, the strength of an electrolyte depends on the percentage of its solute that dissociates if it is ionic or ionizes if it is covalent. In evaluating the electrolytic strength of a substance it is important to know its percent of ion production. Handbooks of chemistry and other sources provide this information, always specifying the molar concentrations of the solutions and the temperature at which the values are valid. Table 2-5 lists the percentages of three strong and three weak electrolytes that produce ions in 0.1-M solutions at a temperature of 25° C. Sodium hydroxide (NaOH) is the only electrovalent compound in the group; 90% dissociates into sodium and hydroxide ions. With hydrochloric acid, 90% of its molecules ionize into hydrogen and chloride ions. In contrast, only 0.01% of molecules of boric acid (H_3BO_3) ionize.

Table 2-5	NaOH	90%	CH_3COOH	1.33%
Percent ion formation	HCl	90%	H_2CO_3	0.207%
of 0.1-M solutions at	HNO_3	90%	H_3BO_3	0.0076%
25°C				

Theoretically, because electrovalent compounds such as sodium chloride, sodium hydroxide, and silver nitrate are 100% ionic in their crystalline forms, they should undergo 100% ionic dissociation in aqueous solution. The same is true of the strong covalent acids. Electrical conductivity measurements of such solutions and less than maximum alteration of freezing and boiling points of water indicate that 100% ion production is not always realized. The term *apparent degree of dissociation,* or *ionization,* as opposed to actual, is used for values such as those in Table 2-5.

The reason for this discrepancy is found in the effect of solute dilution on dissociation and ionization. As stated earlier, the water dipole influences the degree of ion production, and solute concentration is important in determining equilibrium constants. In a concentrated solution there may not be enough water molecules to separate and hydrate the large number of ions of electrovalent compounds or to ionize polar covalent molecules. The closely packed ions of a concentrated solution tend to interfere with each other's activities, and they act as relatively small numbers of groups rather than large numbers of individual ions. Solvent freezing and boiling points are less affected than they would be by a larger number. Diluting a given electrolyte solution reduces interaction among ions and increases the apparent dissociation and ionization. This is one of the reasons for the multiple stages of ionization described and illustrated earlier for sulfuric and phosphoric acids. Diluting a solute may increase the concentration of its ions. Table 2-6 demonstrates the effect on the freezing point of water with increases in dissociation of sodium chloride by increasing the molal dilution tenfold.

As an example, if a quantitative comparison is made between a 0.1-M solution of hydrochloric acid (HCl) with 90% ionization and a 0.1-M solution of carbonic acid (H_2CO_3) with 0.207% ionization, 1 ℓ of each solution will contain 0.1 mole, or 0.1 gmw, of its respective acid solute. Ninety percent of the hydrochloric acid molecules, or 0.90 of 0.1 mole, 0.09 of a mole, dissociate into ions; 0.01 of a mole or gmw remains as intact molecules. Since each dissociating molecule produces one cation and one anion, the concentration, or number per liter of each is the same as the concentration of the dissociating molecules. The ionic and molecular concentrations of the 0.1-M hydrochloric acid solutions would be as follows:

Concentration of H ions = 0.09 mole (or g-ion)/ℓ
Concentration of Cl ions = 0.09 mole (or g-ion)/ℓ
Concentration of HCl molecules = 0.01 mole (or g-mole)/ℓ

Of the 0.1-M solution of carbonic acid, which dissociates into hydrogen (H^+) and bicarbonate (HCO_3^-) ions, 0.00207 of 0.1 of a mole, or 0.000207

Table 2-6
Influence of concentrations of sodium chloride (NaCl) solution on freezing point depression of water

Aqueous molal NaCl concentration	Depression of freezing point (°C) per mole of NaCl
1.00	3.37
0.10	3.48
0.010	3.60
0.0010	3.66
0.00010	3.72

Data from Metcalf, H.C., et al.: Modern chemistry, New York, 1966, Holt, Rinehart & Winston, Inc., and Boylan, P.J., et al.: Elements of chemistry, Boston, 1962, Allyn & Bacon, Inc.

mole of the acid dissociates into ions; 0.9979 of 0.1 mole, or 0.09979 of a mole, remains undissociated. Therefore:

$$\text{Concentration of H ions} = 0.000207 \text{ mole(g-ion)}/\ell$$
$$\text{Concentration of HCO}_3^- \text{ ions} = 0.000207 \text{ mole(g-ion)}/\ell$$
$$\text{Concentration of H}_2\text{CO}_3 \text{ molecules} = 0.09979 \text{ mole(g-mole)}/\ell$$

Furthermore, a 0.1-M solution contains $6.02 \times 10^{23} \times 0.1$, or 6.02×10^{22} molecules/ℓ. Therefore, on the basis of the known percentage of molecules that ionize, the actual number of ions and molecules per liter can be computed as shown in Table 2-7.

Examples of ionization can be expressed in one equation. This relationship holds only for weak electrolytes. The numerators of the following equations are in molar concentrations (moles, or gram ionic, or gram atomic weights per liter) of ions, and the denominators are in molar concentrations (moles or gram molecular weights per liter) of un-ionized molecules of solute.

Brackets indicate concentrations of ions as well as of molecules and undissociated solute. Unless otherwise specified, the concentration implied is moles per liter. Thus $[H^+]$ means moles per liter of hydrogen ions, but the expression gram ions per liter is occasionally encountered; $[HCO_3^-]$ means molar concentration of bicarbonate ions per liter; $[H_2CO_3]$ signifies moles per liter of un-ionized, intact carbonic acid molecules.

(1) Symbolic representation of an acid, HA:
$$\frac{[H^+]\,[A^-]}{[HA]} = K$$

(2) Symbolic representation of a base, BOH:
$$\frac{[B^+]\,[OH^-]}{BOH} = K$$

(3) Acetic acid:
$$\frac{[H^+]\,[CH_3COO^-]}{[CH_3COOH]} = 1.8 \times 10^{-5}$$

(4) Carbonic acid:
$$\frac{[H^+]\,[HCO_3^-]}{H_2CO_3} = 4.3 \times 10^{-7}$$

(5) Boric acid:
$$\frac{[H^+]\,[H_2BO_3^-]}{H_3BO_3} = 5.8 \times 10^{-10}$$

Table 2-7		H$^+$ per liter	Anions per liter	Undissociated molecules per liter
Concentrations of ions and molecules in 0.1-M hydrochloric acid and 0.1-M carbonic acid	0.1-M HCl	5.418 × 10^{22}	5.418 × 10^{22}	6.02 × 10^{21}
	0.1-M H$_2$CO$_3$	1.246 × 10^{20}	1.246 × 10^{20}	6.0074 × 10^{22}

Calculation of ionization (equilibrium) constant

Following is an actual calculation of an ionization constant using acetic acid (CH$_3$COOH). At 25°C, 1.33% of a 0.1 M solution of the acid undergoes ionization, and therefore 98.76% of the molecules do not ionize. Ionization of acetic acid is represented as CH$_3$COOH $\rightleftharpoons$ H$^+$ + CH$_3$COO$^-$.

1. Since 0.1 M solution of acetic acid contains 0.1 gmw of acid per liter, of which 1.33% ionizes, then 0.1 × 0.0133 or 0.00133 of a mole of acid per liter produces ions and 0.1 × 0.9867 of a mole per liter remains un-ionized.

2. Each molecule that ionizes produces two ions, H$^+$ and CH$_3$COO$^-$ (acetate ion), and the concentration of each is the same as that of the ionizing molecules, 0.00133 of a mole of ions per liter. Accordingly, the concentration of un-ionized molecules is 0.09867 of a mole of ions per liter.

3. By definition, K is equal to the ratio between the product of the molar ion concentrations and the molar concentration of the un-ionized molecules, or:

$$\frac{[H^+] \, [CH_3COO^-]}{[CH_3COOH]} = K$$

$$\frac{0.00133 \times 0.00133}{0.09867} = K$$

$$K = 1.8 \times 10^{-5}$$

Exercise 2-8: Calculate the K of the following symbolic acid and base:
A. 0.1-M HA, with 2.5% ionization.
B. 0.5-M BOH, with 1.9% dissociation

Ionization constant of water

The ionization of water is the basis for a system of calibrating acidity and alkalinity that is discussed below. Pure water produces the two ions H$^+$ and OH$^-$, and although its degree of ionization is very minute, it has an important ionization constant. In a sense, water consists of an aqueous solution of H$^+$ and OH$^-$, or it may be considered a solution of these two ions dissolved in molecular water. Its ion/molecule ratio can be expressed as:

$$\frac{[H^+] \, [OH^-]}{[HOH]} = K$$

However, the degree of ionization of water is so small and the concentration of un-ionized molecules is proportionally so large, that any small change in the degree of ionization would not produce a detectable reciprocal change in the concentration of the un-ionized molecules. Therefore, the molar concentration of molecular water does not change significantly and can be considered as another constant in the ratio. The ratio can be rewritten as:

$$\frac{[H^+][OH^-]}{K_2} = K_1$$

and

$$[H^+][OH^-] = K_1 K_2 = K_w$$

The dissociation constant of water, K_w, has been determined to be 1×10^{-14}. Therefore, if

$$[H^+][OH^-] = 10^{-14}$$

then, because there is one H^+ for each OH^-, the concentration of each ion is 10^{-7} moles or gram ions per liter. Pure water is as much acid as it is base, and it is therefore *neutral* in action.

Designation of acidity and alkalinity

Using pure water as a reference point, it can be stated that any solution having a greater hydrogen ion concentration than that of water is acid in its reaction, or any solution with a less concentration of hydroxide ions than water is also acidic. Similarly, a solution with a greater hydroxyl concentration or a lesser hydrogen ion concentration than water is basic. By agreement, the hydrogen ion concentration of pure water has been adopted as the standard by which to compare reactions of other solutions. Electrochemical techniques are used to measure the hydrogen ion concentration of unknown solutions and the degree of their acidity or alkalinity determined by variation of their $[H^+]$ above or below 1×10^{-7}. Therefore, a solution of a $[H^+]$ of 8.2×10^{-4} has a higher $[H^+]$ than water and is acid; one with a $[H^+]$ of 3.6×10^{-8} has less hydrogen ions than water and is alkaline. There are two related techniques for recording acidity and alkalinity of solutions using the hydrogen ion concentration of water as the neutral standard.

Nanomoles per liter of $[H^+]$. The first method reports the actual measured molar concentration of hydrogen ions, which can then be compared to that of water. The $[H^+]$ of water is 1×10^{-7} of a mole per liter. Written as a decimal, it would be 0.0000001, or one ten millionth of a mole. A ten millionth falls into the next thousandth increment of the decimal system, the billionth (prefixed *nano*). Thus one ten millionth equals 100 billionths, and the hydrogen ion concentration of water can be designated as 100 nanomoles (nM)/ℓ. With this as a reference, any solution that has a $[H^+]$ of 100 nM/ℓ is neutral, greater than 100 nM/ℓ acid, and less than 100 nM/ℓ alkaline. The degree of acidity or alkalinity is proportional to the distance of a given $[H^+]$ from the 100 nM/ℓ reference. This system of nomenclature is limited in its use because of the tremendous range of possible $[H^+]$, from the very acid to the very alkaline. It is not feasible to convert all $[H^+]$ values to nanomoles since this does not eliminate all awkward numbers. The system is applicable to needs of cardiopulmonary physiology, however, because the range of hydrogen ion concentrations is very narrow and seldom exceeds values of 20 to 100 nM/ℓ.

pH. To simplify acid-base comparisons, the principle of pH was developed. pH is the "hydrogen ion exponent," the *negative log of the hydrogen ion concentration used as a positive number*. It is derived by converting the entire value for $[H^+]$ to a single negative exponent of 10 by calculating its logarithm. The $[H^+]$ of water is 1×10^{-7}, and since the log of 1×10^{-7} is -7, the pH of water is 7. For example:

(1) $[H^+]$ of 8.2×10^{-4}
   $pH = \log 8.2 \times 10^{-4} = \bar{4}.914 = -3.086 = 3.09$

(2) $[H^+]$ of 4.0×10^{-8}
   $pH = \log 4.0 \times 10^{-8} = \bar{8}.602 = -7.398 = 7.40$

(3) $[H^+]$ of 6.7×10^{-11}
   $pH = \log 6.7 \times 10^{-11} = \bar{11}.826 = -10.174 = 10.17$

Any solution with a pH of 7 is neutral, corresponding to the $[H^+]$ of pure water. As the pH value decreases numerically below 7, it is a negative log and represents an actual $[H^+]$ greater than 7; therefore it is acid. Conversely, pH values greater than 7 represent lower $[H^+]$ and are alkaline. The pH scale is illustrated below.

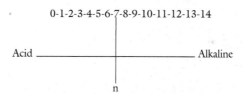

The compactness of the pH scale can be illustrated by comparing its midpoint with two extremes having varying molar concentrations of hydrogen ions:

$$pH = [H^+]$$
$$0 = 10^0 \text{ or } 1.0 \text{ M/}\ell$$
$$7 = 10^{-7} \text{ or } 100 \text{ nM/}\ell$$
$$14 = 10^{-14} \text{ or } 10^{-5} \text{ nM/}\ell$$

Exercise 2-9: Calculate the pH of the following to two decimals:
A. $[H^+] = 7.6 \times 10^{-5}$
B. $[H^+] = 3.04 \times 10^{-2}$
C. $[H^+] = 5.16 \times 10^{-12}$
D. $[H^+] = 1.01 \times 10^{-8}$
E. $[H^+] = 8.66 \times 10^{-10}$

Exercise 2-10: Calculate the $[H^+]$ of the following:

A. pH = 3.21
B. pH = 8.92
C. pH = 5.01
D. pH = 10.26
E. pH = 6.66

Chapter 3 Anatomy of the respiratory system*

DAVID H. DAIL

Proper function of the respiratory system is critical to maintenance of normal gas exchange and, therefore, to life. Since the structure of this system is intimately related to its function, structural abnormalities are quickly expressed in functional terms. To provide a framework for the chapters that follow, this chapter will review the normal anatomy of the respiratory system. The respiratory structures that will be described are the nose, mouth, pharynx, larynx, trachea, lungs, and surrounding chest walls and diaphragms (Fig. 3-1).

Development

A brief review of the development of these structures is helpful. In early embryologic development, one central tube is formed from a grooved inpouching of the surface of the spherical embryo. This tube forms the mainstream of the gastrointestinal tract and its derivatives. Very early in this development, a bud forms from this tube. This bud divides, grows, and becomes the lungs. Partial residual connections in the form of tracheoesophageal fistulas may occur to remind us of these events.

In the head, a transverse septum forms that is destined to become the pal-

*From Shibel, E.M., and Moser, K.M., editors: Respiratory emergencies, St. Louis, 1977, The C.V. Mosby Co.

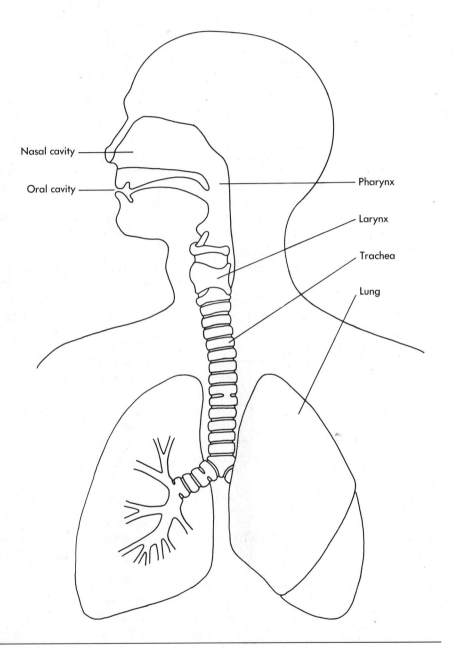

Fig. 3-1   The respiratory tract consists of the nasal cavity, oral cavity, pharynx, larynx, trachea, and lung. The larynx divides the system into the upper and lower respiratory tract.

ate. This divides the intake end of this primitive tube into a nasal passage and an oral cavity (again see Fig. 3-1). The nasal cavity serves a predominantly respiratory function, whereas the oral cavity serves a mixed function, being involved in gastrointestinal function as well as in speech and respiration. Where these divisions rejoin behind the palate, in a space called the pharynx, respiratory and nutritive functions are shared for a short distance until they again separate at the division of the larynx and the pharynx in the upper neck. Food and liquids pass from the mouth anteriorly to posteriorly, whereas air, of course, moves bidirectionally through nose and mouth to the pharynx and larynx. Thus, a crossover of these functions occurs in the pharynx. A flap valve called the epiglottis on the larynx helps direct flow into the proper channels. This critical separating function is normally competent.

The respiratory structures will be considered under groups belonging to the head, neck, and chest. The upper respiratory tract is that portion above the larynx, and the lower respiratory tract consists of the trachea and lungs.

Head

Nasal cavity

The nasal cavity forms the gateway to the respiratory system. It begins as two flexible, flared rubbery entryways called wings, or alae, enclosing a space on each side called the vestibule. The nasal cavities continue more posteriorly as paired air spaces, nasal walls, and protuberances from these walls. The right

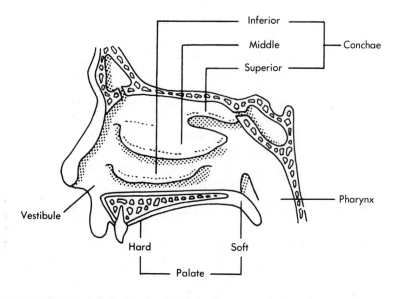

Fig. 3-2   Lateral view of internal structures of nasal cavity. Note three conchal plates extending from lateral walls. The palate with hard and soft portions divides nasal cavity from oral cavity. These two cavities rejoin posteriorly as the pharynx.

side is separated from the left side by a nasal septum. Three bony plates called conchae project into each nasal cavity. These extend in a downward and medial fashion from the lateral walls (Fig. 3-2). The nasal septum deviates to one side or the other to some degree in many people. Posteriorly, the two separate nasal cavities merge together above and behind the soft palate to form the upper portion of the pharynx, or nasopharynx. The entry of the nostril contains strong hairs. These act in a delicate way and the conchal plates act in a gross way to protect the upper respiratory tract from intrusion by foreign material.

Squamous epithelium lines the vestibule as well as the mouth, pharynx, and larynx. The nasal cavities, sinuses, trachea, and larger and smaller conducting airways in the lung are lined by ciliated, tall, pseudocolumnar epithelium. The cilia are fine microscopic hairlike projections extending into the lumens of these tubes. They sway rapidly together in waves. In the lower respiratory tract, this action moves material up out of the lungs to be coughed out or swallowed. In the nasal cavities, material is projected posteriorly to meet the same fate. It is important for the cilia to remain healthy and active to carry out this function. Extensive surgery or other influences such as certain drugs can alter the ciliary action.

Lubrication in the respiratory tract is provided by mucus. This is produced by submucosal glands and by individual cells within the mucosal lining called goblet cells. Goblet cells are so named because they look like the bowls of small goblets. The mucous film helps trap small foreign particles.

Warming and humidification of air begins as soon as it starts its two-way journey through the respiratory tract. Particularly in the nasal cavity, where moving air first enters and "air conditioning" is begun, the mucous membranes are supplied with a large amount of blood flow. This helps to warm the incoming air rapidly. This process continues throughout the respiratory tract. If one considers how brief an alternate inspiration and expiration is and notes how warm and wet the air is on its return to the outside, it is apparent that these processes are very effective. In an extremely dry environment, the wetting function may be overpowered, and a person may note drying of his nose and mouth. Likewise, when a common cold injures this tissue, it responds excessively and the surface weeps resulting in a runny nose.

The other major function of the nasal cavity is to serve as an exposure chamber for the sense of smell. However, since the sense of smell is not pertinent to this book, it will not be considered further.

Sinuses

Connected with the nasal cavities are empty spaces in the facial and skull bones technically called the accessory respiratory sinuses (Fig. 3-3). These are symmetrically paired structures, the most accessible being the frontal and maxillary sinuses. The more anterior ethmoid and more posterior sphenoid sinuses are near the midline above and just behind the nasal cavities. All are named for the bones in which they occur. All open into the nasal cavity, usually under

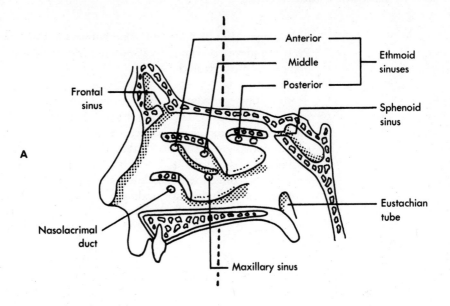

A

Frontal sinus

Nasolacrimal duct

Anterior

Middle

Posterior

Ethmoid sinuses

Sphenoid sinus

Eustachian tube

Maxillary sinus

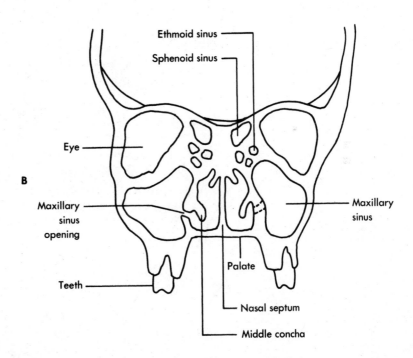

B

Ethmoid sinus

Sphenoid sinus

Eye

Maxillary sinus opening

Teeth

Palate

Nasal septum

Middle concha

Maxillary sinus

Fig. 3-3   The nasal sinuses are named for bones in which they occur. **A,** In lateral view (as in Fig. 3-2) but with chonchae cut away. Note entrances into nasal cavity of various sinuses and their location within these cavities. **B,** Frontal view of face taken at level of dotted line in **A.** Note position of maxillary sinuses in each cheekbone. Sphenoid sinuses are behind ethmoid sinuses, although they appear to be at same level in this frontal view.

the conchae (Fig. 3-3, *A*). No one knows the exact purposes of the sinuses. Problems develop when these become inflamed, obstructed, or when their bony walls are fractured.

Palate

Separating the nasal cavity from the oral cavity is the roof of the mouth, the palate (Fig. 3-2). The anterior two-thirds has a bony skeleton that accounts for its designation, hard palate, whereas the posterior one-third is without such support and is therefore called the soft palate. From the midline portion of the soft palate at the back of the mouth extends the soft, fleshy uvula, which points in the direction of the lower respiratory tract (Fig. 3-4). Its purpose, in coordination with the surrounding walls, is to control flow in eating, drinking, sneezing, coughing, and vomiting.

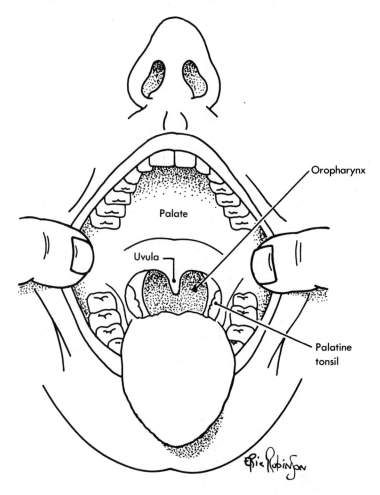

Fig. 3-4   View into opened mouth. Soft midline uvula is seen hanging from fleshy tonsillar pillars. Pharynx is seen at back of mouth.

Oral cavity

The mouth should be considered an accessory respiratory passage. Mouth breathing is used during speech and when nasal obstruction is caused by upper respiratory tract infections or foreign materials. The lips, teeth, tongue, jaw muscles, and spontaneous reflexes help protect the mouth from injury or unwanted intrusion. Care of the mouth and teeth and the quality of chewing are important factors in protection of the lower respiratory tract. The mucosal surfaces here also provide luxuriant wetting and warming qualities for incoming air. Saliva is produced by major and minor salivary glands and provides some moisture for inhaled air. However, it serves two other major functions. It is a wetting agent for food, and it also contains enzymes that start the digestive process while food is being chewed.

The oral cavity ends where a web on each side (posterior palatine pillar) arches toward the midline to join the midline fleshy uvula (Fig. 3-4). Against the front of each of these webs sit the palatine tonsils, more commonly just called tonsils. The tongue is a strong muscular mass used not only for speech but for moving materials about within the mouth. Taste buds are present on its surface. The posterior surface is supplied with many nerve endings that originate reflexes that account for protective gagging. These reflexes must be considered when passing fingers, tubes, instruments, or other objects through the mouth in the conscious or semiconscious patient.

Pharynx

The space behind the nasal cavities and mouth is called the pharynx, from the Greek word for "throat" (Fig. 3-5). It extends to the point where the

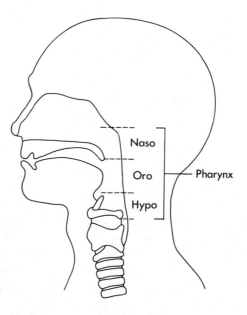

Fig. 3-5   Pharynx is divided into three anatomic subdivisions. These divisions are named for structures in respiratory tract that are in proximity to them.

airway (at the larynx) and the digestive tract (esophagus) separate. The portion behind the nasal cavities is called the nasopharynx as noted above. The Eustachian tubes open into the lateral-posterior-superior nasopharynx walls and connect the nasopharynx with the middle portion of each ear. On the superior posterior wall is the other major lymphoid mass of the upper respiratory tract, the adenoid tonsil, commonly called the adenoids. The two palatine tonsils and one adenoid tonsil comprise the major components of Waldeyer's ring, the so-called guardian ring of lymphoid material surrounding the entries of the respiratory and gastrointestinal tracts.

The portion of the pharynx at the back of the oral cavity is called the oropharynx. This extends from the uvula above to the epiglottis and base of tongue below. Nasotracheal and nasogastric tubes passed through the nose must turn inferiorly at the nasopharynx and continue in that direction through the oropharynx if they are to reach the trachea, lungs, or stomach.

The inferior portion of the pharynx, between the epiglottis and final entries into the larynx and esophagus, is called the hypopharynx (or laryngopharynx). This is a short segment extending into the neck. It corresponds to the height of the epiglottis and is a critical dividing point in separating solids and fluids from air.

Neck

Epiglottis

The epiglottis is a platelike structure that extends from the base of the tongue backward and upward (Figs. 3-1, 3-6, and 3-7). In adults it is 2 to 4 cm long and 2 to 3 cm wide. It is only 2 to 5 mm thick. This structure can at times be seen by looking directly through the mouth. It is more readily seen in babies and children than in adults and is especially noticeable in crying babies. This structure is the flap valve over the entry to the larynx. During routine swallowing, the epiglottis closes in coordination with contraction of the muscular walls in the region, covering the airway and directing the swallowed material into the esophagus. The almost unconscious act of swallowing is a rather remarkable process requiring coordination of multiple neuromuscular functions. When they are hampered, the lower respiratory tract can be violated by aspirated material. A powerful back-up system is the cough reflex. When one is unconscious or has neural or other control problems, these protections may not be sufficiently effective and aspiration of foreign materials into the lungs may occur.

The head and its airways tend to form a roughly 90-degree angle with the pharynx-larynx axis (Fig. 3-6, *B*). With loss of consciousness, the head often droops downward, making this angle 120 degrees or more (Fig. 3-6, *A*), thus partially or completely obstructing the channels connecting the respiratory structures in the head to those in the neck. To help alleviate this obstruction, the head and lower jaw are usually extended so that the head and neck structures can form a straight tube as nearly as is safely allowable (Fig. 3-6, *C*).

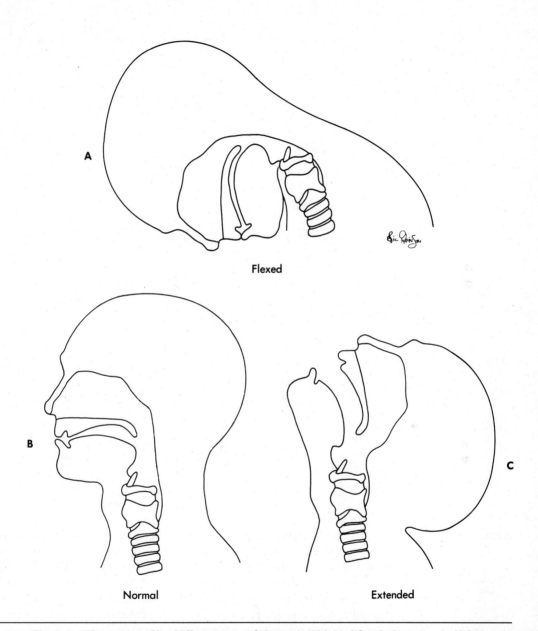

Fig. 3-6   The position of head affects patency of airway. **A,** With head flexed, airway may be kinked, making breathing or intubation difficult. **B,** Normal upright relationship of head and neck to chest. **C,** Extension of head straightens airway, making breathing, clearance of material, or intubation easier.

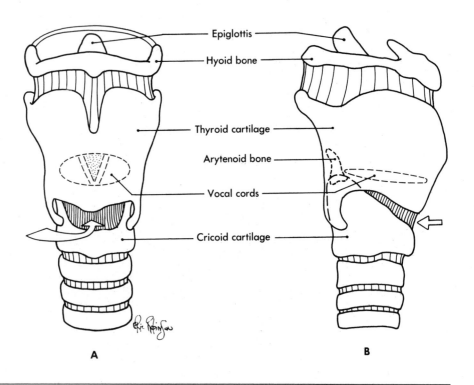

Epiglottis

Hyoid bone

Thyroid cartilage

Arytenoid bone

Vocal cords

Cricoid cartilage

A

B

Fig. 3-7   Larynx is seen in frontal **(A)** and lateral **(B)** views. Note location of vocal cords and relationship of epiglottis to opening of larynx. The arrows refer to notch between larynx and cricoid cartilage referred to in text.

Larynx   The larynx (Adam's apple) is a cartilaginous box below the pharynx. Its major function is sound production, but it is also important as a protective valve because of the narrowing of the air passage at this point (Fig. 3-7). Sounds are produced by vibrating the vocal cords, which extend for variable distances into the midportion of the larynx. The cords appear as white bordered veils. They are drawn apart in inspiration by active muscular contraction, and relax toward midline during expiration (Fig. 3-8). Some fluttering of the cords in the airstream is observed during breathing. During speech, the cords are drawn tightly toward each other so that the vibrations are of higher frequency. The larynx is highly mobile. By changing the length of the cords and by associated change in location in the neck, one may produce high or low

Front

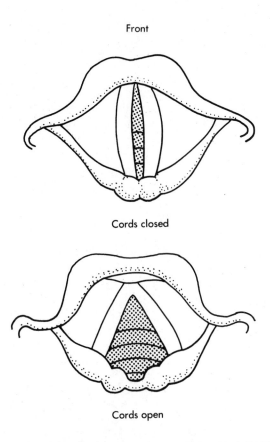

Cords closed

Cords open

Fig. 3-8   View into larynx from back of mouth to the front. Vocal cords vary in tension, length, and relationship to one another. Note open inspiratory position versus expiratory or resting closed position. Inside of trachea with its cartilaginous rings is seen through opening between vocal cords.

pitched sounds. By varying the volumes of air passing these cords, one may vary the intensity of the sounds.

Above the larynx is the hyoid bone, which is important in adjusting phonation (sound) and swallowing. Immediately below the larynx is a thickened cartilaginous ring called the cricoid cartilage. The main anterior protuberance or forward notch of the larynx can be felt externally with the finger. If the finger is allowed to slide down from the larynx into the circular groove immediately under it, the bottom of the laryngeal cartilage will be felt (*arrow* in Fig. 3-7). This is the zone where an emergency tracheostomy tube can be inserted directly with little danger of interfering with major blood supply or other vital functions. Catheters for removal of secretions also are inserted here for "transtracheal aspiration." Surgical tracheostomy is usually placed 1 to 3 cm below the cricoid cartilage when there is adequate time, lighting, equipment, and instrumentation to avoid dangerous complications.

Trachea

The trachea is a tubular structure that begins at the cricoid cartilage. It extends through the neck into the mediastinum to a point behind the junction of the upper and middle thirds of the sternum (breastbone) where it divides into the two main-stem bronchi (Fig. 3-1). It is about 2.0 to 2.5 cm in diameter and about 11 cm long. It contains 16 to 20 U-shaped cartilaginous rings that help to hold it open. Each cartilage is 4 to 5 mm high and not easily felt externally, except in very thin individuals. Posteriorly, there is a thin muscle extending between the open ends of the U (Fig. 3-9). This combined muscular-cartilaginous structure provides support yet allows some variation in diameter during inspiration, expiration, and coughing. A continuous internal membranous coat envelops the rings, the posterior muscle, and the space between the rings. The trachea can be seen on a roentgenogram as an air-filled structure in contrast to the blood vessels and other structures that have a water

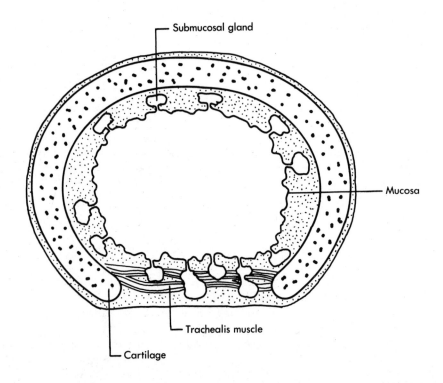

Submucosal gland

Mucosa

Trachealis muscle

Cartilage

Fig. 3-9   Trachea is composed of U-shaped cartilaginous rings connected posteriorly by membrane covering thin trachealis muscle. This arrangement allows variation in tracheal caliber. Note mucosal and submucosal glands lining airway.

density appearance (Fig. 3-10). Therefore, on the usual negative x-ray film, it and other air spaces, including most of the lungs, appear black compared with the grayer or whiter soft tissues. (See Chapter 9.)

Chest

Mediastinum

The mediastinum is the central structure in the chest and contains the trachea, heart, major blood vessels, nerves and that portion of the gastrointestinal tract in the chest, the esophagus. It also contains the thymus gland, lymph nodes, and occassionally part or all of the thyroid or parathyroid glands. The mediastinum occupied the space between the sternum (breastplate) and the spine (Fig. 3-10). The substance surrrounding the mediastinum with its many vital organs is scant. Any compression or invasion of the mediastinum has a high likelihood of compromising some of these life-sustaining structures. Infection spreading in this area can be devastating.

The trachea is almost midline in the neck, but in the superior mediastinum

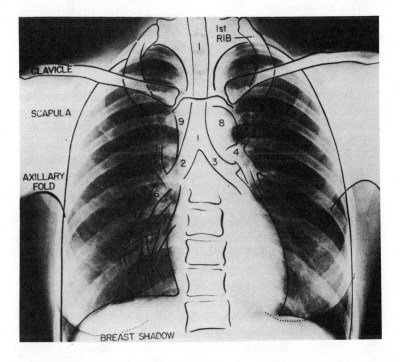

Fig. 3-10   Roentgenogram of mediastinum and lungs. Air-containing structures such as trachea and lungs are dark on this negative. The mediastinum is the central structure between lungs. Note air-filled trachea within this structure *(1)*. Hilus of each lung is its connection with the mediastinum. It contains main stem and first division airways *(2 and 3)* as well as the major pulmonary blood vessels *(4, 5, 6, and 7)*. (From Fraser, R.G., and Paré, J.A.: Structure and function of the lung with emphasis on roentgenology, Philadelphia, 1971, W.B. Saunders Co.)

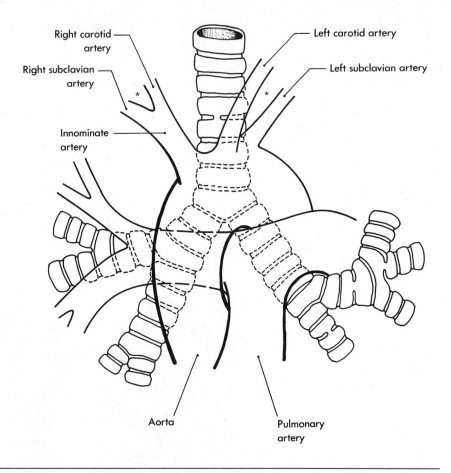

Right carotid artery

Right subclavian artery

Innominate artery

Left carotid artery

Left subclavian artery

Aorta

Pulmonary artery

Fig. 3-11   Diagram of relationship between main pulmonary artery and aorta, with their main branches, as they leave right and left ventricles of heart. Trachea is in background. The aorta arches over main pulmonary artery, which divides into right and left branches that enter the lungs. The aorta supplies oxygenated blood to remainder of body. The asterisk (*) on each side indicates the course of phrenic and vagus nerves as they enter thorax.

it deviates slightly to the right, allowing room for the aorta to pass by on its left side (Fig. 3-11). At the point of tracheal bifurcation in the chest, a sharp dividing cartilage called the carina extends up in midline to help demarcate flow into the right or left side. Very few aspirated objects lodge exactly at this point. The larger ones are stopped at the larynx; the smaller pass into the lungs. The right main stem bronchus angles off at 20 to 30 degrees from the midline, whereas the left angles off more sharply at 45 to 55 degrees (Fig. 3-12). Therefore, aspirated solid objects and fluids have a greater tendency to continue in the straightest course following the right bronchus. This tendency

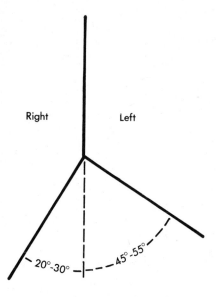

Fig. 3-12   Course of trachea and right and left main stem bronchi. Notice that right main stem bronchus continues on straighter course from midline than left main stem bronchus.

to follow the straightest and most dependent course continues in the airway distribution in the lungs in a predictable manner. Knowing such patterns helps one suggest aspiration from the location (Fig. 3-13). The point of junction between each lung and the mediastinum is called the hilus. This is the region where airways, blood vessels, nerves, and lymphatic channels leave or enter the mediastinum (see Fig. 3-10).

Phrenic and vagus nerves

Two major nerve pathways pass through the mediastinum, the phrenic nerves, which supply the diaphragm, and the vagus nerves, which supply most internal organs of the thorax and abdomen. They enter the chest in front of the subclavian arteries and lateral to the carotid arteries. At this point they diverge.

The phrenic nerves run on each side of the mediastinum anterior to the hilar structures. The left phrenic nerve travels a longer course than the right as it extends around the heart, which projects toward the left. Injury of the phrenic nerve causes paralysis of the diaphragm it innervates.

Each vagus nerve at its entry into the chest sends off a branch that curves back up to the larynx called the recurrent laryngeal nerve. This branch leaves the right side in the low neck. The recurrent branch of the left vagus nerve comes off in the upper portion of the chest. This branch angles under the arch of the aorta on the left side of the mediastinum before it goes back to the left

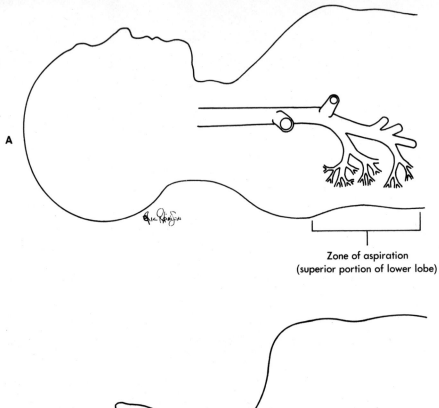

A

Zone of aspiration
(superior portion of lower lobe)

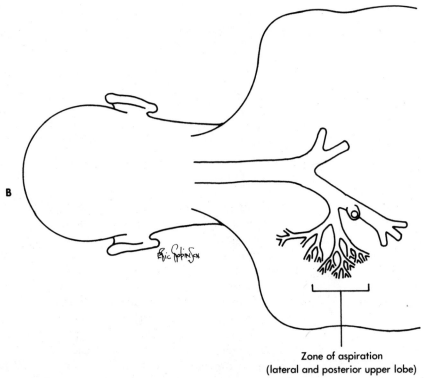

B

Zone of aspiration
(lateral and posterior upper lobe)

Fig. 3-13   Aspirated fluid can be spread about in many portions of lung, but some regions appear most frequently involved out to their most dependent position. If patient is in upright position, such material goes to basal portions of lungs. **A,** When patient is supine, this material involves predominantly the superior portions, especially the superior segment of the lower lobes. **B,** When patient is on one side or the other, this material involves lateral and posterior portions of upper lobe.

side of the larynx. Paralysis of one or both of these nerve can cause hoarseness, since the vocal cords do not close.

Branches of the vagus nerve also provide sympathetic and parasympathetic supply to the lung. These are important in many function, including regulation of airway diameter, cough reflexes, and control of respiration.

Airway divisions

Each main stem bronchus divides into branches supplying each lobe of the lung. The right lung has three lobes in most individuals—the upper, middle, and lower. At a point about 3 cm from the carina, the right mainstem bronchus gives rise to the upper lobe bronchus. The remaining major airway is called the intermediate bronchus. It continues for 3 to 4 cm and then divides into the middle and lower lobe bronchi.

The left lung generally has only two lobes, upper and lower. The left main stem bronchus measures about 5 cm long. It then divides into left upper and lower lobe bronchi. The counterpart to the right middle lobe is a part of the upper lobe in the left lung and is called the lingula. Its bronchus arises from the left upper lobe bronchus. There is no intermediate bronchus on the left.

Bifurcations and trifurcations of the bronchi continue to the periphery of the lung. The lobes are divided into fairly constant divisions called segments. The right and left lungs are similar except as noted in Table 3-1 and Fig. 3-14. The most widely used naming system in North America is that of Jackson and Huber. The number system helps to show which segments on the left correspond to those on the right. Since the right middle lobe and lingular portion of the left upper lobe differ slightly, they are given different names

Table 3-1
Bronchopulmonary
segments*

Segment	Number	Segment	Number
Upper lobe		Left upper lobe	
Apical	1	Upper division	
Posterior	2	Apical-posterior	1 and 2†
Anterior	3	Anterior	3
Right middle lobe		Lower (lingular) division	
Lateral	4	Superior lingula	4
Medial	5	Inferior lingula	5
Right lower lobe		Left lower lobe	
Superior	6	Superior	6
Medial basal	7	Anteromedial	7 and 8†
Anterior basal	8	Lateral basal	9
Lateral basal	9	Posterior basal	10
Posterior basal	10		

*The subdivisions of the lung and bronchial tree are fairly constant. Slight variations between the right and left sides are noted by combined names and numbers.

†*Editor's note:* Some authors feel that the left lung should be numbered such that there are eight segments, where the apical-posterior is numbered 1 and anteromedial is numbered 6.

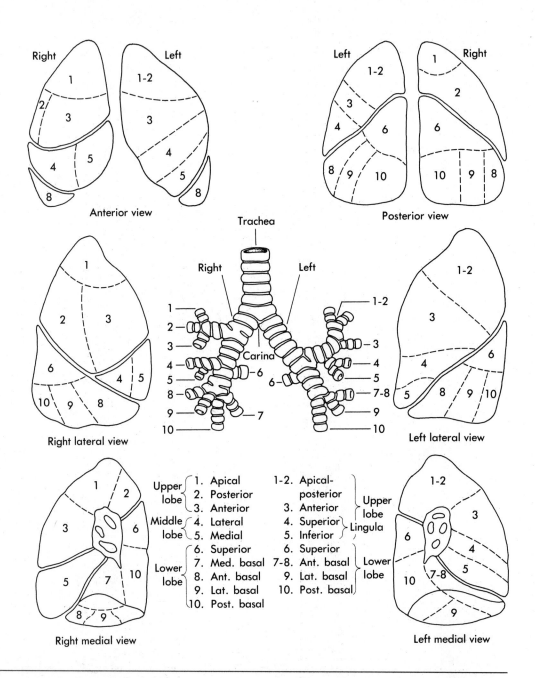

Fig. 3-14   Bronchopulmonary segments diagrammed. Again note similarities, with minor variations, between right and left lungs. (See editor's note for Table 3-1.)

Table 3-2
Bronchial and bronchiolar division

Structure	Generation from			Number	Diameter of individual structures	Total cross-sectional area	
	Trachea	Segmental bronchus	Terminal bronchiole				
Trachea	0			1	2.5 cm	5.0 cm²	Cartilaginous conducting structures
Main bronchi	1			2	11-19 mm	3.2 cm²	
Lobar bronchi	2-3	0		5	4.5-13.5	2.7 cm²	
Segmental	3-6	1		19	4.5-6.5 mm	3.2 cm²	
Subsegmental bronchi	4-7			38	3-6 mm	6.6 cm²	
Bronchi		2-6		Variable	Variable	Variable	
Terminal bronchi		3-7		1,000	1.0 mm	7.9 cm²	
Bronchioles		5-14		Variable	Variable	Variable	No cartilage in walls
Terminal bronchioles		6-15	0	35,000	0.65 mm	116 cm²	
Respiratory bronchioles			1-8	Variable	Variable	Variable	
Terminal respiratory bronchioles			2-9	630,000	0.45 mm	1,000 cm²	
Alveolar ducts and sacs			4-12	14×10^6	0.40	1.71 M²	
Alveoli				300×10^6	0.25-0.30 mm	70 M²	

Note marked increase in numbers of subunits and in cross-sectional surface area as bronchi divide. Bronchi contain cartilage in their walls, whereas bronchioles are smaller and do not have cartilage. (Adapted slightly from Bates, D.V., Macklem, P.T., and Christie, R.V.: Respiratory function in disease, Philadelphia, 1971, W.B. Saunders Company.)

describing their segmental relationships. In the left lung, some segments are combined to form a single segment.

Note Table 3-2. As further divisions occur in the airway system, the total number of bronchi increases tremendously, as does the total surface area. There are 300 million terminal air spaces. The surface area for gas exchange provided by these spaces is gigantic, in the range of 40 to 100 m^2, the average being 70 m^2. This means the lung has 35 times the surface area of the skin in the average person.

The primary function of the lung is gas exchange—absorbing oxygen and excreting carbon dioxide. This exchange takes place in the terminal air units, which are of microscopic size. This region of gas exchange is called the respiratory zone. It begins at approximately the seventeenth division of bronchi (Fig. 3-15). The last seven divisions are very small and short. All previous portions of the respiratory system serve to condition and conduct the gases to and from this respiratory zone and therefore are called the conducting pathways, or conducting zone. Since no gas exchange takes place in the conducting airways, they constitute the respiratory dead space (see Chapter 4). The total volume of the conducting airways is approximately 150 ml in the average adult. One-half of this space is in the upper and the other half in the lower respiratory tract. The lungs effectively have their greatest surface of exposure where gas exchange occurs, and not in the conducting zones (Fig. 3-16).

Very small airways contain no cartilage. The absence of cartilage is the hallmark of the "little bronchus," of bronchiole. Cartilage is present in the walls of airways down to approximately 1.0 mm in diameter (Table 3-2). The strictly conducting bronchioles are called terminal bronchioles (Table 3-2, Figs. 3-15 and 3-16). The bronchioles that open directly into the air spaces are very small and are called respiratory bronchioles (Figs. 3-15 and 3-17). These, together with the alveolar ducts and sacs and alveoli themselves, represent the respiratory zone of the lung (Fig. 3-18). The alveolus is the final air space in this system. It represents the unit of gas exchange.

The highly magnified architecture of the alveolus is shown in Fig. 3-19. Note that it is essentially a pocket of air extensively draped by a thin membrane containing capillaries. The distance between the alveolar air and capillary blood is between 0.35 and 2.5 μ. (For comparison, a red blood cell measures 7 μ in diameter.) This extremely thin wall is necessary for rapid exchange of gases between air and blood. There is a large excess of gas exchange units in the normal resting individual. The transit time for blood passing through the lung capillaries at rest is approximately one-half second. It is estimated that gas exchange is complete when the blood has traversed one-fourth the distance of the capillaries in the normal resting individual. These reserves are important for normal exercise and in disease states.

The presence of a continuous alveolar lining over the capillaries was confirmed in 1953 by early electron microscopy. The two principal cells composing the lining are the very thin flat cells (called type I pneumocytes or membranous pneumocytes because of their thin flat conformation) and more cuboidal cells (type II pneumocytes). The former are fragile and easily injured.

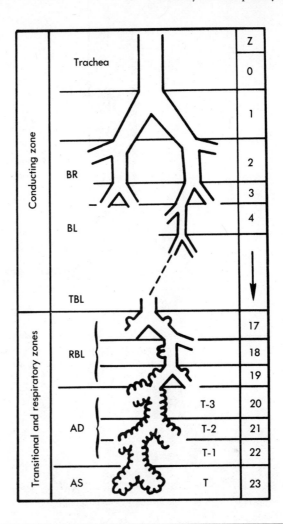

Fig. 3-15 The airways that only conduct gases back and forth are designated the conducting zone of lung. These include approximately the first 17 divisions of the tracheobronchial tree. The unit where gas exchange occurs, from respiratory bronchiole to alveolar space, is called the respiratory zone. *BR* = bronchus, *BL* = bronchiole, *TBL* = terminal bronchiole, *RBL* = respiratory bronchiole, *AD* = alveolar duct, *AS* = alveolar space, *Z* = order of airway division. (From Weibel, E.R.: Morphometry of the human lung, Heidelberg, 1963, Springer-Verlag.)

Type II cells proliferate in cases of injury and give rise to new type I cells. Type II cells also are thought to be the cells of origin in the lungs of a surface-wetting agent, surfactant. This substance decreases surface tension and is important in preventing alveolar collapse.

Vascular supply   The vascular supply of the lungs is composed of two separate systems, pulmonary and bronchial.

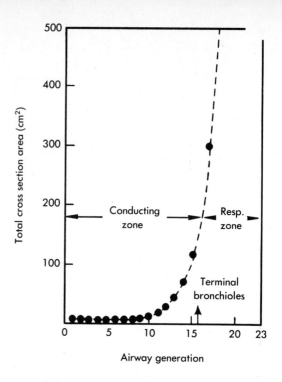

Fig. 3-16 Since no gas exchange takes place in the conducting zone, this region is called the anatomic dead space (see Chapter 4). The gas exchange surface increases markedly at the level of the terminal bronchiole. (From West, J.: Respiratory physiology—the essentials, Baltimore, 1974, The Williams & Wilkins Co.)

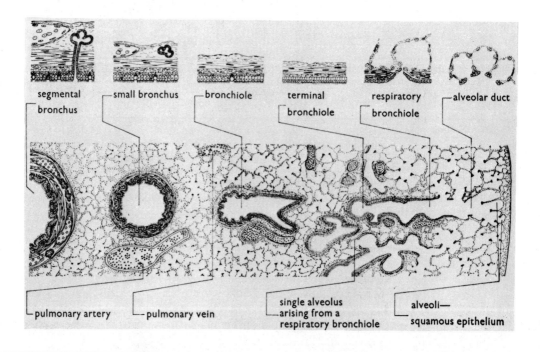

Fig. 3-17 Histologic diagram of airways from segmental bronchus to alveolus. (From Freeman, W.H., and Bracegirdle, B.: An atlas of histology, London, 1966, Heinemann Educational Books Ltd.)

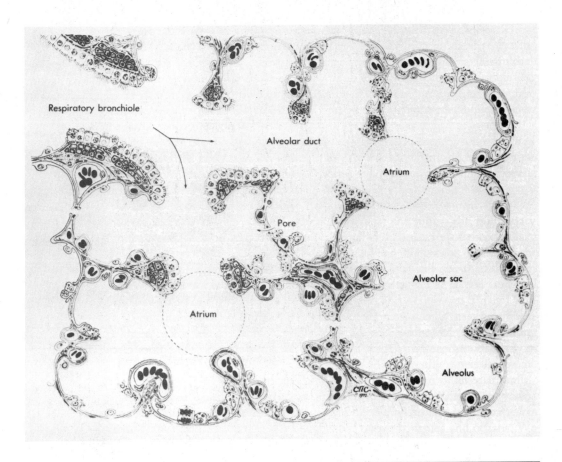

Fig. 3-18   Diagrammed respresentation of microscopic view of terminal airways. These units compose respiratory zone of lung. (From Sorokin, S.P.: The respiratory system. In Greep, R.O., and Weiss, L., editors: Histology, New York, 1973, McGraw-Hill Book Company. Used with permission of McGraw-Hill Book Company.)

The right side of the heart, via the main pulmonary artery, delivers unoxygenated blood to the lungs. The left side of the heart, through the aorta, delivers the freshly oxygenated blood to the body. The main pulmonary artery and aorta exit from the heart and pass superiorly (Fig. 3-11). Just below the point of tracheal division into the right and left mainstem bronchi (the carina), the main pulmonary artery divides into corresponding right and left pulmonary arteries, which accompany respective bronchi. In fact, this companionship continues through all the divisions into the distal air spaces. The branches of the pulmonary artery are always adjacent to the bronchi and bronchioles.

Since blood coming through the pulmonary arteries lacks sufficient oxygen for the metabolism of the lung tissues, a separate arterial supply, called the

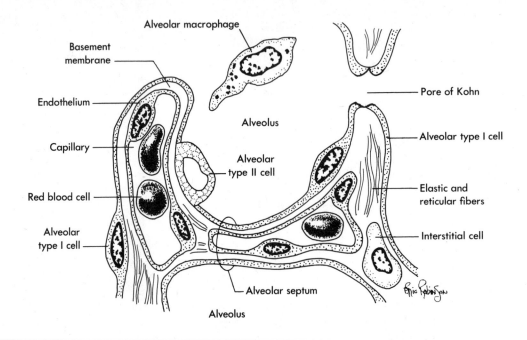

Fig. 3-19   Very high power view of alveolus. Alveolar walls or septae are occupied mainly by capillaries. Basement membrane of capillary is fused with that of alveolar lining. Interstitium contains a few interstitial fibers, composed mostly of reticular support fibers, elastic fibers, and one interstitial cell. An incomplete portion of alveolar septum called a pore of Kohn is shown (see also Fig. 3-27). Type I lining cells are very flat. Small distance between blood and air makes gas exchange remarkably efficient. Type II cells are much less numerous than type I cells. Type II cells are source of surfactant. The alveolar macrophages are mobile phagocytic cells that migrate into alveoli from the bloodstream.

bronchial arteries, also accompanies the bronchi. These branches usually come from the second to fourth thoracic intercostal arteries but can come from the aorta or any of the other nearby systemic arteries. The amount of blood flow required to support the lung tissue is remarkably small, perhaps 5 to 50 ml/min, compared to the 5,000 ml/min of blood traveling through the pulmonary arterial system. In diseased lungs, the bronchial artery supply may increase greatly.

Between each set of accompanying bronchi, bronchioles, pulmonary and bronchial arteries, and arterioles are thin fibrous septa (Fig. 3-20). These septa continue from the pleura to the larger bronchi and pulmonary arteries. Within these septa the venous blood and lymphatics originate as thin streams in and near the pleura. The pulmonary veins accept all of the the blood supplied by the pulmonary arteries and most of that by the bronchial arteries. The bronchial veins within the bronchial walls, however, return a small portion of the bronchial arterial blood to the right atrium. The small pulmonary veins come

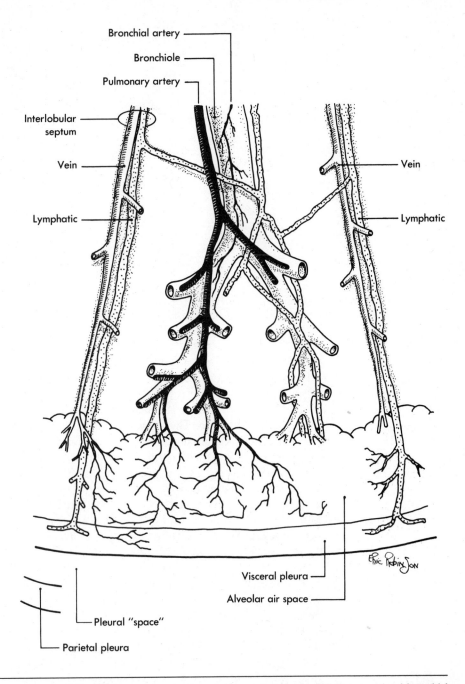

Bronchial artery

Bronchiole

Pulmonary artery

Interlobular
septum

Vein

Lymphatic

Vein

Lymphatic

Visceral pleura

Alveolar air space

Pleural "space"

Parietal pleura

Fig. 3-20   Diagram of distal pulmonary arteries, bronchioles, and air spaces with their associated bronchial arteries. Pulmonary veins lie in fibrous tissue septa between these paired pulmonary arteries and airways. Note that lymphatic channels travel with both sets of structures.

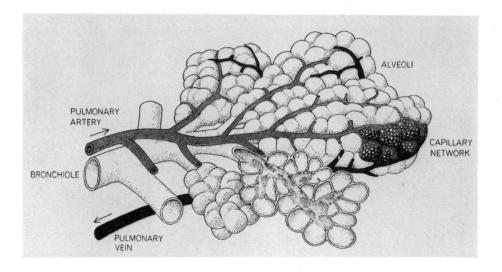

Fig. 3-21   Diagram of capillary bed surrounding alveoli. It is the densest vascular network in body. Capillaries are nearly equal in length and width and very close together. (From The effects of smoking by E.C. Hammond. Copyright © 1962 by Scientific American, Inc. All rights reserved.)

together at each hilus to form two right and two left main pulmonary veins, returning blood to the left atrium of the heart.

Gas exchange   The air-blood interface at the alveolar surface deserves comment. Capillaries in the lung are unique. They represent the most dense capillary network in the body. They are essentially an interweaving network of canals, hardly longer than they are wide, with very little space between them. It has been estimated they are 10 μ long and 7 μ wide. These fine tubes are so interlaced (Fig. 3-21) that the capillary bed should be thought of more as a pool of blood than a series of pipes. This bed is so well structured that the 100 to 300 ml of blood in the capillaries at any one time are spread over most of the 70 m^2 of surface. Considered another way, roughly a teaspoon of blood is spread over 1 m^2 of surface—a remarkable feat.

Lymphatics   Lymphatic channels freely join with each other in the pleura and travel toward the hilar regions, both in the septa accompanying veins and about the bronchi-pulmonary artery complexes (Figs. 3-20 and 3-22). The lymph flow is directed through one or more lymph nodes clustered about each hilus. From there lymph travels through the mediastinum to rejoin the general circulation. These lymphatic channels are not detectable on chest roentgenograms unless they are distended or thickened by disease.

We have considered some of the protective mechanisms in the upper respiratory tract. However, fine particles less than 5 μ in diameter can bypass these mechanisms and can float with the current of air into the terminal air spaces.

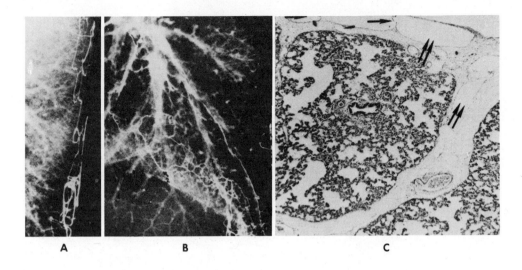

A   B   C

Fig. 3-22 Radiographs of lymphatic channels following their injection with contrast material. The pleural lymphatics are seen in profile in **A**. One lymphatic channel marked with an arrow in **B** is following a pulmonary vein. Tissue section (**C**) shows pleural lymphatics marked with one arrow and septal lymphatics marked with two arrows. (From Heitzman, E.R.: The lung: radiologic-pathologic correlations, St. Louis, 1973, The C.V. Mosby Co.).

These include bacteria and other infective organisms. Circulating scavenger cells called macrophages are an important defense to the lung from these foreign particles. These cells migrate into the air spaces from the passing circulation and clean up debris. Lymphatic drainage and ciliary action exist only to the level of the terminal bronchiole. Therefore, whatever material is to be disposed of at the alveolar level, with or without assistance of macrophages, must find its way to these bronchioles and from there be removed from the lungs via mucous film, cough, or lymphatic drainage.

Lung units and their connections

A moment should be spent considering organization of the peripheral airway structures into groups. The alveolus is the smallest and most basic functioning unit of the lung. It is helpful to think of a larger organizational unit of the lung called a (secondary) lobule. These are the smallest units in the lung surrounded by fibrous tissue septa. These polygonal units vary in size but are from 1 to 2.5 cm on a side and can be observed from the external and cut surface (Fig. 3-23) of the lung. These units correspond to clusters of from three to five terminal bronchioles and contain the distal respiratory zone supplied by these bronchioles. Infection, hemorrhage, and aspiration often, at least temporarily, respect the boundaries between these lobules. Between these (secondary) lobules, interlobular septa are incomplete because some air and fluid does eventually pass into nearby lobules. Fig. 3-24 relates this unit by size to the other basic units of the lung.

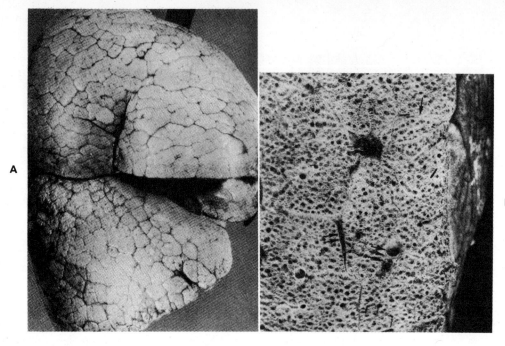

Fig. 3-23 Outer surface (**A**) and cut surface (**B**) of lung. **B,** One arrow marks an interlobular septum, two arrows mark small veins in these septa, and three arrows point to a pulmonary artery and bronchiole near center of secondary lobule. (From Heitzman, E.R.: The lung: radiologic-pathologic correlations, St. Louis, 1973, The C.V. Mosby Co.)

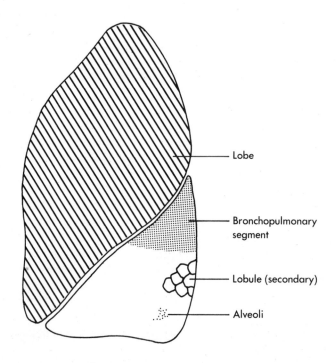

Lobe

Bronchopulmonary segment

Lobule (secondary)

Alveoli

Fig. 3-24 Diagrammatic representation of units of lung. Alveoli are actually microscopic in size.

Other interconnections exist in the lung. Alveolar septa were at one time thought to be entirely intact, but now it is well known that holes exist between them called pores of Kohn (Fig. 3-25). These vary from 5 to 15 μm in diameter. These pores allow collateral air flow between adjacent portions of lung (Fig. 3-26) and help explain why a bronchus might be completely obstructed and yet the tissue beyond the obstruction may remain at least partially aerated.

Connections also exist between lobes in many lungs. The major (interlobular) fissures, which divide the right lung into three lobes and left lung into two lobes, extend completely through to the medial surfaces of the lungs in only 50% of 75% of individual lungs. Therefore, in the 25% to 50% of cases with incomplete interlobular fissures, air or fluid can spread between major lobes through the connections noted above. There are, of course, alternate routes of spread between lobes—via airways, blood, lymph flow, and pleura or pleural cavity. Spread between both lungs can also be by airway, blood, or lymphatic pathways.

Pleura

The surface of the lungs, portions of the major interlobular fissues, the inside of the chest walls composing the chest cavities, and the lateral portions of the mediastinum are covered by a thin mesothelial layer called pleura. That portion covering the lungs and extending onto the hilar bronchi and vessels and into the major fissures is called the visceral pleura. The portion covering the inner surface of the chest wall and the mediastinum is called the parietal pleura (Figs. 3-20 and 3-27). Although the two portions are described by these different names, they are really one continuous lining. The deeper portions of the visceral pleura contain elastic and fibrous fibers and small venules and lymphatics. The interlobular septa are continuous with this layer, and the veins and lymphatics course along these septa, starting as fine caliber vessels in the pleura.

A lubricative mucous solution is produced by the single-layered cuboidal cells lining the pleura and is important in allowing one pleural surface to slip over the other. This slipping or gliding happens to some extent during breathing or coughing in the normal individual. Injury sometimes obliterates this potential space. This obliteration is usually without clinical significance, although it may become important if it is of sufficient degree to inhibit lung expansion.

The chest cavities

If one were to remove both lungs from their positions in the body, one would find empty cavities. In the midline would be the mediastinum with its contents as previously noted. Surrounding these cavities above, behind, and laterally is the chest wall. The chest has, as its basic skeletal structure, the rib cage. This portion of the skeleton does indeed form a peripheral cage (Fig. 3-28). From their attachments at the spine, the ribs extend around and downward in front of the arms. There they turn upward again and continue, not as bone but as cartilages to the sternum. This cartilage is soft and moderately flexible in younger individuals. These qualities are lost as the individual ages

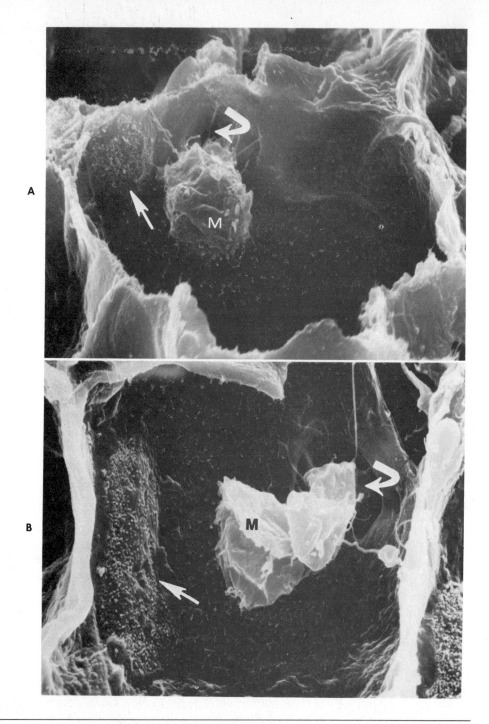

Fig. 3-25 Scanning electron micrographs of alveolar air spaces. **A,** Note thin partitions or septa between adjacent alveoli. The thin platelike type I cells compose most of these. Type II cells have projections off their surfaces that appear dotted or hairy *(straight arrow)*. Alveolar macrophage *(M)* is seen at back partially covering pore of Kohn *(upper curved arrow)*. **B,** Similar view with two or three macrophages passing through pore of Kohn. (Grateful appreciation is given to Mr. Mike Wagner, of San Diego, Calif., for use of the electron micrographs.)

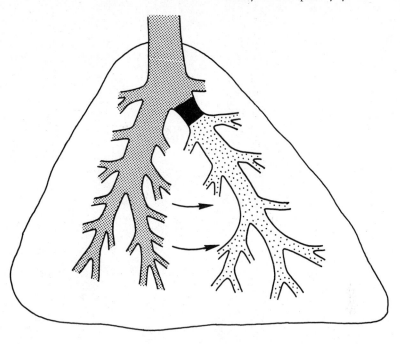

Fig. 3-26   Collateral air flow is possible due to pores of Kohn. Shown in solid black is obstructing plug in airway. Some air flows from nonobstructed airway into obstructed airway beyond site of obstruction.

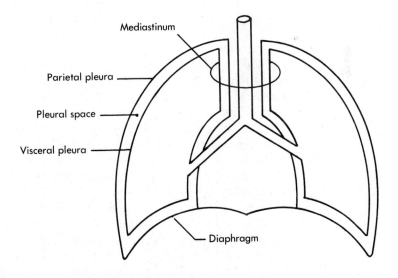

Fig. 3-27   This diagrammatic sketch shows overall relationship of chest organs, cavities, and investments. The mediastinum occupies space between lungs. Each lung sits within its chest cavity. This cavity is lined by parietal pleura, which covers chest cage, diaphragm, and lateral mediastinum, and by visceral pleura, which covers lungs.

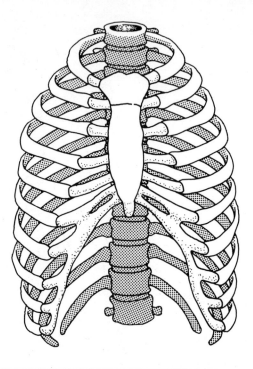

Fig. 3-28   Chest cage. Ribs arch around from vertebral column joining sternum through cartilaginous extensions.

and cartilages usually become calcified. The rib cage then becomes less flexible. This can be noted during closed chest massage in different age groups. During inhalation, the ribs move out and up, especially in the lower portions of the thorax. With advancing age the rib cage may become more fixed in the up and out position, and the chest may become more rounded or barrel-shaped.

Under each rib is an accompanying artery, vein, and nerve. These travel in a groove on the underside of the rib (Fig. 3-29). To avoid these structures when passing needles through the intercostal space, one inserts the needle just above the next lower rib. Thin intercostal muscle sheets connect the ribs to one another.

Attached at the inferior portion of each rib cage and sealing this portion of the chest cavity are the two thin muscle sheets, the diaphragms (Fig. 3-27). These curve up into the lower aspects of each chest cavity as smooth domes. During inspiration, these muscles contract, flatten their domes, and are important in enlarging the chest cavity. During expiration, they relax and ride further into the chest and contribute to decreasing the size of the chest cavity. Thus, inspiration is the portion of respiration requiring active muscle contraction. Normal expiration represents a relaxation of contraction.

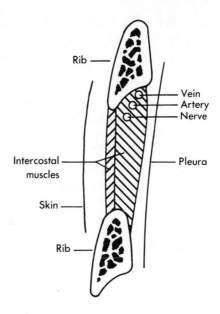

Fig. 3-29   Intercostal muscles fill spaces between ribs. An intercostal artery, veins, and nerve run in groove just beneath lower edge of each rib.

The pleural space and the expanded lung

As noted there is a gliding surface between the visceral and parietal pleural layers that is lubricated by a mucinous substance. This is spoken of as a potential space since in the normal person there is no true space but a fluid-filled surface. If air, fluid, or other substances are introduced into this area, the two pleural surfaces separate easily. The parietal pleura stays relatively fixed in position supported by the bony rib cage, but the lung and the visceral pleura are displaced from the chest wall.

The lung itself has elastic properties. Elastic tissue is woven throughout the lung, following with bronchi and bronchioles, in the media of vessels, in the pleura, and as scattered interstital contractile cells spread in the peripheral interstitial tissue of the lung. The lung always tends to decrease in volume because of this elasticity. These elastic properties are demonstrated clearly when a lung is removed from the chest cavity and quickly collapses into a smaller size, or when air or fluid is introduced into the pleural space. This tendency of the lung to contract is important in the development of negative intrapleural pressure (see Chapter 4). In addition to collapse of an entire lung, it is possible for a portion, such as a lobe, to collapse. The most common cause of a lobar collapse is obstruction of its bronchus. With reabsorption of air behind this obstruction and with inadequate collateral air flow, the tissue decreases in volume. The remaining lobe or lobes expand to fill most of the volume thereby lost. Once such a collapse has occurred, attempts should be undertaken to correct it so that it does not become permanent.

The normal anatomy and protective mechanisms of the respiratory tract have been examined. Physiology of respiration will be considered in the next three chapters.

Bibliography

Fraser, R.G., and Paré, J.A.: Structure and function of the lung with emphasis on roentgenology, Philadelphia, 1971, W.B. Saunders Company.

Heitzman, E.R.: The lung: radiologic-pathologic correlations, St. Louis, 1973, The C.V. Mosby Co., chapter 3.

Murray, J.F.: The normal lung: the basis for diagnosis and treatment of pulmonary disease, Philadelphia, 1976, W.B. Saunders Company.

Chapter 4   Ventilation

The terms *ventilation* and *respiration* are frequently used interchangeably because they are generally synonymous, but to many there is a subtle difference between them. Ventilation may be considered as the mechanical movement of air into and out of the lung in a cyclic fashion, whereas respiration often refers to the exchange of oxygen and carbon dioxide in the lung and at the body cell. The primary function of the lung is respiration, to supply the body with oxygen and to remove the waste product of metabolism, carbon dioxide; but to fulfill this function the lung must have adequate ventilation. Thus we begin our study of cardiopulmonary physiology with a consideration of the first need—aeration of the lung.

Ventilation is a cyclic activity, both automatic and voluntary, and it consists of two components—an inward flow of air, called *inhalation* or inspiration, and an outward flow, called *exhalation* or expiration. The physical forces responsible for this air movement constitute the mechanics of ventilation. The inhalation-exhalation cycle moves a volume of gas, the *tidal volume* (V_T), into and out of the respiratory tract. As students observe their own ventilatory pattern, they will note that both tidal volume and *rate of breathing* (f, for frequency per minute) vary with physical activity. The product of these two factors, and a physiologically important parameter to evaluate, is the *minute volume* ($\dot{V}_E$). This is the amount of gas moved per minute, and although theoretically it should equal the tidal volume times the frequency, for practical reasons it is defined as the volume *exhaled* per minute (indicated by its symbol) and is measured by time-collecting exhaled respiratory gas. The relationships between tidal volume, minute volume, frequency, the nature of the airways through which the gas flows, and the physical forces responsible for gas movement are critical in determining the effectiveness of ventilation, and some of the important factors influencing them are defined and discussed in this chapter.

Dead space (rebreathed volume)

The term *dead space* (V_D) is used preferentially in this text because at this time it is more common than rebreathed volume. *Rebreathed volume* (V_{RB}), however, is a more accurate expression.

The respiratory therapist should understand the concept of *dead space* and the role it plays in ventilation. Dead space is defined as that portion of the respiratory tract that is *ventilated but not perfused by the pulmonary circulation*. *Perfusion* refers to the end point in arterial blood flow, where capillaries and tissue cells come into *intimate* contact for mutual exchange of contents. A review of anatomy will remind the student that the respiratory tract is supplied by two circulations, the systemic and the pulmonary. The conducting airways of the bronchial tree are served by the systemic circulation, and the bronchial and bronchiolar cells (as any other body tissue) are perfused by branches of the bronchial arteries to maintain their viability and function. The alveoli, however, are perfused by capillaries of the pulmonary circulation, and here pulmonary arterial blood bathes the alveolar cells and is but a fraction of a micron away from alveolar air. Only at this level can oxygen and carbon dioxide pass between air and blood. By definition, then, ventilatory dead space consists of the conducting airways down to the level of gas exchange and *any alveoli* that receive less than their normal pulmonary capillary perfusion. Thus, dead space does not contribute to respiration but constitutes a volume that must be filled by ventilation before air can reach perfused alveoli.

Dead space is of three types: *anatomic* (V_D ant), *alveolar* (V_D alv), and *physiologic* (V_D phys). These are illustrated in Fig. 4-1.

1. *Anatomic dead space* consists of the purely conducting airways of the nose and mouth, pharynx, larynx, trachea, bronchi, and bronchioles to the respiratory level.
2. *Alveolar dead space* is a less well-defined volume that consists of a variable number of alveoli whose perfusion is reduced or absent as a result of, among other causes, gravitational shifts in pulmonary blood flow distribution in the normal subject and impaired flow in the diseased.
3. *Physiologic dead space* is the sum of the anatomic and alveolar dead spaces, and its description as "physiologic" implies that it is the functional dead space of ventilation.

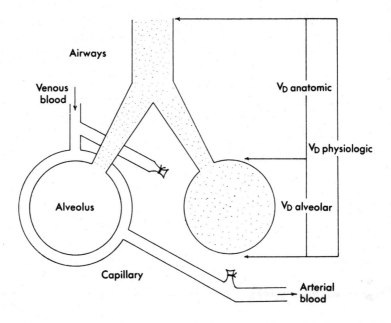

Fig. 4-1   The three types of dead space are shown in this sketch, which schematically represents two alveoli, their supporting airways, and capillaries. One alveolus is normally perfused and ventilated; but the capillary to the other is shown as if it were tied off and removed, so that the alveolus is freely ventilated but not perfused. The relationships of the dead spaces are indicated, as defined in the text.

Measurement of dead spaces can be performed in the cardiopulmonary laboratory by techniques that are discussed here.

In theory, all alveoli should be perfused, with no alveolar dead space. Therefore physiologic and anatomic dead spaces should be identical and in the average adult should measure approximately between 150 and 160 ml. Should there be some alveoli with inadequate perfusion, a small alveolar dead space will exist that will increase the physiologic dead space.

Two points should be emphasized at this time. First, dead space is not dead at all because it is a functional volume that plays an important part in ventilation and is bound by living tissue. Second, it is a volume that is rebreathed. Let us suppose the volume of air exhaled by a subject is 500 ml, and the dead space of the subject is 150 ml. Of the 500 ml of air exhaled, the first 150 ml come from the upper portion of the respiratory tract, the conducting airways, or dead space, and the remaining 350 ml from the alveoli. At the end of exhalation, then, airways are not empty but contain 150 ml of air that have been moved up from the alveoli. With the next inhalation this 150-ml volume of dead space air, which has already been breathed, will be the first of the inspired air to be drawn back down into the alveoli and rebreathed. The student will find this principle of rebreathed volumes of critical importance in the management of patients on mechanical ventilators.

Classification of ventilation

Types of ventilation may be classified as physiologic or clinical ventilation. *Physiologically,* we can consider *total ventilation,* or *minute volume* ($\dot{V}_E$), *dead space ventilation* ($\dot{V}_D$), and *alveolar ventilation* ($\dot{V}_A$). For safe and effective management of patients in ventilatory failure, the respiratory therapist must clearly understand the differences between and the importance of each of these types:

1. *Total ventilation* refers to the amount of air moved into and out of the entire respiratory tract in liters per minute in the resting state. Normally ranging from 5 to 10 ℓ/min, this volume gives only a rough estimation of ventilatory efficiency, since it does not indicate how much air is reaching alveoli.
2. *Dead space ventilation* is the minute volume in liters that ventilates the physiologic dead space. This is also sometimes called *wasted ventilation.*
3. *Alveolar ventilation* is the minute volume in liters that ventilates all the perfused alveoli and obviously is the difference between the total and dead space ventilation. Usually it is between 4 and 5 ℓ/min.

Functionally, only the alveolar ventilation is of importance, since it determines how much air will be available for gas exchange. Perhaps it is already evident that a patient's breathing pattern can be so disturbed that with a rapid rate and a small tidal volume, a large total volume of air may be moved that does little more than ventilate the dead space, leaving only a small amount to reach the alveoli.

Clinically, in the resting state we note *normal ventilation, hypoventilation,* and *hyperventilation:*

1. *Normal ventilation* is that amount of minute ventilation that provides adequate alveolar ventilation at a normal rate and with a minimum of effort. Disruption of easy ventilation by disease, even with satisfactory alveolar aeration, can produce some of the most serious physical disabilities.
2. *Hypoventilation* is that state of impaired breathing whereby the alveoli are inadequately ventilated to fulfill the body's gas exchange needs. Hypoventilation may be the result of either a *pathologic increase in dead space* (as from pulmonary distention, or increased ventilation/perfusion ratios, to be described later) or a *reduction in alveolar minute volume* (as from abnormally small tidal volumes, or retarded breathing frequency). Table 4-1 illustrates theoretic exaggerated examples, with volumes measured in milliliters. To compensate for an increased dead space, the patient must increase either rate or tidal volume, and in each instance the additional muscular effort is disabling. Conditions causing a reduced ventilatory rate usually do not permit voluntary compensation by increasing the tidal volume, although sometimes a patient with restricted volumes can

manage a compensatory rate increase. Again, this is possible only to a certain degree and is physically strenuous. We will see later that the patient with this defect, by virtue of the underlying disease, is usually unable to compensate at all. The respiratory therapist will find that the treatment of hypoventilation will be one of his or her most demanding responsibilities.

3. *Hyperventilation* is an overaeration of the alveoli beyond physiologic needs caused by an increase in tidal volume or rate or both and may be voluntary or involuntary. It can upset respiratory stability and impair circulation, but it is especially important for the therapist to note that hyperventilation is often induced by certain respiratory therapy procedures.

Dead space–to– tidal volume ratio

A variety of diseases and clinical disorders can cause an increase in physiologic dead space. As seen in Table 4-1, when dead space increases, alveolar ventilation can fall. Or, if total ventilation is also increased, alveolar ventilation can be maintained by keeping the *ratio* of dead space to ventilation nearly the same.

This useful index can be expressed by comparing physiologic dead space to the patient's tidal volume as a ratio: V_D/V_T. The values used in Table 4-1 for normal can be used as an example. Here the V_D is 150 ml, and the V_T is 450

Table 4-1
Types of hypoventilation and their compensation methods*

	Normal	Hypoventilation due to increased V_D	Compensation	
V_T	450	450	450	600
V_D	150	300	300	300
f	15	15	30	15
$\dot{V}_E$	6750	6750	13,500	9000
$\dot{V}_D$	2250	4500	9000	4500
V_A	4500	2250	4500	4500

	Normal	Hypoventilation due to reduced V_T	Compensation
V_T	450	225	225
V_D	150	150	150
f	15	15	60
$\dot{V}_E$	6750	3375	13,500
$\dot{V}_D$	2250	2250	9000
V_A	4500	1125	4500

*In each example compensation occurs by changing either tidal volume (V_T) or rate (f) to keep alveolar ventilation ($\dot{V}_A$) the same as normal.

ml. By dividing 150 by 450 the resulting ratio is found to be 0.33. This ratio varies somewhat among individuals and with different tidal volumes, generally ranging from 0.2 to 0.4.

Measuring this ratio can be done by using the modified Bohr equation, which compares an estimate of alveolar carbon dioxide and the average carbon dioxide exhaled. The equation is expressed as:

$$V_D/V_T = \frac{P_{A_{CO_2}} - P\overline{E}_{CO_2}}{P_{A_{CO_2}}}$$

where $P_{A_{CO_2}}$ is the partial pressure of CO_2 in the alveoli, and $P\overline{E}_{CO_2}$ is the average CO_2 in the exhaled air.

The arterial P_{CO_2} ($P_{a_{CO_2}}$) is often substituted in the equation because it is available clinically from arterial blood gas measurements and because it is generally very close to being the same as the alveolar P_{CO_2}. The formula then appears as:

$$V_D/V_T = \frac{P_{a_{CO_2}} - P\overline{E}_{CO_2}}{P_{a_{CO_2}}}$$

At the bedside, a sample of the patient's exhaled air can be collected at the same time arterial blood is drawn. The values for $P_{a_{CO_2}}$ and $P\overline{E}_{CO_2}$ are then obtained from the blood gas laboratory, using standard equipment and the resulting values used in the equation. As an example, if the arterial P_{CO_2} is reported to be 40 mm Hg and the mean exhaled air has a P_{CO_2} of 27 mm Hg then:

$$V_D/V_T = \frac{40 - 27}{40}$$

$$V_D/V_T = \frac{13}{40}$$

$$V_D/V_T = 0.325 \text{ or } 0.33$$

This means that the dead space for this patient makes up about one third of the tidal volume. Carbon dioxide is used since only that air that reaches perfused alveoli can participate in removal of carbon dioxide from the lung. The impact of this relationship is discussed further in later chapters.

Action of ventilatory muscles[1-3]

At this time the student should review the anatomy of the thorax, paying particular attention to the relationships between the skeletal parts, the shape of the ribs, and the thoracic musculature. The thorax is somewhat like a cone, with a wide base bound by the diaphragm and a narrow opening at the top called the *operculum*. The latter is bound by the first ribs and the manubrium of the sternum.

Movements of the thoracic cage

For purposes of discussion the ribs are grouped into three categories—the *first rib*, the *vertebrosternal ribs* (2 to 7), and the *vertebrochondral ribs* (8 to 10):

1. The *first rib* moves about the axis of its neck, raising and lowering the

sternum. Although the motion is slight, it produces some increase in the anteroposterior (A-P) diameter of the chest. During quiet breathing this action is not utilized, but it becomes important under conditions of stress.

2. The six *vertebrosternal ribs* (2 to 7) play an important role in ventilation. In contrast to the first rib, these move simultaneously about the axis of the rib neck and the axis between the angle of the rib and its sternal junction (Fig. 4-2). As they rotate about the axes of their necks (Fig. 4-2, *A*), their sternal ends rise and fall, thus increasing the A-P thoracic diameter. This action is referred to as the "pump handle motion." At the same time these ribs move about the longer axes from their angles to the sternum (Fig. 4-2, *B*), leading to an up-and-down motion of the middle segments of the ribs. This "bucket handle" motion produces an increase and decrease in the transverse diameter of the chest. Thus the compound action of these ribs increases and decreases both A-P and transverse diameters smoothly and synchronously.

3. The *vertebrochondral ribs* (8 to 10) have rotation patterns similar to the vertebrosternal group. However, elevation of the anterior ends of these ribs produces a backward movement of the lower end of the sternum, with *reduction* in thoracic A-P diameter (Fig. 4-3). Outward rotation of the middle portions of the ribs increases the transverse diameter, as do the vertebrosternal ribs.

Some do not believe the ribs rotate about their neck axes but rather *abduct* by a sliding motion. Ribs 11 and 12 are not included in any of the three categories mentioned, since they do not participate in changing the contour of the chest but act as muscular insertion points.

Diaphragm

The diaphragm is one of the two major ventilatory muscles, which, by its location and action, is best able to vary the volume of the thorax to produce the pressure changes needed for ventilation. It arises from three locations, the lumbar vertebrae, the costal margin, and the xiphoid, its fibers converging to interlace into a broad connective tissue sheet called the *central tendon*. The configuration of this muscle is that of a tent or a dome, dividing the chest from the abdomen. It is pierced by several structures, such as the esophagus, the aorta, many nerves, and the vena cava and receives its motor innervation from the *phrenic nerves*. Although the diaphragm is a single anatomic structure, the union of its central tendon with the fibrous pericardium functionally divides its dome into two "leaves." For convenience these are often referred to as the right and left diaphragms, or hemidiaphragms. With the liver immediately below it, the right dome is about 1 cm higher than the left, in the resting position, at the end of a quiet exhalation; and although the movements of both leaves are usually synchronous, because each has its own nerve supply, each may function independently of the other.

The mechanical action of the diaphragm is twofold:

1. Contraction draws down the central tendon, flattening its contour, increasing the volume of the thorax, and lowering intrathoracic pressure.

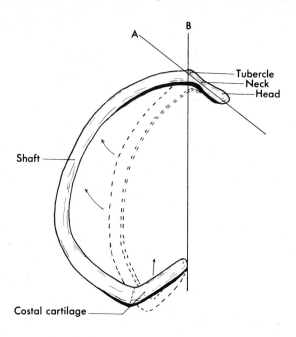

Fig. 4-2   The two axes about which the vertebrosternal ribs rotate during ventilation are indicated by lines *A* and *B*. The former passes through the length of the rib head and neck; the latter follows an A-P direction from the tip of the coastal cartilage to the tubercle. The rib undergoes a compound movement from its starting position *(dotted outline)*, the shaft swinging upward and laterally about axis *B*, and the anterior end moving upward about axis *A*.

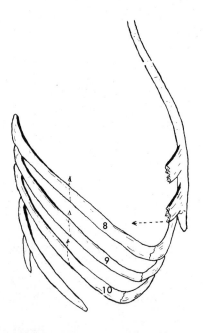

Fig. 4-3   The vertebrochondral ribs, *8* to *10*, have laterosuperior movement ribs 2 to 7, but elevation of their anterior ends retracts the lower end of the sternum, shortening the A-P diameter of the thorax in that plane.

As the diaphragm descends, intraabdominal pressure increases and the muscles of the abdominal wall relax, allowing the upper abdomen to balloon outward. Splinting or rigidity of the abdominal wall interferes with diaphragmatic descent.

2. Contraction of the costal fibers of the diaphragm *raises* and *everts* the costal margin if the dome is intact and intraabdominal pressure is normal. As the abdominal pressure increases during inspiration, this pressure acts as a fulcrum against which continued contraction of the diaphragmatic fibers pull up and out on the costal margin. In Fig. 4-4 the descending diaphragm is opposed by increasing intraabdominal pressure. This pressure finally stabilizes the central portion of the diaphragm so that the force of continued contraction is expended as traction on the costal attachments of the diaphragm. Because of the springlike tension of the ribs and the contour of the thorax at this level, the costal margin is pulled upward and outward, increasing the lateral diameter of the chest.

During inhalation therefore, as the diaphragm contracts, its dome descends and the costal margin of the chest moves outward so that the thorax enlarges both vertically and transversely. It is important to understand and visualize this combined action, since it is easily disturbed in pulmonary disease. Thus, if the diaphragm is abnormally low in position, not only is there a diminished vertical excursion (with a resulting reduction in tidal volume), but contraction of the costal fibers, instead of elevating the costal margin, may even pull in the lower chest boundary and narrow the thorax laterally. Fig. 4-4, *B,* shows an abnormal diaphragm, low in position and relatively flat in contour. Because of its starting position, it can descend very little on contraction, and with loss of its domed shape, contraction tends to pull its fibers centrally on a horizontal plane. This pulls in the costal margin and reduces the diameter of the chest. Much of the little gain in vertical diameter from the limited mobility of the diaphragm is negated by the simultaneous lateral shortening. The diaphragm takes no active part in exhalation and returns to its inspiratory resting position during the passive recoil of the thorax, to be explained later. During forced exhalation, as against resistance, the diaphragm does expel gas from the lung as it is pushed upward by intraabdominal pressure generated by contracting abdominal muscles.

At rest the normal tidal movement of the diaphram is approximately 1.5 cm, and with deep breathing, 6 to 10 cm. With quiet breathing the excursions of both leaves of the diaphragm are about equal, but with a deep inspiration the right diaphragm may move more than the left. In the supine position the total diaphragmatic movement is the same as in the erect position. In a head-down, 45-degree supine tilt, however, the resting level of the diaphragm rises about 6 cm, causing a reduction of the functional residual capacity and the expiratory reserve volume. When the subject lies in a lateral position, the lower diaphragm tends to rise into the chest. Although the diaphragm is the principal ventilatory muscle and the only one used in normal quiet breathing, it is

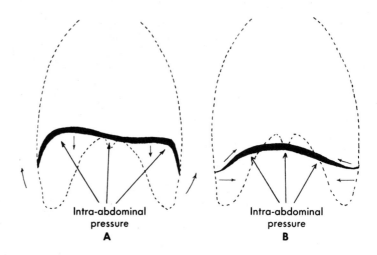

Fig. 4-4   **A,** As the normal diaphragm contracts, it descends, gradually building up pressure in the abdomen until the intraabdominal pressure acts as a fulcrum against which continued contraction everts the costal margin, enlarging the thorax further. **B,** Contraction of the diaphragm, which is abnormally low at the start of inspiration, can only pull in the costal margin, reducing the lower thoracic diameters.

not essential for survival; adequate ventilation is possible even when the diaphragm is completely paralyzed. It is estimated that in the normal adult, each centimeter of vertical movement moves 350 ml of air; thus an excursion of 1.5 cm would effect a tidal volume of 525 ml. This figure does not include the additional increase in thoracic volume from expansion of the lower thorax, which of course would increase the tidal volume.

Affected by paralysis, the diaphragm (either or both leaves) tends to stay at the normal level at rest. During deep inhalation, however, it *rises* as other ventilatory muscles or one normal hemidiaphragm produce a fall in intrathoracic pressure. In quiet breathing the paralyzed leaf may remain immobile or move in either direction. The inspiratory balance of pressure above and below the diaphragm tends to make the paralyzed leaf rise, whereas outward movement of the lower ribs tends to stretch and flatten it, and its final course is the result of these two forces.

Finally, the diaphragm performs important functions other than ventilation. Because it is able to aid in generating high intraabdominal pressure by remaining fixed while the abdominal muscles contract, the diaphragm greatly facilitates defecation, vomiting, coughing and sneezing, and parturition.

Intercostal muscles   The intercostals, the second of the major ventilatory muscles, consist of two sets of muscles filling the gaps between the ribs; they are designated *external* and *internal* (Fig. 4-5):

1. The *external intercostal muscles* arise from the inferior edge of each rib

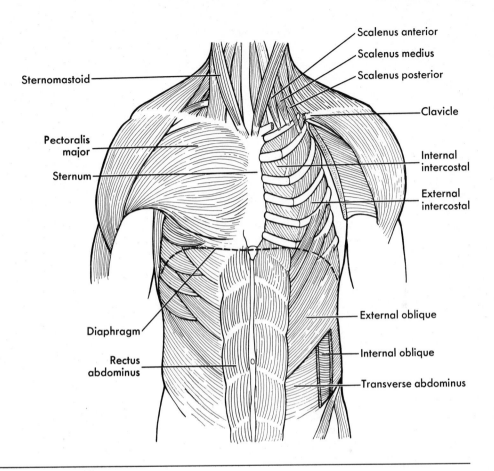

Fig. 4-5   The muscles of ventilation. (See text for description.)

from the rib tubercle to its costochondral junction. The fibers pass inferiorly and anteriorly to insert into the superior edge of the rib below. These muscles are thicker posteriorly than anteriorly and are thicker than the internal intercostals.

2. The *internal intercostal muscles* are located beneath the external intercostals and arise from the inferior edge of each rib from the anterior end of the intercostal space to the rib angles. The fibers pass inferiorly and posteriorly to insert into the superior edge of the rib below. This muscle group is divided into two functional parts:

   a. The *interosseous* portion is located between the sloping parts of the ribs.

   b. The *intercartilaginous* portion is located where the costal cartilages slope superiorly and anteriorly.

Although there is considerable controversy as to the exact mechanism by which the intercostal muscles function, it is well established that by contraction they elevate the ribs, thereby increasing the inspiratory chest volume. This function has been documented by noting its absence during paralysis of muscles. In addition, the muscles solidify and stabilize the chest wall and prevent intercostal bulging or retraction during intrathoracic pressure changes. It is believed that most of the ventilatory effect of the intercostals is produced by the external intercostals and the intercartilaginous portion of the internal intercostals. These muscles contract during inhalation and maintain contraction into early exhalation, by this action elevating the ribs. In the presence of flows up to 40 ℓ/min, the intercostals are quiet during most of exhalation. However, with flows in excess of 50 ℓ/min, the intercostals of the lower spaces contract toward the end of exhalation and also do the same during voluntary maximum exhalation. This action probably gives stability to the chest in the presence of powerful abdominal contraction. As noted above, intercostal contraction continues into early exhalation during quiet breathing, but it then fades as expiratory airflow rises to its maximum. This is not a true exhalation act of the intercostals, for if it were, the peak expiratory airflow would occur at once while lung recoil was also maximal. It is believed that this function of the intercostals is to retard airflow during early exhalation and to facilitate a smoother and less turbulent exhalation. Finally, it appears that contraction of the interosseous portion of the internal intercostals *depresses* the ribs; but the exact role they play in normal ventilation is not clear.

Scalene muscles

The *anterior, medial,* and *posterior* scalene muscles, although individual structures, are considered as a functional unit. Primarily skeletal muscles of the neck, they are also *accessory muscles of ventilation* and play an important role in breathing. The scalenes arise from the transverse processes of the lower five cervical vertebrae and insert into the upper surface of the first rib (anterior and medial scalenes) and the second rib (posterior scalene).

Although the scalenes give support to the neck, we are interested in their ventilatory action. Basically, they elevate and fix firmly the first and second ribs. Their most important function is to aid inhalation under conditions of stress when the diaphragm and intercostal muscles are inadequate to fulfill respiratory needs; this may occur in normal subjects undergoing severe exertion or in patients with pulmonary disease. In a normal subject *static* inspiratory efforts (against a closed glottis or other obstruction, with no movement of air) bring the scalenes into play as intraalveolar pressure drops; and when this pressure reaches -10 cm H_2O, scalenes are active in all subjects. During expiratory efforts the scalene muscles are inactive until intraalveolar pressure reaches 40 cm H_2O, at which point they contract. It is thought that the expiratory function of the scalene muscles is to fix the ribs against the contraction of the abdominal muscles and to prevent herniation of the apex of the lung during coughing.

Sternomastoid muscle

The sternomastoid, designed to rotate the head and support it, is another accessory ventilatory muscle of importance (Fig. 4-5). It arises by two heads from the manubrium of the sternum and the medial end of the clavicle. The heads fuse into a single body that courses superiorly and slightly posteriorly to insert into the mastoid process and occipital bone of the skull. This muscle is usually prominent on each side of the neck of subjects and is especially noticeable with rotary movements of the head.

When functioning to mobilize the head, the sternomastoid pulls from its sternoclavicular origin, rotating the head to the opposite side and turning it slightly upward. However, when the subject fixes the head and neck with other skeletal muscles, the sternomastoid, as a ventilatory muscle, pulls from its skull insertions and elevates the sternum, increasing the A-P diameter of the chest. In all subjects it contracts when intraalveolar pressures reach -10 cm H_2O but has no action during exhalation. In the supine position during normal free breathing, most subjects can attain a volume of 2.5 ℓ and a flow of 60 ℓ/min without use of the sternomastoids. An interesting discrepancy should be noted. During natural, free breathing, normal subjects can move about 2.5 ℓ of air at intraalveolar pressures varying from -25 to -50 cm H_2O with the diaphragm and intercostals alone, and yet under static conditions an intraalveolar pressure of -10 cm H_2O brings the sternomastoid into play. This is not clearly understood.

In chronic pulmonary disease the sternomastoid becomes active in inhalation when the thorax becomes so inflated (elevated resting level) that the low diaphragm loses its efficiency. As the sternomastoids contract and pull up on the sternum, the ribs rotate about their neck axes but not about the rib angle–sternal junction axes. This produces an up-and-down motion with little side expansion. In extreme cases A-P expansion of the thorax may cause the lower ribs to become indrawn, partially negating the increase in chest volume.

Pectoralis major muscle

The third most important accessory ventilatory muscle, the pectoralis major, is a powerful bilateral anterior chest muscle with the primary function of pulling the upper arms into the body in a hugging motion (Fig. 4-5). It is a large, fan-shaped muscle arising from the medial half of the clavicle, the anterior surface of the sternum and the first six costal cartilages, and a fibrous sheath enclosing muscles of the abdominal wall. The muscle fibers converge into a thick tendon that inserts into the upper part of the humerus. The pectoralis major forms the anterior fold of the axilla, and in a muscular individual its outlines are plainly visible beneath the skin.

Like the other accessory ventilatory muscles, the pectoralis pulls in a direction opposite to that of its primary function. If the arms and shoulders are fixed, as by leaning on the elbows or firmly grasping a table, the pectoralis muscle can use its insertion as an origin and pull with great force on the anterior chest, lifting up ribs and sternum and increasing thoracic A-P diameter. The respiratory therapist soon becomes accustomed to seeing patients with chronic pulmonary disease assume characteristic poses for maximum use of the pectoralis. In advanced cases most of the air moved may be the result of the action of this powerful muscle. It aids inhalation only, taking no part in exhalation.

Abdominal muscles

Several muscles make up the abdominal wall, with the obvious purpose of providing support and safety to the abdominal contents (Fig. 4-5). Some of them, however, play an indirect but important role in ventilation and can thus be considered as accessory ventilatory muscles. Four of these will be briefly identified:

1. The *external oblique* arises from the lower eight ribs; posterior fibers insert into the iliac crest, and the rest course obliquely down and forward to insert into a fibrous sheath (aponeurosis) with their counterparts from the other side; the lower edge forms the inguinal ligament in the groin.

2. The *internal oblique* arises from the iliac crest and the inguinal ligament; posterior fibers pass upward to insert into the last three ribs; the rest slope upward and forward to a fibrous aponeurosis.

3. The *transverse abdominal* arises from the costal cartilages of the lower ribs, iliac crest, and lateral part of the inguinal ligament; it passes horizontally forward to an aponeurosis.

4. The *abdominal rectus* arises from the pubic bones, passes upward in a sheath formed by the aponeuroses described above, and inserts into costal cartilages 5 to 7; it is often well defined in a muscular individual.

The abdominals are expiratory muscles with two important actions—to increase intraabdominal pressure and to draw the lower ribs down and medially. In the relaxed supine position the abdominals are inactive during quiet breathing; and they are often inactive in the erect position. With increasing ventilation, they come into play when the expiratory flow reaches 40 ℓ/min. At this level of gas velocity or in the presence of significant resistance to exhalation, or if exhalation is required beyond the preinspiratory resting level (as in inflating a balloon), the elastic recoil of the thorax does not have adequate force to remove enough air in the allotted time. In such circumstances, contraction of the powerful abdominals builds up strong intraabdominal pressure and drives the diaphragm, like a piston, into exhalation. Contraction of these muscles also occurs at the end of voluntary maximum *inhalation* and is a factor limiting the extent of inhalation. In chronic pulmonary disease, especially in the presence of airway obstruction, effective use of the abdominals is often lost, and without these powerful generators of force to push the diaphragm into expiratory action, the patient is at a great disadvantage.

Summary of ventilatory muscle action

Other muscles play varying roles in assisting ventilation and thus can qualify as accessory ventilatory muscles. Most of them are concerned with stabilizing the body to provide better leverage for muscles directly concerned with air movement. However, if the therapist thoroughly understands the function of the muscles just described, he or she will have an adequate foundation for learning some of the therapeutic techniques discussed later. In summary, the function of the ventilatory muscles may be outlined as follows:

1. *Quiet ventilation*
   a. Inspiration
      (1) Diaphragm in all subjects

        (2) Intercostals in most subjects

        (3) Scalenes in some subjects

    b. Expiration—some persistence of contraction of inspiratory muscles early in expiration

2. *Moderately increased ventilation*

    a. For flows up to 50 ℓ/min, same as above

    b. For flows between 50 and 100 ℓ/min, sternomastoid action toward end of inspiration; increased abdominals and intercostals toward end of expiration

3. *Greatly increased ventilation*—above 100 ℓ/min, all inspiratory accessories active, and abdominals active throughout expiration

---

Lung-thorax relationship

Effective ventilation depends on cooperative but reciprocal action between the lung and the thorax, a relationship crudely illustrated by the balloon-in-a-box model in Fig. 4-6, the box represents the thorax, and the balloon the lungs. A review of anatomy will recall that, between the pleura-lined thoracic wall and the pleura-covered lung, there exists the *pleural* or *intrapleural space*. Although in the living subject the approximation of the two pleural surfaces, separated by only a thin film of moisture, makes the space more potential than real, it plays an important role in ventilation. Therefore, for purposes of illustration it is depicted in sketches as a true space.

    The resting level (or resting position of the chest) is the configuration that is assumed at the end of a quiet effortless exhalation and is often referred to as the *end-expiratory position*. In Fig 4-6, *A,* the relations of the lung and thorax are shown at the resting level. The airtight thoracic box encloses a small partial vacuum of about -4 cm H_2O (indicated by the attached manometer), which is maintained by opposing elasticity of the lungs and thorax. This is described

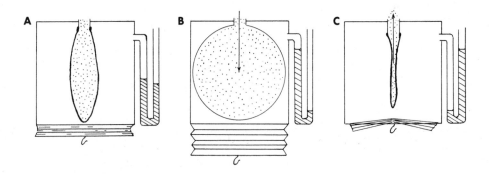

Fig. 4-6   Balloon-in-a-box model of the lung-thorax. **A,** In the resting position, a small negative pressure in the box keeps the balloon slightly distended with air. **B,** As the box expands by dropping its floor, its cavity becomes more negative, and air flows into the balloon. **C,** If the floor of the box is pushed higher than its usual resting level, positive pressure develops in the box, expressing additional air from the balloon but not emptying it.

in more detail below. The pulmonary balloon is suspended in the box, and because it is exposed to and in equilibrium with atmospheric pressure, the surrounding subatmospheric intrathoracic pressure keeps it partially filled with air. Thus at the end of exhalation a considerable amount of air remains in the lungs. The inspiratory flow of air into the lung is brought about by enlargement of the thoracic box through the effort of ventilatory muscles.

Fig 4-6, *B*, shows the accordionlike bottom of the box dropping, enlarging the volume of the box, and simulating the action of the diaphragm. The living thorax, a flexible structure, also expands laterally as muscles act on the ribs. Intrathoracic pressure drops further with the increased volume of the sealed container, the pressure drop is transmitted into the balloon across its flexible wall, intraballoon (intraalveolar) pressure momentarily becomes subatmospheric, and air flows into it. This difference between the higher atmospheric and lower alveolar pressures is called a *pressure gradient* (ΔP). It is a "head of pressure" that allows fluid to flow from the high end of the gradient to the low. The concept of gradients is of great importance in cardiopulmonary physiology and is extensively used later in this text.

During quiet inhalation, intrapleural pressure drops only to about -6 cm H_2O, but a strong inspiratory effort against an obstruction, such as a closed glottis, can drop the pressure to -50 cm H_2O. Exhalation is a passive recoil of the elastic stretch of the lung balloon, made possible by a relaxation of the muscular forces acting on the thoracic box. Air flows from the lung until the resting level is reached to terminate the cycle. Exhalation can be continued below the resting level by bringing into play positive expiratory muscular forces. Principally, this invokes strong contractions of the abdominal muscles to force the diaphragm into the thorax, as illustrated in Fig. 4-6, *C*. With this maneuver the resting negative intrathoracic pressure is replaced by a positive pressure that, against strong resistance, may reach 70 cm H_2O.[4] Although more air is forced from the lungs, they can never be completely emptied.

We have described, in general terms, the basic factors responsible for airflow into and out of the lungs and now consider some of the forces that both initiate and limit air movement. As referred to previously, the ventilatory cycle is the net sum of the action of the opposing forces of the chest and lung, and we now use a different model to illustrate these points, emphasizing that we are not talking about another subject but viewing the same from a slightly different angle.

The thorax (which in our context includes the diaphragm) consists of flexible ribs and muscles; through the intrinsic elastic forces of its tissues, it tends to expand and enlarge, much as a bent bow is under stress to spring straight. Counteracting these chest forces are forces of the lung, whose elastic tissues are stretched and tend to contract and shrink. To understand how these two systems of elastic energy relate to one another, consider the lung-thorax complex as consisting of one set of *bowed flat* springs (thorax) exerting an expansile force tied to a *stretched coiled* spring (lungs) exerting a contractile force, each holding the other in check (Fig. 4-7). Expansion and contraction of the coiled

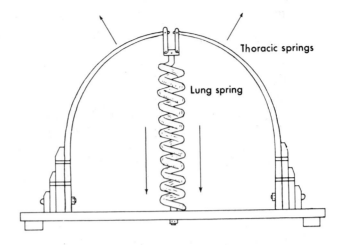

Fig. 4-7   The counteracting forces of the lungs and thorax are schematically represented by two sets of springs. In the resting position, the bowed flat *thoracic springs* are shown as held under bent tension by the coiled *lung spring,* itself partially stretched by the action. *Arrows* indicate the direction each spring tends to move to reach its own position of rest. From the lung-thorax resting position, the thorax can expand or contract, depending on the action of the ventilatory muscles. These muscles can assist the *thoracic springs* to overcome the restraint of the *lung spring,* or they can compress the *thoracic springs* and assist the recoil of the *lung spring.*

spring represent increase and decrease, respectively, in lung volume. At the resting level the chest and lung forces are equal in opposite directions, momentarily in perfect balance, as each prevents the other from following its natural inclination. Although we refer to this brief static period as "resting," it must not be thought that expenditure of energy is wanting, any more than a temporary stalemate in a rope-pull contest can be considered free of physical activity. Indeed, in the airtight balloon-in-a-box structure of the lung-thorax, at the resting position each force is pulling against the other with power equal to that exerted by a 4-cm column of water, developing in the intervening intrapleural "space" a partial vacuum of the same magnitude. This intrapleural subatmospheric pressure holds together the coiled lung spring and the flat, bowed thoracic springs, as the barrel and plunger of a capped syringe are held together by the subatmospheric pressure developing in the syringe barrel in response to attempts to separate the parts.

Inhalation can occur only when the resting level balance between the forces of the lung and thorax is broken by the addition of muscular energy to the elasticity of the thorax. In addition to the effect of diaphragmatic contraction on chest expansion, the intercostal and accessory ventilatory muscles, in a sense, take hold of the bowed "flat springs" of Fig. 4-7 and pull them outward to help them overcome the "coiled spring" of the lung. The depth of inspiration is determined by the amount of chest force applied to overcome lung stretch, and this effort, in turn, is regulated by the mechanism of ventilatory control already discussed. At the end-inspoiratory level necessary to satisfy immediate body gas needs, airflow stops and the chest and lung forces are again in momentary balance. At this point the muscles activating the thorax relax, and the elasticity of the stretched lung, along with the increased intraabdominal pressure, passively returns the lung-thorax system to the resting level. Exhalation against resistance such as obstructive airway disease, in which pulmonary passive recoil lacks the force to move air at a suitable rate, or exhalation below the resting level (Fig. 4-6, *C*), principally uses the abdominal muscles to generate the power necessary to deflate the lung. We can visualize this effort as a force bowing the flat springs of Fig. 4-7. Against obstruction this active expiratory force helps the coiled spring to return the expanded thorax to the resting position. To expel air below the resting level, this force helps the coiled spring to flex the increasing resistance of the flat springs.

Lung volumes   This is an advantageous point at which to introduce the subject of lung volumes, since they depend on the lung-thorax relationship. (The next chapter discusses these more completely.) Fig. 4-8 illustrates the volumetric divisions of the total capacity of the lung; a designated capacity consists of two or more volumes. The *lower dashed line* identifies the end-expiratory resting level, and the *upper line,* the *tidal volume* end-inspiration. Because the chest forces limit collapse of the lung at the end-expiratory resting level, air remains in the lung at this point and is called the *functional residual capacity* (FRC). Forced exhalation, as described previously, can remove air below the resting level by "dipping into" the FRC. This extra air, so expelled, is the *expiratory reserve volume* (ERV). Even after the most strenuous expiratory effort, air still remains in the lung and cannot be removed voluntarily; this is known as the *residual volume* (RV). Thus the FRC is the sum of the ERV and the RV.

If a subject inhales *maximally* from the resting level, then exhales *maximally,* he or she will move a quantity of air known as the *vital capacity* (VC), so called because all the ventilation is within its limits. The VC consists of three volumes: the ERV, the V_T, and the *inspiratory reserve volume* (IRV). The last represents the available expansion of the lung-thorax, beyond resting needs, for exertion or any other demand for deep breathing. The *inspiratory capacity* (IC) measures the total inhalation potential from the resting level. Finally, the sum of the VC and the RV comprises the *total lung capacity* (TLC). All these values can be measured in the cardiopulmonary laboratory by direct or indirect methods (see Chapter 5).

In Fig. 4-7, if we separate the sets of springs, it is apparent that each set will follow its natural tendency—the thoracic flat springs will spring outward, and the lung coiled spring will contract. The same phenomenon will occur if we break the vacuum-sealed intrapleural space, letting it equilibrate with the atmosphere. If the thorax (either side or both) is opened, it will actually ex-

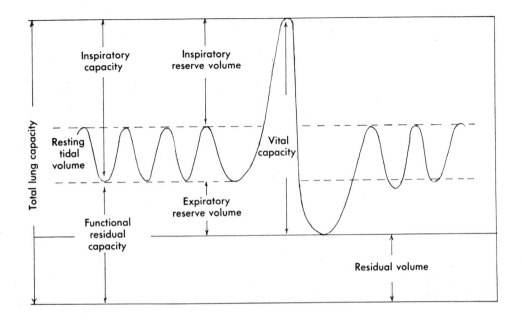

Fig. 4-8   Lung capacities and volumes. Volumetric divisions of the total gas capacity of the lungs. A capacity consists of two or more volumes. (See text for description.)

pand to a larger volume and assume its own *thoracic resting position*. At the same time the lung, freed from its suction adherence to the thoracic wall, will collapse to a smaller volume than the RV of the intact system; but even when exposed to atmospheric pressure, the lung does not become completely airless and still contains a small amount of air called *minimal air*. Fig. 4-9 illustrates the effect of breaking the seal between thorax and lung. In *A,* the lung-thorax is at the resting level, where the lung contains the FRC. *B* depicts the results of equilibrating the intrathoracic space with atmospheric pressure by opening the intact thorax. The lung collapses to its smallest size, the minimal air volume, whereas the thorax enlarges to its unopposed thoracic resting position. *C* is a plot of the *TLC* against *A* and *B,* breaking the *VC* into increments of 20% each. The normal lung-thorax resting position is seen to be at approximately 30% of the *VC,* whereas with disruption of the system the *minimal air* level of the lung is about 40% of the *RV* and the thorax expands to its resting level of some 50% of the *VC.*

Finally, aiding the synchronous movement of lung and thorax is the force of *pleural traction*. In the normal intact lung-thorax complex, both visceral and parietal pleura are in contact during the entire breathing cycle, separated only by the thin film of fluid covering the pleural surfaces. The cohesive force of this fluid layer, working with the intraalveolar pressure gradient, helps to hold together the pleural surfaces so that, as the thorax expands and contracts, the

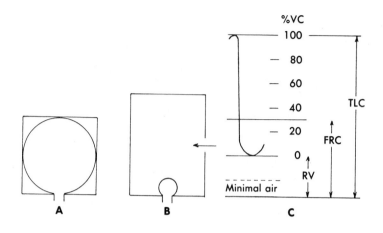

Fig. 4-9   The resting levels of the intact lung-thorax and the separated lung and thorax are plotted against the total lung capacity. **A,** The intact system at its resting level contains the *FRC* and is expanded to about 30% of the *VC*. **B,** The arrow indicates a break in the thoracic wall, exposing the lung to atmosphere and destroying the lung-thorax seal. The lung, containing the *minimal air,* collapses to a new resting level, which is about 40% of the *RV,* and the thorax expands to its own unopposed level of about 50% of the *VC.*

lung accompanies it smoothly. In a sense the lung is partially "dragged" into inflation by the thorax and is held firmly against the inner thoracic wall during exhalation.

Surface tension and ventilation

So far, the collapsing tendency of the lung springs has been attributed only to the elastic fibers in its structure. Augmenting this elastic recoil, however, is another factor that has assumed clinical importance—*surface tension* (ST); a brief review of the principles of surface tension will aid in understanding its role in ventilation.[5-7]

Surface tension may be defined as the force exerted by molecules moving away from the surface and toward the center of a liquid, tending to make a sphere or a curved surface smaller. It occurs at an *interface* or junction between two substances, such as liquid and air, and is best illustrated in a relatively small drop of fluid. Molecules in the mass of a liquid are subjected to physical forces of mutual attraction and are so balanced that they can freely move in all directions. Those molecules on the surface, however, can be attracted only inwardly by their fellow molecules, and the pressure they exert is like to an elastic film tending to contract into a sphere. Fig. 4-10 illustrates the force of mass attraction between liquid molecules. Those molecules at the fluid-air interface have no molecules distally to attract them but are pulled only centrally. This tension over the surface of a drop of liquid keeps it intact in a spherical shape while falling in space or resting on a surface.

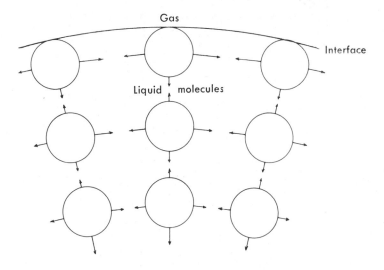

Fig. 4-10   The force of surface tension in a drop of liquid is shown by the action of its fluid molecules. Those molecules within the substance of the drop are mutually attracted to one another *(arrows)* and can move about randomly in a state of balance. Mass attraction can pull the molecules of the outermost layer inward only, creating a centrally directed force, called surface tension, which tends to contract the liquid into a sphere. Pressure within the drop is raised above atmospheric and is expressed by the formula of LaPlace, described in text.

Table 4-2
Examples of
surface tension

Substance	°C	ST in dynes/cm
Water	20	73
Water	37	70
Tissue fluid	37	50
Whole blood	37	58
Plasma	37	73
Ethyl alcohol	20	22
Mercury	17	547

Surface tension is measured in *dynes per linear centimeter across the surface* and may be visualized as the force (in dynes) necessary to produce a tear 1 cm long in the surface layer of a liquid, if one could grasp the surface in the hands and stretch it like a thin rubber sheet until it split.[5] ST is a demonstrable phenomenon that permits an insect to walk on the surface of a pond and enables a needle to float in a glass of water. Surface tensions vary widely among substances and for the same substance vary inversely with temperature. Table 4-2 lists some examples of surface tension values.

The force of ST, like a fist compressing a ball, produces an increase in pressure within a drop of liquid above the ambient. Thus a pressure gradient, or difference in pressure (ΔP), exists across the surface of the drop. The pressure within the drop, dependent on the specific ST and the radius of the drop, is expressed by the formula of LaPlace as:

$$P = \frac{2\ ST}{r}$$

where ST is in dynes/cm, r is the radius in centimeters, and P is in dynes/cm^2. Given a drop with a radius of 2 mm and a ST of 60 dynes/cm, calculate the pressure inside the drop:

$$P = \frac{2 \times 60}{0.2\ cm} = \frac{120}{0.2} = 600\ \text{dynes/cm}^2$$

or

$$P = \frac{600\ \text{dynes/cm}^2}{980} = 6.13 \times 10^{-1}\ \text{g/cm}^2$$

or

$$P = Ht \times D$$
$$\therefore Ht = \frac{P}{D} = \frac{6.13 \times 10^-}{1} = 6.13 \times 10^{-1}\ \text{cm H}_2\text{O}$$

The principle regulating internal pressure of a drop applies equally to a gas bubble in a liquid mass. The gas in the bubble is subject to the same pressure as the center of a drop of the same radius if the substance of the drop has the same ST as the liquid surrounding the bubble. It makes no difference if fluid is surrounded by gas, or gas by fluid; if there is only a single interface, the same radius, and the same ST, the internal compression forces are the same.

For purposes of description the effect of ST on an isolated bubble, can be considered as a spherical volume of gas enclosed in a thin film of fluid. Fig. 4-11 shows that thin though it is, the film contains a finite amount of liquid and

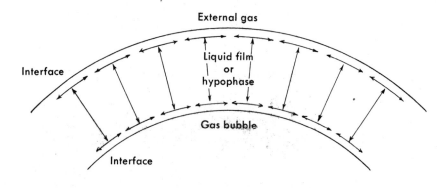

Fig. 4-11   A bubble is a volume of gas enclosed by a thin film of fluid, which has two surfaces. Thus, the forces of surface tension on both surfaces produce a pressure within the bubble twice that in a liquid drop of the same substance and radius.

is called the *hypophase*. Because ST is found only at an interface, and the bubble wall has two gas-fluid interfaces at its two surfaces, the compression force of ST on the enclosed gas is *twice* that exerted by a spherical drop of the same size and substance. Thus the STs of the two surfaces act together to compress the gas bubble. The pressure gradient across a bubble wall can also be expressed by LaPlace's law, with a modification:

$$P = \frac{4\ ST}{r}$$

where *ST* is the surface tension of the liquid in which the bubble is immersed and *r* is the radius of the bubble in centimeters. It is apparent that if the example in the preceding paragraph were a bubble instead of a drop, the pressure would be double the calculated value.

Thus, for a given liquid the *smaller* the drop or bubble, the *greater* the pressure from surface tension. When inflating a balloon, we must use maximum force to *start* inflation, to overcome the initial resistance, then progressively less, up to the capacity of the balloon. Similarly, it would require more pressure to inflate a small bubble than a large one because of the increased pressure of ST in the former. Fig. 4-12 illustrates changes in pressure in an isolated bubble accompanying changes in size and in ST. As the size of the bubble increases from *A* to *B*, the pressure drops, according to LaPlace's law.

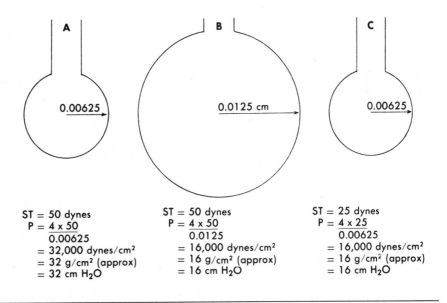

ST = 50 dynes	ST = 50 dynes	ST = 25 dynes
$P = \dfrac{4 \times 50}{0.00625}$	$P = \dfrac{4 \times 50}{0.0125}$	$P = \dfrac{4 \times 25}{0.00625}$
= 32,000 dynes/cm^2	= 16,000 dynes/cm^2	= 16,000 dynes/cm^2
= 32 g/cm^2 (approx)	= 16 g/cm^2 (approx)	= 16 g/cm^2 (approx)
= 32 cm H$_2$O	= 16 cm H$_2$O	= 16 cm H$_2$O

Fig. 4-12   The internal pressure of a single bubble varies with the size of the bubble and the surface tension of its liquid film. An increase in radius from **A** to **B** drops the pressure, but **C** shows that the same pressure drop can accompany a reduction in surface tension, without changing bubble size.

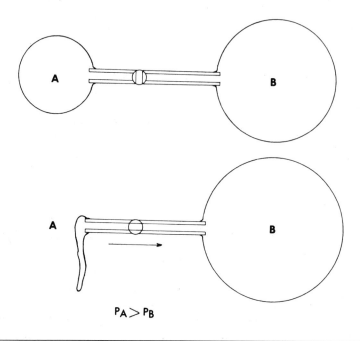

$$P_A > P_B$$

Fig. 4-13   When two bubbles of different sizes, **A** and **B**, but with the same surface tension, are allowed to communicate, the greater pressure in the smaller causes it to empty into the larger.

The bubble at *C* demonstrates that the pressure can remain unchanged if the ST is somehow lowered. Or, viewed differently, Fig. 4-13 shows that if two bubbles of different sizes are allowed to communicate, the smaller will empty into the larger because of the greater pressure in the former.

Bubbles massed together as a foam behave differently than when individually isolated.[8] Fig. 4-14 shows that bubbles in clumps lose their outer air-fluid surfaces and retain only single interfaces, resembling bubbles in a volume of liquid. As a consequence, the internal pressure in grouped bubbles is related to twice the surface tension (2 ST) of the surrounding liquid rather than four time (4 ST), as described previously for single bubbles.

The ability to alter surface tension is a physical phenomenon of great importance to pulmonary physiology, and we now discuss the principle involved before relating it to function. Certain substances can lower ST on contact with fluid surfaces and are called *surfactants*. Soaps and detergents are the most common examples. These agents weaken the molecular bonds at the surface, thus reducing the surface tension and lowering intrabubble pressure. Fig. 4-12, *C,* illustrates this effect. An air bubble in water shrinks and finally disappears under the stress of ST pressure as the pressure hastens the diffusion of air out of the bubble, but the addition of soap to the water, by lowering ST, prolongs or stabilizes the bubble. On the other hand, a surfactant such as a

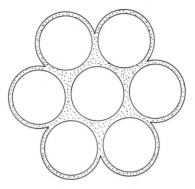

Fig. 4-14 The bubble in the center of the sketch illustrates that while an isolated bubble suspended in air can have two air-fluid interfaces, when it is clumped in a mass of foam, it retains only its inner interface. (See text for the significance of this.)

detergent, by reducing ST, disrupts and disperses small drops of water, making the water "wetter" and increasing its ability to penetrate deeper into fabrics and minute crevices for better removal of dirt.

Let us recall the microscopic structure of the lung, with its millions of alveoli, each one of which is in intimate contact with a thin film of intercellular fluid, and let us view it as a mass of tiny bubbles almost like a foam in interstitial fluid. It is easy now to imagine each of these "alveolar bubbles" as being subjected to forces of tissue fluid surface tension; and indeed, experimental and clinical evidence indicates that ST is an important factor in the mechanics of ventilation. The passive exhalation recoil of the "lung springs" to the resting position is a result of alveolar ST acting with the elastic fibers of the lung. The effect of lung ST is to produce alveolar collapse, and reinflation by inhalation against the ST pressure would be very difficult were it not for the presence of a natural surfactant in the alveoli.

Pulmonary surfactant exists as a single molecule-thick film lining the alveolar walls. Chemically, it is a phospholipid, composed of fatty acids bound to lecithin, and it functions in a most remarkable fashion. Apparently there is a fixed amount of surfactant in each alveolus, and its ability to lower ST depends on a quantitative ratio between it and alveolar surface area. At the ventilatory resting level, because the alveoli are partially deflated, there is a relatively large amount of surfactant in relation to alveolar surface area. Surface tension is lowered, intrapulmonary pressure is lowered, and the alveoli can be easily inflated. As the alveoli distend with inhaled air, their stretched walls present an increasing surface area, the surfactant film becomes stretched and thinned, the ratio of surfactant to surface area falls, and the effect of surfactant decreases. During alveolar distention, the contractile force of ST gradually increases, and at end-inspiration, when muscular inspiratory effort ceases, the combination of

ST and lung elasticity deflates the alveoli to their resting functional residual capacity, completing the breathing cycle. The "half-life" of surfactant is measured in hours (the length of time it takes for half a given mass to disappear in the metabolic process of deterioration), and if its natural replacement is impaired or it is pathologically destroyed faster than it can be replaced, alveolar collapse (atelectasis) rapidly develops.[9] Were it not for the action of pulmonary surfactant, inflating partially collapsed alveoli would require great physical effort, and inhalation would be seriously handicapped. Indeed, in disease states characterized by absence of surfactant, the work of breathing is at times insurmountable. Finally, since at any given time all alveoli are not necessarily identical in size, smaller alveoli tend to empty into larger neighboring alveoli, in accordance with the principle illustrated in Fig. 4-13. This serious interference with even distribution of ventilation is prevented by surfactant which through its varying ratio to surface area, maintains uniform pressure within all alveoli, regardless of size.

Exercise 4-1: Calculate the following:
A. At the resting level, if lung ST is 30 dynes/cm, how many centimeters of water pressure are needed to start inflation of an alveolus with a diameter of 90μ?
B. With a ST of 70 dynes/cm, what is the diameter of a bubble of foam that can be maintained by an inflating pressure of 9 mm Hg?

Elastic resistance to ventilation and measurement of compliance

When discussing the "springs" of the lung and thorax, we described the characteristic of *elasticity,* whereby an object that is stretched by a force tends to recoil to its original shape or position on release of the force. The elasticity of the lung-thorax presents a resistance that must be overcome during inhalation, a resistance that often increases in disease.

A measurement of elasticity, called *compliance,* can be made to evaluate the work of breathing; it gives an estimate of the "stiffness" of the lungs and thorax. Compliance is defined as the *volume change in the lung per unit of pressure change,* and its units are liter per centimeter of water. Measurements must be made under *static* conditions, or at points of *no airflow,* to eliminate other factors such as airflow resistance. As the lungs *lose* their elasticity and become less compliant, or stiffer, the value of this ratio decreases. For a simple analogy, if a balloon contained 1 ℓ of air under a pressure of 15 cm H_2O and it expanded to 1.5 ℓ after the pressure was raised to 20 cm H_2O, its compliance equals $\Delta V \div \Delta P$, or 0.5 ÷ 5, or 0.1 ℓ/cm H_2O.

The pressure-volume relationship of a simple spring is illustrated in Fig. 4-15, where there is a linear response of spring distance to force, up to the limit of stretch. The human ventilatory system, however, is composed of two sets of springs as previously illustrated in Fig. 4-7, and the lung-thorax compliance is obviously the net result of each. Thus ventilatory compliance can be consid-

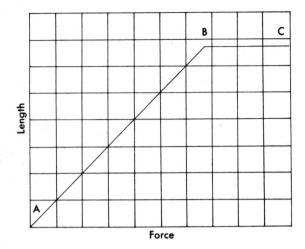

Fig. 4-15   The graph demonstrates compliance of a simple spring (increase in length/increase in force). With increasing force, the spring lengthens in a linear manner, from *A* to *B*, but at the point of maximum stretch further force produces no additional increase in length, *B* to *C*.

ered as a triad of total compliance of lung and thorax (C_{LT}), compliance of the lung alone (C_L), and compliance of the thorax alone (C_T). Compliance of the lung-thorax is *less* than that of either lung or thorax alone; and the student who is acquainted with electrical terminology will recognize that the relationship between total compliance and its two constituents is expressed in the same inverse manner as electrical resistors in parallel:

$$\frac{1}{C_{LT}} = \frac{1}{C_L} + \frac{1^{10}}{C_T}$$

Lung-thorax compliance. Lung-thorax compliance (C_{LT}) can be measured in one of three general ways: (1) The subject, completely relaxed voluntarily or from anesthesia or disease, is placed in a body respirator with head outside at ambient pressure, and ventilation is controlled by the application of negative pressure to the surface of the body (Fig. 4-16). With the subject exhaling into a measuring device such as a spirometer and by varying the negative pressure and correlating this with the volume of air moved, the flexibility of the combined lungs and thorax in terms of liters of air moved per centimeter H_2O pressure exerted can be calculated.[10] (2) A cuffed endotracheal tube placed in an anesthetized subject allows ventilation of the lungs at various delivered *positive* pressures. These values, with their corresponding tidal volumes measured in a spirometer, provide compliance data. Normal C_{LT} by both these methods is about *0.1 ℓ/cm H_2O.* (3) A slightly different technique is the construction of a *relaxation-pressure curve.*[11] With a small pressure-transmitting plastic tube

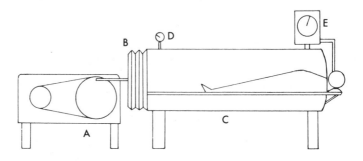

Fig. 4-16   This is a schematic representation of a subject in a body respirator. The motor, *A,* operates bellows, *B,* to create a rhythmic subatmospheric pressure in the cylindrical respirator, *C,* which is recorded by gauge, *D.* As the subject is ventilated by negative pressure applied to his or her body, exhaled air is collected and measured in a meter, *E.* Volume change of the lung-thorax per unit of pressure applied can be determined.

attached to a recording device and placed in his or her nose, the subject inhales a measured amount of air from a spirometer. Then, with tightly closed nose and mouth, the subject relaxes the ventilatory muscles, and the elastic recoil of lung and thorax produces an alveolar pressure recorded by the nasal tube. Repeated at different tidal volume levels, a curve is produced. Compliance by this method is a bit higher than by the above two methods, about *0.12 ℓ/cm* H_2O. Whether the ventilatory pressure is positive or negative makes no difference; for compliance depends on the *absolute* pressure change for each volume change.

Pulmonary compliance. Pulmonary compliance (C_L) is calculated by measuring the *intrapleural pressure* at different levels of end-inspiratory volumes and plotting a pressure-volume curve that is generally linear in the ranges used. Since it is hazardous to invade the pleural cavity, a balloon-tipped catheter is swallowed until the balloon is at a midchest position. The balloon is attached to a pressure-recording device, and the soft-walled esophagus readily transmits surrounding intrapleural pressure to the balloon. The subject inhales to several different levels from a volume recorder (spirometer), and at the peak of each tidal volume (momentarily a static state with no airflow), the corresponding pressure is noted. From these data, liters per centimeter of water can be calculated. An intraesophageal tube records negative intrapleural pressure of a spontaneously breathing subject, but the lungs of a relaxed unconscious or anesthetized subject can be inflated with a positive pressure and the same data obtained. Fig. 4-17 schematically represents the record of three breaths with their corresponding intraesophageal pressures, demonstrating a normal lung compliance of 0.2 ℓ/cm H_2O.

Thoracic compliance. Thoracic compliance (C_T) is determined indirectly by using the inverse relationship described above. If lung-thorax and lung

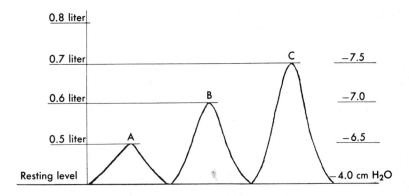

Fig. 4-17   From the resting level with an intrapleural pressure of -4 *cm* H_2O to the static end-inspiratory point A, 0.5 ℓ of air moves with a pressure change of 2.5 cm H_2O. The same p-v relationships exist at B and C. Compliance calculated between any two points is 0.2 ℓ/cm H_2O.

compliances are determined simultaneously, their values can be used to calculate C_T. Thus, if $C_{LT} = 0.1$ ℓ/cm H_2O, and $C_L = 0.2$ ℓ/cm H_2O, then:

$$\frac{1}{C_{LT}} = \frac{1}{C_L} + \frac{1}{C_T} \qquad \frac{1}{C_T} = \frac{1}{0.1} - \frac{1}{0.2}$$

$$\frac{1}{0.1} = \frac{1}{0.2} + \frac{1}{C_T} \qquad C_T = 0.2\ \ell\text{/cm H}_2\text{O}$$

Exercise 4-2: Calculate the thoracic compliance in the following example:

GIVEN: $C_{LT} = 0.072$ ℓ/cm H_2O
                     $C_L\ \ = 0.12$ ℓ/cm H_2O
CALCULATE: C_T

Nonelastic resistance to ventilation	The forces of ventilation must overcome not only elastic tissue tension but also the resistance offered by nonelastic tissue, such as muscle, cartilage, fat, abdominal contents, and the movement of large blood vessels and airways over one another. The inertia of these structures corresponds to the retarding effect of *friction* in any mobile system and modifies the ideal pressure-volume relationship previously described. The work involved in overcoming tissue friction can be illustrated simply as in Fig. 4-18, graphing the stretch of a spring hampered by friction. The uninhibited length response to increasing pressure without friction is recorded as a *dashed line* (similar to Fig. 4-15), whereas the response slowed by friction follows the *solid line*. The latter is curved, as a result of the drag of friction. Area *1* represents the amount of work done to overcome elasticity, and area *2* the additional work to overcome friction.[12]

Fig. 4-18 demonstrates another important characteristic of nonelastic resis-

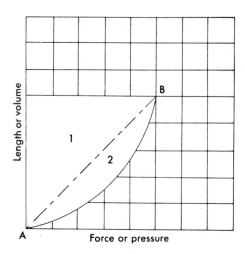

Fig. 4-18 Point *A* is the resting level, and *B* is end-inspiration. *Dashed A-B* represents the pressure-volume relationship of pure elastic resistance, and *curved A-B* the "drag" added by nonelastic friction. At *B*, where airflow momentarily ceases, nonelastic resistance is inactive because it is dependent on movement. The curved line thus disappears, leaving only the elastic resistance of stretch. Areas *1* and *2* represent the work of overcoming elastic nonelastic resistance, respectively.

tance. The tension of elasticity is *continuously* present, once force has been applied to a spring, whether the force is static or changing. In the lung-thorax, once distention has started, elasticity is present whether air is flowing or the lung is at a static breath-holding position. Nonelastic resistance is present *only* during movement, as when force is moving the spring or air if flowing in the lung, and is absent at static positions of no airflow. In Fig. 4-18, point *A* represents the resting position of no airflow and no distention of the lung; point *B* is the end-inspiratory pause with distention but no airflow. At *B*, therefore, only elastic resistance is active. The maximum effect of nonelastic resistance is noted where the two lines are most divergent, the period of greatest rate of airflow.

Airway resistance to ventilation

Flow of gas through airways always encounters resistance that varies with characteristics of the gas and the conducting passages. Resistance (R) is a ratio between the driving pressure responsible for gas movement and the flow of the gas, and it is measured in cm $H_2O/\ell/sec$. The pressure, in cm H_2O, is called the *transairway pressure*, or the *gradient* between the mouth (atmospheric) and the alveolar pressures. It produces the gas flow, which is calibrated in liters per second. During spontaneous inhalation, muscular energy lowers the intrathoracic and alveolar pressures, P_A, below atmospheric or mouth pressure, P_m, while during assisted breathing most ventilators drive gas under pressure into the airways so that P_m exceeds P_A. In either instance there is a pressure gradient from mouth to alveoli allowing airflow into the lung. Thus it makes no difference whether the gradient is positive or negative, since it is the absolute difference that moves air. The relationships between resistance, pressure gradient, and flow are shown in this equation:

$$R = \frac{P_m - P_A}{\dot{V}} = \frac{\Delta P}{\dot{V}}$$

This means that if the resistance remains constant, the *difference* in pressure (pressure drop) from mouth to alveoli will increase if flow is increased and will decrease if flow is decreased.

Let us consider an airway as a tube, the proximal end of which is connected to a gas pressure source (atmosphere, mechanical ventilator), and the distal end closed by a flexible balloon (alveolus). At the moment gas flow starts into the tube, there will be a maximum pressure gradient from mouth to alveoli ($P_m - P_A$) with gas in the tube exerting decreasing lateral pressure down its length, but once gas moves into the alveolus, intraluminal and alveolar pressures will increase, gradually reducing the gradient. When flow stops (end-inspiration), if there is *time,* lateral and alveolar pressures will equilibrate with mouth pressure because at this moment, with no gas flow, pressure will be maximum and uniform throughout the system. For the first time we are emphasizing the importance of time in ventilation, a factor that assumes major proportions in our later discussion of patient management.

The object of breathing, spontaneous or artificially supported, is to deliver a sufficient volume of air to the alveoli within an appropriate time period to satisfy body gas exchange needs. Thus emphasis is on gas volume per unit of time, or flow, and the pressure can be considered as a necessary adjunct to generate this flow. In the preceding equation, if we consider the resistance of a given tube to be constant, we can then look specifically at the critical relationship between pressure and flow. If flow is to be increased, for example, the $P_m - P_A$ difference must be widened, and this can be accomplished in one of two ways: (1) During spontaneous, unassisted breathing, P_m corresponds to atmospheric pressure and can be considered another constant. P_A thus becomes the variable pressure component that must be reduced to increase the gradient, and it is lowered by a more forceful inspiratory effort, generating a larger negative intrathoracic pressure. (2) When breathing is assisted by positive pressure applied to the airway, P_m is the variable factor, and it must be increased to widen the gradient. The obvious conclusion is that gas flow across a conducting system can only be increased or decreased by increasing or decreasing the driving pressure correspondingly. Thus $R = P/\dot{V}$.

The normal airway resistance ranges from *0.6 to 2.4 cm $H_2O/\ell/sec$,* measured at a standard flow rate of *0.5 ℓ/sec.* Suppose pulmonary disease so alters airways by partial obstruction that to overcome the resistance, strong inspiratory efforts are needed, dropping the alveolar pressure to lower values and widening the mouth-alveolar gradient. The following examples compare the data of such a condition with the normal and illustrate the increase in resistance that such a gradient implies:

$$\text{NORMAL: } R = \frac{\Delta P}{\dot{V}} = \frac{1}{0.5} = 2 \text{ cm } H_2O/\ell/\text{sec}$$

$$\text{ABNORMAL: } R = \frac{\Delta P}{\dot{V}} = \frac{5}{0.5} = 10 \text{ cm } H_2O/\ell/\text{sec}$$

Specialized laboratory equipment is available to supply the data needed to calculate airway resistance. Flows are measured with a sensitive apparatus called a *pneumotachograph,* which converts gas velocity into pressure and transmits this pressure to a calibrated recorder, either photographic or electronic, from which final measurements are made. Precise alveolar pressures are best determined by a *body plethysmograph,* an airtight box in which the subject sits or reclines. As the subject breathes, the pressure changes in the alveoli are reciprocated in the space about him or her in the box and relayed to a suitable recorder.

Airway resistance is the result of friction among molecules of flowing gas and between the molecules and the wall of the conducting tube. The two physical gas characteristics contributing to resistance are *density* and *viscosity.* The former has been adequately described earlier, and we now define and discuss the latter. Viscosity of a gas (or liquid) corresponds to friction of a moving solid and varies with individual gases, directly with temperature. The more viscous a gas, the more resistive it is to motion or change of form. It can be visualized as a time-related force exerted by a moving plane surface over a stationary plane surface, expressed in dyne-seconds per square centimeter. A frictional force of 1 dyne over an area of 1 cm^2 for a distance of 1 cm and a period of 1 second is called a *poise.* It should be apparent that viscosity of liquids is greater than that of gases, and the values for both are small enough that they are expressed as fractions of poises. Viscosity of liquids is usually recorded as *centipoises* (10^{-2} poises) and of gases as *micropoises* (10^{-6} poises). A few examples in Table 4-3 illustrate the ranges of these values.

Although the student is not expected to be familiar with the details of this aspect of gas physics, analysis of the formula by which gas viscosity is calculated will reveal some relationships of great importance to the respiratory therapist. *Poiseuille's law* tells us that when gas flows through a tube:

$$n = \frac{\Delta P \pi r^4}{8 l V}$$

where *n* is viscosity, ΔP is a pressure gradient in dynes per square centimeter between the two ends of the tube, *r* is the tube radius in centimeters, *l* is the tube length in centimeters, $\dot{V}$ is gas flow in cubic centimeters per second, and $\pi/8$ is a constant.

The importance of this formula to the general topic of ventilation is the information it gives when manipulated to our purposes. First let us rearrange the equation and equate the two important kinetic ventilatory factors, *pressure* and *flow,* to the others. (*Note:* Unless otherwise specified, our use of the term

Table 4-3
Examples of viscosity
measurements

	Substance	°C	Poises
Liquids	Water	20	1.005×10^{-2}
	Alcohol, ethyl	20	$1.2 \ \ \times 10^{-2}$
	Glycerine	20	1490×10^{-2}
	Oil, castor	10	2420×10^{-2}
Gases	Air	18	182.7×10^{-6}
	Carbon dioxide	20	$148 \ \ \times 10^{-6}$
	Oxygen	19	201.8×10^{-6}
	Helium	20	194.1×10^{-6}

pressure means a pressure recorded on a guage or other device that measures the pressure as above or below ambient atmospheric. Since this implies a "gradient," it is not necessary to use the symbol ΔP, but merely *P*.)

$$P = \frac{n81\dot{V}}{\pi r^4} \qquad \dot{V} = \frac{P\pi r^4}{8ln}$$

If we are not interested in quantitative relationships but only in the general effects of changes in these parameters, one on the other, we can modify the equations by eliminating those factors that would not change significantly under the specified conditions. Pi and 8 are obvious constants; in a given subject the tubing length, 1, representing the airways, is also generally a constant; since a subject breathes but one gas at a time, for any given circumstance gas viscosity is constant. Tube radius, r, is not a constant because in disease airway patency is often a critical variable. Thus the above two equations can be rewritten as simple *proportionalities:*

$$P \cong \frac{V}{r^4} \qquad \dot{V} \cong Pr^4$$

Finally, these two can be combined into a single expression that clearly shows the reciprocal relationships between the three important variables:

$$\frac{Pr^4}{\dot{V}} = k$$

In clinical pulmonary physiology one of the most frequently encountered conditions is that which involves narrowing of the airways through disease. The above ratio tells us that:

1. If the delivery pressure of gas ventilating the lung remains constant, the flow of the gas will vary directly with the *fourth power* of the radius of the airway. We see how a small change in bronchial caliber can effect a tremendous change in the amount of gas reaching alveoli per unit of time.

2. If the flow of the ventilating gas is to remain constant, the delivery pressure must vary inversely with the fourth power of the airway radius. Thus to maintain stable ventilation in the presence of narrowing airways, we may need great increases in driving pressure.

Our use of Poiseuille's law merely reinforces the concept of pressure-flow relationship described at the beginning of this section and quantitates it in terms of airway size. If we consider viscosity (n) as a form of resistance and transform Poiseuille's equation into a proportionality by eliminating the constants, then the two expressions of pressure-flow relationship we have so far encountered are very similar:

$$R = \frac{\Delta P}{\dot{V}} \qquad\qquad n \cong \frac{\Delta P}{\dot{V}}$$

Airflow patterns

In the respiratory tract there are three types of airflow patterns that are related to gas viscosity and density—*laminar, turbulent,* and *tracheobronchial* flow, illustrated in Fig. 4-19.

Laminar flow is a smooth unobstructed flow of gas through a tube of relatively uniform diameter, with few directional changes, and is found mostly in the trachea and main bronchi. Laminar flow is influenced principally by *viscosity* of the gas being moved, at low to moderate flows, and thus the relationships outlined earlier are pertinent in terms of the amount of air moved per unit of time or the pressure needed to move it. In respiratory physiology significant changes in inhaled gas viscosity are rarely of clinical importance. However, uniform narrowing of an airway reduces flow in proportion to the fourth

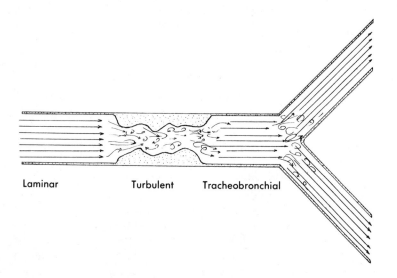

Laminar   Turbulent   Tracheobronchial

Fig 4-19   Three patterns of airflow are found in the respiratory tract. *Laminar* flow is straight and unobstructed, found in the large air passages. *Turbulent* flow is rough and swirling, the result of obstruction and sudden directional changes. *Tracheobronchial* flow is a combination of the two, found in the constantly branching and continuously narrowing airways. (Modified from Comroe, J.H., Jr., et al.: The lung, ed. 2, Chicago, 1962, Year Book Medical Publishers, Inc.)

power of the new radius or requires a similar increase in driving pressure to maintain a steady flow.

Turbulent flow is rough, with much eddy formation, like that of a stream running over a tortuous, rocky bed, and in the airways is generated by sudden changes in direction or acute reduction in diameter. Flow can also be turbulent, even in smooth passages, at high velocity. Ninety percent of the turbulence in the normal respiratory tract occurs in the irregular passages between the nose and trachea, but it is also found in the distal branchings of the small bronchi and bronchioles.[12] It is a factor of great clinical importance in all airways damaged by disease, especially where abnormal secretions, mucosal edema, or structural changes produce abrupt narrowing.

The influence of turbulence on ventilation is best explained by the *Bernoulii effect* (Daniel Bernoulli, 1700-1782), a natural phenomenon widely evident in our daily lives and the functional basis for much of the equipment used in respiratory therapy. Fig. 4-20, *A,* shows the fundamental relationships among pressure, gas flows, and air passage restriction. The derivation of this inverse association of gas pressure and velocity, on which the Bernoulli effect depends, is detailed later in a discussion of the types of fluid energy.

Fig. 4-20, *B,* illustrates a modification of the Bernoulli effect found in a *venturi* (Giovanni Venturi, 1746-1822). The venturi includes a dilation of the gas passage just distal to an obstruction, and if the angulation of the funnel is not over 15 degrees, the gas pressure will be restored nearly to its prerestriction level. Widely used in fluid mechanics, venturis in respiratory therapy equipment are designed to draw in or "entrain" a second gas to mix with the main-flow gas. Such entrainment takes place at the point of low pressure, the distal widening not only permitting pressure restoration but also providing ample space for the increased volume of the mixed gases. Reference will be made later to both the Bernoulli phenomenon and the venturi during discussions of equipment.

A distinction should be made here between the terms *flow* and *velocity*. Flow is a measure of *linear* movement of a fluid *volume* per unit of time, and velocity is a measure of *linear* movement of a fluid per unit of time. For example, in two conducting tubes with different capacities, gases may move at the same velocity but at widely different flows. However, it should be evident that, in a given conducting system operating under a constant delivery pressure, changes in flow entering the system will elicit corresponding qualitative changes in gas velocities through the system. To this limited degree flow and velocity are directly related, but Fig. 4-20, *A,* shows us that the introduction of a restriction in the system necessitates an increase in postobstruction velocity to maintain a steady flow.

Energy is the ability of a substance to perform work, and there are three kinds of energy in a moving fluid:

1. *Potential energy* (PE) is that energy resulting from the force of gravity acting on a volume of fluid elevated above its plane of horizontal flow. Its magnitude is dependent on the weight and height of the fluid, and it

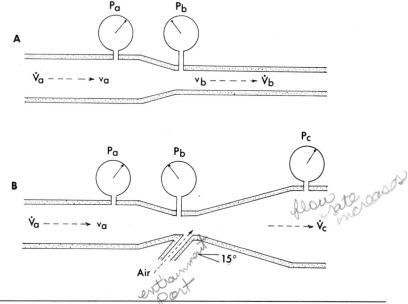

Fig. 4-20   **A,** The Bernoulli effect demonstrates that the *pressure* exerted by a steady flow of gas or liquid in a conducting tube varies *inversely* as the *velocity* of the fluid. With an abrupt narrowing of the passage since the volume of fluid per unit of time leaving (V_b) must equal the time-volume entering the tube (V_a), the linear motion of the fluid per unit of time (velocity, v) must increase as it traverses the structure $(v_b > v_a)$. Thus there is a pressure drop distal to the restriction $(P_b < P_a)$. **B,** The venturi principle states that the pressure drop distal to a restriction can be closely restored to the prerestriction pressure if there is a dilation of the passage immediately distal to the stenosis, with an angle of divergence not exceeding 15 degrees. Thus P_c approximately equals P_a. The venturi is a widely used device to entrain a second gas to mix with the main-flow gas. The subambient pressure distal to the restriction draws in the second gas just past the restriction, and the increased outflow $(\dot{V}_c > \dot{V}_a)$ is accommodated by the widened distal passage.

is best exemplified by a water tower reservoir. Potential energy can also be symbolized as *Hw*, the product of height and weight.

2. *Pressure energy* (P) is the radial force exerted by a moving horizontal fluid and is demonstrated by measuring its lateral pressure while flowing through a pipe.

3. *Kinetic energy* (KE), the energy imparted by the velocity of moving fluid, represents the amount of work performed by matter in motion against a resistive force.

For our purposes we do not need to consider units of measurement as we are interested only in the principles of energy relationships. Thus kinetic energy is expressed as *0.5 × density of the fluid × the square of the velocity of the fluid*, or *0.5 Dv₂*. The derivation of this can be found in standard textbooks of physics.

The Bernoulli theorem for a continuous fluid flow states that the sum of the potential, pressure, and kinetic energies at any given point in the stream will equal the sum of these energies at any other point.[13] However, in our area of interest, since we work with gas flows through tubing circuits under the force of a generated pressure, the factors of elevation and weights of gases are not applicable, and we can ignore potential energy. Thus we can set up an equation in reference to points *a* and *b* in Fig. 4-20, *A*, showing the relationships between pressure and kinetic energies:

$$P_a + 0.5\ Dv_a^2 = P_b + 0.5\ Dv_b^2$$

To make this equation more applicable to our needs in pulmonary physiology, we can alter it and rewrite it as a proportionality. If we assume we are dealing with a single gas, density will be a constant and can be dropped, giving the following proportional expression:

$$P_a - P_b \cong v_b^2 - v_a^2$$

Since the velocity at point *b* is greater than at point *a*, the pressure at *b* must be less than the pressure at *a*. This means that as gas flows through a stricture, its velocity *increases* and its pressure *decreases*, and the magnitude of the pressure drop across the obstruction is proportional to the increase in the *square* of the velocity. Simply, the additional energy expended by the increased velocity reduces the amount of energy available to exert pressure. The implication of this effect is extremely important to the respiratory therapist. If therapeutic gas is applied to the airways of a patient with obstructive disease, the higher the flows delivered at a constant pressure the greater will be the velocities; and with increasing flows the difference between the squares of the preobstruction and postobstruction velocities will be widened. There will be an accompanying decrease in intraluminal pressure distal to the obstruction as the $P_a - P_b$ gradient enlarges.

Earlier it was noted that, given sufficient time, once airflow stops at end-inspiration, mouth, intraluminal, and alveolar pressures will equilibrate. The introduction of a turbulence-producing obstruction interferes with ventilation by hampering pressure equilization. Fig. 4-21 schematically compares laminar with turbulent flow, showing pressure relationships in smooth and obstructed conducting tubes, each of which terminates in an alveolus, *A*, which is inflated by the lateral pressure delivered to it. Fig. 4-21, *A*, depicts the low resistance and small pressure drop of laminar flow, $P_a - P_A$. Alveolar distending pressure is thus not much less than upstream pressure, and at end-inspiration rapid equilibration between P_a and P_A effects maximum alveolar inflation. Time is of relatively little importance. Fig 4-21, *B*, shows that turbulent flow from an obstruction indicates high resistance and is accompanied by a large $P_a - P_A$ drop from the increased postobstruction gas velocity ($P_{b1} - P_{b2}$). Lateral alveolar distending pressure is considerably less than upstream pressure, and at end-inspiration, $P_a - P_A$ will still be large and the alveolus incompletely inflated. Here, time is very important, for if upstream pressure can be held, P_a and P_A will gradually equilibrate to allow completion of alveolar filling. Perhaps the student can now see how the easily equalized pressure gradient from

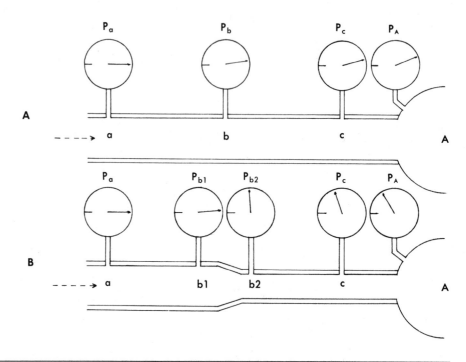

Fig. 4-21   See text.

P_a to P_{b1} might prematurely stop downstream flow and leave the alveolus virtually uninflated.

There is yet another valuable clinical aspect to the Bernoulli phenomenon. Let us rewrite the above proportionality to include the density factor (eliminating the 0.5 as a constant):

$$P_a - P_b \cong D\ (v_b^2 = v_a^2)$$

Inspection shows that with a given increase in velocity the pressure drop across a restriction will be lessened if the gas density is reduced. Thus with obstructed airways, where the Bernoulli effect can be expected to exert a strong influence on the effectiveness of ventilation, distal pressure loss will be minimized with the use of low-density gases. This knowledge makes available to us a very valuable therapeutic tool, and we will see a practical use of the material just discussed when we consider the clinical use of helium.

Tracheobronchial flow is a descriptive term given to the mixture of laminar and turbulent flows found in the normal respiratory tract. Smooth gas flow through short segments of the tract is increasingly broken by the continuous branching of the airways, and even the relatively straight segments become progressively narrower with deeper penetration. Ventilation is thus the net sum of both laminar and turbulent flows, and effective alveolar pressure is related to the gas flow and tube radius in the laminar areas and the square of the gas velocity in the turbulent areas. The body's apparatus for moving air into and out of the lungs is designed to function against a normal balance of these resistances, but when they are increased by disease, the disability that results often requires the skilled services of respiratory therapy.

Relating compliance, rate, flow, and airway resistance	If the therapist's knowledge of compliance, ventilatory frequency, flow, and airway resistance is to have useful clinical meaning, the therapist must see the role played by each in reference to the others. Since the basic function of ventilation is the movement of air, the amount of air moved per unit of energy or pressure exerted determines the efficiency of the system. This, we have already learned, is the description of compliance and is a measure of the elastic resistance of the lung-thorax system. However, we also know that the amount of air moved is dependent on the state of the airways, the degree of their resistance to airflow. Thus, although the elastic resistance determines the pressure necessary to generate a given volume change, flow resistance determines the pressure needed for a given flow. From a practical point of view, then, the overall functional or *measured* lung-thorax compliance is really the net sum of the *actual* compliance of the system and the airway resistance. The general quality of airflow throughout the lungs is dependent on the *uniformity of distribution* of both the elastic properties (actual compliance) in all areas of the lung and the flow-resistive properties (airway resistance) among all the airways. More specifically, it has been determined that, when flows are low, pulmonary air distribution is dependent on lung elasticity and, when flows are high, on airway resistance.[14]

In normal healthy subjects, measured compliance does not vary as much with increased breathing rates as in patients with chronic bronchopulmonary disease, in whom measured compliance progressively drops as frequency increases. Thus the patient with obstructive disease needs increasing effort to move a given volume of air as he or she breathes at higher rates. Although the *actual alveolar compliance may be normal* (a possibility, even in diseased states), the measured compliance, or the volume of air the patient moves per unit of pressure, is depressed. Fig. 4-22 shows the reason for this. For a given volume of air per breath (tidal volume), as the frequency of breathing increases so does the flow, since the volume must be moved faster with each ventilatory excursion. At low frequencies with low flows, the effect of resistance is minimal, and air is equally distributed between two alveoli because the actual compliance of the two pulmonary units determines the distribution of the air. With an increase in breathing frequency, as flow increases, the accompanying flow resistance of the obstruction causes a wide discrepancy in the distribution of flow to the alveoli while increasing the total pressure needed to move the air. Thus, for the overall functional compliance to remain constant in the presence of variable rates of breathing, the distribution of flow must remain constant. This requires that the elastic properties and the flow-resistive properties of all

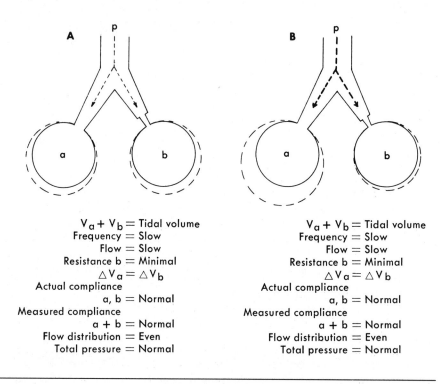

$V_a + V_b =$ Tidal volume
Frequency = Slow
Flow = Slow
Resistance b = Minimal
$\triangle V_a = \triangle V_b$
Actual compliance
a, b = Normal
Measured compliance
a + b = Normal
Flow distribution = Even
Total pressure = Normal

$V_a + V_b =$ Tidal volume
Frequency = Slow
Flow = Slow
Resistance b = Minimal
$\triangle V_a = \triangle V_b$
Actual compliance
a, b = Normal
Measured compliance
a + b = Normal
Flow distribution = Even
Total pressure = Normal

Fig. 4-22 The effect of airway resistance on measured total compliance is shown in sketches where one of each pair of alveoli, with normal actual compliance, is obstructed. The solid-line alveoli are at the resting level, the broken-line at end-tidal inspiration. *P* designates ventilatory pressure. **A,** With a slow frequency, the obstruction has little effect on total ventilation, for the volume changes in the alveoli are equal. **B,** The increased flow reduces the ventilation of alveolus *b*, while *a* compensates by hyperinflating. The increased ventilatory pressure, which attempts to overcome the resistance, lowers the measured, apparent, total compliance.

the pathways of the lung be uniformly distributed, a condition apparently found only in normal lungs. This view of *compliance* gives a more realistic picture of the relation between volumes and pressures than does the classic definition, described earlier.

Exhalation mechanics

Because of its clinical importance, the mechanics of exhalation deserves special consideration. Disturbances in exhalation produce some of the most frequent and severe examples of pulmonary disability. Whereas inhalation is a function of the active contraction of the several muscle groups described earlier, quiet exhalation is the result of *passive recoil* of elastic tissue of the lung, aided by the force of surface tension. At end-inspiration, ventilatory muscles "let go," allowing the lung-thorax to return to the resting level. Under conditions of stress, or in response to airflow obstruction, exhalation may be active

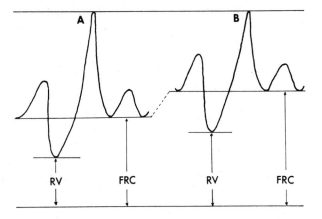

Fig. 4-23 Sketch **A** shows the resting level before, and **B** after, the effect of long-standing airway resistance and/or loss of lung elasticity, as the expansile thoracic springs dominate the pulmonary. Both functional residual capacity and residual volume enlarge. As disease progresses, loss of pulmonary flexibility decreases the expiratory reserve volume, further enlarging the residual volume, and continuing distention may depress the diaphragm to expand the total lung capacity.

through abdominal muscle action, forcing the diaphragm upward for more rapid emptying of the lung. Of critical importance in determining the passivity or activity of exhalation is the element of *time*. If the body's gas exchange needs, for a given level of physical exertion, can be satisfied by an effortless passive exhalation before the succeeding inhalation is triggered, supplementary muscular activity will not be needed; but if there is an increased gas exchange need, or if disease of the respiratory tract is impeding gas flow or uptake, or if there has been loss of lung-thorax elasticity, the body may require additional expiratory effort to move enough air from the lungs in *time* to satisfy the need. This effortful exhalation may be so energy consuming as to produce marked disability.

Airway resistance to exhalation and loss of elasticity are important factors in determining ventilatory patterns. During quiet breathing, airway resistance to inhalation and exhalation in healthy subjects is about the same, even though the negative intrathoracic pressure of inhalation dilates and elongates the bronchioles and the rising pressure of exhalation narrows and shortens them. Forced exhalation, on the other hand, does increase resistance. If exhalation is forced through normally patent airways and against negligible resistance, as in unobstructed hyperventilation, the high velocity of exhaled air creates its own resistance as a result of turbulence, but the expiratory muscular effort responsible is adequate to maintain smooth airflow. However, many pulmonary diseases damage and weaken the walls of the bronchioles. In such circumstances, should airway obstruction or loss of elasticity necessitate a strong expiratory effort to overcome resistance, the excessive positive pressures generated in the thorax may collapse the weakened bronchioles before the alveoli they drain are emptied. This condition of *air trapping* is a common complication of chronic bronchopulmonary disease, often posing a management problem for the respiratory therapist, and is discussed more fully later.

With prolonged airway resistance or loss of elasticity, structural changes may occur in the chest. A major consequence of these disturbances is the gradual elevation of the resting level of the chest, as air trapping and/or inadequate recoil force prevent the lung-thorax from returning to its original, normal end-expiratory position. As shown in Fig. 4-23, this produces an increase in both the functional residual capacity and the residual volume. If uncorrected over a sufficient period of time, there is a progressive increase in the size of the thorax, expecially in its anteroposterior diameter, the deformity descriptively called a "barrel chest." This is a remarkable phenomenon, since it most frequently occurs after the middle years, when the skeleton is well fixed, but it attests to the force exerted by the distended lung, coupled with the traction of accessory ventilatory muscles, to be described later. Because of the elevated resting level, the affected subject gives the appearance of holding the chest in the inspiratory position, a condition frequently seen in pulmonary emphysema.

Introduction to control of ventilation	The rhythmic control of ventilation involves a complex system of chemical receptor sites, blood gases and acid-base influences, muscle innervation, and more. Under normal conditions the amount of ventilation is automatically controlled, such that there are only small changes in arterial blood gases and pH. The determinants of ventilation are composed of both chemoreceptors in blood vessels and in the brain and mechanical or stretch receptors of the lungs and chest wall. Neuron impulses from these receptor sites serve to dictate both inspiratory and expiratory respiratory muscles for moving adequate amounts of air.

The respiratory therapist encounters many patients with disorders affecting this system. Some of the therapy provided has profound effects, as discussed in later chapters. A detailed account of the primary mechanisms for control of ventilation are included in Chapter 6 following discussion of blood gases and acid-base balance. For those interested in the discussion of control of ventilation at this point in their reading, refer to p. 222.

Summary	In good health the respiratory system is able to assure the body of a maximally effective ventilation, with a minimum of effort for any given level of need. Indeed, except under conditions of physical stress, we are generally unaware of the easy rhythmicity of our own breathing until it becomes impaired. Although we have not yet considered details of internal physiologic derangement of blood gas exchange that can upset the normal pattern of breathing,

we should be impressed with the multitude of physical factors that influence ventilation and wonder at the ease with which it is accomplished.

Effective respiratory therapists must be observant. They must be able to judge, at least grossly, the general efficiency of the patient's ventilation on the basis of clinical observation. This means that they must have a clear mental picture of a *normal* breathing pattern for a given individual. They will note, for example, the rate and depth of tidal air exchange and attempt to determine whether the patient is hypoventilating or hyperventilating. They will evaluate the patient's work of breathing by looking for evidence of the use of accessory muscles of ventilation, the resting end-expiratory chest level, signs of inspiratory epigastric retraction or retraction of the costal margins, and evidence of expiratory abdominal contraction. They will observe the time relations between inspiration and expiration to see whether the normal inspiration-longer-than-expiration pattern is reversed. Such information will aid in carrying out, most efficiently and comfortably, the assigned treatment. Many times, of course, effortful breathing or a great effort to breathe is apparent at once. Such a patient can be described as short of breath at rest or at any specified level of activity. Therapists will frequently hear the term *dyspnea* used, and they should understand its real meaning. Dyspnea is a symptom, a subjective feeling experienced only by the patient, not objectively observed by someone else. If a patient states that he or she is having difficulty breathing, then the patient is dyspneic. It means that the patient is uncomfortably aware of the need to work to breathe. The therapist will be surprised at the number of patients who are obviously breathing with effort but who do not complain of it.

Although there are many pathologic aberrations in ventilatory patterns, there is one type with which the therapist should be familiar because of its frequency. This is referred to as *periodic breathing,* and while there are variations of it, the most common is known as *Cheyne-Stokes' respiration.*[15-17] It is characterized by alternating periods of hyperventilation and apnea. Tidal volume excursions get progressively deeper with each breath, reach a maximum, gradually get smaller in amplitude, and then cease completely. Each period of ventilation and apnea can last up to 20 seconds.[15] The "waxing and waning" pattern is characteristic and makes this disorder easy to recognize, even when the apnea may not be complete. Cardiovascular rather than respiratory factors are usually responsible for Cheyne-Stokes' breathing, which is basically the result of cerebral oxygen want caused by a reduced circulatory output of the left ventricle associated with obstructive cerebrovascular disease that reduces blood flow the brain. Despite the apneic intervals, average blood carbon dioxide levels are usually low because of the hyerventilation. We are not concerned with the treatment of this condition, but the therapist should be on the watch for it and call it to the attention of attending medical or nursing personnel whenever it is noted.

A less commonly encountered periodic pattern is *Biot's respiration.* This is somewhat similar to Cheyne-Stokes', except that the hyperventilatory phases are abrupt in onset and termination, without the crescendo-decrescendo character of Cheyne-Stokes'. The respiratory efforts may vary in intensity, and the intervening apneic periods may be unequal and irregular. Biot's breathing is usually the result of severe brain damage, and although the exact mechanism is not known, many believe that there may be a reduced inhibitory action of the higher brain centers on the inspiratory function of the respiratory center, allowing periodic breakthrough of excessive inspiratory efforts.[16]

References

1. Campbell, E.J.M.: The respiratory muscles and the mechanics of breathing, London, 1958, Lloyd-Luke, Ltd.
2. Sinclair, J.D.: In Licht, S., editor: Electro-diagnosis and electromyography, New Haven, Conn., 1961, Elizabeth Licht, Publisher.
3. Agnostoni, E.: In Howell, J.B.L., and Campbell, E.J.M., editors: International Symposium on Breathlessness, Oxford, 1966, Blackwell Scientific Publications.
4. Best, C.H., and Taylor, N.B.: The physiological basis of medical practice, Baltimore, 1943, The Williams & Wilkins Co.
5. McDonald, J.E.: The shape of raindrops, Sci. Am. **190:**64, 1954.
6. Clements, J.A.: Surface tension in lungs, Sci. Am. **207:**121, 1962.
7. Avery, M.E., and Clements, J.A.: Pulmonary surfactants and atelectasis, Physiology, vol. 1, March 1963.
8. Scarpelli, E.M.: The surfactant system of the lung, Philadelphia, 1968, Lea & Febiger.
9. Clements, J.A.: In Liebow, A.A., et al., editors: The lung, Baltimore, 1968, The Williams & Wilkins Co.
10. Rahn, H., Otis, A.B., Chadwick, L.E., and Fenn, W.O.: The pressure-volume diagram of the thorax and lung, Am. J. Physiol. **146:**161, 1946.
11. Fenn, W.O.: Mechanics of respiration, Am. J. Med. **10:**79, 1951.
12. Comroe, J.H., Jr., et al.: The lung, ed. 2, Chicago, 1962, Year Book Medical Publishers, Inc.
13. Black, N.H.: An introductory course in college physics, New York, 1956, The Macmillan Co.
14. Mead, J.: Mechanical properties of the lung, Physiol. Rev. **41:**281, 1961.
15. Bates, D.V., and Christie, R.V.: Respiratory function in disease, Philadelphia, 1964, W.B. Saunders Co.
16. Cherniack, R.M., Cherniack, L., and Naimark, A.: Respiration in health and disease, ed. 2, Philadelphia, 1972, W.B. Saunders Co.
17. Cherniack, N.S.: In Fishman, A.P., editor: Assessment of pulmonary function, New York, 1980, McGraw-Hill Book Co.

Chapter 5

Basic pulmonary function measurements

JOHN W. YOUTSEY

Pulmonary function testing and the clinical application of test results can provide valuable information concerning the status of the cardiopulmonary system. A variety of tests are now available that provide diagnosis and evaluation of respiratory disease.

Pulmonary function testing provides the mechanism to evaluate the ability of the lungs to maintain ventilation and oxygenation. The primary functions of the lung are to oxygenate mixed venous blood entering the pulmonary capillaries from the pulmonary arteries and to remove excess carbon dioxide before the blood returns to the heart via the pulmonary veins. The ability of the lungs to perform these functions is dependent on the integrity of the airways, the function of the diaphragm and thoracic muscles, the status of the cardiovascular system, and the condition of lung tissues themselves.

General considerations

A complete evaluation of pulmonary function requires multiple lung-function studies. Such studies will measure lung volumes and capacities, flow rates, diffusion capacities, and the distribution of ventilation. By using a combination of these tests, a complete and *quantitative* picture of lung function can be developed.

A clinical approach to pulmonary function testing should emphasize both diagnostic and therapeutic information. Too often, pulmonary function tests are used merely to verify the suspected diagnosis. However, pulmonary function testing has both diagnostic and therapeutic roles. General considerations or questions should be addressed concerning the diagnostic and therapeutic aspects of testing and evaluation (Table 5-1).

Uses of pulmonary function tests include the following:
1. *Screening for pulmonary disease.* Screening programs can detect functional or mechanical lung changes caused by disease in the general population and in industrial workers or other high-risk groups.
2. *Preoperative evaluation.* Preoperative evaluation can identify those patients who may have an increased risk of pulmonary complications after surgery.
3. *Assessment of disease progression.* Evaluation can not only help make or verify the initial diagnosis but can also be used as an evaluation of disease progression, the reversibility of the disease, and the evaluation of a rehabilitation protocol such as exercise.

Arterial blood gases

Another method to help evaluate the pulmonary function of a patient is the measurement of arterial blood gases: Pa_{O_2}, Pa_{CO_2}, pH, and HCO_3^- (see Chapter 6 for further description). Blood gases are used most frequently in critical

Table 5-1 Basic questions for clinical pulmonary function testing	**Diagnostic**	**Therapeutic**
	Is lung disease present?	Is the disease reversible?
	What type of lung disease?	To what degree is the disease reversible?
	What degree of lung disease?	Is rehabilitation feasible?
	Single or multiple diseases present?	Can rehabilitation be objectively evaluated?
	Can multiple diseases be separated?	Can rehabilitation be subjectively evaluated?

care units where the patients are supported by mechanical ventilation, constant positive airway pressure (CPAP), or oxygen therapy or during weaning procedures. Blood gases, however, do correlate well with pulmonary function and therefore are a valuable adjunct to pulmonary function testing. Pulmonary shunting and dead space are components of pulmonary diseases and can be identified by measuring a patient's arterial blood gases. When the pulmonary mechanics are altered to the degree that oxygenation and carbon dioxide release can not occur properly, arterial blood gases provide a clinical tool for assessment.

Many disease states demonstrate reliable arterial blood gas *patterns*. However, normal arterial blood gas values do not rule out respiratory disease. Normal blood gas values may be observed when mild to moderate pulmonary disease is present. Also, because of the body's compensatory mechanisms, abnormal blood gases may not always reflect the extent of disease. The use of arterial blood gas measurement complements pulmonary function testing but can not replace it as either a diagnostic or a therapeutic tool. Table 5-2 lists normal and abnormal blood gas values.

Physiologic considerations	The physiologic classification of pulmonary diseases consists of *obstructive* lung diseases, *restrictive* lung diseases, and *combined* lung diseases. Obstructive lung disease is characterized by the patient's decreased ability to exhale maximally. The primary factor in obstructive airway disease is the increase in airway resistance. This is caused by bronchospasm, pulmonary secretions, and/or a breakdown of the structural support system of small airways (bronchioles). As a result, airflow is decreased on inspiration and expiration.

Pulmonary function parameters that signify obstructive disease processes include:

1. Increased airway resistance.
2. Decreased forced expiratory flow rates.
3. Air trapping, exemplified by decreased vital capacity and increased residual volume.

Restrictive lung disease is characterized by a loss in lung volume. The primary factor in restrictive lung disease is a decrease in lung compliance (disten-

Table 5-2 Arterial blood gas values	Measurement	Normal*	Respiratory acidosis†	Respiratory alkalosis†
	Pa_{O2}	80-100 mm Hg	Low	Normal
	Pa_{CO2}	35-45 mm Hg	High	Low
	pH	7.35-7.45	Low	High
	HCO_3^-	22-26 mEq/ℓ	Normal	Normal

*At normal body temperature and standard pressure.
†Simple, noncompensated.

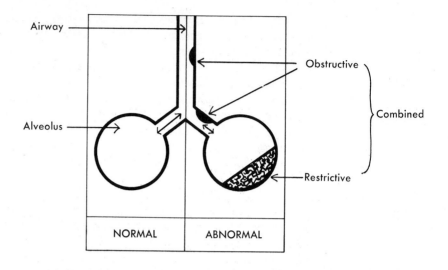

Fig. 5-1   Diagram of the physiologic aspects of pulmonary (lung) disease.

sibility). This can be a result of changes in the lung tissues (parenchyma), the chest wall, or both. This decrease in lung compliance is usually the result of lung inflammation, fibrotic lung disease, neoplasms, kyphoscoliosis, and neuromuscular diseases. As a result, lung volumes are decreased. The only single *diagnostic* parameter for restrictive lung disease is a significant reduction in the total lung capacity.

There are no single parameters that can identify combined lung disease. It is necessary to look at the relationships between those parameters measured and the predicted values. Fig. 5-1 summarizes the physiologic considerations of pulmonary function testing.

Testing overview   Although arbitrary, pulmonary function testing can be divided into two categories: conventional and supplementary. The conventional or clinical spirometry division consists of the measurement of lung volumes and capacities and expiratory flow volumes. Most hospitals have the technical capability for these testing measurements. Furthermore, methods of clinical spirometry have been used for many years and are easily performed. For the majority of patient care situations, the conventional pulmonary function tests provide the essential clinically useful information.

The supplementary pulmonary function tests consist of the measurement of pulmonary compliance, diffusion, lung scans, closing volumes, flow volume curves and loops, and plethysmography. These tests are normally used in specific clinical situations, in pulmonary research, or where conventional testing has not adequately clarified the patient's status.

As stated previously, pulmonary function testing can provide a great deal of information helpful in establishing the patient diagnosis. Furthermore, these tests can determine the type of disease process (obstructive, restrictive, combined), the degree or extent of the disease process, and the potential reversibility of disease.

Pulmonary function tests can be divided into two further categories: those tests that measure *volumes* (and *capacities*) and those tests that measure *flow rates*. Specific tests under each category can provide the information necessary to evaluate the lungs' ability to maintain ventilation and oxygenation.

Conventional pulmonary function tests	The lung can be subdivided into separate *volumes* of gas. These volumes can be added together in various combinations called lung *capacities*. A lung capacity must contain at least two lung volumes. There are four lung volume measurements and four lung capacities. These volumes and capacities are shown in Fig. 5-2. The majority of lung volumes are recorded and measured through simple spirometry; however, the *residual volume* and therefore the *total lung capacity* and the *functional residual capacity* cannot be measured directly during simple spirometry.
Lung volume and capacity tests	

Definitions

tidal volume (TV or V_T) is the volume of air that is inhaled or exhaled from the lungs during quiet breathing.

inspiratory reserve volume (IRV) is the maximum volume of air that can be inhaled following a normal quiet inspiration.

inspiratory capacity (IC) is the sum of the tidal volume and the inspiratory reserve volume (IC = TV + IRV). It is the maximum amount of gas that can be inhaled following a quiet exhalation.

expiratory reserve volume (ERV) is the amount of gas that can be exhaled from the lung following a quiet exhalation.

vital capacity (VC) is the sum of the inspiratory reserve volume, the tidal volume, and the expiratory reserve volume (VC = ERV + TV + IRV). It is the maximum amount of gas that can be inhaled following a maximum exhalation of gas, or the maximum amount of gas that can be exhaled following a maximum inhalation.

The following lung volumes and capacities cannot be measured directly from a simple spirogram.

residual volume (RV) is the volume of gas remaining in the lungs after a complete exhalation.

functional residual capacity (FRC) is the sum of the residual volume and the expiratory reserve volume (FRC = RV + ERV). It is the maximum amount of gas in the lungs following a normal quiet exhalation (also known as resting expiratory level).

total lung capacity (TLC) is the sum of the vital capacity and the residual volume (TLC = VC + RV). It is the maximum volume of gas in the lungs at the end of a maximum inhalation.

Clinical test procedures

Tidal volume. The tidal volume is easily measured directly from a simple spirogram (Fig. 5-2). The patient is asked to breathe normally into a spirometer or other appropriate instrument that has either a kymograph or similar

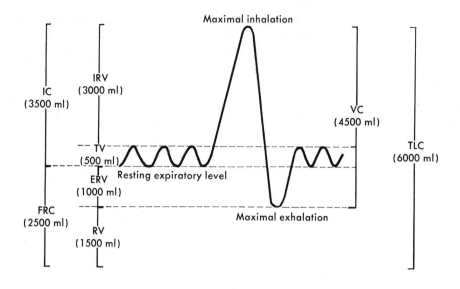

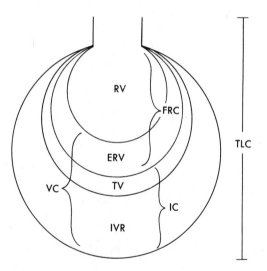

Fig. 5-2   Lung volumes and capacities. Representation of a normal spirogram and the divisions of lung volumes and capacities. Numbers shown are for comparison for an average sized, young adult.

recording device attached. For the purpose of test validity and standardization, the patient should be in a sitting position, and a nose clip should be used. The patient breathes through a tight-fitting mouthpiece until a normal rhythm is established. It generally takes the patient 2 to 3 minutes to *adjust* to the nose clip and mouthpiece. Since the tidal volume will vary normally from breath to breath, an average tidal volume is a more reliable measurement. The total volume of air ($\dot{V}$) moved during either inhalation *or* exhalation for a period of time (usually 1 minute) should be measured. This total volume is then divided by the ventilatory rate (f). The following formula can be used to calculate the tidal volume:

$$V_T = \dot{V}/f$$

where *f* is the ventilatory rate or frequency and $\dot{V}$ is the volume of air inhaled or exhaled in a given time period (usually 1 minute).

The normal tidal volume is approximately 500 ml for the average healthy adult with a range of about 100 ml. There is a great deal of variation in the normal population, and measurements beyond the normal range (400 ml to 600 ml) are not necessarily indicative of a disease process. Normal tidal volume values are often observed in both restrictive and obstructive lung diseases. Therefore, the tidal volume alone is not a valid indicator of lung disease.

Inspiratory capacity. The inspiratory capacity is also measured directly from a spirogram. The patient is asked to breathe in maximally at the end of a normal exhalation. Fig. 5-2 demonstrates that the inspiratory capacity is composed of two lung volumes: the tidal volume and the inspiratory reserve volume. The following formula demonstrates this relationship between lung volumes and capacities:

$$IC = TV + IRV$$

The normal inspiratory capacity is approximately 3000 ml to 4000 ml, again with a significant variation in the normal population. The inspiratory capacity will represent around 75% to 80% of the vital capacity and around 55% to 60% of the total lung capacity. Like the tidal volume measurements, normal values can be observed in both obstructive and restrictive lung diseases. However, generally the inspiratory capacity will be reduced in both restrictive and obstructive lung diseases. Increases usually mean that the patient was not truly at the *resting expiratory level* when the test was performed.

Inspiratory reserve volume. Inspiratory reserve volume, a component of the inspiratory capacity, is usually not measured during spirometry. Like both the tidal volume and the inspiratory capacity, it can be normal in both restrictive and obstructive diseases. It is not a significant clinical measure of lung mechanics.

Expiratory reserve volume. The expiratory reserve volume is measured directly from the spirogram. The patient is asked to breathe normally for a few breaths and then exhale maximally. The expiratory reserve volume is that volume of air exhaled between the resting expiratory level and the maximum exhalation level on the spirogram.

The normal expiratory reserve volume is approximately 1000 ml and represents around 20% to 25% of the vital capacity. It can be either normal or reduced in obstructive and restrictive lung diseases.

Vital capacity. The vital capacity is measured from the spirogram by having the patient inhale as deeply as possible and then exhale fully, taking all the time that is necessary to exhale completely. A similar test called the forced vital capacity (FVC) requires the patient to complete the same maneuver; however, the patient must exhale as forcibly and quickly as possible.

The normal range for vital capacity is 4000 ml to 5000 ml and represents approximately 80% of the total lung capacity. Normal values can vary signifi-

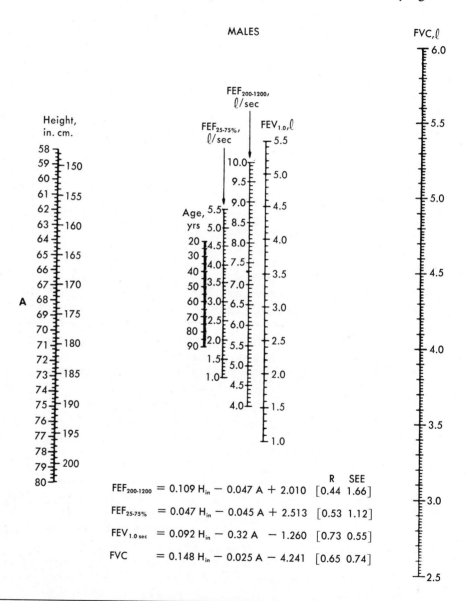

$$FEF_{200\text{-}1200} = 0.109\ H_{in} - 0.047\ A + 2.010\ [0.44\ 1.66]$$

$$FEF_{25\text{-}75\%} = 0.047\ H_{in} - 0.045\ A + 2.513\ [0.53\ 1.12]$$

$$FEV_{1.0\ sec} = 0.092\ H_{in} - 0.32\ A - 1.260\ [0.73\ 0.55]$$

$$FVC = 0.148\ H_{in} - 0.025\ A - 4.241\ [0.65\ 0.74]$$

Fig. 5-3   Spirometric standards for, **A,** males and, **B,** females (BTPS). (From Morris, J.F., Koski, W.A., and Johnson, L.C.: Am. Rev. Resp. Dis. **103**(1):57, 1971.)

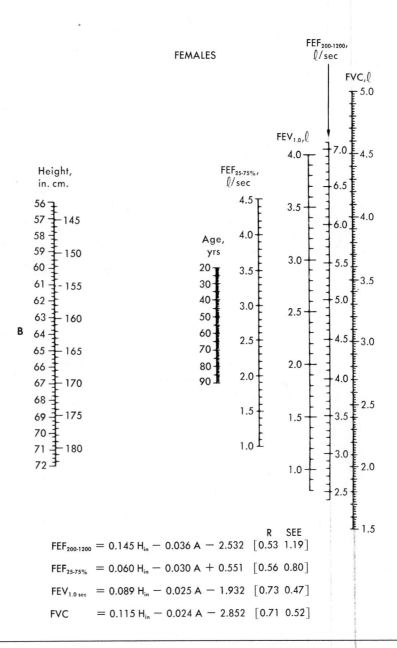

FEF$_{200-1200}$ = 0.145 H$_{in}$ − 0.036 A − 2.532 [0.53 1.19]

FEF$_{25-75\%}$ = 0.060 H$_{in}$ − 0.030 A + 0.551 [0.56 0.80]

FEV$_{1.0\ sec}$ = 0.089 H$_{in}$ − 0.025 A − 1.932 [0.73 0.47]

FVC = 0.115 H$_{in}$ − 0.024 A − 2.852 [0.71 0.52]

Fig. 5-3, cont'd For legend see opposite page.

cantly depending on age, sex, and test position. Weight is not a factor in predicting normal values. Because of this, various nomograms are available for predicting normal values. Fig. 5-3 represents typical nomograms for predicting spirometric values for men and women.

A decrease in vital capacity occurs in restrictive lung diseases. In early to moderate obstructive lung diseases, the vital capacity may be normal or reduced. In severe obstructive lung disease, the vital capacity is generally reduced. A reduction can occur in two ways: (1) reduction in total lung capacity, which is observed in restrictive lung diseases, and/or (2) increase in residual volume, which is observed in obstructive lung diseases.

A forced vital capacity will generally be significantly less than a normal vital capacity in patients with obstructive lung disease. This is primarily a result of airway collapse during the forced expiration and the trapping of air that results. To be significant, the difference between the vital capacity and the forced vital capacity should be greater than about 10%.

Residual volume and functional residual capacity. The residual volume does not represent a direct measurement that can be taken from a simple spirogram; it can only be measured indirectly. Residual volume is a very important test in pulmonary mechanics. It is usually elevated in obstructive lung diseases. The normal residual volume is approximately 1500 ml and represents 33% of the vital capacity and 25% of the total lung capacity. In fact, the residual volume must be known in order to measure the total lung capacity and the functional residual capacity. Most indirect pulmonary function tests actually measure the functional residual capacity, and by using the formula RV = FRC − ERV, one is able to calculate the residual volume.

The three most commonly used tests for the measurement of the residual volume are helium dilution, nitrogen washout, and body plethysmography.

Helium dilution test. This test is also called the *closed-circuit method.* The principle is based on the dilution of helium in a closed-spirometer system. A known volume and concentration of helium (He) are introduced into the spirometer system. Following a normal exhalation, the patient is connected to the system. While the patient is connected, carbon dioxide is eliminated through a carbon dioxide absorbent, and oxygen is added at a rate equal to the oxygen consumption. The patient rebreathes the gas in the system until an equilibrium is reached. This usually takes less than 7 minutes; however, in patients with severe lung disease this can take up to 30 minutes before equilibrium of the helium between the patient and the spirometer system occurs (Fig. 5-4).

Two major calculations are necessary before the residual volume itself is calculated:

1. The volume in the spirometer system must be known:

$$V = \frac{\text{He added (ml)}}{\%\text{He (1st reading)}}$$

2. The functional residual capacity must be calculated:

$$FRC = \frac{(He_1 - He_2)}{He_2} \times V \times BTPS \text{ correction factor}$$

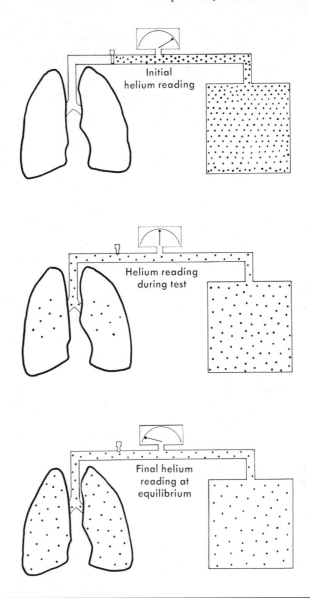

Fig. 5-4   Indirect spirometric method for measuring the functional residual capacity and the residual volume. Helium dilution method.

where FRC is the functional residual capacity; V is the volume in the spirometer system; He_1 is the initial concentration of helium before patient added to system; He_2 is the final equilibrated concentration of helium; and *BTPS correction factor* is the conversion factor to change volume to body temperature and pressure saturated. The expiratory reserve volume is then subtracted from the functional reserve volume because of the following relationship:

$$FRC - ERV = RV$$

The end-expiratory level or FRC is a more reliable point from which to measure as compared to the RV, since starting the test at RV requires maximal expiratory effort by the patient.

Nitrogen washout test. Also called the *open-circuit method,* this test is based on the principle that the patient inhales pure oxygen from the spirometer system and *washes* the nitrogen from the lungs. It is assumed that the nitrogen concentration in the lungs is in equilibrium with the atmosphere (approximately 79%). The patient's exhaled gas is monitored and its volume and nitrogen percent measured. The patient breathes 100% oxygen for approximately 7 minutes, until *washout* occurs (Fig. 5-5). The test must occur in a completely closed system since the leakage of room air would alter the measured nitrogen percent. Like the helium dilution test, the patient is connected to the system at the end-expiratory level. In this way an accurate functional residual capacity is achieved.

The following formula is used to determine the functional residual capacity by the nitrogen washout method:

$$V_1 N_1 = V_2 N_2$$

or

$$V_1 = \frac{V_2 N_2}{N_1}$$

where V_1 is FRC, the volume of gas in the lungs at end-expiratory level; N_1 is nitrogen percent in the lungs at the beginning of the test; V_2 is expired volume; and N_2 is nitrogen percent in the spirometer at the end of the test. The expiratory reserve volume is then subtracted from the functional residual capacity again because of the relationship $FRC - ERV = RV$.

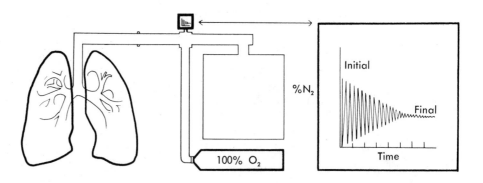

Fig. 5-5   Indirect spirometric method for measuring the functional residual capacity and residual volume. Nitrogen washout method.

Body plethysmography. The plethysmograph uses Boyle's law ($k = V \times P$), which states that at a constant temperature, the product of the pressure (P) and the volume (V) of a system is constant (k); therefore, pressure varies inversely with volume. The plethysmograph measures the total gas volume within the chest. The functional residual capacity is measured by placing the patient in a sealed chamber. Manometers measure the airway pressure and the chamber pressure. An electronically controlled shutter occludes the airway periodically for only an instant. Pressure changes are measured under conditions of no airflow via the transducer at the mouth. Pressures are measured in the thorax (airway) and in the chamber. Volume changes in the thorax create volume changes in the chamber, which in turn are reflected by pressure changes in the chamber.

When conducting the test, the patient is placed in the chamber, connected to the mouthpiece, and asked to breathe normally through the mouthpiece (Fig. 5-6). At end-inspiration and end-expiration there is no airflow, and the

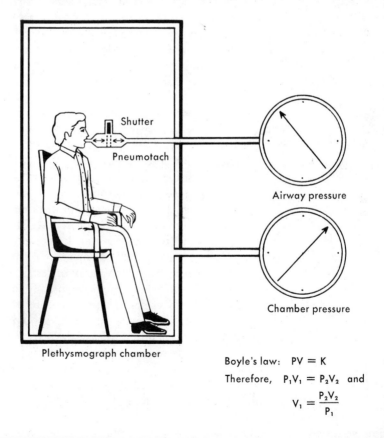

Boyle's law: $PV = K$

Therefore, $P_1V_1 = P_2V_2$ and

$$V_1 = \frac{P_2V_2}{P_1}$$

Fig. 5-6   Body plethysmography method for measuring lung volumes. *P₁*, initial alveolar pressure; *V₁*, initial thoracic gas volume (unknown); *P₂*, test alveolar pressure (shutter closed); *V₂*, test thoracic gas volume (shutter closed).

alveolar pressure is equal to the airway pressure at that time. At a specific time (end-expiration, for example) the shutter is occluded, and the various volume and pressure values are measured. The formula k = VP for Boyle's law can be rewritten as follows:

$$P_1V_1 = P_2V_2$$

where P_1 is initial alveolar pressure; V_1 is initial thoracic gas volume; P_2 is test alveolar pressure; and V_2 is test thoracic volume.

By solving for V_1, the equation can be rearranged:

$$V_1 = \frac{P_2V_2}{P_1}$$

If the shutter is closed at the resting expiratory level, then V_1 = FRC.

Total lung capacity. The total lung capacity is the sum of the vital capacity and the residual volume. Each can be measured as described previously. The total lung capacity is the only truly *diagnostic* single parameter in spirometry. It is always elevated in obstructive lung diseases and reduced in restrictive lung diseases. Certain disorders such as pulmonary edema, atelectasis, consolidation, etc., will cause a reduction. Although a reduced total lung capacity is always observed in restrictive lung diseases, a reduced total lung capacity does not necessarily mean that a restrictive lung disease exists.

Interpretation of lung volumes and capacities. When interpreting lung volumes and capacities, as well as all pulmonary function testing results, several factors should be considered:

1. *Patient history.* A patient history should include age, sex, height, weight, weight gains or losses, and vital signs. A family history of pulmonary or cardiac diseases should be ascertained. The patient should be questioned concerning allergies, current medications, recent illnesses, and general information about the home and work environment.

2. *Patient cooperation.* All test procedures should be explained thoroughly before actual testing is begun. It should be determined if the patient is capable either physically or mentally of full cooperation. This is important in determining the validity of certain test results.

3. *Predicted values.* Test results are usually reported in relationship to normal predicted values. These values are based on the patient's age, sex, and height. Test results, however, should also be evaluated against the total patient picture. Over reliance on nomograms, for example, can be misleading in some patient situations.

In addition, the various lung volumes and capacities should be looked at collectively. Table 5-3 summarizes lung volume and capacity changes that occur in obstructive and restrictive lung diseases.

Airflow volume tests

The simple spirogram along with predicted average or normal values can provide *clues* as to the type of respiratory disorder (restrictive, obstructive, or combined). With the exception of the total lung capacity, which is diagnostic of disease, the other values alone do not provide sufficient information.

Table 5-3
Lung volumes and
capacities in
pulmonary disease

Test	Obstructive disease	Restrictive disease
Tidal volume (V_T)	Normal or elevated	Normal or reduced
Inspiratory capacity (IC)	Normal or reduced	Normal or reduced
Expiratory reserve volume (ERV)	Normal or reduced	Normal or reduced
Vital capacity (VC)	Normal or reduced	Reduced
Residual volume (RV)	Increased	Normal or reduced
Functional residual capacity (FRC)	Increased	Normal or reduced
Total lung capacity (TLC)	Increased	Reduced

Tests that measure airflow volumes provide important information relating to the actual function of the lungs, the degree of impairment, and often the general location (e.g., large airways, small airways, etc.) of the primary problem. In order to gather this additional information, tests that measure the actual pulmonary mechanisms are needed. Timed forced expiratory volumes (FEV_t) provide a great deal of information. Such tests measure the ability of the patient to maximally exhale as much as possible and in the shortest period of time. FEV_t tests are recorded on spirometry equipment. In recent years, the use of electronic instruments and computers has simplified the calculation of the various FEV_t tests.

Definitions

forced vital capacity (FVC) is the maximum volume of gas that the patient can exhale as forcefully and as quickly as possible. It will be lower than the normal slow vital capacity (SVC) when airway collapse and air trapping are present. The forced vital capacity is usually measured in liters (see p. 175).

forced expiratory volume, half second ($FEV_{0.5}$) is the maximum volume of gas that the patient can exhale during the first half second during a forced vital capacity maneuver.

forced expiratory volume, 1 second (FEV_1) is the maximum volume of gas that the patient can exhale during the first second during a forced vital capacity maneuver.

forced expiratory volume, 3 seconds (FEV_3) is the maximum volume of gas that the patient can exhale during the first 3 seconds during a forced vital capacity maneuver.

forced expiratory volume percent (FEV%) is the precent of the *measured* forced vital capacity that a given FEV_t represents.

The following are not actually forced expiratory volumes timed but are included under the section of airflow volumes.

forced expiratory flow, 200-1200 ($FEF_{200-1200}$) is a measure of the average expiratory flow during early phase of exhalation. Specifically, it is a measure of the flow rate for the 1000 ml of expired gas immediately following the first 200 ml of expired gas. Originally this test was called the maximum expiratory flow rate (MEFR). The test is recorded in liters per minute or liters per second.

forced expiratory flow, 25%-75% (FEF_{25-75}) is a measure of the average expiratory flow rate during the middle 50% phase of exhalation. The first quarter and the last quarter of the exhalation is ignored. The flow rate of the middle 50% is thus measured. The test is recorded in liters per minute or liters per second.

maximum voluntary ventilation (MVV) is the maximum volume of gas that a patient can move during 1 minute. Previously it was called the maximum breathing capacity (MBC). The results are expressed in liters per minute. The test is usually run for 10, 12, or 15 seconds and a liters per minute value calculated.

peak expiratory flow (PEF) is the maximum flow rate at which a patient can exhale during a forced expiration. The tests results are recorded in liters per second or liters per minute.

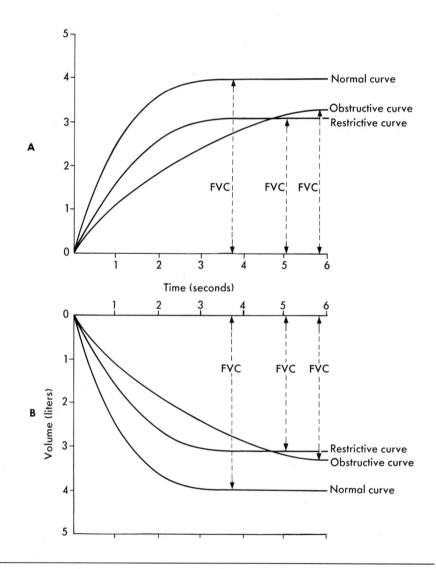

Fig. 5-7   Forced vital capacity curves comparing normal, obstructive, and restrictive disorders. **A** shows curves as they appear on commonly available spirometers with tracings beginning at the bottom left corner. **B** shows same curves as they appear on some spirometers that begin tracings at upper left corner.

Clinical test procedures

Forced vital capacity. The forced vital capacity is easily measured with simple spirometry as well as electronic devices. The patient is asked to exhale as forcibly and as quickly as possible into the spirometer or pneumotachometer. The patient should breathe in maximally and exhale as quickly as possible. Coaching the patient is necessary to achieve the maximum exhalation possible for the particular patient. The significance of this test has already been discussed. Fig. 5-7 demonstrates forced vital capacities from common bedside spirometer tracings for the normal, obstructive, and restrictive states. The forced vital capacities in both the obstructed and restricted curves are shown reduced below the normal. The primary difference between the curve in the restricted patient as compared to the obstructed patient is the *slope* of the curve.

Forced expiratory volume timed. The forced expiratory volume during a specified time interval (0.5, 1, or 3 seconds) determines the maximum volume of gas that can be exhaled during the forced vital capacity maneuver in those time intervals. The patient is asked to perform a forced vital capacity as previously described. The spirometer drum moves at a preset speed. With the horizontal axis as the time interval, the exhaled volume can be measured directly from the spirometer for a specific time period (Fig. 5-8). The volume must be corrected to BTPS. The predicted values for the FEV_1 can be calculated from Fig. 5-3.

It is more clinically valuable to look at the FEV_t as it is related to the patient's forced vital capacity. Therefore,

$$FEV\% = \frac{FEV_t}{FVC \times 100\%}$$

Normal values for the FEV% are listed in Table 5-4. Patients with obstructive pulmonary disease will show a reduction in the $FEV_t\%$, while patients with restrictive disorders will generally show normal $FEV_t\%$ when compared to their *measured* forced vital capacity. However, if compared to normal prediction values, the FEV_t, expressed as a volume, will be reduced.

Forced expiratory flows, 200-1200 and 25%-75%. The $FEF_{200\text{-}1200}$ and $FEF_{25\text{-}75}$ represent average flow rates that occur during specific intervals on the forced vital capacity curve. These flows were originally described as maximum expiratory flow rates, and therefore the $FEF_{200\text{-}1200}$ was called the *maxi-*

	Test (FEV%)*	Normal clinical range†
Table 5-4	$FEV_{0.5}$	50%-70%
Normal clinical ranges	FEV_1	70%-83%
for forced expiratory	FEV_2	84%-93%
volumes timed (FEV_t)	FEV_3	94%-97%

*FEV_t/FVC × 100.
†Decreases with age.

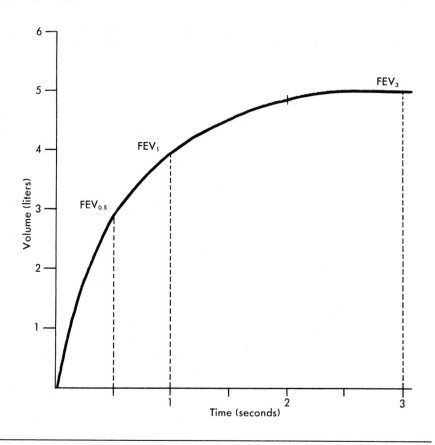

Fig. 5-8   Forced expiratory volumes for 0.5, 1, and 3 seconds.

mum expiratory flow rate (MEFR) and the FEF_{25-75} was called the *maximum mid-expiratory flow* (MMF).

Both measures can be made on a simple spirogram where a timed forced vital capacity is recorded. For the $FEF_{200-1200}$ test, the time interval is marked between the 200-ml point and the 1200-ml point. A straight line is drawn between these points, and the line is extended to intersect two 1-second time lines (Fig. 5-9). The volume of air measured between the two time lines can be read from the spirogram and is recorded as a flow rate in liters per second. The volume measured must be corrected to BTPS.

The FEF_{25-75} is a measure of the flow rate during the middle portion of the forced vital capacity, or the time necessary to exhale the middle 50%. The only limitation is that the first 25% and last 25% of the forced vital capacity are ignored. A straight line is drawn between the points that represent 25% and 75%. Again, the line is extended through two 1-second lines and the volume measured and corrected to BTPS (Fig. 5-10).

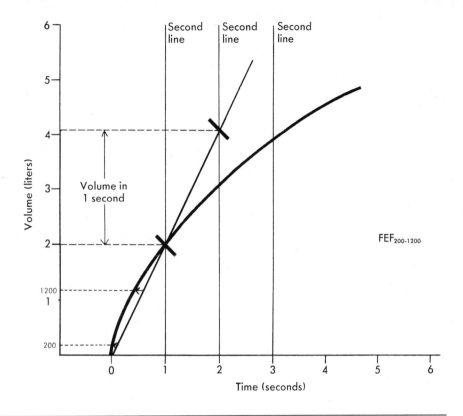

Fig. 5-9   Forced expiratory flow, 200-1200.

Both the FEF_{25-75} and the $FEF_{200-1200}$ measure the *average* flow rate in a specific time period. The *difference* between the two depends on *where,* during the forced vital capacity curve, the measurement is made. The normal $FEF_{200-1200}$ is usually greater than 5 ℓ/sec (300 ℓ/min). Since the test is done at initial high lung volumes (early forced expiration), it is a measure of the integrity and function of the large airways. This test is also a very good indicator of patient effort. A reduced $FEF_{200-1200}$ will be observed in patients with significant obstructive lung disease and in many patients with severe restriction. The $FEF_{200-1200}$ is both independent of the forced vital capacity and most responsive to bronchodilator therapy.

The normal FEF_{25-75} is approximately 4 ℓ/sec (240 ℓ/min). This test is a good measure of small or distal airway function. Since it measures lung function at lower lung volumes it is relatively independent of patient effort. A reduced FEF_{25-75} will be observed in patients with obstructive lung disease. The test is also sensitive to the early changes that occur in the obstructive lung disease process. Because of this, the FEF_{25-75} may detect changes in the lung function that are not apparent from the $FEF_{200-1200}$.

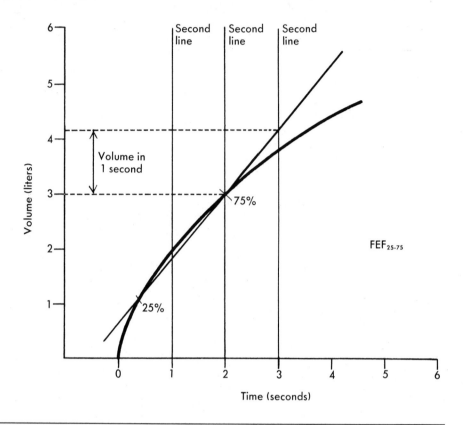

Fig. 5-10   Forced expiratory flow, 25%-75%.

Maximum voluntary ventilation. The maximum voluntary ventilation test is an index of the integrity and function of the lung-thorax relationship. Therefore it includes measures of the airway resistance, status of the respiratory muscles, and integrity of the lung parenchyma. This test is *extremely* dependent on patient effort.

The patient usually takes a standing position (with support if necessary) and is instructed to breathe as rapidly and deeply as possible for 10, 12, or 15 seconds. The patient volumes are measured on a spirogram (Fig. 5-11) or electronically for the specific period of time. The volumes are then extrapolated to liters per minute. For example:

Volume of air moved in 10 sec: 30 ℓ
BTPS correction factor to liters per minute: 60 sec $\div$ 10 = 6
MVV = 30 × 6 = 180 ℓ/min

The use of a ventilometer pen on many spirometers simplifies the measurement of the volume of gas moved in the specific time period. The ventilometer simply adds all inspiratory volumes in a period of time. Once corrected for the

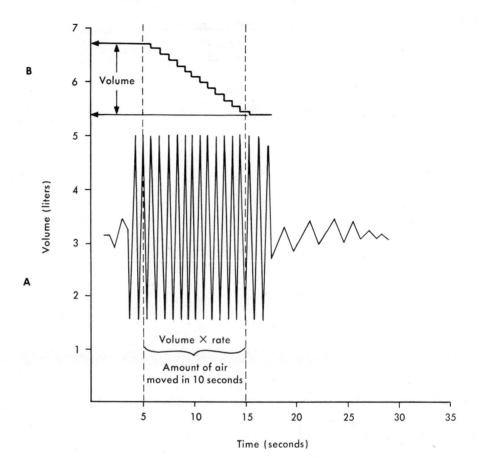

Fig. 5-11 Maximum voluntary ventilation tracing. **A,** Actual ventilations recorded during a 10-second period. **B,** Summation recording (addition of inspiratory volume) measured during the 10 seconds. Summation volume times correction factor (e.g., 25 for Collins spirometer) equals actual volume.

gear train reduction, it provides an easy way to measure the volume of gas moved (Fig. 5-11):

> Volume of air moved in 10 sec: 1.2 ℓ
> BTPS correction factor to liters per minute: 60 sec ÷ 10 = 6
> Gear reduction factor: 25
> MVV = 1.2 × 25 × 6 = 180 ℓ/min

As with all volumes measured on a water-sealed spirometer, the recorded values are corrected to BTPS.

Predicted maximum voluntary ventilation values are based on sex, age, and body surface area. Normal values vary significantly (25% to 30%) in the population; therefore, only major reductions in the values are clinically significant.

The maximum voluntary ventilation is greatly reduced in patients with moderate and severe airway obstruction. Generally, a measured value less than 75% of the predicted is significant. The normal for males is about 160 to 180 ℓ/min; it is slightly lower in females. In restrictive lung disease the maximum voluntary ventilation value may be normal or only slightly reduced. The maximum voluntary ventilation was previously called the *maximum breathing capacity* (MBC).

Peak expiratory flow. The peak flow (PEF) is the maximum flow rate that occurs at any point in time during the forced vital capacity. It is measured by drawing a line against the steepest portion of the forced vital capacity curve. Normal peak flows average 9 to 10 ℓ/sec. Because of such high flows, it is difficult to measure accurate peak flows from a spirogram. In this instance, the electronic measuring devices (pneumotachometers) are preferable because of their accuracy.

The reliability of peak expiratory flow as a clinical tool for evaluating lung mechanics is limited because of the initial high flow rates that can occur even in obstructive disorders. Decreased peak flows are reflective of nonspecific mechanical problems of the lung, patient cooperation, and effort. Table 5-5 provides a summary of spirometric values and airflow volume values in normal, obstructive, and restrictive disorders.

Supplementary pulmonary function tests

The pulmonary function tests discussed here are classified as *supplementary* because they do not constitute part of clinical spirometry. Supplementary testing provides the additional information that is sometimes necessary to better define a patient's pulmonary disease process.

Table 5-5
Spirometric and airflow volume measurements

Measurement	Normal*	Obstructive	Restrictive
TV	500 ml	N ↑	N ↓
IC	3500 ml	N ↓	N ↓
ERV	1000 ml	N ↓	N ↓
VC	4500 ml	N ↓	↓
FVC	4500 ml	N ↓	↓
RV	1500 ml	N ↑	N ↓
FRC	2500 ml	N ↑	N ↓
TLC	6000 ml	N ↑	↓
$FEV_{0.5}$	>50% FVC†	↓	N
FEV_1	>70% FVC†	↓	N
FEV_2	>83% FVC†	↓	N
FEV_3	>93% FVC†	↓	N
$FEF_{200-1200}$	>5 ℓ/sec (300 ℓ/min)	↓	N ↓
FEF_{25-75}	>4 ℓ/sec (240 ℓ/min)	↓	N ↓
MVV	160-180 ℓ/min (±25%)	↓	N ↓
PEF	9-10 ℓ/sec	N ↓	N ↓

*Examples for young healthy male of average size.
†FVC = measured, *not* predicted.

Definitions

airway resistance (R_{aw}) is the driving pressure necessary to move a volume of gas in a specific period of time. Mathematically, it is the ratio of the driving pressure to the flow and is expressed in cm $H_2O/\ell/sec$.

compliance (C) is a measure of the distensibility of the chest and/or lungs; that is, it is the volume change in the lung per unit pressure change and is expressed in $\ell/cm\ H_2O$.

closing volume (CV) is a measure of the volume of gas remaining in the lung when the small airways presumably begin to close during a controlled maximum exhalation.

closing capacity (CC) is the sum of the closing volume and the residual volume: CC = CV + RV.

flow volume curve or loop is the graphic relationship between flow rates and resultant volumes during a forced vital capacity and subsequent forced inspiratory volume maneuver.

ventilation and perfusion scans are lung function studies using radioactive materials to assess gas distribution and blood flow in the lungs.

Clinical test procedures

Airway resistance. The most common method for measurement of airway resistance is body plethysmography. Airway resistance is the ratio of the driving pressure to the airflow and can be represented with the following formula:

$$R_{aw} = \frac{\Delta P}{V}$$

Where R_{aw} is airway resistance; ΔP is driving pressure ($P_1 - P_2$); and $\dot{V}$ is airflow.

The driving pressure (ΔP) is equal to the atmospheric pressure (P_1) minus the alveolar pressure (P_2). In order to measure the driving pressure, the body plethysmograph is used. The patient is placed in the sealed plethysmograph. Volume changes in the thorax will create volume changes in the chamber, which in turn are reflected by changes in the chamber pressure. During inspiration, the lung increases in size. This creates a subatmospheric pressure in the alveoli, and air moves into the lung because of the pressure gradient. At the same time, the increased size of the thorax is compressing the gas in the chamber, and a reciprocal increase in chamber pressure results (Boyle's law). During exhalation the opposite occurs. Recording the pressure in the plethysmograph (P_p) during this time provides a value for one variable in the formula used to calculate the airway resistance. In the absence of airflow, airway pressure at the mouth is equal to the alveolar pressure (P_A). While the patient is breathing, an electronic shutter momentarily closes. This creates a no-flow situation, and the alveolar pressure can be determined. During this time, if one measures the airflow ($\dot{V}$) with a pneumotachometer, the airway pressure can be calculated by the following formula:

$$R_{aw} = \frac{P_A/P_p}{\dot{V}/P_p}$$

where R_{aw} is airway resistance; P_A is alveolar pressure; P_p is plethysmograph pressure; and V is airflow. This formula actually describes the relationship between two sets of ratios: changes in the alveolar pressure and pressure in the plethysmograph (P_A/P_p) and changes between flow rate and pressure in the plethysmograph ($\dot{V}/P_p$). The test is usually done by having the patient pant at tidal volumes of approximately 100 to 200 ml at high rates, usually greater than 100 breaths/min. Panting reduces many of the artifacts that would otherwise interfere with the test results. Fig. 5-12 shows the measurement of airway resistance in the body plethysmograph.

Airway resistance is normally between 0.5 and 3 cm H_2O/ℓ/sec, measured at a standardized flow rate of 0.5 ℓ/sec. It is lower during inspiration and higher during exhalation. In addition, airway resistance decreases with increasing lung volumes primarily because of the increasing airway caliber. Any factor that reduces the caliber of the airway will cause an increase in airway resistance. Such factors include edema, bronchial secretions, bronchoconstriction, and vascular congestion (inflammation). A loss of lung elasticity will also cause an increase. Therefore, such disorders as asthma, emphysema, bronchitis, etc., will cause increases in airway resistance.

Compliance. Compliance is a measure of the distensibility of the lungs (C_L), the thorax (C_T), or both (C_{LT}). In essence, it measures the *ease* with which the lung volume is changed. It is expressed in ℓ/cm H_2O (BTPS). Increased com-

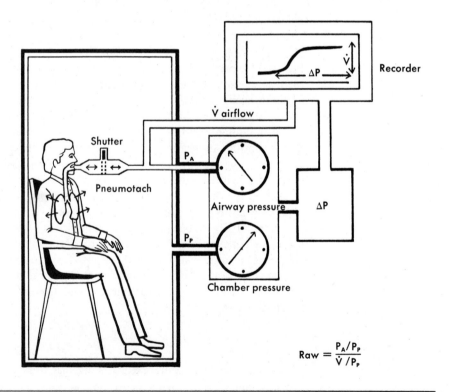

$$Raw = \frac{P_A/P_P}{\dot{V}/P_P}$$

Fig. 5-12   Measurement of airway resistance in the body plethysmograph (see text).

pliance means a greater increase in lung volume per centimeter of water pressure; likewise, a reduced compliance means a smaller change in lung volume per centimeter of water.

When determining the C_{LT}, it is necessary to know the transpulmonary pressure and the specific lung volumes at each pressure. In doing this, a pressure-volume curve is generated (Fig. 5-13). The transpulmonary pressure (P_L) is the difference between the intrapleural pressure (P_{Pl}) and the alveolar pressure (P_{Alv}): $P_L = P_{Pl} - P_{Alv}$. When compliance is measured under static conditions (static compliance) the alveolar pressure is equal to the atmospheric pressure (P_{atm}). In this case, the atmospheric pressure is assumed to be equal to zero by standard; therefore, the transpulmonary pressure is equal to the intrapleural pressure: $P_L = P_{Pl}$.

The formula for calculating the static lung compliance (C_L) is:

$$C_L = \frac{\Delta V}{\Delta P}$$

where ΔP is the pressure gradient or ΔP_L. Since $P_L = P_{Pl}$, $\Delta P_L = \Delta P_{Pl}$. Therefore:

$$C_L = \frac{\Delta V}{\Delta P_{Pl}}$$

Measurement of the lung compliance is done by having the patient swallow a balloon catheter. The catheter is positioned in the lower third of the esophagus and connected to a manometer to measure pressure. At this point, the

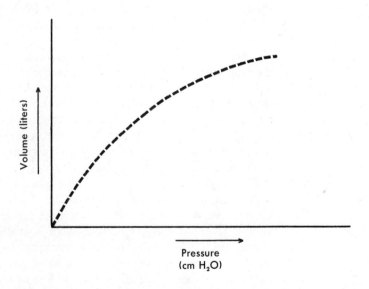

Fig. 5-13   Pressure-volume curve demonstrating compliance.

esophageal pressure is equal to the intrapleural pressure. Pressure changes can be plotted against various lung volumes (Fig. 5-13). Normal lung compliance is approximately 0.2 ℓ/cm H_2O.

The lung-thorax compliance (C_{LT}) can be measured with body plethysmography. By serially reducing pressures within the chambers and measuring the resulting changes in volume, a pressure-volume curve can be plotted. The lung-thorax compliance is equal to 0.1 ℓ/cm H_2O. Given these two values, one can easily calculate the thoracic compliance:

$$\frac{1}{C_L} + \frac{1}{C_T} = \frac{1}{C_{LT}}$$

$$\frac{1}{0.2} + \frac{1}{0.2} = \frac{1}{0.1} \; \ell \; cm/H_2O$$

$$\therefore C_{LT} = 0.1 \; \ell/cm \; H_2O$$

The total lung-thorax compliance is about one half of either the lung or thorax compliance alone. This is a result of the opposing forces of the lung and thorax.

When compliance measurements are made during the breathing cycle, *dynamic compliance* is measured. In the normal lung, the dynamic compliance (C_{dyn}) is equal to the lung compliance because of the opposing forces between the lungs and the thorax.

Changes in lung and chest wall compliance occur in several disease processes. Lung compliance is most affected by bronchopulmonary diseases, whereas chest wall compliance is most affected by diseases of the thoracic nerves, joints, and muscles and obesity. Restrictive lung diseases reduce lung compliance as a result of the stiffness of the lung tissue. In obstructive lung diseases such as pulmonary emphysema, the lung compliance is high because of destruction of the lung support tissues and parenchyma.

Closing volume. Closing volume measures the amount of gas remaining in the lung when the small airways presumably begin to close during exhalation. A modification of the single-breath nitrogen test is used to calculate this volume. The closing volume is measured and often expressed as a ratio to the vital capacity (CV/VC). A second measurement often made is called the closing capacity. The closing capacity is the sum of the closing volume and the residual volume: CC = CV + RV. The closing capacity is expressed as a ratio to the total lung capacity (CC/TLC).

The single-breath nitrogen washout procedure often used is also called the *resident gas* technique. The patient is allowed to sit quietly and breathe room air for several minutes. The patient then exhales completely to the residual volume level. At this point the patient is switched to a 100% oxygen gas source and inhales to the total lung capacity. The patient then exhales slowly into a spirometer system, which measures the nitrogen content of the exhaled gas as well as exhaled volumes. Fig. 5-14 represents a typical recording for the single-breath nitrogen test to measure closing volume. As the patient exhales into the spirometry system, the larger airways (which now hold 100% oxygen)

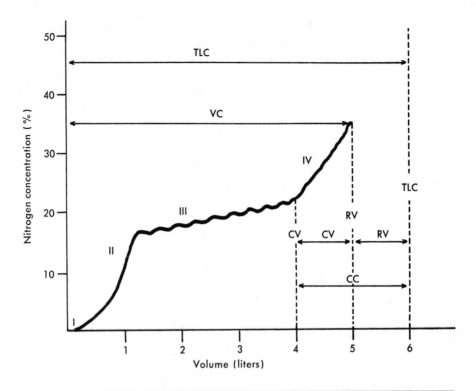

Fig. 5-14   Single-breath nitrogen test curve for measuring closing volume and capacity. *Phase I,* expired dead space gas; *phase II,* mixed dead space and alveolar gas; *phase III,* alveolar plateau; *phase IV,* airway closure.

empty first, followed by the smaller distal airways. These airways tend to collapse in the basal regions of the lung at which point the nitrogen percent of the exhaled air rises abruptly. The volume expired after this rise is the closing volume (phase IV). The increase in nitrogen percent results from the fact that when the basal airways close, exhaled gas will contain a large portion of alveolar gas from the apical lung regions (high nitrogen percent).

Early obstructive airway disease, smoking, and increasing age increase the closing volume above the 15% to 20% of the vital capacity found in normal young adults. The closing capacity usually represents about 30% to 40% of the total lung capacity in healthy adults.

The closing volume can also be increased in patients with moderate to severe restrictive disorders where the closing volume exceeds the functional residual capacity.

Flow volume loops. The flow volume loop is not really a new pulmonary function test but rather a new graphic representation of a maximum forced expiratory flow volume (MEFV) followed by a maximum inspiratory flow volume (MIFV). These are also called peak expiratory flow (PEF) and peak inspiratory flow (PIF), respectively.

The flow volume loops and curves have developed with the use of electronic spirometry in clinical practice. The patient is instructed to perform an expiratory forced vital capacity maneuver followed by an inspiratory forced vital capacity maneuver. The electronic transducer then measures the flow rate and volume simultaneously (see Fig. 5-15).

The initial portion of the MEFV is *effort dependent;* however, after the first third of the expiratory curve, the curve is *effort independent* and reproducible. The effort-independent portion follows the peak expiratory flow rate and is altered in disease changes of both restriction and obstruction (Fig. 5-16).

The predicted values for forced vital capacity, FEV_t, peak flow, etc., are the same as with the conventional values. The expired flows increase rapidly to a peak and then decrease in a somewhat linear fashion.

Patients with obstructive lung disease show low flows. This is true in absolute terms as well as in percent predicted. The inspiratory portion of the curve is more sensitive to central airway obstruction, while the expiratory por-

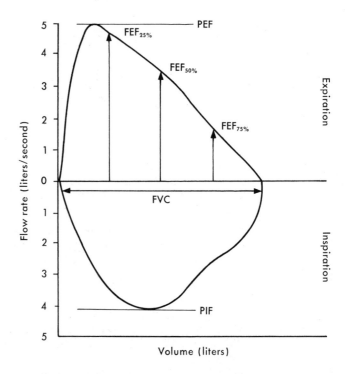

Fig. 5-15   Flow volume loop. *PEF,* peak expiratory flow; *PIF,* peak inspiratory flow; *FEF%,* forced expiratory flow at x% of FVC; *FVC,* forced vital capacity.

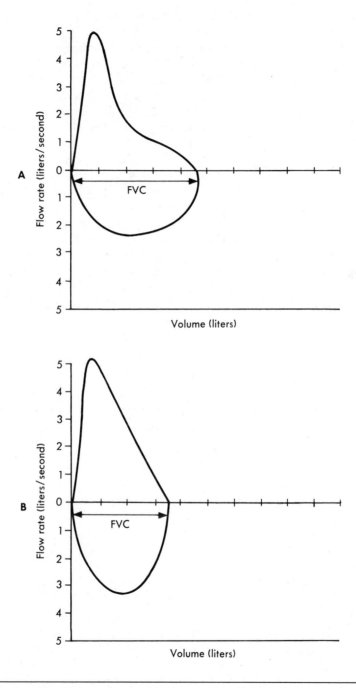

Fig. 5-16   Flow volume loops comparing, **A,** obstructive and, **B,** restrictive disorders.

tion of the curve is more sensitive to peripheral airway obstruction and restrictive disease processes.

The restrictive lung disease processes will show near normal peak expiratory flow volume (FEV$_t$) when compared to the percent forced vital capacity (%FEV$_t$/FVC).

It is debatable whether the flow volume curve (loop) offers new information over that that can be had from the FEV$_t$ and forced expiratory flow tests. The primary advantage is the graphic representation, which may promote an increased understanding of lung function and the related ease of superimposing measurements to evaluate bronchodilator therapy and progression of the disease process (Fig. 5-17).

Diffusing capacity of carbon dioxide (DL$_{CO}$). The diffusing capacity of the lung provides a measure of the amount of functioning pulmonary capillary bed in contact with functioning alveoli. It is a clinical assessment tool to evaluate the lung's gas exchange mechanism. This method of evaluating the movement of gas across the alveolar capillary membrane into the pulmonary blood flow is more a measure of the integrity of the functional lung unit rather than pulmonary mechanics. The *diffusing capacity* is the number of milliliters of a gas that enter the pulmonary blood flow per minute for each mm Hg partial pres-

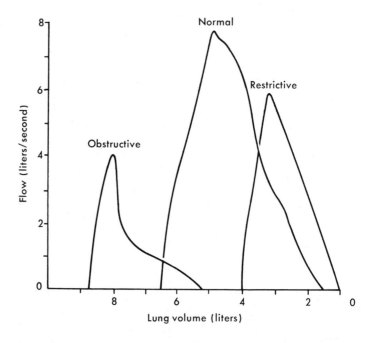

Fig. 5-17   Maximum expiratory flow volume curve example comparing normal with obstructive and restrictive disorders. Displayed as flows at actual lung volumes.

sure difference between the alveoli and pulmonary blood. The diffusing capacity is expressed in ml/min/mm Hg.

Carbon monoxide (CO) has a very high affinity for the hemoglobin molecule and diffuses rapidly into the pulmonary blood flow. In fact, it has an affinity nearly 210 times greater than oxygen for hemoglobin. This high affinity keeps the capillary partial pressure of carbon monoxide very low. As a result, its movement across the alveolar capillary membrane is diffusion limited and *not* limited by a reduction in the ΔP_{CO} diffusion gradient. Clinically, a reduction in the diffusion of carbon monoxide will occur as a result of two major factors: (1) increased "thickness"* of the alveolar capillary membrane and/or (2) decreased functional surface area available for diffusion. In addition, other factors should also be taken into consideration since these can also influence the DL_{CO} measurement:

1. Distribution of inspired gas.
2. PA_{O_2} and PA_{CO_2}.
3. Hematocrit.
4. Pulmonary capillary blood volume.
5. Pulmonary capillary blood flow.

The DL_{CO} is a measure of the transfer of carbon monoxide from the alveoli to the pulmonary blood flow and can be described by the following formula:

$$DL_{CO} = \frac{\text{ml CO transferred/min}}{\text{A-a gradient of CO (mmHg)}}$$

Although several tests can be used to measure diffusing capacity, the single-breath technique is most commonly used. The patient is required to inhale a deep breath of a 0.3% carbon monoxide and 10% helium gas mixture. The patient must inhale from the residual volume level. The patient must hold his or her breath for 10 seconds and exhale. The amount of carbon monoxide that diffuses into the patient's lungs is the difference in the concentration of carbon

Editor's note: Whether actual thickening occurs is debated; however, the membrane does not transfer the gas normally, making it act as though it had an increased distance across from one side to the other.

Table 5-6 Effect of various factors on the diffusing capacity of carbon monoxide	Factor	Diffusing capacity
	↑ Hematocrit (↓)	↑ (↓)
	↑ Pulmonary blood flow (↓)	↑ (↓)
	↑ Exercise level	↑
	↑ Alveolar volume (V_A) (↓)	↑ (↓)
	Diffuse pulmonary fibrosis	↓
	Emphysema	↓
	Pulmonary embolism	↓
	Pulmonary hypertension	↓
	↑ PA_{O_2}	↓
	↑ PA_{CO_2}	↑
	Supine body position	↑

monoxide in the alveolar gas at the end of the 10-second interval and the beginning concentration. Normal diffusing capacity of carbon monoxide is 25 ml/min/mm Hg. As stated before, several factors can alter the DL_{CO} above or below the normal value; a summary of such factors and their influence is provided in Table 5-6.

Further study of the DL_{CO} and the relationship to alveolar volume (V_A) can provide interesting insights into gas exchange and pulmonary pathology. For example, the DL_{CO} is usually reduced in pulmonary emphysema but not chronic bronchitis. This is because of the loss of the alveolar-capillary bed that occurs in emphysema. In chronic bronchitis, the loss of lung parenchyma is minimal and does not alter the DL_{CO}.

Ventilation and perfusion scans. Various ventilation and perfusion studies ($\dot{V}/\dot{Q}$ scans) can be used to measure the gas distribution and pulmonary blood flow in the lungs. The radioxenon (^{133}Xe) method is used to measure regional distribution of ventilation. The patient performs the test in a supine or sitting position. The patient then inhales a normal tidal volume from a closed system containing a specific volume or concentration of ^{133}Xe. The patient holds his or her breath for a 10- to 20-second period of time during which photoscintograms are made over the lung field (Fig. 5-18).

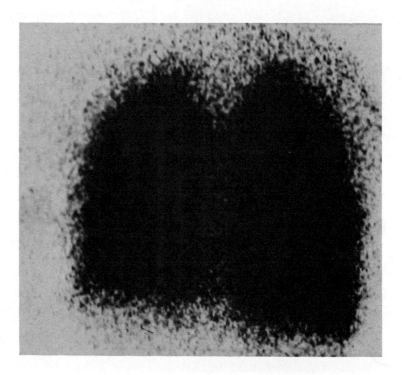

Fig. 5-18 ^{133}Xe ventilation scan showing normal regional distribution of ventilation.

Serial photoscintograms can also be made over a 10- to 15-minute period using a rebreathing technique. This is helpful in determining the rate of equilibrium of gas in the lung. Finally, the patient may be returned to atmospheric breathing and serial photoscintograms made to determine the *washout* of the ^{133}Xe.

Lung perfusion can be studied using microaggregated aluminum particles *tagged* with radioactive iodine (^{131}I). The patient is injected with the iodine preparation and serial photoscintograms are made over the lung fields (Fig. 5-19) as the blood perfuses the lungs.

The ventilation and perfusion scans provide maximum information when used together. Scintilation counters can be used to *quantify* the ventilation and perfusion information. The information describes how the alveolar ventilation and pulmonary perfusion are matched in the patient. In the normal individual, the V/Q scans will show greater ventilation and perfusion in the bases of the lung and less ventilation and perfusion in the apices. The scans can identify areas of the lung not receiving ventilation and/or adequate perfusion.

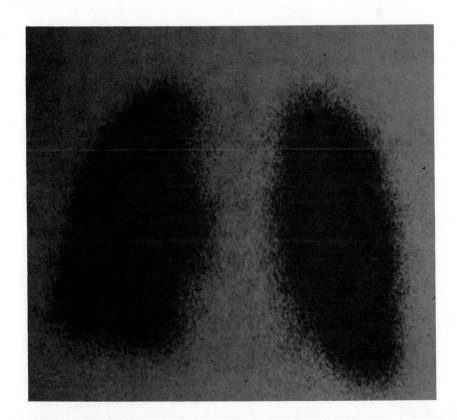

Fig. 5-19 ^{131}I perfusion scan showing normal regional perfusion in the lung.

General interpretation of pulmonary function tests

When interpretating pulmonary function test results, it is imperative to relate the principle of the test to the normal physiology of the lung. For example, the forced expiratory flow tests measure the maximum flow rates during a certain phase of the forced vital capacity maneuver. In essence, one is measuring how fast a gas is moving through a tube, or series of tubes, during a specific time. Those factors that would alter the flow of gas become critical in understanding how and why certain pulmonary disorders will alter the results. The forced expiratory flow will always be reduced in significant obstructive disease processes and yet may be normal in many restrictive lung disorders, because those factors that normally obstruct flow do not exist in many restrictive disorders. However, if the restrictive disease is very severe, the patient may not be able to create sufficient force in the stiff lung to expel gas at a normal rate. Here, the reduced forced expiratory flow is not really a result of obstruction but rather caused by the restricted (stiff) lung. Unless one can reason through *why* certain results are obtained, interpretation can become a confusing and frustrating process. Furthermore, one would not be able to evaluate the validity of the test results. The following section develops a logic format to provide an overall view of pulmonary function test interpretation and the reasoning process involved.

Lung volumes and capacities

In Fig. 5-20, the *vital capacity* can be reduced in both restrictive and obstructive disease processes. Therefore, since the *total lung capacity* is the differential *diagnostic* test, it is included. A normal vital capacity does not rule out early obstructive processes; therefore, the forced vital capacity will test for air trapping, which occurs in early airway disease. In this case, the vital capacity, the forced vital capacity, and the total lung capacity will establish either a normal lung or the primary disease process (obstruction, restriction). In addition, depending on the degree of alteration, combined disease processes can be present.

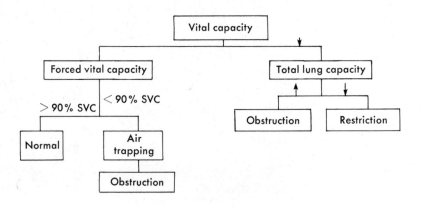

Fig. 5-20 Schematic of lung volumes and capacities. ↓ = decreased or less than normal; ↑ = increased or above normal.

Forced expiratory volumes timed

The FEV_t helps measure the *degree* or severity of the lung malfunction as a result of the underlying pulmonary disease. FEV_t describes the severity of obstructive defects while the vital capacity, forced vital capacity, total lung capacity, and DL_{CO} measure the severity of restrictive processes.

In Fig. 5-21, a normal *FEV_1/FVC* ratio does not rule out either an early or mild airway obstruction, while a decreased ratio does identify the obstruction. The degree of obstruction will depend on the percent of the forced vital capacity the FEV_1 measures. The FEF_{25-75} is specific for the middle to small (peripheral) airways; therefore a reduction in the FEF_{25-75} when the FEV_1/FVC is normal signifies peripheral airway obstruction and disease. Remember that in restrictive disorders the FEV_t values often are within normal range; therefore, the FVC% predicted becomes an important indicator. A normal FEV_1/FVC will usually rule out significant airway and large airway obstruction but *not* early airway disease nor mild peripheral airway obstruction. In pul-

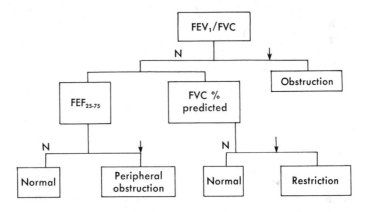

Fig. 5-21   Schematic of forced expiratory volumes timed. N = normal; ↓ = decreased or less than normal.

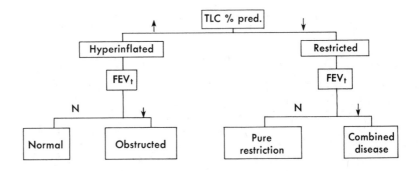

Fig. 5-22   Schematic of total lung capacity as percent of predicted. N = normal; ↓ = decreased or less than normal; ↑ = increased or above normal.

monary function test interpretation the disease process is relatively easy to classify as primarily obstructive or restrictive. However, the role of each disease is difficult to appraise in combined disease processes. For this reason, the total lung capacity expressed as a percent of predicted (TLC% pred.) is probably the most clinically powerful measure in pulmonary function testing.

In Fig. 5-22, the decreased TLC% pred. identified the primary problem as restrictive but did not rule out an obstructive component. By putting together the decreased TLC% pred. and the decreased FEV_t, an interpretation of a combined disease process is apparent.

Bibliography

Ayers, L.N., et al.: A guide to the interpretation of pulmonary function tests, ed. 2, Upper Montclair, N.J., 1978, Projects in Health, Inc.

Bates, D.V., Macklem, P.T., and Christie, R.V.: Respiratory function in disease, ed. 2, Philadelphia, 1971, W.B. Saunders Co.

Blair, H.T.: Clinical indications and usefulness of pulmonary function testing. Medical Grand Rounds, Baylor College of Medicine, Aug. 1975.

Comroe, J.H., et al.: The lung, ed. 2, Chicago, 1962, Year Book Medical Publishers, Inc.

Cotes, J.E.: Lung function: assessment and application in medicine, ed. 4, Oxford, England, 1979, Blackwell Scientific Publications.

Craig, D.B., et al.: Closing volume and its relationship to gas exchange in seated and supine positions, J. Appl. Physiol. **31**:717, 1971.

Fishman, A., editor: Assessment of pulmonary function, New York, 1980, McGraw-Hill Book Co.

Hunsinger, D.L., et al.: Respiratory technology: a procedure manual, ed. 2, Reston, Va., 1976, Reston Publishing Co., Inc.

Morris, J.F., et al.: Prediction nomogram (BTPS), spirometric values in normal males and females, Am. Rev. Resp. Dis. **103**:57, 1971.

Petty, T.L.: Pulmonary diagnostic techniques, Philadelphia, 1975, Lea & Febiger.

Rarey, K.P., and Youtsey, J.W.: Respiratory patient care, Englewood Cliffs, N.J., 1981, Prentice-Hall, Inc.

Ruppel, G.: Manual of pulmonary function testing, ed. 2, St. Louis, 1979, The C.V. Mosby Co.

Seaton, A.N., et al.: Lung perfusion scanning in coal workers pneumoconiosis, Am. Rev. Resp. Dis. **103**:338-348, 1971.

Slonim, N.B., and Hamilton, L.H.: Respiratory physiology, ed. 4, St. Louis, 1981, The C.V. Mosby Co.

West, J.B.: Pulmonary pathophysiology: the essentials, Baltimore, 1977, The Williams & Wilkins Co.

Chapter 6 — Blood gases, control of ventilation, and acid-base balance

---

The natural mechanisms of ventilation in good health and the techniques of respiratory therapy in the treatment of disease are designed to provide the circulating blood with sufficient oxygen for general cellular needs and to remove excess carbon dioxide. Failure to satisfy these two requirements subjects the blood to a reduced oxygen content *(hypoxemia)*, deprives tissue cells of oxygen *(hypoxia)*, and allows abnormal amounts of carbon dioxide to accumulate in the blood *(hypercapnia)*. Excessive ventilation or therapy, on the other hand, can overload the body with oxygen *(hyperoxemia, hyperoxia)* and reduce blood carbon dioxide to abnormally low levels *(hypocapnia)*.

In this chapter we review the principles governing the actual movement of respiratory gases into and out of the circulation, the transportation systems that carry the gases between lung and body, and the intricate neurochemical mechanism that regulates spontaneous breathing. The influence of respiratory gases on the stability of the acid-base balance of the body is also included as an integral part of the overall study of blood gases.

Mechanics of diffusion

Our study of the physiology of the respiratory tract has brought us to that critically vital structure, the perfused alveolus. So far we have been concerned with factors responsible for the mass movement of air from the atmosphere into the conducting airways. With air in the alveoli, we now consider the mechanisms by which oxygen is extracted and made available to the body in exchange for carbon dioxide. For this we have to think microscopically, for we are dealing with gases at the molecular level and with the physical and chemical reactions in which they take part in their travels to and from body cells. We first review the manner in which the respiratory gases overcome the boundary between the "inside" and the "outside" of the body, the alveolar wall, by the process of diffusion.

Diffusion is the movement of gas molecules from an area of relatively high partial pressure of the gas to one of low partial pressure. As all motion requires some driving force, so diffusion depends on a pressure gradient. The two gases with which we are concerned, oxygen and carbon dioxide, not only must diffuse from one anatomic area to another but must also move through formidable obstructions—the alveolar wall–pulmonary capillary barrier (sometimes called the alveolar-capillary [A-C] membrane) and the body cell wall–systemic capillary barrier.[1] Thus, for gases to pass between the alveoli and the pulmonary capillary blood, there must exist a pressure gradient for each gas across this barrier. The production and magnitude of these gradients are of great concern to us from here on. Fig. 6-1 illustrates the nature and structure of the A-C barrier, and if we keep in mind the minuscule size of a molecule of gas, we must be impressed with the task facing it in making the obstacle-ridden trip between alveolus and blood, and blood and tissue cell.

Since the A-C membrane is essentially a fluid barrier, the ability of gases to diffuse through it depends on two physical laws governing the passage of gas through liquid:

1. *Henry's law* states that the weight of a gas dissolving in a liquid at a given temperature is proportional to the partial pressure of the gas. The amount of gas that can be dissolved by 1 ml of a given liquid at standard pressure and specified temperature is called its *solubility coefficient* and varies *inversely* with the temperature. The solubility coefficient of oxygen in plasma, at 37°C and 760 mm Hg pressure, is 0.023 ml, and for carbon dioxide is 0.510 ml.

2. *Graham's law* states that the rate of diffusion (D) of a gas through liquid is directly proportional to its solubility coefficient and inversely proportional to the square root of its density (or gram molecular weight). The number of milliliters of a gas that will diffuse a distance of 0.001 mm (1μ), over a square centimeter surface per minute, at 1 atm of pressure, is the *diffusion coefficient* of the gas.

Combining these two properties, we can say that the relative rates of diffusion of two gases are directly proportional to the ratio of their solubilities and inversely proportional to the ratio of the square roots of their densities or gram molecular weights. To illustrate this, let us compare the relative diffusi-

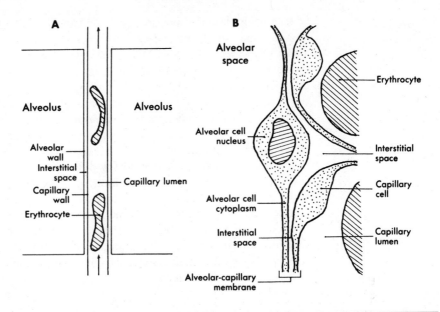

Fig. 6-1   **A** diagrams the relationship between the components of the alveolar-capillary (A-C) membrane, and **B** is a magnification sketch of a section through the structure. The *alveolar wall* is a cytoplasmic extension of the alveolar epithelial cells; it is separated from the adjacent capillary epithelial cells by a space, which may be real or potential, called the *interstitial* or intermembranous space. This space may contain tissue fibrils, and the accumulation of fluid here is of great clinical importance. The thickness of the A-C membrane varies from 0.4μ to 2.0μ, depending on the contents of the space. (Modified from Divertie, M.D., and Brown, A.L., Jr.: J.A.M.A. **187**:938, 1964.)

bility of carbon dioxide with oxygen or, to state it another way, determine how much more or less diffusible is carbon dioxide than oxygen:

$$\text{Diffusibility of CO}_2 \cong \frac{\text{Sol coef CO}_2 \times \sqrt{\text{gmw O}_2}}{\text{Sol coef O}_2 \times \sqrt{\text{gmw CO}_2}}$$

$$\cong \frac{0.510 \times \sqrt{32}}{0.023 \times \sqrt{44}}$$

$$\cong \frac{0.510 \times 5.657}{0.023 \times 6.663}$$

$$\cong \frac{19}{1}$$

In other words, carbon dioxide is 19 times as diffusible as oxygen.

Exercise 6-1: Given the following data, what is the diffusibility of gas B compared with gas A?

	Gas A	Gas B
Sol coef	0.25	0.65
gmw	30	50

In cardiopulmonary physiology, knowledge of the diffusing capacity of the lung is sometimes helpful in evaluating pathologic conditions. The expression *diffusion capacity of the lung* (D_L) is defined as the number of milliliters of a specific gas that diffuse from the lung across the A-C membrane into the bloodstream each minute, for each mm Hg difference in the pressure gradient across the membrane. The two most common gases used to measure this function are low-concentration carbon *monoxide* (CO) and oxygen, and in reporting values obtained we must identify the gas used. Thus average normal values are $D_{L_{CO}}$ = 17 ml/min/mm Hg and $D_{L_{O_2}}$ = 20 ml/min/mm Hg.[2]

Disease of the lung, if it modifies diffusion at all, almost always reduces diffusion. This implies that some abnormality has made it difficult for gas molecules to cross the A-C membrane in a reasonable period of time, in response to a normal pressure gradient. Some rare causes of elevated diffusion capacity have occurred with polycythemia rubra vera, with people born and living at high altitude, many years after a pneumonectomy (one lung removed), and questionably with certain asthmatics. The clinical implications of this fact are discussed further in Chapter 8.

Diffusion gradients

The pressure gradient across the A-C membrane is essential for gas diffusion. It is dependent on the concentrations of the gases in the inspired air and alveoli, as well as in the blood. Since there is a continuous interchange in the alveoli of oxygen and carbon dioxide, each diluting the other, the alveolar concentrations of these gases are considerably different from their atmospheric concentrations. Table 6-1 presents some average normal values for *dry* inspired, alveolar, and exhaled air.

Corrected for the saturated state of these gases in the alveoli, their alveolar partial pressures (P_A) at 1 atm are about:

O_2	CO_2	N_2	H_2O
100 mm Hg	40 mm Hg	573 mm Hg	47 mm Hg

At the circulatory end of the gradient, the respiratory gases in the blood also exert their own partial pressures. Although the transportation and utilization of the gases have not yet been discussed, we know that venous blood returning to the lung has less oxygen and more carbon dioxide than does arterial blood. Therefore the partial pressures will differ between the types of blood. The average normal venous (Pv) and arterial (Pa) partial pressures are

Table 6-1 Composition of dry inspired, alveolar, and exhaled air		**%O₂**	**%CO₂**	**%N₂, etc.**[3]
	Inspired air	20.95	0.03	79.02
	Alveolar air	14.0	5.6	80.4
	Exhaled air	16.3	4.5	79.2

shown in Table 6-2. If reference is made to oxygen or carbon dioxide tension in blood generally, without regard for its arterial or venous character, gas tensions may be symbolized as PO_2 or PCO_2.

An explanation is in order for the 90 to 100 mm Hg range of arterial oxygen tension listed in Table 6-2. The average Pa_{O_2} of a large number of normal subjects would probably fall at about 95 *mm Hg*, in a range that would extend from 90 mm Hg to perhaps 103 mm Hg. If the lung were a "perfect" organ, every alveolus would have exactly the same PO_2 and the arterial blood leaving each alveolus would, through the process of diffusion to be described below, have exactly the same PO_2 as each alveolus, about 100 mm Hg. The lung, however, is not perfect, and normally there are slight discrepancies between the ratios of ventilation to perfusion among the many A-C units. As a result, a sample of mixed arterial blood (blood from all areas of the lung returning to the heart for distribution through the systemic circulation) often has an oxygen tension less than that of an air sample taken from the lungs as a whole. For the sake of uniformity, mixed arterial blood will be assumed to have an oxygen tension of 95 mm Hg, the 5 mm Hg difference between it and alveolar oxygen tension constituting a normal *alveolar-arterial oxygen tension gradient*. This term is used again later, with both normal and abnormal connotations. However, when describing physiologic events at the level of a single alveolus and its capillary, we will assume in the interest of simplicity that the A-C unit is "perfect" unless otherwise specified and that the local capillary-arterial oxygen tension is 100 mm Hg.

It should be noted that blood values for nitrogen partial pressure were not included. This by no means indicates that such a pressure does not exist. However, as far as the physiology of respiration is concerned, nitrogen is an *inert* gas in that it takes no part in metabolic gas exchange. It can be considered as a filler, taking up whatever space is not used by the two respiratory gases. Nitrogen diffuses readily between alveoli and blood, and the partial pressure it exerts is the difference between (1) the sum of the respiratory gas pressures and the atmospheric pressure and (2) the water vapor pressure. Nitrogen is of medical importance under certain circumstances and is discussed further when indicated.

We can now correlate the above data on partial pressures and show how they make up gradients to promote a continuous and relatively smooth diffusion of respiratory gases. Consider the alveolus as a small pump that is constantly drawing in oxygen (air) and expelling carbon dioxide, thus maintaining alveolar partial pressures at *average* levels as described previously. At any given moment the pressures in the alveolus will vary according to the time of the

Table 6-2				
Gas partial pressures in venous and arterial blood	Pv_{O_2}	40 mm Hg	Pa_{O_2}	90-100 mm Hg
	Pv_{CO_2}	46 mm Hg	Pa_{CO_2}	40 mm Hg

ventilatory cycle (or cycling of the alveolar pump), but samples of alveolar air over many cycles determine these average partial pressures. Two pressure gradient systems are established, one between alveolar oxygen (100 mm Hg) and venous oxygen (40 mm Hg) and a smaller one between venous carbon dioxide (46 mm Hg) and alveolar carbon dioxide (40 mm Hg). Oxygen, with its partial pressure maintained through the alveolar pump, diffuses from the alveolus into the pulmonary blood, *equilibrating* the PO_2 of the blood with that of the alveolus. As the blood flows past the alveolus, it thus takes up oxygen and leaves the capillary as *arterialized* blood, with a PO_2 in equilibrium with the alveolar oxygen, around 100 mm Hg. Simultaneously, carbon dioxide flows from the pulmonary capillary with its PCO_2 of 46 mm Hg into the alveolus with its average PCO_2 of 40 mm Hg. Again, the alveolar pump, by the regulated exhalation of carbon dioxide, maintains the gradient until the capillary blood has equilibrated with the alveolus, and the arterialized blood leaves the capillary with a PCO_2 of 40 mm Hg. Fig. 6-2 illustrates the "perfect" diffusion gradients across the A-C membrane and the manner in which venous blood becomes arterialized.

The element of time is a critical factor in the diffusion of oxygen, although it is not directly related to the ability of the A-C membrane to exchange the gas. For blood to leave the pulmonary capillary adequately oxygenated, not only is the integrity of the membrane important but the blood must spend sufficient time in contact with the membrane to permit maximum diffusion. In

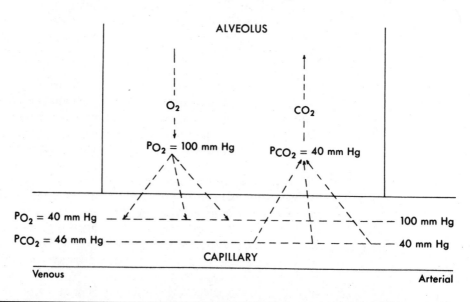

Fig. 6-2   Ventilation maintains the mean alveolar gas tensions as noted in the sketch. As blood enters the venous end of the pulmonary capillary, it loses its carbon dioxide and takes up oxygen, until these two gases are in equilibrium with the mean alveolar tensions, and it leaves the capillary as arterial blood.

the normal subject at rest, it takes about 0.75 second for a given point in the bloodstream to traverse the pulmonary capillary, and with the increased velocity of heavy exercise, about 0.34 second.[4] Most oxygen diffusion occurs at the beginning of the capillary; thus it would require a very severe diffusion defect to be solely responsible for inadequate oxygenation. However, since such pathologic conditions as fever, acute blood loss, and certain cardiac irregularities can increase the cardiac output and blood velocity, it is reasonable to suppose that when associated with sufficient pulmonary disease, the rapid flow of blood through the pulmonary capillaries might be a significant contributing factor to incomplete oxygenation.

Our discussion of gradients so far has centered about the A-C membrane, but for a clear picture of diffusion we must include the equally important gradients at the tissue cellular level, for it is to service the cells that the ventilation-transportation system exists. The respiratory gas gradients at the cell can be visualized as the reverse of those in the lung. As the metabolism of the cell depletes its store of oxygen, the intracellular PO_2 drops below that of the blood entering the arterial end of the systemic capillary, and oxygen diffuses into the cell. At the same time the carbon dioxide diffuses from its higher pressure level in the cell into the capillary blood, and the blood becomes venous, returning to the lung to repeat its circuit. In a sense we are dealing with two sets of gradients (alveolar-blood and blood-cell, for both oxygen and carbon dioxide) that provide gas transportation between the extremes of the two wider gradients of alveolus-cell for oxygen and cell-alveolus for carbon dioxide.

Oxygen transportation	The mechanism by which oxygen is carried between the alveolus and the body cell is discussed first, followed by a description of the transportation of carbon dioxide. It must be clearly understood that these two processes occur simultaneously, and it is only for convenience and clarity that we are separating them. Both gases are carried in the blood by virtue of their abilities to dissolve in blood or to combine with some of the elements of blood. An understanding of basic principles of gas transportation is essential for the safe and intelligent treatment of cardiopulmonary defects. Oxygen is carried in the blood in two "compartments." One is the blood plasma, in which oxygen is dissolved in very small but important amounts, and the other is the hemoglobin of the erythrocyte, which carries the bulk of the load.
Dissolved oxygen	As oxygen molecules diffuse into the blood, some go directly into solution in the plasma, and when this compartment is filled, the rest continue into the erythrocytes. The amount of oxygen that dissolves depends on the solubility coefficient of oxygen in plasma at body temperature. Thus for every 760 mm Hg pressure, 0.023 ml of oxygen dissolves in each milliliter of plasma. It is customary to refer to dissolved blood gases in terms of *volume percent* (vol%), which means so many *milliliters of gas per 100 ml of plasma*. Ml/dl could also be

used, but vol% is more common. Therefore for every 760 mm Hg pressure, there are 2.3 vol% of dissolved oxygen, and this can be reduced to the basic factor of 0.003 vol% for *each* millimeter of mercury PO_2. Calculation of the amount of oxygen that dissolves in plasma at any PO_2 is simply: *Vol% = PO_2 × 0.003*. In average normal arterial blood, with its PaO_2 of 95 to 100 mm Hg, the dissolved oxygen equals 0.3 ml of oxygen for each 100 ml of plasma. However, the PaO_2 of a subject breathing pure oxygen theoretically could reach 673 mm Hg, with dissolved oxygen of 2.02 vol%. The value of 673 is reached as follows: Recalling that physiologic gases are calculated in the dry state and assuming complete alveolar-arterial equilibrium with no PO_2 gradient, we can calculate that the alveolar gases of a subject breathing pure oxygen at 1 atm have a pressure of 760 − 47 = 713 mm Hg (atmospheric pressure − water vapor pressure). After a subject has breathed 100% oxygen for several minutes, nitrogen that was in the alveoli during air breathing is completely washed out, leaving only oxygen and carbon dioxide. With a carbon dioxide tension of 40 mm Hg, alveolar (and presumably arterial) oxygen tension equals 713 − 40, or 673 mm Hg. A method of estimating PA_{O_2} at

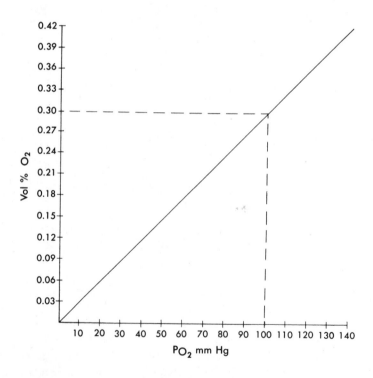

Fig. 6-3   The relationship between the number of milliliters of oxygen dissolved in blood and its consequent partial pressure is linear. Each 0.003 ml of oxygen dissolved in 100 ml of blood (vol% of O_2) exerts a pressure of 1 mm Hg. The *dashed line* emphasizes the fact that arterial blood, with an average PO_2 of 100 mm Hg, has 0.3 ml of oxygen dissolved in each 100 ml.

any concentration of inhaled oxygen employs the *alveolar air equation,* which is not considered at this time (see Appendix 12). Fig. 6-3 illustrates, by graph, the linear relationship between partial pressure of oxygen and volume percent of oxygen dissolved in the plasma.

Combined oxygen   Most of the oxygen in the body is carried physically bound to or combined with the *hemoglobin* (Hb) of the erythrocytes. Hemoglobin is the "red stuff" of the blood, giving to blood its characteristic colors, and except in abnormal conditions, it is always confined to the erythrocyte. Should disease or disturbed physiology produce rupture of the red cells, the spillage of hemoglobin into the plasma is referred to as *hemolysis* of the cell with subsequent *hemoglobinemia.* Hemoglobin is a protein, *globin,* combined with an iron-containing compound called *heme.* The large and heavy molecule has a *physical* molecular weight of 66,700, but in its respiratory function its *physiologic* molecular weight is considered to be only 16,700. There are many different kinds of hemoglobin, designated by letters A, C, E, F, G, H, I, J, K, and S. Some of these types are variants of the normal; others are clinically pathologic. The differences in the hemoglobin types lie in the structure of the globin portion, which is made up of many amino acids derived from diet.

We will soon see that the transportation of oxygen and of carbon dioxide in the erythrocyte are mutually dependent on one another, since they alternate in using hemoglobin as a carrier; but first we consider oxygen alone and then relate the two systems.

Venous blood leaving the body cells still contains some oxygen, enough to maintain a partial pressure of about 40 mm Hg, but because of its depleted oxygen supply, most of its hemoglobin is called *reduced hemoglobin.* This is often symbolized simply as *Hb* or more properly as *HHb,* since it has acquired a hydrogen ion in its participation in the transport of carbon dioxide from the cells. In the pulmonary capillaries, immediately on release of carbon dioxide, the HHb converts to the potassium salt, *KHb.* In this form hemoglobin combines with oxygen molecules diffusing into the erythrocytes, becoming *oxyhemoglobin,* Hb_{O_2}, or better, KHb_{O_2}. One gram-molecular weight of oxygen, 32 g, can combine with 16,700 g of hemoglobin, and this factor determines the physiologic molecular weight of hemoglobin as noted above. Because

$$\frac{1 \text{ mole } O_2}{16,700 \text{ g Hb}} = \frac{22,400 \text{ ml } O_2}{16,700 \text{ g Hb}} = \frac{1.34 \text{ ml } O_2}{\text{g Hb}}$$

each gram of hemoglobin is able to take up and carry 1.34 ml of oxygen.* If we assume a normal hemoglobin concentration of 15 g/dl blood, the combined oxygen *capacity* is 1.34 × 15 = 20.1 ml O_2/dl blood, or *20.1 vol%,* and is directly related to the amount and quality of available hemoglobin.

*Editor's note: Some controversy exists concerning the amount of oxygen that can combine with hemoglobin. Some investigators believe that the theoretic maximum is 1.39 ml/g hemoglobin, although in practice this number was not obtained.[5,6] The value of 1.34 is still commonly used and, therefore, retained for this section.[7-10]

However, the quantity or content of oxygen actually carried is dependent on the hemoglobin *saturation*. This refers to the amount of oxygen combined with hemoglobin in proportion to the amount of oxygen the hemoglobin is capable of carrying if it has its full load. It is expressed as a percentage from the ratio content/capacity. Although the capacity can be calculated as above if the presence of abnormal or inactive hemoglobin is suspected, in the laboratory the oxygen content can be chemically analyzed in volume percent; then by exposing the sample to air to allow it to combine maximally with oxygen, we can determine its capacity. If the content is one half the capacity, the saturation is reported as 50%. Because the lung is not a "perfect" organ, in the normal subject breathing room air at 1 atm pressure, the average saturation of mixed arterial blood ($S\bar{a}_{O_2}$) is about 97%, and the average saturation of mixed venous blood entering the lung through the pulmonary circulation ($S\bar{v}_{O_2}$) is about 70% to 75%. *Unsaturation* is the converse of saturation and refers to the degree to which blood is not saturated. Thus normal arterial blood may be considered to be 3% unsaturated, and venous blood, 30% unsaturated. Since saturation equals content/capacity, then content equals capacity times saturation, and the amount of oxygen combined with hemoglobin in average normal arterial blood with 15 g/dl hemoglobin equals:

$$1.34 \times 15 \times 0.97 = 19.5 \text{ vol\%}$$

It is worth our while to spend a moment here to clarify the mechanisms responsible for the normal 97% hemoglobin oxygen saturation of mixed arterial blood leaving the lungs. When there is no impediment to the diffusion of a normal amount of oxygen under normal pressure across the alveolar-capillary membrane, failure of mixed arterial blood to show 100% saturation of its available hemoglobin is the result of venous blood mixing with it. This combination is called a *venous admixture,* and it may be the result of a physical or anatomic shunt or a *ventilation/perfusion imbalance.*

Shunt. A condition whereby venous blood physically bypasses the lung without perfusing ventilated alveoli is termed a *right-* (venous blood) *to-left* (arterial blood) *shunt.* The mixed venous-arterial blood has a lower oxygen content and saturation than does pure arterial blood. Two normal anatomic shunts contribute to the 3% arterial unsaturation, and they are referred to as physiologic because they are not a result of pathologic conditions.[5]

Thebesian venous drainage. Thebesian veins are very small vessels that drain the myocardium and empty through minute openings into both atria. Those that communicate with the left atrium mix venous blood with arterial and may provide a major part of the normal arterial unsaturation.

Bronchial venous drainage. The airways, like all other body tissues, are perfused by the systemic circulation through the bronchial arteries and veins. Bronchial venous drainage, however, is quite unorthodox, and most of it enters the pulmonary veins (arterialized blood) directly, with only a few identifiable bronchial veins joining azygous and intercostal venous systems. Here, then, is another source of venous admixture to keep arterial oxygen saturation below 100%.

Ventilation/perfusion imbalance. Positional underventilation in proportion to perfusion of some alveoli may find venous blood perfusing incompletely ventilated lung tissue. Thus partially unsaturated blood mixes with fully saturated blood from other areas, creating a venous admixture. Such a phenomenon is likely to be found in dependent lung segments, especially during periods of relatively shallow breathing.

Pathologic shunts and ventilation/perfusion ratios are considered in Chapter 8.

Determinants of oxygen saturation	Let us now consider those factors responsible for determining the degree of arterial oxygen saturation—*partial pressure of arterial oxygen, hydrogen ion concentration of the blood (pH), body temperature, organic phosphates, and fetal hemoglobin.* One of the most important fundamentals of pulmonary physiology is the relationship between oxygen saturation and these factors, graphically illustrated in the *oxygen dissociation curves,* which indicate the physiologic conditions under which oxygen combines with or dissociates from its hemoglobin carrier. When all the elements of ventilation, pulmonary air distribution, ventilation/perfusion ratio, and alveolar diffusion are able to achieve a PO_2 or 100 mm Hg in arterial blood with a normal pH of 7.40 at body temperature, the arterial oxygen saturation will be approximately 97%.

Partial pressure of oxygen. Fig. 6-4 is the dissociation curve of blood at 37°C, showing the important relationship between PO_2 and SO_2 at three pH values. For the moment we will concern ourselves only with the middle curve. The dissociation curve is not linear like that of the dissolved oxygen graph but is doubly curved. The upper end of the curve slopes gently downward to the left for a distance and then becomes steep in its middle segment. The line at PO_2 of 100 mm Hg meets the normal pH 7.40 curve at a point corresponding to a SO_2 or 97%. Even if some abnormality reduced the PO_2 to 65 mm Hg, arterial blood would still be 90% saturated, but if the curve were linear, the SO_2 would be only about 64%. The relatively flat upper part of the curve prevents wide fluctuations in saturation (and thus in content) in the presence of oxygen tension drop resulting from disease or environmental abnormalities, but below PO_2 of 50 mm Hg, the drop in saturation becomes precipitous.

When arterial blood perfuses body tissues and equilibrates with the oxygen-poor cells, its PO_2 drops to the venous level of about 40 mm Hg and its saturation to approximately 73%, but on its return to the lung, where it equilibrates with the alveolar PA_{O_2} of about 100 mm Hg, it again becomes 97% saturated. This portion of the curve, between PO_2 of 100 mm Hg and 40 mm Hg, represents the loading and unloading of oxygen in the lung and at the body cell. If we stipulate a hemoglobin content of 15 g/dl, assume complete oxygen equilibration between blood and both lung and tissue cell, and assume that the pH remains at 7.40 (actually there is a slight shift of about 0.03 pH unit as blood varies between venous and arterial), we can calculate the total

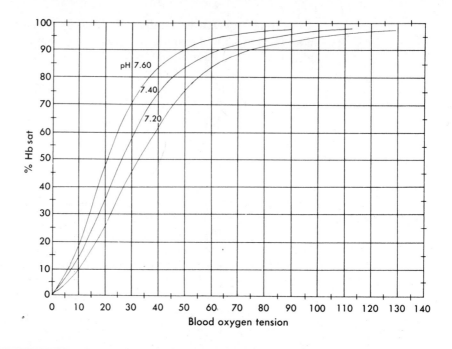

Fig. 6-4   Oxygen dissociation curve of blood at 37°C, showing variations at three pH levels. For a given oxygen tension, the higher the blood pH, the more the hemoglobin holds onto its oxygen, maintaining a higher saturation.

Table 6-3
Oxygen content of arterial and venous blood

	Vol% arterial O_2	Vol% venous O_2
Combined O_2 (1.34 × 15 × Sat)	19.5	14.7
Dissolved O_2 (Po_2 × 0.003)	0.3	0.1
TOTAL O_2 CONTENT	19.8	14.8

volumes percent of oxygen (combined plus dissolved) in both arterial and venous blood, as in Table 6-3.

This arterial-venous (a-v) difference of 5 vol% represents the amount of oxygen given up to tissue cells and is referred to as the *average oxygen uptake.* Obviously, the uptake of all body cells at one time is not the same, but the blood reflects the mean of the body as a whole. When physiologic abnormalities cause a low Pa_{O_2} breathing room air, the resulting drop in arterial saturation can often be corrected by so elevating the alveolar Po_2 with high oxygen concentrations that the Pa_{O_2} will rise toward the upper end of the dissociation curve. Because of the continuing flattening of the upper curve, increasing Pa_{O_2} values produce reducing increments of increase in saturation of hemoglobin, and 100% saturation is finally reached at Pa_{O_2} of about 340 mm Hg.

Hydrogen ion concentration of the blood (pH). The mechanism and clinical significance of blood pH changes are discussed later, but it should be explained here that the path and shape of the oxygen dissociation curve depend on pH as well as on blood oxygen tension and saturation. An increase in $[H^+]$ (drop in pH) moves the curve to the right, and a decrease (rise in pH) moves it to the left, an immediate effect of the direct action of hydrogen ions on the hemoglobin molecule. This is known as the *Bohr effect,* and it demonstrates that hydrogen ions decrease the ability of hemoglobin to hold onto oxygen. Thus, as blood pH drops (increase in $[H^+]$), oxygen is released to the cells, and saturation at a given PO_2 is lowered. Conversely, with a rising pH (decrease in $[H^+]$) the affinity of hemoglobin for oxygen is increased, saturation remains high, and oxygen is less available to the cells.

Even within the narrow range in which blood alternates between arterial and venous, the Bohr effect has physiologic importance. As noted previously, blood pH varies about 0.03 pH unit between venous and arterial, and this is illustrated in Fig. 6-5, which shows a segment of the normal dissociation curve. As blood becomes venous, ⓥ, its increased carbon dioxide content raises $[H^+]$ and lowers pH by a mechanism described in the next section. As a result, the oxygen curve moves slightly to the right, and at a given PO_2 shows a lower SO_2 than does the pH 7.40 curve, indicating release to the tissues of a greater volume of oxygen. In the lung, arterialized blood, ⓐ, loses carbon dioxide, its pH rises, and it has an increased affinity for oxygen. The Bohr effect thus facilitates pulmonary uptake and tissue delivery of oxygen.

Fig. 6-5 illustrates variation in the shape and position of the oxygen dissociation curve with wide ranges of pH. Given a Pa_{O_2} of 50 mm Hg, there is a difference of 15% saturation between pH 7.20 and 7.60. Variations in blood pH alone, with no change in oxygenation, can modify the oxygen content/

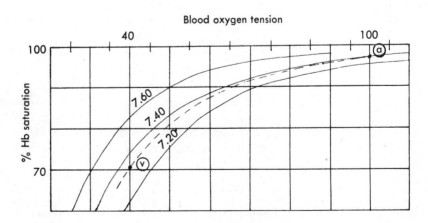

Fig. 6-5   Bohr effect. The *dashed line* indicates the physiologic shift in oxygen dissociation curve as changing blood carbon dioxide content alters blood pH between arterial, ⓐ, and venous, ⓥ, points.

capacity ratio of hemoglobin; or, to put it another way, the affinity of hemoglobin for oxygen is dependent on the pH of the blood. For example, in acidosis, the curve shows us that severe unsaturation of hemoglobin with oxygen may exist even with a near normal PO_2. A clinically important observation can be made from the effects of the pH shifts of the dissociation curve. For a given PO_2, because the blood is able to maintain a higher oxygen saturation in a state of alkalosis than in acidosis, alkalosis might seem to be a distinct advantage to the body economy and suggest the desirability of that state as a preventative of hypoxemia. However, let us compare the performances of both the pH 7.60 and pH 7.20 dissociation curves in a hypothetical situation. We again assume a hemoglobin concentration of 15 g/dl and complete oxygen equilibration at PO_2 of 100 mm Hg and 40 mm Hg, for arterial and venous blood, respectively. From the dissociation curves, we read oxygen saturations of 98% for arterial blood and 84% for venous blood at pH of 7.60 and corresponding saturations of 94% and 62% at pH of 7.20. We can now compute the a-v oxygen difference between the alveoli and tissue cells for each abnormal pH value, comparing them with the normal, as outlined in Table 6-4.

There is less than 1 vol% of oxygen difference between alkalotic and acidotic arterial blood, but after tissue perfusion the a-v oxygen difference of acidotic blood is more than double that for alkalotic. The important inference here is that alkalotic blood does not dissociate readily but rather holds onto its oxygen, making the oxygen less available to body cells than does normal or acidotic blood. This does not mean that acidosis is beneficial just because it releases oxygen more freely, for we will see that the acidotic state is generally a very unwholesome condition for the entire body physiology. Close inspection of the dissociation curves shows that if the arterial blood has a very low oxygen tension (40 to 50 mm Hg), the oxygen uptake difference between alkalotic and acidotic blood, at venous levels of 10 to 20 mm Hg PO_2, is much less than at normal arterial values, but acidotic blood still releases more oxygen. The objective of respiratory therapy treatment is to restore physiology as close to normal as possible.

P_{50}. Shifting positions of the oxygen dissociation curve are sometimes referred to as changes in the P_{50}. This is the partial pressure of blood oxygen that half saturates hemoglobin, providing 10 vol% of oxygen bound to hemoglobin. As shown in Fig. 6-4, the P_{50} of the normal middle curve is *26.5 mm Hg*. In contrast, the P_{50} of blood with a pH of 7.60 is about 20.5 mm Hg and with a pH of 7.20, about 32 mm Hg. A dissociation curve that shifts to the left is said to have a low P_{50} and to the right, a high P_{50}. A low value

Table 6-4		Total vol% arterial O_2	Total vol% venous O_2	a-v vol% O_2
Arterial-venous oxygen difference at three pH levels	pH 7.60	20.0	17.0	3.0
	pH 7.40	19.8	14.8	5.0
	pH 7.20	19.2	12.6	6.6

tells us that something has happened to increase the affinity of hemoglobin for oxygen. The hemoglobin holds the oxygen more firmly than normal, and less pressure is needed to bind the two. It is harder for oxygen to dissociate from hemoglobin, thus its availability to tissues is reduced. A high P_{50} tells us that something has weakened hemoglobin's intrinsic ability to hold on to oxygen and that a higher gas pressure is needed for binding. Oxygen escapes hemoglobin more easily and is more readily available to tissues. We can say therefore that a high pH, or a low [H^+], produces a low P_{50} oxygen dissociation curve (leftward shift), and a low pH, or high [H^+], produces a high P_{50} curve (rightward shift).

Body temperature. Fig. 6-6 illustrates the influence of body temperature on oxygen saturation and dissociation. It is customary to measure oxygen tension at a temperature of 37°C, then by the use of tabulated factors or nomograms, correct tension and saturation to the patient's actual temperature. Many combinations of pH and temperature can produce a host of possible curves. The therapeutic use of low body temperature (hypothermia) employs the principle of reduced oxygen need and utilization under conditions of cooling. This effect is evident in the lower a-v oxygen differences shown on the low-temperature dissociation curve. (Compare with pH effect described previously.)

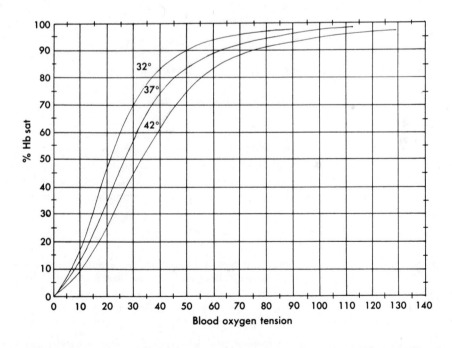

Fig. 6-6   Oxygen dissociation curve of blood at a pH of 7.40, showing variations at three temperatures. For a given oxygen tension, the lower the temperature, the more the hemoglobin holds onto its oxygen, maintaining a higher saturation.

Organic phosphates. In the area of general metabolism, organic phosphate compounds play vital roles in many cellular biochemical reactions and are essential to the transfer of energy on which cellular function depends. Within the past few years, attention has been directed to the involvement of phosphates in respiration. The two most significant organic phosphates in this reference are *2,3-diphosphoglycerate (DPG)* and *adenosine triphosphate (ATP)*. In the interest of brevity and because of its relatively greater importance, we describe DPG as the prototype.[11-17]

DPG is found *in the erythrocyte,* where it is formed as one of the chief end products of glucose metabolism, and it is bound to unsaturated hemoglobin. Like hydrogen ions, *DPG decreases the affinity of hemoglobin for oxygen,* high levels expediting oxygen release and low levels its retention by hemoglobin. By chemical measurement, its normal concentration is 4.0 to 5.25 mEq/ℓ of erythrocytes.

DPG shifts the oxygen dissociation curve to the right (high P_{50}) to promote oxygen unloading at the tissues. Three factors modify the action of DPG:

Hypoxia. DPG concentration increases with hypoxia ot any cause, shifting the dissociation curve to the right to make up for the hypoxia by increasing the availability of oxygen to the tissues.

Anemia. As hemoglobin concentration drops, DPG increases about 0.23 for each gram per deciliter loss of hemoglobin. This response may compensate for up to half the oxygen deficit caused by the anemia and may account for the lack of hypoxic symptoms, so frequent even in severe anemia.

Blood pH. DPG concentration varies directly, about 5%, with each 0.01 pH unit change. Thus a shift of the dissociation curve caused by the Bohr effect is countered, to some degree, by a reverse shift from DPG action.

Fetal hemoglobin. During fetal life and for up to 1 year after birth, the body has *hemoglobin F* or fetal hemoglobin. Because of the chemical differences between fetal and adult hemoglobin, the oxygen dissociation curve is shifted to the left for hemoglobin F. While the fetus is developing in the mother with a low P_{O_2}, this leftward shift is particularly advantageous for the fetus to pick up oxygen from the mother's blood. After birth, however, the shift is less advantageous, and the fetal hemoglobin is eventually replaced by the adult type.

Carbon dioxide transportation

As oxygen diffuses from the blood into the body cells, carbon dioxide moves from cells to blood and is transported to the lung for excretion. However, all of the carbon dioxide carried in venous blood to the lung is not removed; enough remains to exert a partial pressure of 40 mm Hg in the arterial blood. Carbon dioxide transportation is more complicated than that of oxygen but must be understood clearly, for the amount of carbon dioxide in transit is one of the major determinants of the acid-base balance of the body. From 50 to 60 vol% of carbon dioxide are carried in three plasma and three erythrocyte compartments: *in plasma*—bound to protein, as bicarbonate, and in physical solution; *in erythrocytes*—dissolved in erythrocyte water, combined with hemoglobin, and as *carbonic acid*.

Fig. 6-7 diagrams both carbon dioxide and oxygen transport in the blood, and their exchange at body cell and the lung. The *horizontal rectangle* represents an erythrocyte suspended in plasma. The left side of the diagram shows the alveolar-capillary barrier and gas exchange in the lung, and the right side, the diffusion of gases across the cellular membrane. *Solid arrows* indicate the direction of gas movement, the molecules or ions that react with one another, and the products of their reactions. *Dashed-line arrows* identify the dissociation of compounds into molecules or ions. *Circled numbers* on the right index horizontal reactions for reference in the following discussion.

Because our primary interest is with carbon dioxide, we only note in passing the basic elements of oxygen transport, shown at the *top* of the diagram. Oxygen diffuses from alveolus into plasma, on the left, and some goes directly into solution. This is only a small volume, and when the perfusing blood is quickly saturated, the remaining oxygen enters the erythrocyte, where it reacts with reduced potassium hemoglobin made available by the dissociation of potassium bicarbonate of the carbon dioxide system. When the erythrocyte reaches a systemic capillary (right half of Fig. 6-7), the oxyhemoglobin separates into reduced potassium hemoglobin and oxygen. The latter diffuses out of the erythrocyte, into plasma solution and then into the cell, leaving a smaller amount dissolved in the plasma after cellular perfusion than after alveolar. The reduced hemoglobin is now ready to participate in carbon dioxide carriage.

Plasma transport of carbon dioxide

Bound to protein. As carbon dioxide leaves the cell, ⑩, a very small amount of it combines with plasma protein to form a complex called a *carbamino compound*, ①. This fraction of the carbon dioxide in the blood is relatively insignificant, comprising only 1.12 vol% of the total.

More of the carbon dioxide goes into physical solution in the plasma, ③, but once dissolved, follows two different pathways.

Bound as bicarbonate. In solution one fraction of the carbon dioxide reacts with plasma water, ②. By hydrolysis the carbon dioxide and water form carbonic acid, which at once is ionized into hydrogen and bicarbonate ions. These hydrogen ions are an important and significant portion of the total circulating hydrogen ion concentration that governs our acid-base balance. The bicarbonate ion becomes part of the *alkaline reserve* of the body, also important in acid-base regulation.

Dissolved in plasma. The other fraction of dissolved carbon dioxide remains in physical solution, unchanged, ④. This dissolved volume of carbon dioxide is about 1000 times as great as that which hydrolyzes into carbonic acid, a proportion that remains remarkably constant. This ratio is exceedingly useful to us. While we would like to be able to measure the concentration of the hydrogen ions from carbonic acid ionization, this is not technically feasible for clinical use. We can measure the amount of dissolved carbon dioxide very

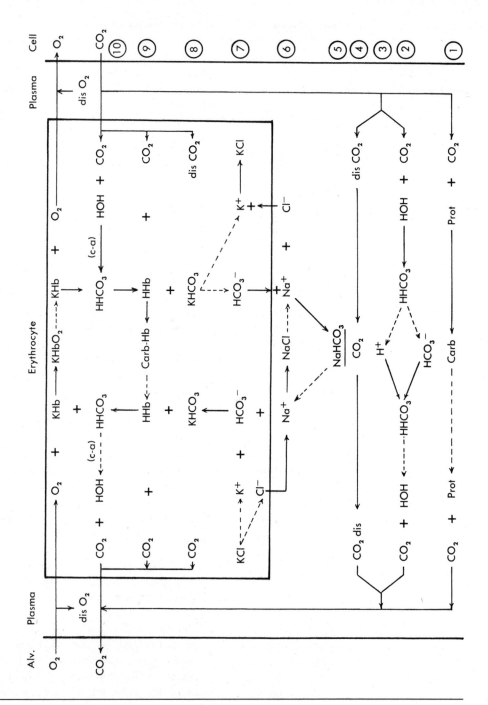

Fig. 6-7   Blood transport routes of oxygen and carbon dioxide. (See text for detailed description.)

easily, however, and because of the ratio of carbon dioxide to hydrogen ions, can deduce concentrations of the latter.

Erythrocyte transport of carbon dioxide

Dissolved in erythrocyte. Another insignificant portion of carbon dioxide after it has diffused through the erythrocyte membrane, goes into physical solution in the erythrocyte water and is noted here only for completeness, ⑧.

Combined with hemoglobin. A larger fraction of the gas combines with the *reduced acid* hemoglobin (HHb), made available by the release of oxygen to the tissues and, because hemoglobin is a protein, forms carbamino-hemoglobin, ⑨, somewhat similar to its combination with plasma protein. This is a very rapid reaction, and since the combining power of reduced hemoglobin with carbon dioxide is greater than that of oxyhemoglobin, the gas is readily picked up at the cell and discharged at the lung. The carbamino-hemoglobin constitutes from 8% to 10% of the total carbon dioxide transported but 20% to 25% of the carbon dioxide released in the lung.

As carbonic acid. The major portion of the transported carbon dioxide is hydrated in the red cell to carbonic acid, a normally slow process that is speeded up by an enzyme catalyst called *carbonic anhydrase* (c-a). The following sequence of steps then takes place: The carbonic acid immediately ionizes, as it does in the plasma. The reduced potassium hemoglobin, available after the release of oxygen, reacts with the newly formed carbonic acid (shown vertically on the diagram) to produce reduced hemoglobin (HHb), and potassium bicarbonate ($KHCO_3$), ⑨ and ⑧. As soon as the potassium bicarbonate is formed, it ionizes and the bicarbonate ion *diffuses out of the erythrocyte* into the plasma, as part of an interesting maneuver known as the "chloride shift," or the Hamburger phenomenon. To maintain ionic equilibrium, if one ion leaves the red cell, another must enter to replace it. Large amounts of sodium chloride are present in plasma, and as the bicarbonate ions leave the red cell, chloride ions enter in exchange, ⑥. The sodium of the plasma sodium chloride then combines with the bicarbonate from the red cell to form sodium bicarbonate; ⑤, and the released potassium in the erythrocyte combines with the shifted chloride from the plasma to produce potassium chloride, ⑦.

The remainder of Fig. 6-7 shows reversal of the reactions just described, as blood reaches the lung and carbon dioxide is moved from blood to alveolus in exchange for oxygen from alveolus to blood. Later in the text we discuss another ratio shown in the diagram, that between sodium bicarbonate and dissolved carbon dioxide at lines ④ and ⑤. Our clinical understanding and evaluation of acid-base balance is built on this approximately 20:1 relationship.

Just as there is a relationship between blood PO_2 and oxygen saturation of hemoglobin, expressed by the oxygen dissociation curves, so there is a relationship between blood PCO_2 and whole blood content of carbon dioxide, calculated in volumes percent. This too can be graphically demonstrated in so-called *carbon dioxide dissociation curves,* as shown in Fig. 6-8. The first point to note is the influence of oxygen saturation on the PCO_2 content ratio. We know that carbon dioxide levels modify the oxygen dissociation curve (Bohr effect), and we now see that SO_2 determines the course of carbon dioxide dissociation. This is called the *Haldane effect*. Fig. 6-8, *A*, shows the curves of carbon dioxide dissociation for three levels of blood oxygen saturation, two of which are physiologic values, and the third an extreme for contrast. These might be called "laboratory curves," since they are experimentally determined by subjecting samples of whole blood to various oxygen saturations and measuring the carbon dioxide content of each at different carbon dioxide tension exposures.

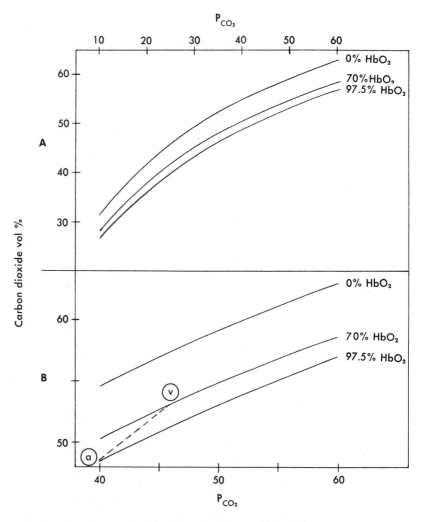

Fig. 6-8   Haldane effect and carbon dioxide dissociation curves. **A,** The relationship between carbon dioxide content and tension at three levels of hemoglobin saturation. **B,** Close-up of the curves between P_{CO_2} of 40 mm Hg and 60 mm Hg (see text for details). (Modified from Comroe, J.H., Jr., et al.: The lung, ed. 2, Chicago, 1962, Year Book Medical Publishers, Inc.)

The purpose of the curves is to show how carbon dioxide dissociates from, or leaves, the blood as its partial pressure drops or, contrarily, the increasing amounts of carbon dioxide accumulating in the blood as tension rises. The graphs indicate how this relationship depends on oxygen saturation. Fig. 6-8, *B,* shows selected segments of the curves to include the physiologic range of PCO_2, from the arterial point, ⓐ, with a PCO_2 of 40 mm Hg, SO_2 of 97.5% and carbon dioxide content of 48 vol%, to the venous point ⓥ, with a PCO_2 of 46 mm Hg, SO_2 of 70%, and carbon dioxide content of 53 vol%. Since oxygen saturation changes from arterial to venous blood, the true physiologic carbon dioxide dissociation curve must lie somewhere between the two "laboratory curves" for arterial and venous saturation, and such a curve is shown as a *dashed line* in Fig. 6-8, *B.* The student can see that at ⓐ, with its high SO_2, the capacity for a PCO_2 of 40 mm Hg is low, thus encouraging the excretion of the gas in the lung. At ⓥ, with its lower SO_2, the capacity of the blood to hold carbon dioxide at a given partial pressure increases, facilitating the removal of the gas from tissue cells. It is at this venous point, ⓥ, that the dissociation of oxyhemoglobin takes place, indicated in the RBC rectangle of Fig. 6-7, whereby oxygen is released, and reduced potassium hemoglobin is made available to react with carbonic acid.

In summarizing respiratory gas transportation, let us remember that the many processes described do not take place in intermittent stages but occur rapidly, simultaneously, and continuously. The close correlation and interdependence between oxygen and carbon dioxide transportation is evidenced by the Bohr and Haldane effects. Also, although Fig. 6-7 is limited to only half of the carbon dioxide circuit, in the interest of economy, it can also illustrate reactions that occur when blood reaches the lung, by visualizing the same processes with the directions of the arrows turned about.

Most of the carbon dioxide is carried in the plasma but must pass through the erythrocyte as bicarbonate ion by the chloride shift mechanism. Of critical importance is the relationship between the carbon dioxide that is carried as the compound sodium bicarbonate and that which is in physical solution in the plasma. The former is referred to as the *bound* carbon dioxide , and the latter as the *dissolved.* Under normal conditions the ratio of the bound to the dissolved carbon dioxide is remarkably constant at 20:1. Such a ratio is essential to maintain normal acid-base balance of the blood. The amount of physically dissolved carbon dioxide is directly proportional to the amount of carbon dioxide that is hydrolyzed in the plasma to carbonic acid; thus the dissolved carbon dioxide represents the amount of this acid present in plasma. The 20:1 proportion of combined to dissolved carbon dioxide is therefore a ratio between an *acid salt* and a *weak acid,* an important concept of buffering to be discussed with acid-base balance.

Because the carriage of carbon dioxide involves chemical reactions, the chemical quantitative expression of *millimoles per liter* (mM/ℓ) or *milliequivilents per liter* (mEq/ℓ) is more frequently used than volumes percent (vol%) to indicate amounts of the gas in the blood. The calibration is 1 gmw $\times$ 10^{-3} of

Table 6-5		Arterial		Venous	
Carbon dioxide content of arterial and venous blood		**Vol%**	**mEq/ℓ**	**Vol%**	**mEq/ℓ**
	Combined CO_2	53.5	24.0	60.4	27.1
	Dissolved CO_2	2.7	1.2	3.1	1.4
	Total CO_2	56.2	25.2	63.5	28.5
	P_{CO_2}	40 mm Hg		46 mm Hg	

carbon dioxide per liter of plasma. The actual measurement of blood carbon dioxide in the laboratory is done as volumes percent but is converted to millimoles per liter according to the following principle (as noted on p. 7, the molar volume of carbon dioxide to be used here is $22.3\ell)^{17}$:

(1) Vol% = ml CO_2/100 ml plasma
(2) 1 mM CO_2 = 1 gmw CO_2/1000 = 22,300 ml/1000 = 22.3 ml
(3) 1 mM CO_2/ℓ = 22.3 ml CO_2/1000 ml plasma = 2.23 ml CO_2/100 ml plasma
(4) Therefore, *mM CO_2/ℓ = vol%* ÷ 2.23
(5) Since 1 mMCO_2/ℓ = 1 mEqCO_2/ℓ, mEqCO_2/ℓ = vol.% ÷ 2.23 also.

Average values for carbon dioxide of venous and arterial blood are listed in Table 6-5, and since mEq/ℓ is more common in medicine, it is used instead of mM/ℓ.

Acid-base balance

For optimum function of the body cells, the chemical reactions of their environment (body fluids and blood) must remain within a specific narrow range. Deviations of a body pH above and below the normal range interfere with cellular metabolism and at extreme levels cause death of the cells. Survival is unlikely when pH drops below 7 or when it exceeds 7.80. The net result of all the interreactions of substances in the body should produce a hydrogen ion cencentration $[H^+]$ to maintain a blood pH of 7.35 to 7.45 with an average normal of *7.40 for arterial blood,* just slightly alkaline. The pH is influenced by food, drink, and disease, but the body has a great capacity for maintaining a normal reaction in the face of factors that would change it. Maintaining a normal acid-base balance is one of the body's more important functions and one in which respiration plays a major role. Should the blood pH fall below the normal range, becoming *less* alkaline, a state of *acidemia* is said to exist; should it rise above the range, becoming more alkaline, *alkalemia* exists. This terminology is in keeping with the recommendations of a select committee representing the American College of Chest Physicians, and the American Thoracic Society.[18] They define acidemia as a state of the blood with a pH less than normal, and alkalemia as a state with a pH greater than normal. Other acid-base terms are defined later. At this point we describe physiologic buffers and their importance to acid-base chemistry.

Buffers and the Henderson-Hasselbalch equation

A "buffer system" is a combination of a *weak acid* and a *salt* of that acid, and when introduced into a chemical reaction, it limits or buffers large changes in hydrogen ion concentration to prevent wide swings in pH. Although the industrial use of buffers is extensive, we are interested only in a few biologic systems, among which the following are worth identifying:

In plasma
    Carbonic acid/sodium bicarbonate $H_2CO_3/NaHCO_3$
    Sodium *acid* phosphate/sodium *alkaline* phosphate $NaH_2PO_4/NaHPO_4$
    Acid proteinate/sodium proteinate   HProt/NaProt
In erythrocytes
    Acid hemoglobin/potassium hemoglobin   HHb/KHb
    Potassium *acid* phosphate/potassium *alkaline* phosphate KH_2PO_4/K_2HPO_4

The carbonic acid/sodium bicarbonate is by far the most important of all the buffers and is used exclusively in the following to describe the detailed function of a buffer.

If a *strong* acid is added to a buffer pair, the chemical reaction will yield a *weak* acid and a neutral salt, and a *strong* alkali will yield a *weakly* alkaline salt and water. Thus, if hydrogen chloride is added to the carbonic acid/sodium bicarbonate mixture, the strong acid will react with the bicarbonate of the buffer:

$$HCl + \frac{HHCO_3}{NaHCO_3} \rightarrow HHCO_3 + NaCl$$

This converts the strong acidity of hydrogen chloride to the relatively weak acidity of carbonic acid, and the increase in $[H^+]$ is slight. Similarly, if sodium hydroxide is added to the same buffer, it will react with the carbonic acid of the mixture:

$$NaOH + \frac{HHCO_3}{NaHCO_3} \rightarrow NaHCO_3 + HOH$$

The strong alkalinity of sodium hydroxide is "buffered" into the relatively weak alkalinity of sodium bicarbonate. Eventually the buffer will be used up, but in the meantime the $[H^+]$ of the reaction, and thus the pH, will change gradually rather than abruptly.

In a buffer pair the weak acid is slightly ionized, whereas its accompanying salt is almost completely ionized, and the $[H^+]$ of the buffer system is proportional to the ratio between the concentration (in moles per liter) of the free acid and the acid "bound" by base as the salt. The $[H^+]$ and pH of any buffer pair can be calculated if the concentration composition of the mixture and the equilibirum (ionization) constant of the weak electrolyte (the acid) are known. Using the simple expression for the ionization of a weak acid, we will demonstrate how it can be modified to determine the reaction of the buffer. The dissociation of carbonic acid (written as $HHCO_3$) is:

$$HHCO_3 \rightleftharpoons H^+ + HCO_3^- \quad \text{(very slight ionization)}$$

thus

$$\frac{[H^+][HCO_3^-]}{[HHCO_3]} = K_{ac}$$

and

$$[H^+] = K_{ac}\frac{[HHCO_3]}{[HCO_3^-]}$$

In this buffer mixture, since most of the acid is un-ionized ($[H^+]$ is very minute), the molar concentration of un-ionized acid in the numerator of the preceding ratio for all practical purposes is the same as the known acid concentration that was used to prepare the buffer. On the other hand, because the salt sodium bicarbonate is almost completely ionized:

$$NaHCO_3 \rightleftharpoons Na^+ \times HCO_3^- \qquad (complete\ ionization)$$

the value of the bicarbonate ion in the above denominator is approximately the same as the total molar concentration of the salt used in the buffer. Thus, the above ionization equation for a weak acid can be rephrased to express the ionization of a buffer system, of which it is a part, by substituting molar concentration of the buffer *salt* in place of the bicarbonate ion:

$$Molar\ concentration\ H^+ = K_{acid} \times \frac{Molar\ concentration\ HHCO_3}{Molar\ concentration\ NaHCO_3}$$

From the foregoing is derived the *Henderson-Hasselbalch equation,* which is a cornerstone of the clinical application of the principles of acid-base balance. Since pH is the negative log of the hydrogen ion concentration used as a positive number, the buffer ionization equation can be rewritten to allow calculation of the pH:

$$H^+ = K_{ac} \times \frac{acid}{salt}$$

$$\log H^+ = \log\left[K_{ac} \times \frac{acid}{salt}\right]$$

$$\log H^+ = \log K_{ac} + \log\left[\frac{acid}{salt}\right]$$

$$pH = -\log K_{ac} - \log\left[\frac{acid}{salt}\right]$$

$$pH = pK + \log\left[\frac{salt}{acid}\right]$$

$$pH = pK_{ac} + \log\left[\frac{NaHCO_3}{H_2CO_3}\right]$$

Note the use of the term *pK.* Similarly to pH, pK means the *negative log of the equilibrium constant of the acid component of the buffer system,* used as a positive number. Because laboratory techniques make it easier to determine the amount of *dissolved* carbon dioxide in the blood than the carbonic acid content and because the dissolved carbon dioxide is directly proportional to the blood carbonic acid, the concentration of dissolved carbon dioxide is used in the equation in place of the *acid,* with a compensatory change in the ionization constant. Under physiologic conditions the carbonic acid ionization K has a value of 7.85×10^{-7}, which is easily converted by calculation into a pK of *6.1.* Also, the importance of the numerator of the equation, usually referred to as "base" rather than salt, lies in the bicarbonate ion, since it represents and includes "bound" acid. Finally, because of the small quantities involved, it is convenient to calibrate concentrations as milliequivalents per liter. The Henderson-Hasselbalch (H-H) equation, as it applies to the carbonic acid/sodium bicarbonate buffer system for determination of blood pH, can be summarized as follows:

(1) $\quad pH = 6.1 + \log \left[\dfrac{m \ Eq/\ell \ \text{of bicarbonate}}{m \ Eq/\ell \ \text{of dissolved } CO_2} \right]$

(2) $\quad pH = 6.1 + \log \left[\dfrac{[HCO_3^-]}{[\text{dissolved } CO_2]} \right]$

Application of the H-H equation

Since carbon dioxide, both dissolved in solution and combined as bicarbonate, is intimately involved in acid-base balance, it is easy to see why ventilation is so important in regulating this balance and why a clear understanding of this relationship is necessary for those treating respiratory diseases. We now discuss in some detail those factors involved in the acid-base equation and learn to use the equation for better understanding of acid-base physiology.

For our purposes the term *acid-base balance* refers to the ratio between carbonic acid and its salt, the base sodium bicarbonate. In evaluating this balance, we can measure in the laboratory certain blood values, which we then apply to the equation for whatever information is desired. First we must be acquainted with some of the terms used. *Total carbon dioxide content* means all the carbon dioxide that can be chemically extracted and measured from a blood sample. This includes the *sum* of the combined carbon dioxide (as bicarbonate) and the dissolved carbon dioxide; and it is measured as volumes percent and converted to milliequivalents per liter as described earlier. The *dissolved carbon dioxide* is that fraction of the blood gas that is in solution in the blood plasma. The *combined carbon dioxide,* also called *bound carbon dioxide, base,* and *bicarbonate,* refers to that portion of the total carbon dioxide that is contained in the blood bicarbonate. This can be measured directly by chemical analysis (not clinically applicable), computed as the difference between the total **and** the dissolved carbon dioxide, or calculated from the H-H equation.

Laboratory technology makes it easy and quick to measure directly the partial pressure of carbon dioxide in a blood sample. The P_{CO_2} can be converted to milliequivalents per liter very simply by a factor, the derivation of which is demonstrated below:

(1) 1 mole CO_2 = 22,300 ml at 760 mm Hg pressure
(2) 1 mM CO_2 = 22.3 ml
(3) Sol coef CO_2 at 760 mm Hg = 0.51 ml CO_2/ml plasma

(4) Thus the ml CO_2/ml plasma at any P_{CO_2} $= \dfrac{P_{CO_2} \times 0.51}{760}$

(5) The ml CO_2/ℓ plasma $= \dfrac{P_{CO_2} \times 0.51 \times 1000}{760}$

(6) The mM CO_2/ℓ plasma $= \dfrac{P_{CO_2} \times 0.51 \times 1000}{760 \times 22.3} = P_{CO_2} \times 0.03014$

(7) Or, using mEq/ℓ instead of mM/ℓ, the mEq CO_2/ℓ plasma $= P_{CO_2} \times 0.03014$.

The normal arterial P_{CO_2} value of 40 mm Hg multiplied by the factor 0.03 gives a concentration of dissolved carbon dioxide of 1.2 mEq/ℓ.

Let us assume that an arterial blood sample yields a total carbon dioxide content of 56.2 vol%, which converts to a concentration of 25.2 mEq/ℓ, and the P_{CO_2} is 40 mm Hg, or 1.2 mEq/ℓ. The bicarbonate value is the *difference* between these, or 24 mEq/ℓ. The H-H equation can now be used to determine the arterial pH:

$$\text{pH} = 6.1 + \log \left[\frac{24}{1.2}\right]$$
$$= 6.1 + \log 20$$
$$= 6.1 + 1.301$$
$$= 7.40$$

A critical point to learn here is that the blood pH depends on the *ratio* of the bicarbonate to dissolved carbon dioxide rather than on the absolute value of each. As long as the ratio is 20:1, the pH will always be 7.40. The values could be 12:0.6 or 48:2.4 or any other combination to yield 20. Reference is made to this in the discussion of carbon dioxide transportation, and the student should now be starting to understand the true meaning of "acid-base balance."

The total carbon dioxide blood content plays no role in contemporary blood gas or acid-base evaluation. Before the days of current instrumentation, volumetric measurement of the milliliters of carbon dioxide per 100 ml of blood was the only readily available clinical technique, and although it indicated some abnormalities, it was far from adequate. The importance of evaluating bicarbonate and dissolved carbon dioxide individually is emphasized a little later. Since total carbon dioxide includes both of these fractions, variations in it do not differentiate between them. For example, because the bicarbonate/carbon dioxide ratio has such a relatively high numerator, an increase in bicarbonate of 50% gives a total carbon dioxide of 37.2 mEq/ℓ, or 82.9 vol%, noticeably greater than the normals of 25.2 mEq/ℓ, or 56.2 vol%. Yet an equally significant 50% increase in dissolved carbon dioxide is reflected in a small total carbon dioxide change to 25.8 mEq/ℓ, or 57.5 vol%. Despite its clinical uselessness, total carbon dioxide is included in exercises later to enhance the student's understanding of the relationships of all the factors involved in acid-base balance and to show how this volumetric procedure may be used as a backup in the laboratory should equipment failure prevent direct measurement of one of the H-H equation variables.

Of the three variables in the H-H equation, any one obviously can be calculated if the other two are known. In actual cardiopulmonary practice, compact equipment now available makes it convenient to measure pH, P_{CO_2}, and P_{O_2} on the same blood sample, a procedure much easier than the chemical analyses of total carbon dioxide and bicarbonate. Nomograms and charts are also available to show the relation among the various factors. However, to understand fully these relationships the student should know how to use the H-H equation to solve for an unknown, given two known variables. For practice in performing such exercises, the following equations are listed for reference. Some merely represent differences between calculated values, and others are algebraic rearrangements of the H-H equation, one example of which is detailed in Appendix 10.

(1) $mEq/\ell = vol\% \div 2.23$

(2) Dissolved CO_2 in $mEq/\ell = P_{CO_2} \times 0.03$

(3) $P_{CO_2} = \dfrac{\text{Total } CO_2 \text{ in } mEq/\ell}{0.03 \times [1 + \text{antilog (pH} - 6.1)]}$

(4) Total CO_2 in $mEq/\ell = HCO_3$ in mEq/ℓ + dissolved CO_2 in mEq/ℓ
$= P_{CO_2} \times 0.03 \times [1 + \text{antilog (pH} - 6.1)]$

(5) HCO_3 in $mEq/\ell = $ Total CO_2 in mEq/ℓ − dissolved CO_2 in mEq/ℓ
$= P_{CO_2} \times 0.03 \times [\text{antilog (pH} - 6.1)]$

Following are examples of acid-base calculations:

Example 1:
GIVEN: Arterial $P_{CO_2} = 52$ mm Hg, and total arterial CO_2 content $= 62$ vol%
CALCULATE: Arterial pH

Solution: Dissolved $CO_2 = 0.03 \times 52 = 1.56$ mEq/ℓ
Total $CO_2 = 62 \div 2.23 = 27.8$ mEq/ℓ
$HCO_3 = 27.8 - 1.56 = 26.24$ mEq/ℓ

$$pH = 6.1 + \log\left[\frac{26.24}{1.56}\right] = 6.1 + 1.225$$

$$pH = 7.33$$

Example 2:
GIVEN: Arterial pH $= 7.24$, and arterial $P_{CO_2} = 56$ mm Hg
CALCULATE: Dissolved CO_2, total CO_2, HCO_3

Solution: Dissolved $CO_2 = 0.03 \times 56$ $= 1.68$ mEq/ℓ
Total $CO_2 = 1.68 \times [1 + \text{antilog (7.24} - 6.1)]$
$= 1.68 \times [1 + \text{antilog (1.14)}]$
$= 1.68 \times 14.8$ $= 24.9$ mEq/ℓ
$HCO_3 = 24.9 - 1.68$ $= 23.2$ mEq/ℓ

Example 3:
GIVEN: Arterial pH $= 7.58$, and total arterial CO_2 content $= 19.2$
CALCULATE: P_{CO_2}

Solution: $P_{CO_2} = \dfrac{19.2}{0.03 \times [1 + \text{antilog (7.58-6.1)}]}$

$= \dfrac{19.2}{0.03 \times [1 + \text{antilog (1.48)}]}$

$= \dfrac{19.2}{0.03 \times 31.2}$

$= 20.3$ mm Hg

The answers to such calculations can be checked by fitting them into the H-H equation (p. 219) to see whether the equation balances.

Exercise 6-2:

GIVEN		CALCULATE
A. P_{CO_2} = 32 mm Hg	Total CO_2 = 55 vol%	pH
B. P_{CO_2} = 56 mm Hg	Total CO_2 = 66 vol%	pH
C. P_{CO_2} = 72 mm Hg	Total CO_2 = 30 vol%	pH
D. Total CO_2 = 55 vol%	pH = 7.26	P_{CO_2}
E. Total CO_2 = 44 vol%	pH = 7.55	P_{CO_2}
F. Total CO_2 = 30 vol%	pH = 7.35	P_{CO_2}
G. P_{CO_2} = 55 mm Hg	pH = 7.41	Total CO_2; HCO_3
H. P_{CO_2} = 38 mm Hg	pH = 7.52	Total CO_2; HCO_3
I. P_{CO_2} = 26 mm Hg	pH = 7.30	Total CO_2; HCO_3

Control of ventilation

Although the general principles of ventilation are covered in Chapter 4, a discussion of the factors regulating it is included at this point. Because ventilation is as deeply involved with the body's acid-base homeostasis as it is with the mechanics of air movement, we believe that the student should first be exposed to the fundamentals of blood gas transport and acid-base balance. Also, this sequence will make for a smooth transition into the discussion of clinical acid-base problems with which this chapter closes.

Until fairly recently, the central control of ventilation was believed to rest in a single *respiratory center* located in the medulla of the brain. It was further thought that as arterial blood perfused the highly specialized cells of the center, the partial pressure of its contained carbon dioxide was sensed by the cells, and if the P_{CO_2} was higher than normal, impulses from the center stimulated the ventilatory muscles to blow off excess carbon dioxide; if the pressure was low, ventilation was depressed to allow the gas to be retained. Similarly, oxygen lack and excess supposedly increased and decreased breathing, respectively. Contemporary studies of the mechanics of the ventilatory system, however, have made it clear that its control is exceedingly complex, and our knowledge of it is incomplete and often speculative. The problem of trying to present a clear picture of this vital process is further complicated by conflicting and contradictory data and opinions. We now briefly discuss those factors that seem to be most generally accepted as the prime determinants of ventilation and consider one possible pattern of their interrelationships.

The neural and chemical structures that control ventilation are divided into the two categories of *peripheral* and *central,* depending on their location outside or within the brain; Fig. 6-9 outlines their various roles.

Instead of one cerebral respiratory center, there are at least three, one in the medulla and two in the pons. In addition, there is a less well-located area in the medulla containing *chemoreceptors,* which is described below. Similar che-

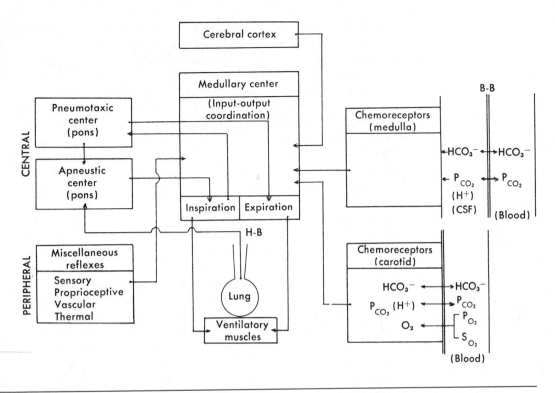

Fig. 6-9   Ventilatory control. Diagram of relationships between *central* and *peripheral* factors regulating breathing. (See text for details.)

moreceptors are found among the peripheral stimulators, along with reflexes from the lung and a variety of other organs and tissues.[19] As we discuss the relationships among these factors, we will not necessarily confine ourselves to a sequence depending on their central or peripheral locations.

The *medullary center* can be considered to have two major functions. First, it acts as a coordinator for stimuli reaching it from all other areas involved in ventilatory control. These stimuli carry information concerning the somatic gas exchange needs and the data from sensory, chemical, and other factors that can modify breathing. The medullary center's task is to match these needs and influences and to determine the ventilatory pattern most useful to the body as a whole, on a breath-to-breath basis. Second, the medullary center sends its nerve impulses to the muscles of ventilation through two subcenters that individually control the inspiratory and expiratory phases of breathing. Thus, instead of acting as the sole regulator of ventilation, responding directly to carbon dioxide and oxygen levels as once believed, the medullary center is more of a final determinant of breathing patterns, responding to autonomic stimuli as well as to the voluntary stimuli of the higher centers of the cerebral cortex, which can override them all.

Chemoreceptors are groups of specialized nerve cells that can differentiate between concentrations of hydrogen ions and oxygen in the fluid perfusing them. There are two sets of chemoreceptors, one diffusely distributed in the medulla of the brain, known as *medullary* or *central chemoreceptors,* and the other located in the bifurcations of both carotid arteries, called *peripheral chemoreceptors,* or *carotid bodies.* Similar structures are located in the arch of the aorta, the *aortic bodies,* but since these are more concerned with cardiovascular than with ventilatory control, we will use the carotid bodies as representative of peripheral receptors for our discussion.[20,21] As indicated in Fig. 6-9, both central and peripheral chemoreceptors send impulses to the medullary center, and while there are similarities in their functions, there are also significant differences. We consider first the effect of hydrogen ions on chemoreceptors, then the effect of oxygen.

Circulating hydrogen ions come from two sources: (1) dissolved carbon dioxide that hydrolyzes into carbonic acid and that in turn dissociates into hydrogen and bicarbonate ions; and (2) ionization of other acids in the blood, both normal and abnormal. We know that the hydrogen ion concentration is directly proportional to the ratio of the concentrations of dissolved carbon dioxide, reflected as P_{CO_2}, and the bicarbonate ion: thus $[H^+] \cong P_{CO_2}/HCO_3^-$. The membrane of the peripheral chemoreceptor cell is only slightly permeable to ions such as hydrogen and bicarbonate so that they move slowly across this barrier, but it readily allows passage of the un-ionized dissolved carbon dioxide. Therefore, should the blood carbon dioxide level rise because of increased metabolic production or because of inhalation of the gas, its rapid diffusion quickly raises carotid receptor intracellular carbon dioxide, increases the CO_2/HCO_3^- ratio, and elevates the hydrogen ion concentration. This increase in cellular hydrogen ion concentration triggers nerve impulses from the chemoreceptor to the medullary center, indicating the need to step up ventilation to blow off excess carbon dioxide. Conversely, an excessive removal of blood carbon dioxide, as by a period of voluntary hyperventilation, leaves a relative surplus of intracellular bicarbonate ion over carbon dioxide, and when overbreathing ceases, the lowered hydrogen ion concentration causes an interval of apnea as the medullary center is instructed to reduce breathing and allow a buildup of blood carbon dioxide to normal.

These responses to carbon dioxide tension changes, mediated through the carotid bodies and the medullary center, are of course dependent on a reactive and functional ventilatory system. Hypercapnia or hypocapnia caused by pulmonary abnormalities, which manifest as hypoventilation or hyperventilation, may cause hydrogen ion changes as described, but because of pulmonary disease there will be no ventilatory system responses. Further, the influence of the central chemoreceptors, described below, on chronic states of carbon dioxide changes, or in conditions of primary ventilation defects, is probably more important than is that of the peripheral sensors.

In contrast, peripheral chemoreceptor reaction to changes in blood hydrogen ions as a result of fluctuations in bicarbonate levels is slow because of the poor diffusibility of the ion across the cell membrane. Metabolic (nonrespiratory) disturbances such as increases in fixed or abnormal acids circulating in the blood can deplete the available bicarbonate ions and, by thus increasing the blood PCO_2/HCO_3^- ratio, raise its $[H^+]$. This sets up a bicarbonate concentration gradient from chemoreceptor to blood, and although diffusion of the ion is slow, bicarbonate eventually leaves the cell, increasing the intracellular PCO_2/HCO_3^- ratio, elevating $[H^+]$, and stimulating hyperventilation. The increased breathing in turn depletes blood carbon dioxide, lowers the PCO_2/HCO_3^- ratio, and tends to return the blood hydrogen ion concentration toward normal. On the other hand, metabolic increases in blood bicarbonate, as by ingestion or infusion of the ion, or relative increases, as from renal or emetic loss of fixed normal acids, can reverse the bicarbonate ion gradient and eventually lower the hydrogen ion concentration within the receptor cells. Reduced ventilation then retains carbon dioxide in the blood to balance the elevated bicarbonate and normalize the $[H^+]$.

There is an interesting difference between the operation of the central chemoreceptors and the carotid bodies, although the principles described for the latter generally apply to the former.[22] Where the peripheral chemical sensors are perfused directly by the blood, the medullary cells are separated from the blood by circulating *cerebrospinal fluid (CSF),* and between these two systems there is a semipermeable membrane referred to as the *blood-brain barrier (B-B* in Fig. 6-9). Anatomically, this is found at surfaces where perfusing capillaries are in contact with the CSF in the arachnoid space of the brain. The barrier is nearly, if not completely, impermeable to many ions, including hydrogen and bicarbonate, but is rapidly permeable to undissociated dissolved carbon dioxide. Also, the CSF is not simply a filtrate of blood plasma, since it may contain concentrations of ions not in equilibrium with the blood. Exchange across the blood-brain barrier, in addition to the pressure gradient diffusion of readily diffusible substances like carbon dioxide, also involves a physiochemical process known as *active transport* for substances to which the barrier is impermeable by diffusion. Active transport is a phenomenon found in other body systems that basically uses cellular energy to move substances through biologic membranes in the face of opposing concentration gradients across such barriers. Thus bicarbonate can cross the blood-brain barrier by the active transport mechanism without dependence on a pressure difference across the membrane. While this process is not as fast as the rapid movement of diffusible carbon dioxide, it gives the central receptors considerable versatility in adjusting to blood chemical needs more quickly than would reliance on the slow diffusion of the ion.

The role of the medullary chemoreceptors in regulating ventilation to acute carbon dioxide changes (other than those caused by mechanical ventilatory disorders) is the same as that described for the carotid mechanism, and the two systems function in concert. Variations in blood carbon dioxide are quickly answered by the responses of CSF hydrogen ion concentrations, since carbon dioxide easily crosses the blood-brain barrier. Because hydrogen ions, like bicarbonate, diffuse poorly across cell membranes, it is probable that the central chemical sensors are activated by the hydrogen ions bathing their surfaces, rather than by ions generated within them. At any rate a high concentration of hydrogen ions in the CSF causes the central chemoreceptors to stimulate the medullary center into increased ventilation, and a low concentration retards it. Like its peripheral counterpart, the central chemoreceptor cannot correct a malfunctioning ventilatory system.

An example of the combined action of both sets of chemoreceptors in response to metabolic acidosis will best illustrate how the function of the central receptors differs from the peripheral receptors. Let us imagine the incursion of a disease-generated acid into the blood, and consider in an artificial stepwise sequence some of the subsequent events. First, the excessive number of hydrogen ions depletes much of the circulating bicarbonate buffer, creating gradients for bicarbonate from CSF and carotid body cells to the blood. As bicarbonate leaves the cells and CSF, cellular and CSF PCO_2/HCO_3^- ratios and $[H^+]$ are raised, and the medullary center is signalled to stimulate hyperventilation. The increased breathing, however, gradually eliminates some of the blood carbon dioxide, initiating diffusion of the gas from carotid cells and CSF, dropping their hydrogen ion concentrations and retarding the hyperventilation. The active transport mechanism of the blood-brain barrier now becomes active, moving more bicarbonate out of the CSF to raise the hydrogen ion concentration and reestablish hyperventilation. Metabolic alkalosis can provoke a mirror image response of this sequence, with reactions moving in opposite directions. We can generalize by stating that in the face of metabolic hydrogen ion changes in the blood, both central and peripheral chemoreceptors work together to effect rapid ventilatory correction, but the central sensors, through the energy of the blood-brain barrier active transport, better stabilize responses for prolonged action.

The effect of oxygen on ventilation is mediated almost entirely through the peripheral carotid bodies, another difference between the two sets of chemical sensors.[23] The carotid bodies are sensitive to both blood oxygen tension and content, a reduction in either stimulating the medullary center to increase ventilation, and a combination of subnormal tension and amount of gas having an additive effect on the amplitude of breathing. Conversely, high oxygen tensions can reduce ventilation. Finally, the maximum stimulation to breathing results from a combination of hypoxemia and hypercapnia acting together on the chemoreceptors.

The reaction of the peripheral chemoreceptors to hypoxemia is modified by the effect of hydrogen ion concentration on the receptors, in a paradoxic manner. Responding to a drop in oxygen tension, the carotid bodies stimulate the medullary center to increase ventilation. However, the resulting hyperventilation reduces blood carbon dioxide, setting up a diffusion gradient that moves carbon dioxide from both peripheral and medullary chemoreceptors, lowering their hydrogen ion concentrations and retarding ventilation despite the hypoxemic stimulus. Given sufficient time, the active transport will move bicarbonate ions out of the CSF, elevating the hydrogen ion concentration and improving ventilation. This phenomenon is responsible for a sequence sometimes seen in prolonged oxygen deficit, in which initial hyperventilation is followed by depressed breathing and finally by the return of hyperventilation.

Another relationship between the simultaneous effects on ventilation of oxygen and hydrogen ions is illustrated by the state of chronic hypoventilation. If hypercapnia, with its elevated blood and chemoreceptor hydrogen ion concentration, is of long standing, the active transport of the blood-brain barrier will have time to move bicarbonate ions into the CSF and restore the latter's hydrogen ion concentration to normal. This removes the usual stimulating effect on breathing of a high carbon dioxide level and leaves ventilatory drive almost entirely to the low blood level of oxygen, which is also a product of hypoventilation. Sustained spontaneous ventilation is thus dependent on a degree of hypoxia, the therapeutic correction of which may lead to the cessation of breathing.

The *apneustic center* is located in the lower portion of the pons and is referred to as a pontine center. Apneusis is a condition in which ventilation stops in the inspiratory position. In such instances the resting level is end-inspiratory rather than end-expiratory, although the apneustic level is at the end of *full* inspiration. The apneustic center, if unrestrained, promotes deep and prolonged inspiration, but normally it is controlled by the *pneumotaxic center* and *inflation reflexes (Hering-Breuer)* from the lung. Disease of the pons leading to abnormal stimulation of the apneustic center can produce apneustic breathing, a gasping type of ventilation with maximum inspiration.

The *pneumotaxic center* is also in the pons, located slightly higher than the apneustic. As noted previously, it controls the effect of the apneustic center and encourages a rhythmic ventilation. It has been suggested that the pneumotaxic center receives impulses from the medullary inspiratory subcenter and in turn sends impulses to the medullary expiratory subcenter, thus limiting the extent of inhalation.

An *inflation reflex*, commonly called the Hering-Breuer reflex (*H-B* in Fig. 6-9), carries impulses from the lung to the brain through the vagus nerve. Sensory receptors in the lung or bronchioles respond to the stretch of the distending lung and relay inhibitory impulses to the central control through the apneustic center, inhibiting the latter's function and limiting further inflation. By restricting unnecessary inhalation, the inflation reflex assists the respiratory system in moving a volume of air adequate to supply the alveoli, with a minimum of energy expenditure.

There are several *miscellaneous reflexes,* widely scattered sensing devices that contribute to the total data on which the medullary center depends. Included are reflexes that respond to pain, temperature, tissue pressure and stretch, and circulatory dynamics. These are detailed in this text, but the student is encouraged to study them elsewhere in order to have the broadest possible view of this important feedback system.

In summary we can say that the *medullary center* receives nerve impulses from a wide variety of sources throughout the body, analyzes them, determines the necessary level of breathing, and through inspiratory and expiratory sub-centers stimulates the ventilatory muscles into appropriate action. In the back-ground, the pontine *apneustic center,* with its inherent ability to produce a full and sustained inhalation, acts as a sort of guarantee against failure of the lung to expand. The *pneumotaxic center,* also in the pons, keeps the apneustic center in check, and in addition correlates inspiratory and expiratory impulses from the medullary center and helps to maintain a rhythmic ventilation. The *Hering-Breuer stretch reflex,* originating in bronchiolar or alveolar walls, modifies the apneustic center's action by limiting inhalation and helps the medullary center establish a smooth and easy combination of tidal volume and rate. A large number of miscellaneous stimuli bring sensory, pressure, thermal, circulatory, and probably other information to the medullary center for the latter's consideration of ventilatory needs. The greatest influences, however come from blood and CSF hydrogen ion concentration and oxygen content stimulation of medullary and carotid chemoreceptors. These help correlate ventilation with acid-base balance as well as with gas exchange needs. Finally, the entire autonomic ventilatory control complex is subject to voluntary override by the higher areas of the cerebral cortex. Such a summary is oversimplified and, because of knowledge gaps, may be inaccurate in some details, but it does present a practical picture of at least the major factors responsible for control of ventilation.

Clinical acid-base states

When we consider the acid-base balance from a clinical, or patient-oriented, point of view rather than seeing it only as a chemical reaction in blood, we speak of *acidosis* and *alkalosis.* The suffix *-osis* is "a word termination denoting a process, especially a disease or morbid process, and sometimes conveying the meaning of abnormal increase."[24] Thus acidosis is a pathologic state that can, but does not necessarily, produce acidemia, and alkalosis a state that may include alkalemia. Acidosis is characterized by *hypercapnia* (elevated arterial carbon dioxide tension) when it is caused by respiratory disease, and *hypobasemia* (lowered arterial bicarbonate concentration) when it is caused by metabolic or nonrespiratory causes. Alkalosis is characterized by *hypocapnia* (lowered arterial carbon dioxide tension) when it is a result of respiratory disease, and *hyperbasemia* (elevated arterial bicarbonate concentration) when it is caused by metabolic or nonrespiratory causes.[18] In the pages immediately following, we differentiate in some detail between acidosis and alkalosis, and in each of these categories, between respiratory and metabolic. We also introduce the very important concept of *compensation.*

Perhaps the student is still not clear about proper uses of the "emias" and the "oses" in acid-base communication. This is understandable, and in many instances analyzing the subtleties of definitions may be more time consuming than it is worth. From habit, if nothing else, when talking generally about clinical states and problems we use the "oses" and reserve the "emias" for specific references to blood pH levels.

Let us now consider the nine fundamental acid-base conditions and their chemical characteristics, as listed in Table 6-6.

The analysis of acid-base abnormalities by blood gases has become more sophisticated through the years, and new concepts have developed that increase the ease and accuracy of the analysis. Such concepts as the base excess (BE) and standard bicarbonate are examples.

The BE concept is a way of quantifying the *metabolic* contribution of acid-base disturbance and helps fine tune the analyses when mixed disorders or compensation occurs. The normal range is 0 ± 2 mEq/ℓ of base. When a negative number is seen (-3 or less), this is called a base *deficit,* and a metabolic source of acid is contributing to the acid-base abnormality.

Table 6-6 Table of acid-base states	**Normal balance**	$\dfrac{24\ \text{mEq}/\ell}{1.2\ \text{mEq}/\ell}$ (40 mm Hg)	Ratio $\dfrac{20}{1}$	**mEq/ℓH$^+$** 40	**pH** 7.40
	Respiratory acidosis	$\dfrac{24\ \text{mEq}/\ell}{2.4\ \text{mEq}/\ell}$ (80 mm Hg)	$\dfrac{10}{1}$	80	7.10
	Respiratory acidosis (compensated)	$\dfrac{48\ \text{mEq}/\ell}{2.4\ \text{mEq}/\ell}$ (80 mm Hg)	$\dfrac{20}{1}$	40	7.40
	Respiratory alkalosis	$\dfrac{24\ \text{mEq}/\ell}{0.6\ \text{mEq}/\ell}$ (20 mm Hg)	$\dfrac{40}{1}$	20	7.70
	Respiratory alkalosis (compensated)	$\dfrac{12\ \text{mEq}/\ell}{0.6\ \text{mEq}/\ell}$ (20 mm Hg)	$\dfrac{20}{1}$	40	7.40
	Metabolic acidosis	$\dfrac{12\ \text{mEq}/\ell}{1.2\ \text{mEq}/\ell}$ (40 mm Hg)	$\dfrac{10}{1}$	80	7.10
	Metabolic acidosis (compensated)	$\dfrac{12\ \text{mEq}/\ell}{0.6\ \text{mEq}/\ell}$ (20 mm Hg)	$\dfrac{20}{1}$	40	7.40
	Metabolic alkalosis	$\dfrac{48\ \text{mEq}/\ell}{1.2\ \text{mEq}/\ell}$ (40 mm Hg)	$\dfrac{40}{1}$	20	7.70
	Metabolic alkalosis (compensated)	$\dfrac{48\ \text{mEq}/\ell}{2.4\ \text{mEq}/\ell}$ (80 mm Hg)	$\dfrac{20}{1}$	40	7.40

When a positive number greater than $+2$ is seen, there is a base excess, and either acid is being lost by metabolic or nonrespiratory routes (e.g., vomiting) or base is being excessively generated via metabolic means and being added to the acid-base problems.

The base excess is a number obtained from the Siggaard-Andersen nonogram. In order to use the nonogram one must first obtain the pH, Pa_{CO_2}, plasma bicarbonate, and hemoglobin.

The standard bicarbonate is similar to the *plasma* bicarbonate and is important because it eliminates the effects of a natural phenomena that can cause an inaccurate determination of the bicarbonate level. It therefore is a way of actually accessing the *metabolic* impact of bicarbonate alone. As indicated earlier:

$$CO_2 + H_2O \rightarrow H^+ + HCO_3^-$$

If high levels of carbon dioxide are found in the blood the equation is driven to the right by mass action alone and results in a higher bicarbonate level. This falsely suggests a metabolic source of bicarbonate greater than what actually is in operation.

By allowing the blood sample to equilibrate at a *standard* carbon dioxide tension of 40 mm Hg, the excess carbon dioxide is removed from the blood and the sample is then analyzed for bicarbonate content.

In acute respiratory failure with carbon dioxide retention, the plasma bicarbonate will be increasingly in excess of the standard bicarbonate as the patient's carbon dioxide retention worsens. Because of practical limitations of this test, it is most useful in eliminating errors in bicarbonate determination caused by hypercapnia.

When several factors work together to maintain a physiologic balance and one of the factors behaves abnormally to threaten the equilibrium, the other factors readjust their levels of function in an attempt to make up for the deficiency and maintain stability of the system. This is called *physiologic compensation*. Thus each of the four types of acid-base upsets can exist as uncompensated or compensated. The differentiation is not as clear-cut as indicated in the table, which is exaggerated for emphasis. Compensation actually starts as soon as the balance is upset, and although we have shown the disturbances in equilibrium and their compensation as isolated stages purely for demonstration purposes, these processes occur simultaneously. Finally, compensation is often incomplete, becoming less effective as the imbalance increases until it eventually breaks down. For the severe levels of decompensation shown, full physiologic compensation would be impossible, and all degrees of partial compensation could be found in a real clinical situation.

The following general rule will help to keep acid-base disturbances in a reasonable mental order: *Respiratory* disorders upset the *denominator* of the acid-base ratio because ventilation regulates the blood carbon dioxide, and compensation attempts to adjust the numerator to restore a 20:1 ratio; *metabolic* disorders upset the *numerator* of the ratio as bicarbonate is either increased or decreased, and compensation attempts to adjust the denominator.

The dissolved carbon dioxide can be changed, either primarily or as a secondary compensation, only by modifying the ventilatory pattern with hypoventilation or hyperventilation. The bicarbonate compensates by an increase in production or by varying the amounts excreted in the urine.

Respiratory acidosis

Respiratory acidosis is *always* the result of *alveolar hypoventilation* with its retention of carbon dioxide in the arterial blood. The hypoventilation may be a result of (1) chronic cardiopulmonary disease with failure of the ventilatory control system, (2) neuromuscular or skeletal disease with inadequate ventilatory muscular action, or (3) the action of drugs such as narcotics and sedatives, which depress respiratory center action. Regardless of cause, there is an increase in the partial pressure of arterial carbon dioxide and, depending on the state of compensation, a drop in arterial pH.

Compensation begins as soon as the carbon dioxide starts to accumulate and is a major function of the kidney. The body attempts to increase the amount of bicarbonate, keeping pace with the rising dissolved carbon dioxide, to maintain the necessary 20:1 ratio for a pH of 7.40. Reference to Fig. 6-7 will recall the mechanism of the chloride shift, whereby as the amount of carbon dioxide increases in the blood, chloride moves out of the plasma into the erythrocyte in exchange for bicarbonate. As a result, during the compensation for respiratory acidosis, the level of plasma chloride drops and the bicarbonate increases. Here the action of the kidney is of extreme importance, for the kidney uses two mechanisms to regulate the essential electrolyte levels. First, it selectively rejects the excretion of the bicarbonate ion in the urine, conserving it in the plasma for its use as a blood buffer. At the same time it reduces the excretion of sodium, retaining it to combine with the increased amounts of bicarbonate. The additional amounts of sodium bicarbonate thus made available to counter the increasing retained carbon dioxide are referred to as the *alkaline reserve*. Second, in place of sodium the kidney removes from the blood increasing amounts of hydrogen ion, as hydrogen chloride and ammonium chloride (NH_4Cl). This serves the dual purpose of maintaining electrolyte balance, by substituting one positive ion for another in the urine, and most important, for the health of the body, it reduces the overall acidity of the blood. In a sense the perceptive kidney, recognizing that retained carbon dioxide represents increasing amounts of carbonic acid, removes as many hydrogen ions as it can from the blood to "compensate" for the respiratory-induced acidity. If the onset of respiratory acidosis is rapid and acute, renal compensation may not be able to keep up with the rising carbon dioxide on a minute-by-minute basis, and the compensatory exchange of hydrogen for bicarbonate may not reach its maximum efficiency for 3 or 4 days. In slowly developing acidosis, as is often seen with chronic pulmonary disease when repeated infections and the progressive lung destruction span months or years, the compensatory process may adjust proportionately to the acidosis. In such instances pH levels may be maintained stable, within the normal range, not less than 7.35. It should be emphasized that because kidney action can prevent a serious drop in pH, this does not mean that acidosis is absent. Examination of arterial blood would reveal an elevated P_{CO_2}, and this is conclusive evidence of respiratory acidosis in a patient with ventilatory failure, but an acidosis compensated by renal action.

There is a limit to which the body can compensate an acid-base upset, beyond which there is a "break" in compensation. This point varies considerably among patients, and in uncomplicated chronic respiratory disease the kidney can often maintain a normal arterial pH in the face of a high P_{CO_2}. One study concluded that renal compensation was rarely complete for a CO_2 tension greater than 70 mm Hg,[25] while another cites compensation for, and good tolerance of, tensions up to 90 mm Hg.[26] The therapist will see many patients with varying degrees of hypercapnia and accompanying acidemia, and frequently they will have associated conditions that influence acid-base balance, especially metabolic disorders and cardiac failure.

In pulmonary emphysema, for example, slowly progressive alveolar hypoventilation can produce a chronic hypercapnia that may be countered by a migration of bicarbonate ions into the CSF, maintaining there a normal $[H^+]$ bathing the medullary chemoreceptors. This same hypoventilation also fails to supply the alveoli with adequate oxygen so that hypercapnia is accompanied by hypoxemia and cellular hypoxia. Under such a circumstance the most active stimulus to ventilation is the low arterial P_{O_2}, mediated through the carotid bodies and referred to as the *hypoxic drive*. This is not an efficient mechanism, for it requires a steady state of hypoxia to perpetuate a tidal air exchange. Should the hypoxia manage to effect enough ventilation to improve oxygen uptake, a simultaneous drop in blood carbon dioxide would draw carbon dioxide from the CSF, leaving there an excess of bicarbonate, which in turn would stop the drive. This paradoxic antagonism between these two important components of the respiratory control system, which places the patient in great jeopardy, may be one of the most important physiologic casualties of chronic respiratory failure. Hypoxia must be present for the chemoreceptor drive to function, and this function ceases when hypoxia is corrected. In this circumstance, **indiscriminate use of oxygen can be fatal.** In ventilatory failure, respiratory exchange is inadequate for prolonged survival, but *some* ventilation is better than *none,* even though it maintains a state of hypercapnia and hypoxia. Should the patient be given oxygen to relieve hypoxia, the chemoreceptors can cease to function, and *breathing can stop.* In this state of apnea, acidemia and cellular acidosis can rapidly increase to a fatal level, and the patient can expire, often with a paradoxically healthy-appearing pink complexion. This is a very real risk in the treatment of patients in failure and must be guarded against by all those involved in the patient's management. Safe and effective techniques are discussed in Chapter 12.

The patient in respiratory acidosis will manifest hypoventilation in one of two ways. The tidal volume will be small, sometimes with barely perceptible chest and epigastric motion, or the patient will be tachypneic, with rapid shallow movements that accomplish little more than ventilation of the dead space.

Laboratory examinations will show a low pH, an elevated P_{CO_2} and bicarbonate, a low serum chloride, and an acid urine. If acid-base compensation is poor, the patient's mental state will be obtunded or he or she may be in a coma, and almost always the ventilation is enough impaired that hypoxia produces visible cyanosis. Although much of the management is directed toward the underlying disease, the most critical treatment is the correction of hypoventilation, usually best accomplished by assisting the patient with mechanical ventilators or controlling breathing completely. *While being given adequate ventilation,* the patient can be given oxygen as needed to correct hypoxia, blood gas and pH determinations being used frequently to monitor the effectiveness of therapy.

Example 4: respiratory acidosis (acute). The patient is a 60-year-old white man with long-standing chronic bronchitis. He is in the emergency ward with severe respiratory distress. On 1 ℓ of nasal flow blood gases show:

pH: 7.33 Pa_{CO_2}: 55 mm Hg HCO_3^-: 28 mEq/ℓ
                  Pa_{O_2}: 54 mm Hg   BE: +1 mEq/ℓ

Example 5: compensated respiratory acidosis. This 54-year-old woman has had asthma for many years. She was hospitalized 1 week ago, now feels improved, and is to be discharged. Before discharge this blood gas is obtained while the patient breathed room air:

pH: 7.35 Pa_{CO_2}: 71 mm Hg HCO_3^-: 38 mEq/ℓ
                  Pa_{O_2}: 79 mm Hg   BE: +11 mEq/ℓ

Respiratory alkalosis

Alveolar hyperventilation removes carbon dioxide from the blood, dropping the P_{CO_2} to low levels and elevating the pH. The respiratory center can be stimulated to excessive activity by brain injury or a tumor's increasing pressure on the center, excessive salicylate ingestion, fever, inflammation of the brain, or emotional stimuli. Of immediate concern to the respiratory therapist, however, is the hyperventilation that *he or she* can induce by the use of mechanical ventilators. Artificial ventilation of a patient with a normal respiratory tract can easily be overdone and the patient caused to hyperventilate into respiratory alkalosis. The therapist must watch carefully to prevent this development.

Compensation is accomplished by an increased renal excretion of bicarbonate, retention of chloride, and reduction in both the formation of ammonia and excretion of acid salts. This lowers the blood bicarbonate level, bringing the acid-base ratio back toward 20:1 and reducing the pH.

Alkalosis is as hazardous to the patient as is acidosis. He or she is seen to be breathing deeply, and blood shows an elevated pH, a depressed P_{CO_2}, and depending on the degree of compensation, low bicarbonate and total carbon dioxide levels. Serum chloride may be slightly elevated, and the urine alkaline. The patient may complain of *paresthesias* of the extremities, a sensation of "pins and needles" or of the extremities being "asleep." Reflexes are hyperactive, true tetanic contractions may occur, and somnolence increasing to coma may develop. One of the major complications of alkalosis is its impairment of cerebral circulation, as a rapid decrease in P_{CO_2} produces a contraction of cerebral arterioles, with a reduction in blood flow to the brain. This can be severe enough to cause speech difficulty and muscular paralysis, which may be permanent. Hypocapnia also predisposes the patient to serious disturbance in cardiac rhythm (arrhythmia), which may lead to arrest. Treatment is usually directed toward the underlying cause, but symptomatic relief can often be obtained by the use of sedation to suppress the respiratory center and by the inhalation of carbon dioxide to build up the blood P_{CO_2}.

Example 6: respiratory alkalosis. A distraught 77-year-old man comes to the hospital and is found to have been ingesting large doses of aspirin (acetylsalicylic acid) in a suicide attempt. It is known that aspirin ingestion has two distinct phases as it relates to blood gas abnormality. First, early in the digestion the aspirin stimulates the ventilatory centers so the patient breathes faster and thus blows off carbon dioxide, resulting in a respiratory alkalosis. Next a metabolic acidosis results. This patient's blood gases on room air showed:

pH: 7.52	Pa_{CO_2}: 26 mm Hg	HCO_3^-: 21 mEq/ℓ
	Pa_{CO_2}: 69 mm Hg	BE: −1 mEq/ℓ

Metabolic acidosis   In metabolic disorders, acid-base balance is dependent on the electrolytic balance in the body, or the relation between the positively charged ions (cations) and the negatively charged ions (anions).[27,28] The former consist of sodium, calcium, potassium, and magnesium; the latter, bicarbonate, protein, (serum protein and hemoglobin), phosphate, chloride, sulfate, and organic acids. The bicarbonate, protein, and phosphate ions we already know comprise the buffer systems of the body and are appropriately named *buffer anions*. The remaining anions are designated as *fixed anions*. The cations are combined with a variety of anions, and those that are in combination with the buffer anions (mostly sodium as $NaHCO_3$, but small amounts of the other cations as well) are termed *buffer cations,* and sometimes *buffer base* or *total body buffer*. The remaining cations, combined with other than buffer anions, may be considered as *fixed cations*. The sum of the anions must equal the sum of the cations, and they are usually measured in mEq/ℓ.

The total ionic content of plasma in concentration per liter is depicted in Fig. 6-10. Here, two columns contain the *cations* and *anions,* and their average normal values are indicated. Carbonic acid dissociates so little that it is indicated in both columns as mEq/ℓ of H_2CO_3. The buffer anions are clearly delineated from the fixed anions; the buffer cations are not different cations from the fixed cations but rather are portions of the latter that are combined with buffer anions. It can be seen, for example, that if chloride should decrease in amount, the buffer anions would increase to keep the total unchanged. Also, it is easy to visualize a loss of sodium, with an accompanying loss of bicarbonate, and chloride expanding to replace the bicarbonate. Thus the interchanges between the electrolytes as a result of metabolic reactions modify the buffer anions and through changes, especially in the bicarbonate, regulate pH. Although the metabolic relation to acid-base balance is not of primary concern to the respiratory therapist, a general understanding of the basic principles should be of interest, since many patients will have systemic diseases associated with the respiratory.

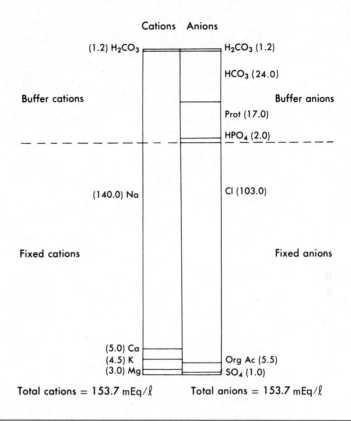

Cations   Anions

(1.2) H₂CO₃ ——— H₂CO₃ (1.2)

HCO₃ (24.0)

Buffer cations   Buffer anions

Prot (17.0)

HPO₄ (2.0)

(140.0) Na   Cl (103.0)

Fixed cations   Fixed anions

(5.0) Ca
(4.5) K
(3.0) Mg   Org Ac (5.5)
                     SO₄ (1.0)

Total cations = 153.7 mEq/ℓ   Total anions = 153.7 mEq/ℓ

Fig. 6-10   Balance between fixed and buffer electrolytes of plasma.

Any systemic disease that causes a depletion of the fixed cations or buffer base, or an increase in the fixed anions, can produce metabolic acidosis. The production of abnormal acids in the blood, or the retention of acids through failure of the kidney to excrete them, will replace buffer anions. This may be viewed as the depletion of the buffer ions while neutralizing the acids. Again, in the plasma, bicarbonate is the major anion involved, since the most prevalent protein, hemoglobin, is found only in the erythrocyte, and phosphate is present in only small amounts. Keeping in mind the H-H equation, we can conveniently visualize an abnormal buildup of acids in the body (especially organic) with which the plasma bicarbonate reacts to neutralize the acidity. This effort depletes the available bicarbonate, lowering the numerator of the H-H equation and reducing blood pH. Retention of chloride, incident to an excessive intake of this ion, will replace some of the bicarbonate in the anion column, lowering the blood pH. Surprisingly, and somewhat paradoxically, loss of potassium, which might be expected to produce acidosis, raises the pH. This is the result of a complex chain of electrolytic exchanges by which there is, in the presence of potassium loss, a disproportionately larger renal loss of chloride so that the net result in an increase in bicarbonate.

Compensation for metabolic acidosis is by an increase in the respiratory removal of carbon dioxide proportionately to the bicarbonate through the mechanism of hyperventilation. In Table 6-6, from the blood findings alone it is not possible to distinguish between *compensated* respiratory alkalosis and *compensated* metabolic acidosis. In this case the clinical picture of the patient's condition will be the deciding factor. The treatment of metabolic acidosis is obviously that of the underlying disease, since the respiratory abnormality is a compensatory act and not a reflection of respiratory disease.

Example 7: metabolic acidosis (acute). A 19-year-old college student is brought to the emergency room comatose and cyanotic. Needles and syringes were found in his room. Needle marks are seen on his skin. Heroin addiction is suspected but because of the information obtained from his blood gases while he breathed an unknown oxygen concentration, a serum glucose level is obtained that showed he has diabetic ketoacidosis. Here are the gases:

pH: 7.29 Pa_{CO_2}: 34 mm Hg HCO_3^-: 17 mEq/ℓ
            Pa_{CO_2}: 97 mm Hg   BE: -9 mEq/ℓ

Note the high Pa_{O_2}. It is elevated because the patient is hyperventilating to blow off his carbon dioxide to get rid of hydrogen, which allows for a higher alveolar PO_2 and arterial PO_2 (see Appendix 12).

Example 8: compensated metabolic acidosis. A 38-year-old man has severe diarrhea and has suffered for weeks without medical attention. Because of the diarrhea, he has lost pancreatic fluid, which contained large amounts of bicarbonate. When excreted through the bowels this results in an enormous bicarbonate loss.

pH: 7.37 Pa_{CO_2}: 35 mm Hg HCO_3^-: 19 mEq/ℓ
            Pa_{O_2}: 102 mm Hg   BE: -5 mEq/ℓ

Metabolic alkalosis   Metabolic alkalosis is the product of any systemic disease that causes an excess of buffer through a relative increase of fixed cations over fixed anions. This can be the result of the loss of chloride of gastric hydrogen chloride in protracted vomiting, the retention of large amounts of sodium by the ingestion of alkalis (the sodium thus combining with additional bicarbonate), the disproportionate loss of chloride over sodium common with use of diuretics, or the effect of potassium loss just mentioned. (This is often found in potassium loss that occurs with intubation and drainage of the bowel, long-term use of corticosteroids, or a reduced potassium intake.) Compensation is attempted by a conservation of carbonic acid through hypoventilation to raise the acid denominator of the H-H equation and to restore a 20:1 ratio. Again note that *compensated* metabolic alkalosis is indistinguishable chemically from *compensated* respiratory acidosis, which emphasizes the fact that diagnostic reliance cannot be placed completely on the laboratory.

Example 9: metabolic alkalosis. A 83-year-old white woman with heart disease has been taking a powerful diuretic to remove excess edema fluid from her legs and help keep her free of pulmonary edema. She is hospitalized because of vomiting and muscle cramps. Her blood gases on 3 ℓ/min nasal oxygen shows the results of losing chloride and potassium in her urine because of the effects of the diuretic:

pH: 7.48 Pa_{CO_2}: 43 mm Hg HCO_3^-: 31 mEq/ℓ
                Pa_{O_2}: 71 mm Hg   BE: +8 mEq/ℓ

Example 10: compensated metabolic alkalosis. A 63-year-old man shows typical blood gas and acid-base changes seen in compensating for metabolic alkalosis. Note the hypoventilation resulting in an elevated Pa_{CO_2}. The fact that the pH is on the high side of normal suggests the basic abnormality is an alkalosis, not a respiratory acidosis caused by retained carbon dioxide. In compensation, the body never compensates beyond the midpoint of 7.40.

pH: 7.43 Pa_{CO_2}: 50 mm Hg HCO_3^-: 32 mEq/ℓ
                Pa_{O_2}: 94 mm Hg   BE: 7 mEq/ℓ

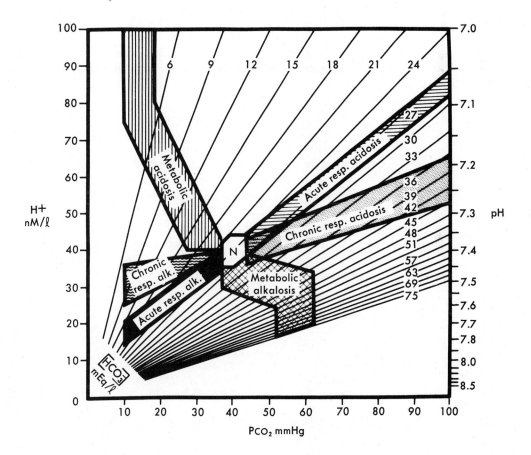

Fig. 6-11   Acid-base map. (See text for description.) (Reprinted from Goldberg, M., et al.: The Journal of the American Medical Association, Jan. 15, 1973, Vol. 223. Copyright 1973, American Medical Association.)

Mixed acid-base states

It is obvious that combinations of disorders may occur in the same patient.[29,30] Any of the four respiratory states may coexist with any of the four metabolic states, and patients with simultaneous respiratory and metabolic diseases often present complicated pictures. Referred to earlier, and emphasized again, is the patient with respiratory acidosis who swings rapidly into respiratory alkalosis because of too vigorous therapy and thus demonstrates not simultaneous but alternating acid-base disorders. A respiratory imbalance in one direction can theoretically be offset by a metabolic imbalance in the other, with a resulting normal pH. Differentiation between these possibilities is a medical problem requiring the finest diagnostic acumen and intelligent use of the laboratory, and the difficulties encountered should be appreciated by the respiratory therapist.

When acid-base status is very labile, responding to both metabolic and respiratory stimuli, it is sometimes helpful to monitor the blood gas changes with a so-called *acid-base map*. Many formats are available, one example of which is illustrated in Fig. 6-11. The areas of acid-base abnormalities surrounding a central normal axis were plotted as 95% confidence bands or limits, based on the clinical and statistical analysis of a large number of patients with a wide variety of acid-base imbalances. Such a confidence limit simply means that in all probability, of 100 patients whose arterial blood gas data projection lines intersect in a given designated area, 95 have that disorder. Intersects outside the mapped areas indicate mixed acid-base problems.

Such a device gives no information not available in a simple flow chart, is no substitute for a solid understanding of acid-base physiology, and does not provide an automatic, foolproof diagnosis. However, it gives a visual running account of sequential relationships between blood gas values and the probable clinical states they represent. Each student must decide whether or not a learning tool such as this is best for him or her.

Other examples of blood gas and pH values can be found elsewhere in the medical literature, and students are encouraged to seek these out for further information and practice.[9,31-33]

References

1. Divertie, M.B., and Brown, A.L., Jr.: The fine structure of the normal alveolocapillary membrane, J.A.M.A. **187**:938, 1964.

2. Comroe, J.H., Jr., et al.: The lung, ed. 2, Chicago, 1962, Year Book Medical Publishers, Inc.

3. Dittmer, D.S., and Grebe, R.M., editors: Handbook of respiration, Philadelphia, 1958, W.B. Saunders Co.

4. Roughton, F.J.W.: The average time spent by the blood in the human lung capillary, and its relation to the rates of carbon monoxide uptake and elimination in man, Am. J. Physiol. **143**:621, 1945.

5. Nunn, J.F.: Applied respiratory physiology, ed 2., Kent, England, 1977, Butterworth & Co.

6. Gregory, I.C.: The oxygen and carbon dioxide capacities of fetal and adult hemoglobin, J. Physiol. (Lond.) **236**:625, 1974.

7. Murray, J.F.: The normal lung, Philadelphia, 1976, W.B. Saunders Co.

8. Fishman, A.P., editor: Assessment of pulmonary function, New York, 1980, McGraw-Hill Book Co.

9. Shapiro, B.A., Harrison, R.A., and Walton, J.R.: Clinical application of blood

gases, ed. 2, Chicago, 1977, Year Book Medical Publishers, Inc.

10. Comroe, J.H.: Physiology of respiration, ed. 2, Chicago, 1974, Year Book Medical Publishers, Inc.,

11. Benesch, R., and Benesch, R.E.: Intracellular organic phosphates as regulators of oxygen release by haemoglobin, Nature **221:**618, 1969.

12. Astrup, P.: Red-cell pH and oxygen affinity of hemoglobin, N. Engl. J. Med. **283:**202, 1970.

13. Oski, F.A., et al.: Red-cell 2,3-diphosphoglycerate levels in subjects with chronic hypoxemia, N. Engl. J. Med. **280:**1165, 1969.

14. Torrance, J., et al.: Intraerythrocyte adaptation to anemia, N. Engl. J. Med. **283:**165, 1970.

15. Lichtman, M.A., et al.: Reduced red cell glycolysis, 2,3-diphosphoglycerate and adenosine triphosphate concentration, and increased hemoglobin-oxygen affinity caused by hypophosphatemia, Ann. Intern. Med. **74:**562, 1971.

16. Klocke, R.A.: Oxygen transport and 2,3-diphosphoglycerate (DPG), Chest **62** (suppl.):79s, 1972.

17. Peters, J.P., and Van Slyke, D.D.: Quantitative clinical chemistry, vol. 2, Baltimore, 1931, The Williams & Wilkins Co.

18. ACCP-ATS Joint Committee on Pulmonary Nomenclature: Pulmonary terms and symbols, Chest **67:**583, 1975.

19. Dejours, P.: Respiration, Oxford, England, 1966, Oxford University Press.

20. Winterstein, H.: Chemical control of pulmonary ventilation, N. Engl. J. Med. **255:**331, 1956.

21. Winterstein, H.: Chemical control of pulmonary ventilation, N. Engl. J. Med. **255:**216, 1956.

22. Peters, R.M.: The mechanical basis of respiration, Boston, 1969, Little, Brown & Co.

23. Lugliani, R., et al.: Effect of bilateral carotid-body resection on ventilatory control at rest and during exercise in man, N. Engl. J. Med. **285:**1105, 1971.

24. Dorland's illustrated medical dictionary, ed. 25, Philadelphia, 1974, W.B. Saunders Co.

25. Refsum, H.E.: Acid-base disturbances in chronic pulmonary disease, Ann. N.Y. Acad. Sci. **133:**142, 1966.

26. Petty, T.L., and Neff, T.A.: Renal function in respiratory failure, J.A.M.A. **217:**82, 1971.

27. Snively, W.D., et al.: Systematic approach to fluid balance, part 1, G.P. **13:**74, Jan. 1956.

28. Snively, W.D., et al.: Systematic approach to fluid balance, part 2, G.P. **13:**74, Feb. 1956.

29. Fordham, C.C., III, and Relman, A.J.: Mixed respiratory and metabolic acidosis, N. Engl. J. Med. **256:**698, 1957.

30. Robin, E.D.: Abnormalities of acid-base regulation in chronic pulmonary disease, with special reference to hypercapnia and extracellular alkalosis, N. Engl. J. Med. **268:**917, 1963.

31. Burton, G.G., Gee, G.L., and Hodgkin, J.E., editors: Respiratory care: a guide to clinical practice, Philadelphia, 1977, J.B. Lippincott Co.

32. Jones, N.L.: Blood gases and acid-base physiology, New York, 1980, Thieme-Stratton, Inc.

33. Rose B.D.: Clinical physiology of acid-base and electrolyte disorders, New York, 1977, McGraw-Hill Book Co.

Chapter 7   Cardiovascular system

In view of the many texts written on the structure, function, and pathology of the heart, it is unnecessary for us to undertake a comprehensive review of cardiology. However, because the functions of the heart and lungs are so interrelated, a brief explanation of some selected features of the cardiovascular system is pertinent, with emphasis on those aspects relating most directly to principles and practice of respiratory therapy. From references already made, it should be apparent that the therapist will frequently be called on to treat patients with both pulmonary and cardiac diseases and should always be aware of *cardiopulmonary* function.

Fundamental anatomy

The heart is a muscular organ located in the chest cavity behind the sternum (Fig. 7-1). About two thirds of the heart is to the left of the sternum's midline, and the heart is bordered inferiorly by the diaphragm.

The *pericardium* is the serouslike sac that surrounds the outside of the heart next to the outer wall, the *epicardium*. The *endocardium* is the inner wall of the heart. The heart muscle, the *myocardium,* is made of laminated layers of specialized cardiac muscle fibers. These muscle fibers provide the heart with the

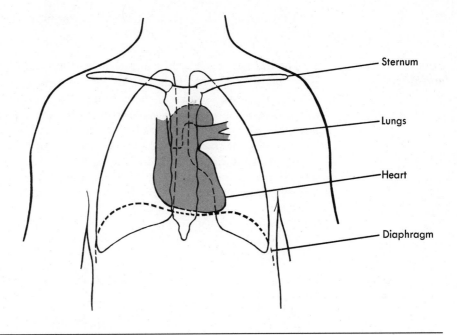

Fig. 7-1   The heart lies in chest behind sternum, toward left side, and rests on diaphragm.

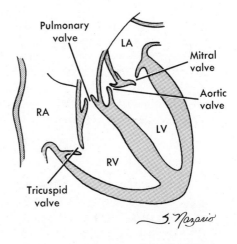

Fig. 7-2   Schematic of heart chambers and valves. *RA,* right atrium; *RV,* right ventricle; *LA,* left atrium; *LV,* left ventricle.

ability to change the size of its chambers during contraction and relaxation, creating a pumplike action.

Heart chambers and valves

The heart is comprised of four chambers and can be thought of as a dual-sided pump. Each side, right and left, has an *atrium* and a *ventricle* (Fig. 7-2). The atria receive blood and pump it into the ventricles. The right ventricle pumps blood into the *pulmonary circuit,* while the left ventricle pumps blood into the *systemic circuit.* The right side of the heart is separated from the left by a *septum*; the *interatrial* portion and the *interventricular* portion.

Between the right atrium and the right ventricle is a one-way valve called the *tricuspid valve* (Fig. 7-2). This three-leafed valve directs blood flow from the atrium to the ventricle without allowing backflow to occur when the ven-

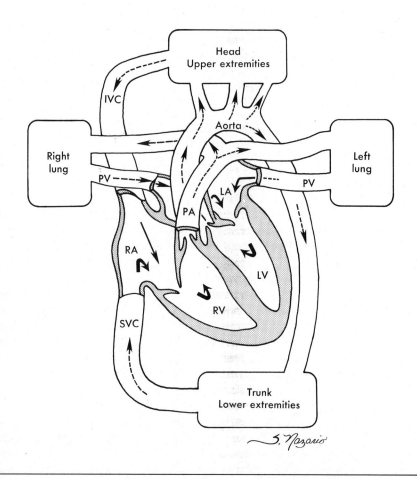

Fig. 7-3   Schematic of plan of circulation. *RA,* right atrium; *RV,* right ventricle; *LA,* left atrium; *LV,* left ventricle; *IVC,* inferior vena cava; *SVC,* superior vena cava; *PA,* pulmonary artery; *PV,* pulmonary vein.

tricle contracts. The *pulmonary valve* is a semilunar valve at the outflow of the right ventricle, which allows blood to flow from the ventricle into the pulmonary artery.

The *biscuspid* or *mitral valve* separates the left atrium from the left ventricle. When the left ventricle contracts, the mitral valve prevents backflow to the atrium. Instead, blood flows from the left ventricle through the *aortic valve* and into the aorta. The aortic valve is another semilunar, one-way valve.

Plan of circulation   Fig. 7-3 represents the basic plan of blood flow to and from the heart. Venous or "deoxygenated" blood from the head and upper extremities enters the right atrium from the *superior vena cava* while blood from the lower body and extremities enters from the *inferior vena cava.* From there blood flows through the tricuspid valve into the right ventricle. The right ventricle pumps blood through the pulmonary valve, into the pulmonary arteries, and on to the lungs. Oxygenated blood returns to the left atrium through the pulmonary veins. The left atrium pumps blood through the mitral valve into the left ventricle, where it is pumped through the aortic valve and into the aorta. From the aorta the blood flows out to the tissues of the upper and lower body and extremities. From the various body tissues, venous blood returns to the vena cavae.

Cardiac cycle   In the performance of its function as a pump, the heart works through a ceaseless series of cycles, from the prenatal period to the moment of death. Each cardiac cycle is composed of a contraction of the myocardial fibers, followed by a period of rest. Contraction of the involuntary muscle is achieved by a forceful shortening of each fiber so that as the total muscle mass contracts, it builds up a pressure in the cavities it encloses, reduces their volumes, and expresses their contents into the cardiac outflow tracts. Nerve impulses from the higher centers of the central nervous system are carried to the heart by the vagus nerve, which contains parasympathetic fibers, and by sympathetic nerves arising from the upper thoracic segments of the spinal cord. The former inhibit heart action, the latter stimulate it, and the net sum of the constant barrage of impulses through these channels determines the final controlling influence.

Within the heart itself, a highly specialized system of conducting tissue is responsible for the precisely timed distribution of impulses to all parts of the myocardium. Under suitable conditions the intact heart removed from all nerve connections can continue to beat for a period of time, which demonstrates that despite its control over cardiac contraction, the central nervous innervation is not essential for heart action. There must be, therefore, an automatic stimulus in the heart capable of maintaining contraction but, in the intact subject, greatly influenced by the central nervous system. This is labeled the *conduction system* of the heart. Fig. 7-4 illustrates the major portions of this system: *the sinoatrial node* (sinus node), the *atrioventricular node* (A-V node), the *atrioventricular bundle* (bundle of His), and the *bundle branches* and *Pur-*

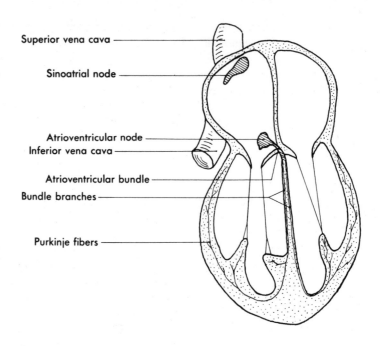

Superior vena cava

Sinoatrial node

Atrioventricular node
Inferior vena cava

Atrioventricular bundle
Bundle branches

Purkinje fibers

Fig. 7-4   Conduction system of the heart. (See text for description.)

kinje fibers. The histology of the conduction system is that of highly specialized muscle fibers rather than nerve fibers but capable of conducting muscle-stimulating impulses.

Sinoatrial node (sinus node). The sinus node is called the *pacemaker* of the heart and is a small nodule of conducting tissue, about ³/₄ inch long, located in the muscle of the right atrium just in front of the opening of the superior vena cava. The sinus node initiates electrical impulses (described later), which radiate from it in the fashion of circular ripples from a stone dropped into water. Traveling at a rate of 1000 mm/sec, these impulses are discharged at variable rates, from 50 to 90/min but average about 70/min at rest. They excite the atrial myocardium to contract, both atria functioning simultaneously. The discharge rate of the sinus node is modified by nervous control, increased by the sympathetic nerves, and inhibited by the parasympathetic through vagal innervation. Cardiac rate can be increased by excessive stimulation of sympathetic nerves or by drugs simulating sympathetic action, and the heart can be slowed or stopped by parasympathetic action, especially through the action of certain reflexes carried by the vagus nerve. Both effects are of considerable clinical importance.

Atrioventricular node (A-V node). Similar in structure to the sinus node, the A-V node is located in the right atrium on the lower part of the interatrial septum just above the septal leaf of the tricuspid valve. It functions as a pickup and relay station for sinus impulses. With no structural connection to the sinus node, the A-V node is stimulated by the radiating sinus impulses, and it relays these onward into the ventricles. Should the sinus node fail to function because of disease, the A-V node then assumes the duties of pacemaker, but it is less effective than the sinus node.

Atrioventricular bundle (bundle of His). A well-defined bundle of muscular tissue originates at the A-V node and runs horizontally forward over the septal tricuspid valve leaf to the upper part of the interventricular septum. The sinus impulse received by the A-V node is transmitted through the bundle and is thus carried to the myocardium of the ventricular chambers. This is the only conduction link between atria and ventricles, and when it is damaged or destroyed by disease, a condition of *block* is said to exist, a cardiac condition commonly encountered in clinical medicine.

Bundle branches and Purkinje fibers. On the upper part of the interventricular septum, the A-V bundle terminates by dividing into two *bundle branches,* the right and left, each going to its respective ventricle. The bundles pass down the septum, beneath the endocardium, giving off branches to the papillary muscles, and then continue into the ventricles, where they divide into innumerable fine filaments and form a network (Purkinje fibers) interlacing the depths of the ventricular muscle. The impulse, originating in the sinus node, is carried at a rate of some 5000 mm/sec to every portion of the ventricles, in effect stimulating all myocardial fibers simultaneously, for uniform contraction of both ventricles.

The sequence of the cardiac cycle is contraction of both atria, driving blood into the ventricles, followed by contraction of both ventricles, which expels the blood into the cardiac outflow tracts. These phases of muscular contraction are respectively called atrial and ventricular *systole.* After systole both sets of chambers enter a period of rest and muscular relaxation called *diastole.* Because systole and diastole of the two sets of chambers are not of uniform duration, there is some overlapping, illustrated in Fig. 7-5, which shows the start of a cardiac cycle with ventricular systole, as a matter of convenience. Note that the atria spend most of their time in diastole, during which time blood flows into these chambers from the venae cavae and pulmonary veins and, with the tricuspid and mitral valves closed, the atria distend with blood. After about 0.3 second of atrial diastole, a point corresponding to the end of ventricular systole, the atrioventricular valves open and atrial blood flows into the ventricles. Then, at 0.7 second, atrial systole occurs for a brief 0.1 second, forcibly ejecting the last of the atrial blood into the ventricles. During atrial diastole, ventricular systole takes place, for about 0.3 second; then as the A-V valves open, the semilunar valves close and the ventricles enter their diastolic phase. For approximately 0.4 second, atrial and ventricular diastoles coincide and the entire heart is quiet, as blood is flowing by gravity from atria into ventricles. The myocardium has a peculiar quality that assures the heart of maximum contractile effort. Once systolic contraction begins, the fibers are *refractory,* or resistant to further stimulation, until they have had time to recover and regain their energy. This means that repeated stimuli cannot maintain them in a state of

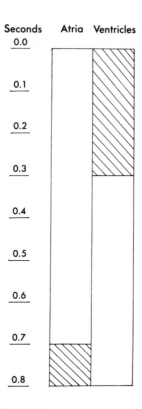

Fig. 7-5   The duration and relationships of the systolic *(shaded)* and diastolic *(clear)* components of the cardiac cycle are shown for a rate of 75 beats/min.

continued contraction, which would eventually lead to serious fatigue. The refractory period of the myocardium is maintained through systole and for an additional period of time approximately equal to the duration of systole, when it once again is responsive to stimuli.

The heartbeat, as palpated through the chest wall and at the peripheral arterial pulses, reflects the force of ventricular systole only, since the contraction of the atria is not sufficiently strong to be transmitted. The pause between beats consists of ventricular diastole, the last part of atrial diastole, and the unnoticed atrial systole. As the heart rate varies, the duration of the cycle segments will vary inversely. Thus rapid rates (tachycardia) often associated with disease not only reduce the rest periods of the myocardium but also, by shortening filling time, can reduce the cardiac output per beat (stroke volume).

Electrophysiology of the heart

As with other muscles, contraction of myocardial fibers is an electrical phenomenon consisting of the buildup and discharge of a minute electrical current. A strip of muscle fiber may be visualized as covered with positive and negative charges, these charges being equally distributed throughout the strip so that in the resting state the net electrical charge is neutral. With an electrical potential present, the muscle strip is polarized and is neither predominately positive nor negative. Should a portion of a muscle strip become excited or activated, or suffer injury, the area so affected becomes electronegative in relation to the rest of the muscle, as the zinc electrode of a battery is electronegative to the copper electrode. With this disruption in the even distribution of the electric charges, zones of opposite polarity are formed, and a current flows from the positive to the negative zone. The muscle strip undergoes a process of *depolarization,* whereby all of the charges are used up in the current flow, until the strip is completely depolarized, or without electric potential. Functionally, this is the stage of muscle contraction, or cardiac systole. During diastole the muscle strip undergoes *repolarization,* with reestablishment of the original polarity. This process proceeds in the reverse direction from depolarization, starting with the end of the strip most recently depolarized, and since it involves zones of opposite polarity, a current is also produced during repolarization. Fig. 7-6 demonstrates those two important phenomena. The *rectangles* represent muscle strips; those fully shaded at the top of the left column and the bottom of the right column are in the resting, polarized state, with equal numbers of positive and negative charges. Over the center of each strip is an electrode to pick up current flow and lead it to a recording device that will translate the flow into a curve. The recorder is so designed that when the electrode is opposite positively charged tissue, an upright curve is written, and when opposite negative, a downslope. Representative curves are illustrated adjacent to each rectangle.

Because the polarized strip in the left column has a net neutral charge evenly distributed about it, no current flows and the electrode records a straight, or *isoelectric* line. After a suitable stimulus, depolarization begins as a zone of negativity at the left end of the strip, and this depolarized area is delineated in the illustrations from the remainder of the still polarized muscle by a vertical boundary line. The opposite side of the boundary is positively charged, and the direction of current flow is depicted by arrows. As depolarization progresses, the electrode is faced with the approaching positive charge and records an upstroke. When the boundary is directly beneath the electrode, because it is neither positive nor negative, the curve drops to the isoelectric line. Almost at once, strong negative charges are recorded, the curve drops sharply below the baseline, and as the negativity moves gradually away from the electrode, its influence wanes, the curve returning up to the baseline. At this point the strip is completely depolarized, and charges are absent. The right column shows the repolarization proceeding in the opposite direction, recording curves that are the reverse of those of depolarization.

The preceding principles are widely used in diagnostic electrocardiography and in monitoring devices for the continued observation of cardiac action in acutely ill patients. The electrical characteristics of the intact heart are more

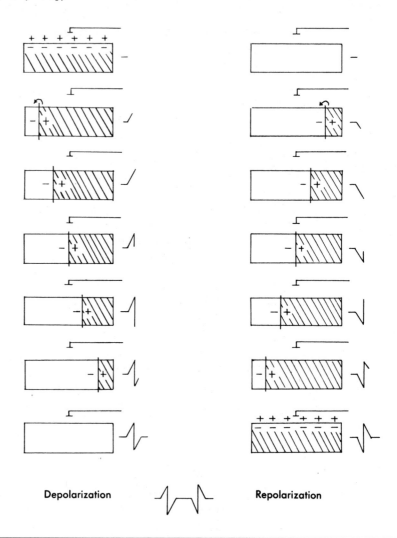

Fig. 7-6 Schematic representation of depolarization and repolarization of heart muscle. (See text for description.) (Modified from Barker, J.M.: The unipolar electrocardiogram, New York, 1952, Appleton-Century-Crofts.)

complex than those of the isolated muscle strip, and the currents recorded by the electrodes are the net sums of many currents in the areas being explored. It is not intended to present a course in electrocardiographic interpretation but only to describe the basic major features of this important diagnostic tool.[1] Fig. 7-7 represents a typical "average" electrocardiographic segment, showing the characteristic curves recorded from a normal heart. The electrocardiographic machine amplifies the small electric currents brought to it by the electrode leads and passes them through a *galvanometer,* in which is located a pivoted

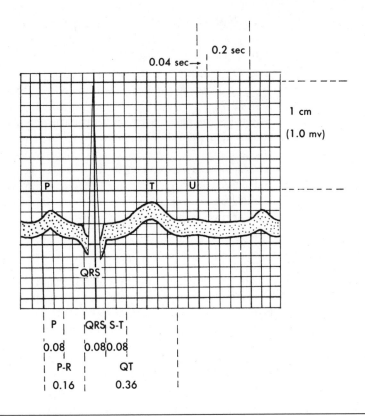

Fig. 7-7   Sketch of a normal electrocardiographic pattern. (See text for description.)

writing arm called a *stylus*. Depending on the polarity of the current passing through the galvanometer, the stylus is attracted to one or the other pole of the galvanometer magnet. By convention, positive deflections move the stylus upward, and negative deflections downward. The movements are recorded on specially calibrated graph paper, which moves at a fixed speed, and the curves thus written can be measured in terms of voltage (vertical amplitude) and time (horizontal distance). Many different leads are used to give various electric "views" of the heart. For monitoring purposes one lead is employed and the current projected through a cathode tube onto a fluorescent screen, where the record of each heartbeat can be seen as it is formed. Such an instrument is called an *oscilloscope*.

Although the contour of each lead differs from the others, the major components of an electrocardiographic tracing are illustrated in Fig. 7-7. The *bold vertical lines* represent time intervals of 0.2 second, subdivided into increments of 0.04 second. *Bold horizontal lines* are 1 cm apart, measuring an amplitude of 1.0 millivolt (mv), and each interval between represents 0.1 mv. Some normal values of amplitude and duration are indicated in the illustration. The *P* wave records the electrical activity of atrial systole, whereas the *QRS* complex represents ventricular depolarization. The *P-R* interval (actually, the P-QRS interval) is the length of time taken by the atrial impulse to reach the ventricles. The *QT* time is referred to as electrical ventricular systole (not mechanical systole). Diastole extends from the end of *T* to the next *P* and often contains a small *U* wave, the significance of which is not well understood. The *S-T* interval is the pause between ventricular depolarization and repolarization and represents a period of *absolute* ventricular refractoriness, during which the ventricles cannot be stimulated, since they have not yet become polarized. Ventricular repolarization records the *T* wave, during which time the ventricles are only relatively refractory, since they can respond to stimuli in proportion to the degree that repolarization has been completed. After the T, of course, ventricular myocardium is fully responsive.

Cardiac arrhythmias

The importance of the cardiac arrhythmias lies not so much in their relation to respiratory therapy directly as in the frequency with which they occur in the hospital population most apt to be serviced by respiratory therapy. In the performance of duties, the respiratory therapist will see and hear much attention directed to this class of cardiac disorders, and especially in critical care units he or she will see visual evidence of them on oscilloscope monitor screens. We outline here the minimal features of arrhythmias most commonly encountered in hospital practice, ignoring the more bizarre, and leave it to the individual therapist to supplement this material with independent reading.

Although *dysrhythmia* (a malfunctioning rhythm) is probably more accurate, *arrhythmia* has become the standard expression for a cardiac rhythm that deviates from the usual and natural pattern, interrupting the automatic rhythmic heart action that was initiated before birth. Many of the rhythm disturbances can be diagnosed with certainty only by the electrocardiogram, others can be readily detected clinically, and the presence of yet others may be highly suspected. The presence of an abnormal heart rhythm is not necessarily a bad omen, since many of them are innocuous and occur in normal hearts; but others may indicate serious underlying pathologic conditions, and a few signify imminent death. A simple physiologic concept must be understood if one is to appreciate the great variety of abnormal rhythms to which the heart is subject. We have already established that the sinus node is the normal focus for the start of cardiac contraction, but any site in the myocardium or the conducting system is capable of initiating excitation. It is as though an almost infinite number of trigger points are kept subdued by the normal action of the dominant sinus node but express themselves when some factor causes the latter to lose its tight control. We briefly describe the following, all of which the therapist may expect to see in the general hospital: sinus arrhythmia, premature contractions, paroxysmal tachycardia, atrial flutter, atrial fibrillation, ventricular fibrillation, atrioventricular block, and sinus arrest.[2,3]

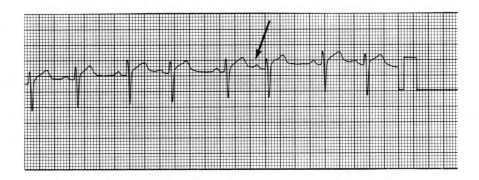

Fig. 7-8   Sinus arrhythmia. *Arrow* denotes early P wave.

Sinus arrhythmia
(Fig. 7-8)

The most frequent and least harmful of all the arrhythmias, sinus arrhythmia, is a normal variant in the young but can be found at almost any age. It is characterized by a change in cardiac rate synchronous with the respiratory cycle, as the heart rate increases during inspiration and decreases with expiration. It can be exaggerated by inspiratory breath holding and eliminated by exercise. The mechanism for its presence is an alteration in the strength of vagal (parasympathetic) influence on the normal pacemaker. Presumably, during inspiration the increased vagal impulses brought into play by the Hering-Breuer reflex quantitatively detract from the vagal impulses serving the sinus node. With lessened parasympathetic inhibition during this phase of respiration, the excitation rate of the node increases with a similar response by the ventricles. This condition has no pathologic implications, and no treatment is indicated.

Premature
contractions
(Figs. 7-9 to 7-11)

Localized areas of the atria, A-V node, and ventricular myocardium may initiate an excitation impulse independently of the sinus node. Because they occur away from the normal focus of stimulation, they are referred to as *ectopic foci.* Premature contractions may be prognostically benign or serious, since they can occur in both normal and diseased hearts. They result from the irritation of some spot in the myocardium or conducting system by a variety of stimulants, among which the following are frequent offenders: excitement, anxiety, smoking, alcohol ingestion, fatigue, gastrointestinal disturbances, and procedures such as thoracic surgery, cardiac catheterization, and digitalis (a vital drug used in the treatment of heart failure but which can irritate the myocardium).

The premature contraction is an "extra" beat and is so named because it is activated before a normal beat would be expected, inserting itself between two normal contractions. If the stimulus is great enough or there is more than one stimulus, there may be a short string of premature contractions. Also, in pathologic states different stimuli may generate impulses from more than one ectopic focus. There are three general types of premature contractions: atrial nodal, and ventricular. In the first an ectopic atrial impulse follows the usual

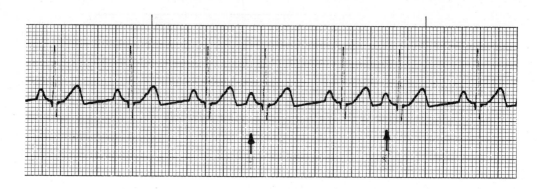

Fig. 7-9   Atrial premature contraction. The prematurely triggered complexes are shown by the arrows.

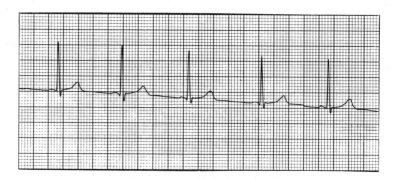

Fig. 7-10   Nodal (junctional) rhythm. Note slow rate (63) and absent P-R interval.

path, and the extra beat cannot be distinguished from a normal (Fig. 7-9). A nodal premature contraction starts in the A-V node (not the sinus node) and also follows the usual path into the ventricles, but because it travels a shorter distance than a sinus impulse, characteristic time measurements on the electrocardiogram identify it (Fig. 7-10). Since a ventricular premature contraction (Fig. 7-11) starts at the opposite end of the excitation chain, its path through the ventricular muscle is grossly abnormal, and the electrocardiographic configuration is often quite bizarre. Ventricular extra systoles may occur with regularity, alternating with normal sinus beats, producing a coupled rhythm referred to as *bigeminy*.

An interesting characteristic of premature contractions, which can sometimes be noted clinically and usually by the electrocardiograph, is the slightly longer than normal refractory period of myocardial fibers. Because the extra ectopic stimulus occurs out of phase, it interferes with the usual sequence of excitability and refractoriness and causes a lag before the next following contraction. This is called a *compensatory pause*. In an atrial premature contraction

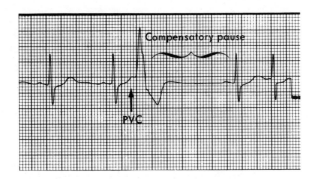

Fig. 7-11   Premature ventricular contraction (PVC).

the ectopic impulse encompasses the sinus node, which must wait until it recovers before it can initiate its own normal beat. Thus the interval between the premature beat and the next normal one is longer than the interval between two normal beats. After ventricular extra contractions, and usually nodal ones as well, the ventricles are refractory to the next normal sinus impulse, leading to a longer pause that is designated as "fully compensated." In this instance the time interval between the normal beats preceding and following the ectopic is exactly twice the time interval between any two other normal beats.

The clinical significance of premature contractions generally depends on the patient's tolerance of them, their frequency, and the presence or absence of underlying disease. Symptoms may be absent, or the patient may complain of "palpitations" or a "thumping" in the chest. The patient is actually aware of the *absence* of heart action during the compensatory pause as well as the difference in contractile force between normal and some abnormal beats. Sometimes dizziness and a sense of fullness in the chest or neck are bothersome.

Paroxysmal tachycardia

Chains or bursts of atrial, nodal, or ventricular premature contractions constitute paroxysmal tachycardia, which may last for prolonged periods of time. During an attack, the cardiac rate may range from 160 to 240/min. The rhythm is usually regular, is not affected by breathing or exercise, and may terminate abruptly. Atrial and nodal paroxysms can often be stopped by strong vagal stimuli, accomplished by exerting pressure on the eyeballs or carotid sinus, or by gagging. Ventricular ectopic foci will not respond to these maneuvers, since the ventricular myocardium is less influenced by vagal innervation than is the atrial.

From a clinical point of view, this abnormality may be functional (not caused by organic disease) or a result of cardiac disease. It often produces weakness and dizziness, and if prolonged, there will be a drop in cardiac output because of the sharp reduction in diastolic filling time from the rapid rate.

A diseased heart may be thrown into congestive failure, and shock is a real threat. There is also the risk that paroxysmal tachycardia will progress to the very grave ventricular fibrillation, on p. 000. Its presence is always an indication for careful observation, and drug therapy of the arrhythmia is a usual precaution.

Atrial flutter
(Fig. 7-12)

In atrial flutter, there is either a rapid circular movement of a stimulus or a repetitive single ectopic focus exciting the atria at rates of 200 to 350/min, with a clocklike regularity. The atrial flutter is named from the flutterlike contraction imparted to the atria. The refractoriness of the A-V node does not usually permit it to transmit more than 180 impulses/min, so many of the atrial signals are blocked. The ratio of blocked to transmitted impulses may be constant in a given instance, such as 2:1, 3:1, 4:1, etc.

Flutter is usually caused by disease, and even with a partial block the ventricular rate is still high enough to compromise cardiac filling and output.

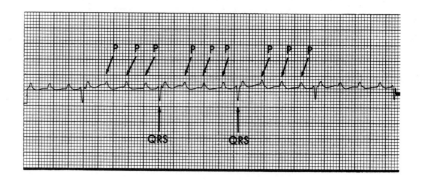

Fig. 7-12   Atrial flutter. Note that there are three atrial contractions to one ventricular contraction (3:1 response).

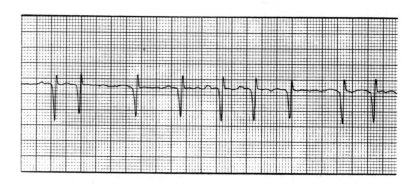

Fig. 7-13   Atrial fibrillation. Rate of ventricular contraction is irregular and greater than 100. No P waves are seen, and the baseline is wavy.

Because of the fixed atrioventricular ratio, the cardiac rate does not increase with exercise, even in those instances in which the block may permit a nearly normal rate. This interferes with the normal cardiac reserve and its response to exercise.

Atrial fibrillation
(Fig. 7-13)

Atrial fibrillation is the most common of the significant abnormal rhythm disturbances and is the usual end point of a preexisting flutter, although a flutter is not a prerequisite. Fibrillation always means cardiac pathologic conditions. The atria are subjected to a completely uncontrolled, randomly irregular barrage of impulses at rates of 350 to 500/min (Fig. 7-13). The A-V node transmits as many of these as it can, and the result is a chaotic ventricular response of grossly irregular contractions of varying intensities. Some of the contractions are too weak to be palpated in the peripheral pulses, and this leads to a *pulse deficit,* a discrepancy between the cardiac rate as counted over the chest and the rate of arterial pulsations.

The therapist will see many patients with this defect, since its causes span the extremes of life. It is a common sequela to such childhood diseases as rheumatic fever and is often seen with degenerative cardiac diseases of later years. Fairly normal activity is not incompatible with it, and many people carry it for years. However, the fibrillation (weak, shaky, ineffectual contraction) of the atria promotes poor atrial emptying, with the retention of blood in these chambers and the subsequent risk of intraatrial thrombus formation, often a source of future emboli. For this reason attempts are usually made to convert such hearts to a normal rhythm. Atrial fibrillation is readily detected by physical examination, but its electrocardiographic picture is characteristic, with the absence of definitive P waves and their replacement by an irregularly wavy baseline.

Ventricular fibrillation
(Fig. 7-14)

So grave as to be imminently fatal if not quickly corrected, ventricular fibrillation consists of a rapid tremulous shaking of the ventricular myocardium completely incompatible with any useful cardiac output. Frequently preceded

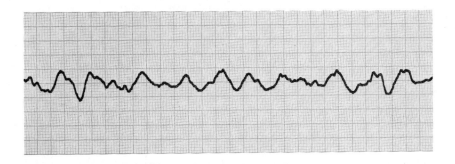

Fig. 7-14   Ventricular fibrillation.

by persistent or recurring ventricular paroxysmal tachycardia, fibrillation can be caused by many conditions, among which are electric shock, anesthesia, mechanical irritation of the heart, severe hypoxia, myocardial infarction, and large doses of digitalis or epinephrine. The rapid drop in cardiac output produces an acute cerebral hypoxia, often manifested by convulsions, and death ensues within a few minutes. From a functional viewpoint, ventricular fibrillation may be considered a form of "cardiac arrest," for although there is some ventricular activity, it is of no value. This abnormality, like sinus arrest, constitutes a true emergency situation, with survival dependent on the immediate application of the techniques of emergency resuscitation.

Atrioventricular block (Fig. 7-15)

Disorders of the myocardium such as inflammations, infarction or arteriosclerotic ischemia, and digitalis toxicity can reduce or destroy the ability of the A-V node or the bundle of His to transmit the sinus impulse to the ventricles.

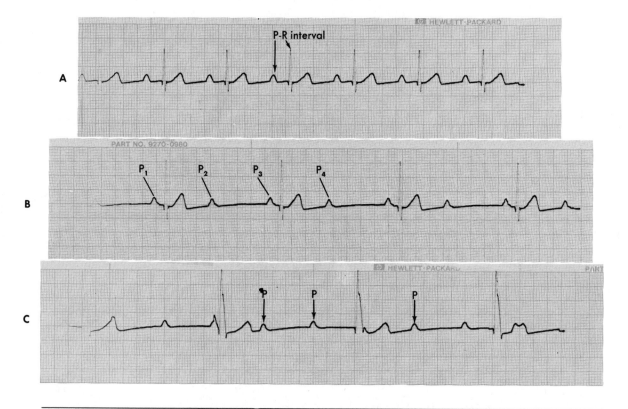

Fig. 7-15   **A,** First-degree A-V block. P-R interval is greater than 0.2 sec (about 0.26). **B,** Second-degree A-V block (Type II Mobility). Note P_1 has conducted QRS following it, as does P_3. P_2 and P_4 have no QRS and are therefore "blocked." **C,** Third-degree A-V block (complete heart block). Note P waves are firing at their own rate, completely independent of the P wave, both in rate and QRS configuration.

If every impulse is conducted but with a prolonged time (prolonged P-R interval on the electrocardiogram), the block is considered as *first degree*. If some impulses are conducted but others dropped, the block is *second degree*. If no atrial impulses are conducted to the ventricles, the block is *third degree*, or "complete." The last is the most important, for with no sinus impulse the ventricles must develop their own pacemaker and are able to do so only at very slow rates of between 25 and 45/min. Under conditions of stress, or in the presence of other arrhythmias, the bradycardia may be inadequate for cerebral blood flow, and the heart may even stop for several seconds. Acute unconsciousness may occur without warning, the so-called *Stokes-Adams syncope* (fainting). Convulsions and death may accompany such episodes. The disability of complete heart block is obvious and the need for treatment urgent.

Some patients with bradycardia, heart block, or arrhythmias that interfere with cardiac function respond to medical therapy, whereas others are realizing new leases on life with the use of electronic pacemakers, or pulse generators, permanently implanted in their bodies. Therapists will frequently serve patients with cardiac problems and should know at least the general nature of pacemakers. Fundamentally, an artificial pacemaker is a battery-operated device that emits an electrical charge, which is carried by a conducting catheter (electrode) into the right atrium or ventricle. Usually the catheter is firmly impacted against the right ventricular wall, and the generated signal stimulates the myocardium into contraction. The therapist may see temporary pacemakers placed in patients during acute episodes of block. For use limited to only a few days, the temporary pulse generator is kept outside the body, a small boxlike unit attached to or near the patient by pins, tape, or other means. The electrode catheter is often introduced into the heart through a jugular vein of the neck. Once cardiac stability is achieved, the temporary unit is removed and the patient continued on other therapy, or it is replaced by a permanent implanted instrument.

Permanent pacemakers are placed in a subcutaneous pocket usually just below either clavicle, and can be easily recognized by a prominent bulge with an overlying scar. The electrode follows one of the large veins into the heart. Occasionally, the pulse generator pocket may be on the upper abdominal wall with the electrode traveling subcutaneously to its attachment on the external surface of the heart, but these are less common than the intracardiac type. Some pulse generators need replacement for battery failure after 2 or more years, while others can be recharged regularly by the patient for longer battery life.

Respiratory therapists should know also that pacemakers can be programed a number of ways; some have preset rates at which they stimulate the heart, while others function on demand in case of failure of the natural spontaneous mechanism.

Sinus arrest

Like ventricular fibrillation, sinus arrest is a second cause of sudden cardiac standstill. The basic defect is failure of the sinus node to initiate an impulse and may be considered a suppression of the node by overwhelming vagal impulses. An ectopic pacemaker may compensate, but often the entire stimulus production of the heart is adversely affected, and no contraction occurs. Death is obvious unless excitation can be resumed. Sinus arrest is likely to accompany the early stages of anesthesia or certain bodily manipulations that are able to set up a strong vagal reflex. These include instrumentation during such examination of body cavities as cystoscopy, bronchoscopy, or pharyngeal probing and occasionally traction on thoracic organs during surgery. Many hearts so affected are perfectly normal and need only a stimulus such as massage or a sharp blow to the sternum to set them back into rhythmic activity.

• • •

Of special interest to the respiratory therapist are three factors related to cardiac arrhythmias, summarized briefly here. Prolonged deep hypoxia can stimulate the production of ectopic foci of excitation and precipitate conduction block in a myocardium already partially ischemic. Physical manipulation of the body can trigger vagal reflexes that are able to arrest heart action by inhibiting the sinus node. Although such incidents are uncommon, presumably moving the head or neck of some patients or initating pharyngeal vagal stimuli by instrumentation are among maneuvers with this potential risk. Finally, high blood levels of carbon dioxide in themselves, or because of the accompanying reduced blood pH, can activate ectopic focal activity. It is also believed that a sudden reduction in a previously elevated carbon dioxide tension can stimulate ventricular arrhythmias.[4,5] These points must be kept in mind in the treatment of patients with ventilatory failure.

Systemic blood flow

With each ventricular systole approximately 60 to 70 ml of blood leave each ventricle so that the stroke volume of the heart is 120 to 140 ml. Obviously, the minute volume, or cardiac output, will depend on the stroke volume and the cardiac rate, a situation analogous to the relation between the ventilatory tidal volume, rate, and minute volume. The speed and power with which systemic arterial blood will disseminate to all parts of the body depend on a balance between two forces—that of left ventricular contraction and that of the resistance of the arterial tree. The latter is referred to as the *peripheral vascular resistance,* an important factor in determining systemic blood flow.

Peripheral vascular resistance may be defined as the resistive force against which the left ventricle has to pump. It is produced by the "tone" of the arterial tree. It should be recalled that arteries contain both elastic and muscle fibers in their structure, and the arterial system as a whole is a continuously branching and narrowing arborization of channels. The elastic recoil of the larger arteries provides the initial resistance to the bolus of blood expelled from the left ventricle, whereas the tone of the muscle fibers of the smaller vessels maintains resistance distally. The apposition of the forces of ventricular contraction and peripheral resistance makes for a relatively smooth flow of blood with a minimal surge effect, which would result if a strong jet of blood were propelled into a rigid conducting system. If the system were flaccid, the ejection force would be dissipated before the stream reached the distal vessels, and again the flow would be uneven. Under the impact of the left ventricular blood, the proximal aorta stretches across its diameter to accommodate the blood volume; then as the aortic valve closes, the elastic aorta recoils. The recoil force is exerted against the column of blood in the arterial system and, since the valve does not yield, forces the blood distally. A wave of expansion and contraction, gradually diminishing, thus carries the blood through the major arteries, with no significant loss of velocity. The smaller arteries and arterioles maintain resistance and also determine the quantity of distal blood flow by appropriate contraction and relaxation of their muscle fibers. The function of these fibers, which is under reflex nervous control, ensures adequate blood supply to those areas of the body in greatest need.

Systemic blood pressure. Each left ventricular contraction must be of sufficient force to impel the systemic column of blood in a continuous circuit, carrying the venous blood back to the right heart, much of the way against gravity. This force is called the left ventricular systolic pressure. Direct measurement of this pressure can be made only by the technique of threading a catheter into the chamber, attaching the proximal end to a pressure recording device. However, an excellent approximation of this ejection force can be reached by measuring the pulsatile force transmitted to the column of blood in the brachial artery. This is the measurement of the familiar *blood pressure*. An inflatable cuff is secured about the upper arm and is connected by a rubber tube to a mercury manometer. By means of a hand bulb, the cuff is inflated until the brachial arterial flow is occluded, the inflating pressure being transmitted to the manometer. The cuff pressure is gradually released until blood just starts to flow again in the artery, and at this precise moment the manometer pressure is noted. At this point the force of left ventricular contraction is enough to overcome (or is equal to) the pressure in the cuff as recorded by the manometer. It is reported as so many millimeters of mercury. In practice, the escape of blood past the occlusion of the cuff is determined by listening with a stethoscope over the artery in the antecubital fossa, at which time a characteristic sound is heard. This is the *systolic* blood pressure, with a wide range of normal from about *90 to 150 mm Hg* and an average in the adult of approximately *120 mm Hg*. After noting the systolic pressure, if the examiner continues to listen while still releasing cuff pressure slowly, he or she will hear a rather abrupt and definite muffling of the arterial sound and finally a disappearance of the sound. The muffling is generally considered to coincide with the elastic recoil of the artery on the blood column and with the closure of the aortic valve. The pressure noted at this time is called the *diastolic* blood pressure and has a normal range of *70 to 90 mm Hg* with an average of 80 mm Hg. Some consider the true diastolic point to be the pressure at the disappearance of the sound. A blood pressure reading should properly include three components, one systolic and two possible diastolic pressures, as for example, 120/80/68. The third figure is rarely used in common practice, however, and only the systolic and first diastolic pressures are recorded, as 120/80.

The physiologic significance of blood pressure values can be summarized in a simplified manner as follows:

Elevated systolic pressure implies an increase in the resistance of the arterial tree, such as occurs with pathologic thickening of arterial or arteriolar walls or reduction in their elasticity.

Reduced systolic pressure indicates a drop in conducting system resistance, as may result from peripheral vascular collapse, a state of shock, or weakness of the left ventricular myocardium.

Elevated diastolic pressure is consistent with an increase in peripheral resistance, often accompanying systolic pressure increase, but it usually implies more advanced resistance than does a systolic increase alone.

Reduced diastolic pressure is found with a loss of resistance or myocardial weakness, as described previously, but also occurs with an incompetent aortic valve, which allows retrograde flow of blood back into the left ventricle during diastolic recoil.

Venous return. Although much of the systolic thrust of the left ventricle has been dissipated by the time capillary blood has perfused tissue cells, the return venous circulation is under a significant head of pressure. Venous return is dependent on the impetus of the arterial flow, aided by the "milking" effect exerted on the veins by surrounding muscles (especially of the lower extremity), the tone of the abdominal musculature, and the negative inspiratory intrathoracic pressure. Thus venous return from the lower limbs is more effective when leg muscles are active than when at rest, a matter of some practical importance, whereas return flow from the head and neck is dependent on gravity and the intrathoracic negative pressure. The effect of intrathoracic pressure on venous return to the heart is of considerable importance to respiratory therapists, as it relates directly to their work. Spontaneous natural breathing is characterized by a relatively long inhalation followed by a short exhalation, so that the time interval of falling intrathoracic pressure is greater than the time of rising pressure; and we know that except under conditions of forced exhalation, thoracic pressure never exceeds ambient.

The thorax thus acts like a large suction pump, aiding the venous blood in its return to the heart, and by virtue of the ventilatory pattern, maximum return occurs during inhalation. It can be properly inferred, then, that any condition that raises the mean intrathoracic pressure will impede the venous return; and it readily follows that if the volume of blood returning to the heart is reduced, the cardiac output will drop. We can easily demonstrate the effect on venous flow of increased intrathoracic pressure by holding the breath, straining, and then observing the color changes in the face from stasis of blood in the veins. Under some conditions we can note marked distention of the superficial veins of the neck. If such a buildup of thoracic pressure is significant and prolonged, venous blood unable to return to the heart will pool in venous reservoirs of the liver and abdominal circulation.

One of the major tools of respiratory therapy, the positive-pressure ventilator, is a potential prime offender in this regard, a matter that is discussed in detail later. Because the venous pressure varies greatly in different parts of the body and with position of the body, its measurement is made under standard conditions. A vein in the antecubital fossa is chosen as the site, and the patient is placed in a flat supine position with the arm supported so that the antecubital fossa is at the same level as the right atrium of the heart. A needle is inserted into the vein and is attached to a special manometer so that the pressure of the column of blood in the vein is balanced against a column of *saline* in the manometer. The normal range of venous pressure is very wide, from 50 to 110 mm of *water*.

Venous pressure measurements have been used for many years to evaluate the retarding effects on venous return of weakness of the right ventricle. In some circumstances elevated venous pressure is readily apparent by visible distention of cervical veins, an important clinical sign. Because peripheral venous pressure (in an extremity) is difficult to measure uniformly, is subject to so many influences, and has such a wide normal range, it has generally been replaced by measurement of the central venous pressure, which is described later in a discussion of acute circulatory failure.

Pulmonary blood flow

The pulmonary circulation, when compared with the systemic circulation, is a low-pressure system. The total circuit distance from right ventricle to left atrium is short, and the pulmonary capillary bed is extensive so that relatively low pressures suffice for blood flow. As an average, the pulmonary artery pressure is about 25/8 mm Hg. Recording pulmonary pressure is not as simple as measuring the systemic pressure and can only be accomplished by means of intracardiac catheterization. By this technique it is possible to measure pressures in the right atrium, the right ventricle, and for a considerable distance into the pulmonary arteries. Such serial readings make it possible to differentiate between lesions, for example, stenotic heart valves, which lead to increased pressures within the heart in the presence of a normal pulmonary system, and an actual increase in the peripheral resistance of the pulmonary arterial tree. Many of the diseases with which the respiratory therapist will have contact produce thickening and/or narrowing of the pulmonary vessels, the resulting increased resistance requiring added ejection force of the right ventricle. Also, destruction of a sufficient portion of the pulmonary capillary bed by disease of the lung, even in the presence of normal remaining vessels, may produce resistance to right heart output, since the same output is forced through a smaller cross-sectional capillary bed. Whenever resistance to pulmonary flow is present, the right ventricle is put under strain, which, if persistent, leads to weakening of the right ventricle. If this is caused by pulmonary disease, the effect on the heart is called *cor pulmonale,* or "pulmonary heart."

Despite the vital importance of the pulmonary arterial blood supply, we cannot overlook the systemic component of the total pulmonary blood flow.[6] The student is encouraged to review the anatomic relationships of the bronchial arteries and note that whereas the pulmonary arteries give off no visceral branches before the level of the alveoli, the bronchial vessels supply the entire length of the bronchial tree to the bronchioles with oxygenated blood. The returning bronchial venous blood follows an interesting variety of routes, which have some clinical significance. The accompanying bronchial veins are imperfect and irregular and can probably accommodate no more than one third of the bronchial venous blood as they empty into the azygos vein. From the distal portions of the airways, bronchial venous blood drains into the *pulmonary veins* (arterialized blood) and thus contributes to the normal small degree of unsaturation of the systemic arterial blood. At the capillary level there are microscopic communications between bronchial and pulmonary capillaries. Here there is a mixture of arterialized systemic blood (bronchial capillaries) with venous blood (pulmonary capillaries). This relationship is unimportant under normal circumstances, but in certain disease states in which there is interruption of pulmonary arterial flow, these communications may become grossly enlarged and provide a significant volume of blood perfusing alveoli, even though it is arterial. This so-called *bronchial collateral flow* can reach tremendous proportions in destructive pulmonary diseases, best exemplified by bronchiectasis.

At this point we describe the essentials of *acute pulmonary edema* because edema of the lung involves a serious disruption of the pulmonary circulation and marked interference with pulmonary gas exchange. It can provoke an acute, life-threatening, clinical situation frequently encountered not only in the hospital emergency room but also in inpatient divisions, and the respiratory therapist plays an important role in its treatment. Theoretically, edema of the lung can be of three types: intracellular, interstitial, and alveolar, but our present interest is centered about the alveolar edema.[7]

Acute pulmonary edema is a condition in which there is a rapid movement of some or all of the blood components across the pulmonary capillary wall into the minute pericapillary space, from which they flow into the alveoli, alveolar ducts, and bronchial tree. Among the many factors that determine the degree of edema are (1) the net osmotic pressure across the capillary wall, between the blood and interstitial lung fluid, (2) the permeability (ease of penetration) of both capillary and alveolar walls, and (3) the capacity of the pulmonary lymphatic drainage, or the ease with which the lymphatics can remove excess interstitial fluid. An upset of the physiologic balance among these factors, whatever the cause, can produce an outpouring of fluid (transudation) into the lungs in a matter of minutes. Despite the frequency with which acute pulmonary edema occurs, little is known about the exact mechanism responsible for it. Presumably a precipitating underlying disease stimulates some autonomic nervous system reflexes that enhance alveolar-capillary permeability. Afferent autonomic nerve endings are found in many organs (heart, vessels, lungs, hollow viscera of the abdomen) that communicate through brain centers with efferent nerves supplying peripheral and pulmonary blood vessels. Abnormal reflexes can be initiated that upset the usual balanced vasomotor tone responsible for smoothly related pulmonary flow and hydrostatic pressure.[8]

Acute pulmonary edema is more a clinical syndrome than a disease entity and accompanies a variety of specific diseases. Among the latter, in which acute edema may play a significant role, are cardiovascular disease, especially coronary heart disease, heart failure, valvular disease, lung diseases, severe infections, brain injury, metabolic disorders, extensive surface burns, and severe body trauma. The acute edema itself may be responsible for the loss of a great enough volume of circulating fluid to precipitate a serious state of shock (see Acute Circulatory Failure later in this chapter), but the outstanding signs and symptoms are the result of the extensive obstruction of airways and alveoli, with resulting hypoxemia and impaired ventilation. Often the onset of acute pulmonary edema may be preceded by a sense of anxiety and then openly manifest itself by sudden dyspnea. The fluid permeating the respiratory tract is churned into a froth by the rapidly moving tidal air exchange, is often pink or frankly blood tinged, and may be of such quantity as to bubble from the mouth under the stress of the patient's strenuous breathing. The neck veins may be markedly distended, and frequently the blood pressure is elevated, unless shock is present. Air passing through the edema fluid produces bubbling sounds known as *rales,* which often can be heard by the unaided ear as well as by the stethoscope, and not rarely the wheezing sounds of air moving through narrow passages are also present. The patient labors hard to breathe and is usually severely cyanotic from severe obstructive hypoxemia. The treatment of acute pulmonary edema is discussed later, but the student can certainly perceive that therapy will be of a dual nature—that of the underlying disease and of the edema itself.

Coronary blood flow	Although we are not concerned with specific diseases at this point, because of the great prevalence of coronary heart disease—especially in the age group comprising the bulk of patients receiving respiratory therapy—a few observations should be made regarding this important segment of the cardiovascular system. Reviewing the anatomy of the heart, the student will recall that the myocardium receives its blood supply through the coronary arteries and that these vessels are the first branches of the aorta, thus ensuring that perfusion of the myocardial cells will be supported by the maximum delivery pressure of the left ventricle. Not only is the contractility of the heart muscle dependent on an adequate blood flow, but the conducting system of the heart is very sensitive to circulatory interference. Because the work demand of the heart is so variable and the organ's response to demand must be prompt, the circula-

tory system of the heart must be flexible and able to adjust blood flow from moment to moment. As long as the coronary vessels are normal in structure, this presents no problem; but when diseased, they subject the function of the entire body to a serious hazard.

From the middle years on, the incidence of impaired coronary circulation increases, yet despite the prevalence of coronary artery disease, relatively little is known about its specific causes. It is believed that the vessels may respond to unknown stimuli, neurogenic or humoral, by a spastic contraction of their muscle fibers. Such episodes reduce the blood flow to the myocardium, often with drastic but usually transient effects, most frequently manifested by acute chest pain. A recurring condition, it is clinically referred to as *angina pectoris* (literally, "pain in the chest"). The coronary vessels are also subject to the same sclerosis, or hardening process, that so often affects the general arterial tree. Attributed to such factors as the degeneration of aging, toxic effects of nicotine directly or indirectly, cholesterol ingestion, neurogenic stimuli, and many others, thickening of the coronary arterial walls effectively and permanently reduces their caliber and elasticity. Such vessels are unable to respond to myocardial need for a rapid increase in cellular perfusion and seriously handicap the cardiac function. Further, the arteries, whether already damaged or not, are subject to the formation of thromboses (blood clots) from causes that again are not clear, with acute or gradual occlusion of their lumens. The respiratory therapist will have frequent occasion to see patients suffering from acute coronary occlusion, many of whom are ill enough to require the services of specialized care units in the hospital.

Interference with myocardial perfusion damages the muscle cells, and when such damage is severe enough to be permanent, the affected myocardium is replaced with fibrosis. Over a period of time the accumulation of fibrosis can reach a point at which there is not enough normal-functioning myocardium for adequate cardiac function, and heart failure develops. Also, should myocardial circulatory insufficiency involve a segment of the conducting system of the heart, rate and rhythm disturbances will be an important part of the clinical picture. The term *infarction* is given to a localized area of the heart where myocardial cells have been replaced by scarring, and *diffuse myocardial fibrosis* to a more generalized distribution of fibrous replacement.

The myocardium is very susceptible to hypoxia, and the coronary vessels, to a sudden drop in arterial carbon dioxide tension. These facts must be kept in mind by the respiratory therapist. Although he or she may be treating a patient primarily for a respiratory ailment, the therapist should also be acquainted with the general state of the patient's myocardial health.

Cardiovascular failure

The respiratory therapist will have constant contact with patients with heart failure and must be aware of the basic physiologic defects involved. Heart failure is considered to be when a heart can no longer fulfill its function of ensuring adequate cellular perfusion to all parts of the body without assistance. Such a state is called *cardiac decompensation*. With its underlying disease still present but its function restored by supportive therapy (digitalis, bed rest, etc.), the heart is said to be in a state of *compensation,* full or partial. A heart may decompensate because of an increase in the work load imposed on it (increased resistance in the circulation, defective function of the cardiac valves), a decrease in the ventricular contractile power (myocardial damage from fibrosis, infection, toxins), or a combination of both. There are a host of classifications of cardiac and vascular functional derangements, based on physiologic and clinical criteria, but it would be inappropriate to attempt to summarize briefly, with any degree of clarity in these few pages, that which is not done with much uniformity in large texts. Because our purpose is to provide the respiratory therapist with a basic orientation to those forms of disease relative to his or her work, we describe only two types of cardiovascular incompetence that are of great importance to the therapist: *congestive heart failure* and *acute circulatory failure*.

Congestive heart failure

The term *congestive* implies an overcrowding and refers to a packing of vessels with blood as a result of a backup of circulation. In this type of failure, since the forward flow of blood is reduced, the blood backlogs in the return vessels, which become distended, and pooling occurs in venous and capillary reservoirs. Velocity is reduced, and there is interference with cellular gas exchange. There are two types of congestive failure, which need differentiation, *left ventricular congestive failure* and *right ventricular congestive failure*.

Left ventricular failure. Strong though it is, the left ventricle can fail if it is opposed by increasing resistance in the systemic circulation or if the myocardium is weakened by disease. Blood returning to the left heart from the lung cannot be ejected rapidly enough, and it backs up in the pulmonary circulation. Vessels in the lung, especially the arterioles, capillaries, and veins, become "passively" congested. Often pressure in these channels increases to the point that blood water is forced from them into the pulmonary pericapillary and interstitial spaces and the alveoli. Although this state justifies the title of pulmonary edema, some important differential points separate it clinically from the acute pulmonary edema discussed previously. The edema produced by left ventricular failure is of a passive nature, because of the increased hydrostatic pressure of blood stasis in the pulmonary circulation. This is entirely different from the "active" acute edema, which is the result of dynamic changes in the A-C membrane and its environment, mediated through nerve reflexes in response to disease that may be remote from the lung. In addition to etiologic and physiologic differences, the functional impairments of these two types of edema vary. However, a patient with passive pulmonary congestion and edema may also be subject to a superimposed acute edema, a not infrequent occurrence. We have already noted that acute pulmonary edema generally has an abrupt onset, runs a stormy course, and is of relatively short duration. Passive edema, on the other hand, is always a result of heart disease and is chronic.

The extravasation of fluid into the lung is of much smaller volume than that of acute edema, and its clinical and physiologic effects on ventilation are of different quality.

Whereas the functional impairment in respiration of acute pulmonary edema is generally obstructive, that of passive congestion and edema is less easily categorized. The congested pulmonary vessels and edema fluid are space occupying and encroach on alveolar air space, with reduction especially noted in the vital capacity. With engorgement of the vessels and perivascular and interstitial fluid increased, the lung becomes less flexible, and loss of pulmonary compliance is an important sequela to left heart failure. The congested vessels also offer increased resistance to the work of the right ventricle, putting it under strain. Of great significance is the combined effect of pulmonary congestion and edema to disrupt normal ventilation-perfusion relationships, interfere with alveolar gas exchange, and produce hypoxia. It is reasonable to suppose that if sufficient edema fluid should accumulate in alveoli and perhaps terminal bronchioles, it would obstruct airflow to the alveoli. In this respect, chronic passive edema may simulate, but to a lesser degree, the effect of acute edema. However, much of the edema of passive congestion may be interstitial, exerting its influence by increasing the thickness of the A-C membrane, creating a "diffusion defect" for oxygen rather than an obstruction to ventilation. It is very probable that both obstruction and diffusion interference play simultaneous or reciprocating roles, depending on the exact dynamics of the congestion at any given time. Because the quantity of pulmonary blood flow can be variable in left heart failure, depending on the degree of compensation or decompensation, its relation to ventilation will also be an important determinant in effective gas exchange. Thus obstruction, diffusion defect, and disturbed ventilation-perfusion relationships may all be important effects of chronic passive edema. These conditions are described more generally, individually, in the next chapter. Finally, the hydrostatic pressure in the congested lung vessels and in the lymphatics of the thorax may reach such heights that fluid will escape into the pleural space, producing a hydrothorax (literally, "water in the chest"). Up to several liters may accumulate here, and because of the obvious effect of lung compression by the fluid, we see that restriction of lung expansion is also a potential risk of left heart failure.

Right ventricular failure. The most frequent cause of failure of the right ventricle is preexisting failure of the left ventricle, and we have already noted that increased back pressure in the pulmonary circulation can produce a pulmonary hypertension, the resistance of which can strain the capacity of the right ventricle beyond its normal compensation. In addition, other intrinsic cardiac diseases, valvular and congenital, can overburden the right heart, but we are interested in a specific type of right failure—that caused by pulmonary disease. *Cor pulmonale* implies compromise of the right ventricle, by the effects of intrapulmonary pathologic conditions, and is characterized by right ventricular enlargement (hypertrophy, a thickening of the myocardial wall; or dilation, an enlargement of the chamber caused by stretching of the myocardial fibers; or both) associated with pulmonary disease known to interfere with right ventricular function.[9] The disease so affecting the right heart usually produces an elevated pressure in the pulmonary circulation, but pulmonary hypertension itself does not constitute cor pulmonale.

Cor pulmonale is most commonly seen and has been best documented in the disease complex obstructive bronchitis–pulmonary emphysema. (This condition is described in more detail in Chapter 8.) Studies of this condition, along with others characterized by ventilatory failure, indicate that the most important elements in the genesis of cor pulmonale are probably bronchiolar obstruction, alveolar hypoventilation, and hypoxia.[10] The exact interrelation of these factors is not entirely clear, but it has been suggested that hypoxia may exert its influence directly on the myocardium. On the other hand, the effect of chronic hypoxia may be more indirect, perhaps initiating a rise in cardiac output and a subsequent elevation of pulmonary arterial pressure. Others place more emphasis on the prerequisite of chronic airway obstruction as a prime mover in the development of right heart strain but with hypoxia and hypercapnia as necessary factors.[11] Whatever the mechanism, the right ventricle is subjected to increasing resistance in providing pulmonary perfusion, and it responds by increasing its mass of myocardial tissue for greater contractile force (hypertrophy) or by elongating its myocardial fibers for greater contractile leverage, enlarging the ventricular cavity (dilation); or the two may exist together. The right side of the heart becomes prominent by x-ray examination and shows certain electrocardiographic patterns suggesting enlargement.

When the right ventricle fails, it can no longer maintain an adequate output (although the early signs of impending failure may be an increased output), and stasis or congestion occurs in the systemic circulation that supplies it. Pooling of blood occurs in the veins of the lower extremities and in the venous and capillary beds of the abdominal viscera, especially in the liver. Again, with the weakened right ventricle unable to accommodate the returning venous blood, hydrostatic pressure in the veins promotes the escape of fluid into surrounding tissues, producing edema of the feet and legs, demonstrable swelling of the liver (hepatomegaly), and the outpouring of fluid into the abdominal cavity (ascites). With pure right failure there may be no signs of circulatory embarrassment of the lung, only evidence of its underlying disease. Distention of the superficial neck veins, especially in the supine position, may be a prominent feature of right heart failure, and there will be an expected elevation of peripheral venous pressure.

In summary, because the heart is a mated pair of pumps, each with its own circuit but with each circuit interacting with the other, it is easy to see that each pump is subject to individual failure. Because of the relationship of the two pumps, we can see how the right can fail without materially affecting the left but that failure of the left will eventually strain the right to the point of decompensation. The therapist will see many patients with diseases of the cardiovascular system who will have both left and right congestive heart failure and who will demonstrate to varying degrees any or all of the signs and symptoms characteristic of each.

Acute circulatory failure

Acute circulatory failure is a term that embodies a large number of different diseases and conditions with a variety of causes, but they all have one thing in common—a serious drop in cardiac output resulting from either cardiac or noncardiac causes, with subsequent tissue hypoxia. In contrast to the reduction in cardiac output found in the congestive heart failures previously discussed, that which characterizes acute circulatory failure occurs rapidly, allowing the body little time to adjust to the acute change. The student will encounter this condition frequently, will often be part of the therapeutic team involved in its management, and will soon get accustomed to hearing it referred to as "shock." The name *shock* is not a precise one, since it may have different connotations for different people, and although some have recommended its discontinuance, a name once established is difficult to change.[12] Shock involves many interacting physiologic phenomena of great complexity, and there is no unanimity on classification, either clinical or physiologic. Since we do not wish to get embroiled in controversial theories but rather wish to develop a practical clinical appreciation of this significant condition, we will describe the cardinal features of shock as a composite of those characteristics most frequently accepted.[13-15]

We will avoid the complex classifications of shock that involve the many specific causes and describe it as an abnormal physiologic state with a disproportion between the circulating blood volume and the size of the vascular bed, which leads to circulatory failure (the inability to maintain an adequate minute volume of blood flow for tissue needs) and cellular hypoxia. The three important factors in its genesis are the *blood volume,* the *effectiveness of the cardiac pump,* and the *"tone" of the peripheral vasculature.* Should one or more of these fail, shock will develop if the remainder cannot compensate for the deficiency. With the major component of the shock syndrome a reduced cardiac output, we can rightfully expect there to be an accompanying drop in arterial blood pressure. These two factors subject the body tissues to the risk of hypoxia, since adequate cellular gas exchange requires both a minimum blood volume and a perfusing pressure. In the presence of this threat, the body must protect its most hypoxia-sensitive vital organs, the brain and heart, from oxygen want.

Compensation consists of redistributing the arterial circulation to ensure adequate cerebral and cardiac perfusion, even at the expense of other tissues, especially the abdominal organs and peripheral areas (skin). This is accomplished by widespread vasoconstriction to shift the available blood flow to the two vital structures and also to maintain suitable blood pressure through an increase in peripheral resistance. The blood pressure may continue to fall, a characteristic of shock, but cerebral and cardiac perfusion can remain ample for a long time. Should the shock state progress into what is termed *irreversible shock,* compensation will fail, and vasoconstriction may give way to vasodilation at the capillary and venular levels, with the pooling of large volumes of blood in the capillary beds. This further reduces the circulating blood volume (hypovolemia) and initiates a vicious cycle that may continue to death.

Some types of acute circulatory failure initially show vasodilation rather than vasoconstriction, and in these the underlying disease prevents the constrictor compensation just described. There can be a period of imminent or potential shock before the classical symptoms of hypotension warn of falling cardiac output. Patients suspected of having conditions predisposing to shock are carefully observed for its signs.

We can summarize in a brief outline the major causes of reduction in cardiac output:

1. *Reduction in blood volume*
    a. Loss of blood by hemorrhage
    b. Extravasation of blood or plasma from vessels into intercellular spaces, as a result of damage to capillaries and larger vessels by trauma and surgery
    c. Dehydration, with loss of fluid through skin, kidney, and gastrointestinal tract
2. *Reduced venous return from capillary and venular pooling*
    a. Vasodilation, caused by loss of vasomotor stimuli from toxins (bacterial sepsis)
    b. Vasodilation, caused by loss of vasoconstrictor action, as from spinal anesthesia
3. *Failure of cardiac pump action*
    a. Cardiac filling defect, as from tamponade (compression of heart from pericardial fluid) and tachycardia (insufficient diastolic filling time because of rapid rate)
    b. Cardiac emptying defect, as from an obstructing intracardiac thrombus or large pulmonary embolus
    c. Impaired cardiac function, especially from myocardial infarct

From a practical point of view, the respiratory therapist will see patients go into shock mostly as the result of severe trauma (automobile or industrial accidents, gunshot wounds), extensive surgery (manipulation of viscera, loss of blood and plasma), massive acute blood loss, and overwhelming sepsis (blood invasion by bacteria). Two special circumstances of shock are of particular interest to the therapist. First is the circulatory failure that can follow a disturbance in intrathoracic pressure. Any disorder that can produce a significant elevation in intrapleural pressure, elevating the mean pressure from the negative to the positive range, by virtue of interfering with venous return through the thoracic vessels and by restricting diastolic filling of the heart, can generate shock. It cannot be emphasized too frequently or too strongly that this is an inherent risk in the use of positive pressure ventilating equipment. Second, a condition sometimes referred to as "shock lung," but more properly called adult respiratory distress syndrome, is a serious pulmonary consequence of acute circulatory collapse. It is dealt with in more detail in our consideration of ventilatory failure but is noted here to emphasize the need for respiratory therapists to learn as much about shock as they can.

The clinical picture of shock will be a familiar one to the therapist in a general hospital. The patient may be restless or apathetic and lethargic, but he or she will show marked physical weakness. The skin will be pale, cold, and moist or will show a grayish cyanosis. The superficial veins will be collapsed and difficult to find, a point of considerable therapeutic concern. The blood pressure will be low, at least less than 80 mm Hg, systolic, and in severe states may be so weak as to be unobtainable, and the peripheral pulse will be faint or "thready" and rapid. Urinary output falls off as kidney perfusion is seriously compromised. Body temperature is often below normal. It is beyond the scope of this text to detail the particulars of therapy, which frequently taxes the ingenuity of the medical attendants, but among all the necessary supportive measures the administration of oxygen is of prime importance. The alert therapist will observe the other techniques employed to maintain maximum tissue perfusion, including the "shock position," fluid and blood replacement, and cardiovascular stimulants.

Of high priority in the management of the acutely ill patient whose cardiovascular status is in doubt or who is in frank shock, is the measurement of *central venous pressure* (CVP).[16,17] As the name implies, CVP is the pressure in the large veins within the body as opposed to the pressure in a single extremity earlier described as peripheral venous pressure. CVP is measured by a water manometer often attached at a proper height to the head of the patient's bed. The manometer is in line with a catheter introduced into antecubital, internal jugular, or subclavian veins percutaneously (threaded through a needle inserted in a vein) or by cutdown (directly into a vein exposed by surgical incision of the skin). It is advanced until its tip is in the superior vena cava (Fig. 7-16).

CVP reflects the sum of the action of the pumping heart, the circulating blood volume, and peripheral vascular tone. Its normal range is 8 to 12 cm of water. Venous flow is controlled by cardiac output, and a deficit in cardiac contractibility causes blood to backlog in venous reservoirs, elevating the CVP providing the blood volume remains stable. If the heart is normal, CVP will drop with a decrease in circulating volume, or when peripheral vasodilation causes venous pooling and a reduced venous return. It is thus an aid in the differentiation between cardiac failure and shock and is a good guide to fluid replacement therapy.

In addition to pressure in the central venous system, the vena cava indwelling line allows serial sampling of blood for determination of *central venous oxygen saturation (CVSO₂)*. Blood in the vena cava is pooled blood, a mixture from all parts of the body, representative of average metabolic activity from the body as a whole. $CVSO_2$ is a much more accurate reflection of general oxygen use than is saturation from a peripheral vein and is useful in estimating cardiac output. As cardiac output falls, less blood per unit of time perfuses cells. With a slowing of blood flow, blood-cell contact time increases, and

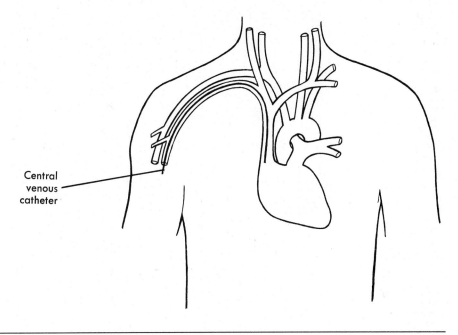

Fig. 7-16   Diagram of placement of central venous catheter.

more oxygen than normal is extracted from the perfusate. Mixed venous blood sampled from the superior vena cava thus has a low oxygen saturation. This is a very useful tool to monitor the progress of myocardial infarction, since experimentation has demonstrated that a drop of $CVSO_2$ below 55% indicates a beginning fall in cardiac output and probable early complicating cardiac failure.[18,19]

Increasing use is being made of another, but similar, technique for cardiovascular evaluation and monitoring, which might be considered a third generation development from the relatively simple and crude peripheral venous pressure measurement. The *Swan-Ganz catheter* represents a sophisticated, electronically monitored complex version of the central venous catheter.[20-23] The basic Swan-Ganz catheter itself is double walled with one channel open at the distal end and the other terminating at an inflatable balloon just before the tip. Proximally, the catheter is attached to a heparinized saline flush reservoir by a flow control unit, and through special pressure tubing, to a pressure transducer. Output from the transducer is carried to a monitor capable of at least two tracer recordings, the cardiac beat and intravascular pressures.

The Swan-Ganz catheter is introduced into a peripheral vein by surgical cutdown under strict asepsis and is advanced into the right atrium or ventricle. Pressure wave forms on the oscilloscope monitor enable the operator to plot the position. Air is instilled in the balloon, and the catheter is literally floated

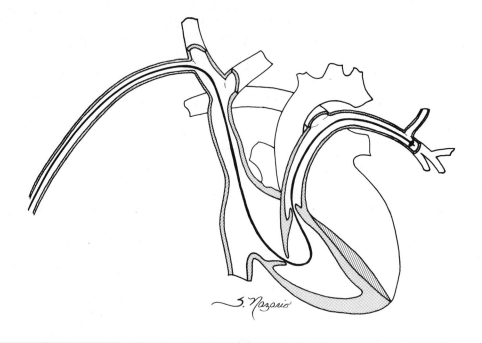

Fig. 7-17 Diagram of balloon-tipped flotation catheter in wedge position in pulmonary artery.

through the pulmonic valve into a pulmonary artery with the blood flow, until it wedges and can go no farther (Fig. 7-17). The balloon is deflated to avoid obstructing blood flow to the surrounding lung.

To attempt to withdraw blood samples through a Swan-Ganz catheter is not as easy or as desirable as through a simple CVP line because of the risk of clotting the lumen. The prime value of this elaborate procedure is its ability to transmit the so-called *pulmonary capillary wedge pressure* (PCW). With the tip of the catheter advanced until the caliber of the pulmonary artery branch stops it, if the balloon is momentarily inflated, the pressure recorded in this wedged position is the pressure across the pulmonary capillary from the pulmonary venous system. It has been shown to reflect two important cardiac forces: (1) the mean left atrial pressure (average of the systolic and diastolic pressures in the left atrium over each cardiac cycle), and (2) the left ventricular end-diastolic pressure (pressure in the blood-filled left ventricle just before its systolic contraction).[24] The PCW, when elevated, is the major signal of the development or presence of pulmonary congestion and edema, since it relates directly to the volume of blood in the pulmonary venous bed. Thus anything impeding the flow of blood out of the left ventricle will cause a back pressure (as long as the mitral valve is patent) through the left atrium and the pulmonary veins to the tip of the catheter wedged into a small vessel on the arterial side of the pulmonary capillary.

Studies comparing the effectiveness of CVP with PCW have shown that

CVP does not accurately reflect pulmonary venous distending pressure in patients with myocardial infarction and does not correlate with x-ray evidence of left ventricular failure as well as does the PCW.[25] Which monitoring technique is used, if any, for a given patient is a clinical decision of the responsible attending physician.

In summary, pulmonary venous pressure measurements are employed to detect signs of left ventricular failure, especially in the early stages of myocardial infarction, and to determine the adequacy of circulating blood volume. In the latter circumstance CVP or PCW catheters are useful in the management of shock and in fluid replacement therapy of any acutely ill patient. The therapist will see some patients on mechanical ventilation monitored with CVP or PCW pressure measurement, especially those whose ventilatory failure is complicated by shock, cardiac disease, or fluid-electrolyte problems.

Congenital heart disease	No attempt is made here to classify and describe this large and important group of cardiac abnormalities, for the number of texts and articles in the literature on the subject are so vast that the student can find material to any desired depth of sophistication. A few principles are discussed that should make further pursuit of the subject more meaningful.

Congenitally deformed hearts are the victims of incomplete or erroneous prenatal development, occasionally the result of maternal disease, but most often result from some unknown cause. The scope of defects ranges from the slight, compatible with normal life, to the severe, incompatible with more than a few minutes of survival. Most defects are detected during childhood or adolescence, and because many are increasingly benefited by surgery, every attempt is made to establish an accurate diagnosis and prognosis. The respiratory therapist in a hospital actively engaged in cardiac surgery will have occasion to see many patients with congenital heart disease, since many of them have associated respiratory problems, and postoperative care often uses respiratory therapy services.

The two broad classifications of congenital disease that concern us here are *acyanotic* (absence of cyanosis) and *cyanotic* congenital defects. The differentiation between the two depends on whether significant amounts of unsaturated blood mix with arterialized blood to produce cyanosis. Many congenital defects consist of communications between the two sides of the heart through septal defects, or openings in the interatrial and interventricular septa. These are called *intracardiac shunts,* since blood can pass from one side of the heart to the other without following the usual channels. Because the pressure in the left heart is greater than in the right, an uncomplicated septal defect will shunt blood from the left to the right. In other words, variable amounts of left heart blood, depending on the size of the imperfection, will pass directly into the right heart, mixing arterialized blood with venous. This, of course, does not produce cyanosis. However, the increased load of blood perfusing the lung, some of which is coming back for a second round, increases the pressure in the pulmonary circulation. Physical exercise may further raise the pulmonary pressure temporarily to a level that exceeds the systemic pressure, reversing the pressure gradient across the septum and converting the shunt from a left-to-right to a right-to-left. During this interval, venous blood will mix with arterial and may produce cyanosis. Also, progressive pulmonary hypertension may strain the right ventricle to the point of failure, and an interatrial shunt may be reversed to cause cyanosis. If narrowing of the pulmonary valve or the pulmonary artery is part of the cardiac defect complex, cyanosis will be present from the early stages in the presence of associated septal openings because of initial pulmonary hypertension.

There are conditions that permit cyanosis even in the absence of pulmonary hypertension, for example, septal defects so large that venous blood mixes with arterial even without a reverse gradient, or an aorta that arises from the right ventricle. Generally speaking, however, the presence or absence of cyanosis in septal cardiac defects depends on the presence or absence of high pressure in the pulmonary circulation.

References

1. Scher, A.M.: The electrocardiogram, Sci. Am. **205**:137, 1961.
2. Smith, R.E.: In Watson, C.J., editor: Outlines of internal medicine, Dubuque, Iowa, 1958, William C. Brown Co., Publishers.
3. Rushmer, R.F.: Cardiac diagnosis, Philadelphia, 1955, W.B. Saunders Co.
4. Price, H.L.: Effects of carbon dioxide on the cardiovascular system, Anesthesiology **21**:652, 1960.
5. Hoffman, B.F., et al.: Physiological basis of cardiac arrhythmias, Mod. Concepts Cardiovas. Dis. **35**:103, 1966.
6. Bjurstedt, H.: In Luisada, A., editor: Cardiovascular functions, New York, 1962, McGraw-Hill Book Co.
7. Visscher, M.B., et al.: The physiology and pharmacology of lung edema, Pharmacol. Rev. **8**:389, 1956.
8. Egan, D.F.: Management of acute pulmonary edema, Hosp. Med. **2**:20, 1966.
9. Ferrer, M.E., and Harvey, R.M.: In Adams, W.R., and Vieth, I., editors: Pulmonary circulation: an international symposium, New York, 1959, Grune & Stratton, Inc.
10. Steinborn, K.E., et al.: Chronic cor pulmonale in the respiratory poliomyelitis patient, Arch. Intern. Med. **110**:249, 1962.
11. Stuart-Harris, C.H.: Pulmonary hypertension and chronic obstructive bronchitis, Am. Rev. Respir. Dis. **97**:9, 1968.
12. Rushmer, R.F., et al.: In Bock, K.D., editor: Essential hypertension symposium on shock, Berlin, 1962, Springer-Verlag.
13. Friedberg, C.H.: Diseases of the heart, Philadelphia, 1956, W.B. Saunders Co.
14. Bordicks, K.J.: Patterns of shock, New York, 1965, The Macmillan Co.
15. Warren, R.: Surgery, Philadelphia, 1963, W.B. Saunders Co.
16. Central venous monitoring in shock (editorial), Conn. Med. **32**:79, 1968.
17. Jernigan, W.R., et al.: The internal jugular vein for access to the central venous system, J.A.M.A., **218**:97, 1971.
18. Goldman, R.H., et al.: The use of central venous oxygen saturation measurements in a coronary care unit, Ann. Intern. Med. **68**:1280, 1968.
19. Hutter, A.M., Jr., and Moss, A.J.: Central venous oxygen saturation, J.A.M.A. **212**:299, 1970.
20. Swan, H.J.C., and Ganz, W.: Catheterization of the heart in man with the use of flow-directed balloon-tipped catheter, N. Engl. J. Med. **283**:447, 1970.
21. Bolognini, V.: The Swan-Ganz, pulmo-

nary artery catheter: implications for nursing, Heart Lung **3**:976, 1974.

22. Armstrong, P.W., and Baigrie, R.S.:
Hemodynamic monitoring in the critically
ill, New York, 1980, Harper & Row, Publishers, Inc.

23. Daily, E.K., and Schroeder, J.S.: Techniques in bedside hemodynamic monitoring, ed. 2, St. Louis, 1980, The C.V.
Mosby Co.

24. Rackley, C.E., et al.: Left ventricular function in acute myocardial infarction and its
clinical significance, Circulation **45**:231,
1972.

25. Forrester, J.S., et al.: Filling pressures in
the right and left sides of the heart in acute
myocardial infarction, N. Engl. J. Med.
285:190, 1971.

Chapter 8   Clinical cardiopulmonary pathology

In this chapter we consider some of the disturbances in cardiopulmonary physiology with which the respiratory therapist can be expected to come into frequent contact. The topics discussed do not constitute specific disease entities but rather consist of some of the major physiologic changes that underlie the common respiratory disorders. This might be a good point to mention a basic philosophy of respiratory therapy. Generally speaking, respiratory therapy is not directed toward the cure of disease in the sense of removing a specific cause. A surgeon removes an inflamed appendix and cures the clinical condition of acute appendicitis; a physician administers an antibiotic and cures a disease by destroying the causative organism. In contrast, respiratory therapy is fundamentally supportive or symptomatic in nature. In the former instance, therapy helps to maintain respiratory and cardiac integrity until more etiologically specific treatment can be effective, and in the latter, it attempts to counter the effects of disease and to help restore maximum function. In a broad sense, then, and with some obvious exceptions, the technology of respiratory therapy is concerned not so much with what the disease under treatment is as with what the disease has done to cardiopulmonary physiology. Although it is important that an effective therapist have a practical working knowledge of relevant clinical diseases, it is far more important that he or she understands the malfunction of respiration brought about by these diseases.

With this in mind, we now discuss major features of five pathologic conditions, some or all of which are common to cardiopulmonary disease in general—hypoxia, airway obstruction, pulmonary distention, pulmonary restriction, and ventilation-perfusion imbalance. Hypoxia can be caused by many factors, including the other four pathologic states here listed. Because it is a consequence of so many abnormalities, perhaps hypoxia should not be discussed parallel with the others. However, its importance as the greatest hazard of all oxygen-dependent creatures, and as the prime object of our therapy, gives hypoxia top priority and our attention first.

Hypoxia and hypoxemia	*Hypoxia* is a general term that means an inadequate availability of oxygen for cell function, whereas *hypoxemia* refers to a diminution in the actual content of oxygen in blood and implies tissue hypoxia but does not indicate what tissue or to what degree.[1-3] Although there is an obvious difference in their meanings, the two are frequently used interchangeably, and as a matter of convenience, the shorter term, *hypoxia,* is used in the following text. It is assumed that the reader can make a mental differentiation between them according to usage of the terms. It is even more important that the student clearly understand the difference between two quantitative expressions of blood *oxygen content, arterial oxygen saturation* (Sa_{O_2}) and *arterial oxygen tension* (Pa_{O_2}).

Since a major step in the process of oxygen transport is the union of oxygen with hemoglobin, the degree to which hemoglobin is saturated with oxygen is a valuable indication of the efficiency of the hemoglobin carriage. The question frequently arises as to which is the better gauge of oxygenation—hemoglobin saturation with oxygen or blood oxygen tension. Neither tells us what we would really like to know—the level of oxygen in tissue cells. Both tell us only of oxygen's availability in the circulating arterial blood or give us a rough idea of its use by the body if measured in mixed venous blood.

Hemoglobin oxygen saturation is an implied quantitative measure of volumes of oxygen per volumes of blood and might seem to be more relevant to our needs than oxygen tension. It is clinically important and useful information but in itself is incomplete without knowledge of the hemoglobin concentration, the grams of hemoglobin per 100 ml of blood. Two subjects, one with 15 g/dl and the other with 7.5 g/dl, may both be 96% saturated with oxygen, but obviously 96% of 15 g of hemoglobin per deciliter of blood represents more oxygen than does 96% of 7.5 g. The product of hemoglobin concentration, hemoglobin oxygen saturation, and the factor 1.34 allows a rapid estimation of the actual volume of oxygen in 100 ml of blood. (See Chapter 6.)

Blood oxygen partial pressure is widely used in determining hemoglobin oxygen saturation. Saturation can be measured directly by time-consuming chemical analysis, but it is much more easily measured from the blood oxygen tension and an oxygen dissociation curve, properly adjusted for pH and temperature. At the upper end of the dissociation curves, saturation changes very slightly with changes in PO_2. As a result, a drop in saturation of only 3% between two samples might seem no cause for alarm, but it can represent a tension drop of 20 mm Hg or more, certainly indicative of some abnormality. PO_2 measurements avoid overlooking slight but significant oxygen content changes.

Finally, because partial pressure is a kinetic parameter, it gives us some idea of the molecular force available to oxygen in its diffusion efforts across physiologic barriers. A useful index of abnormal oxygen transport as a cause of hypoxemia is a comparison of oxygen tensions in alveolar gas and arterial blood, called the alveolar-arterial oxygen tension gradient. The clinical use of this measurement is discussed later, but it obviously requires use of tension rather than saturation data.

Therefore there is no single better way of metering blood oxygen content. Both saturation and tension values give the most complete picture so far available to us when combined with values for hemoglobin.

Causes of hypoxia and hypoxemia

A variety of classifications for causes of hypoxia have been proposed. The following includes the majority of factors that lead to (1) hypoxemia and/or (2) tissue hypoxia.

Reduced alveolar oxygen. Reduced alveolar oxygen can result from either low ambient PO_2 or hypoventilation.

Low ambient PO_2. Breathing a mixture with a low concentration of oxygen at atmosphere, or normal oxygen at subatmosphere, provides an inadequate alveolar oxygen tension for normal diffusion into pulmonary blood. A common example of this problem is encountered during travel to high altitudes, where the unaccustomed visitor often suffers ill effects of hypoxia for several days, the so-called mountain sickness, or hypobarism.

Hypoventilation. Always associated with hypercapnia, hypoventilation reduces the amount of air ventilating the alveoli so that there is not enough oxygen available for normal arterial saturation.

Impaired alveolar-capillary diffusion (diffusion defect). Faced with pathologic changes in any of the structures of the A-C membrane, such as fibrosis, granuloma, proliferation of connective tissue, or interstitial edema, fewer oxygen molecules will be able to penetrate the barrier even with normal alveolar gas tension, and the arterial tension will be considerably less than the alveolar. The student may see this condition referred to in the literature as *alveolar-capillary block,* but in current terminology it is more properly called a *diffusion defect.* A pure diffusion defect is relatively uncommon, and because it is often absent in some conditions in which the pathology would seem to make it probable, much is not known about its exact mechanism. The diagnosis of impared diffusion is basically a laboratory procedure is further discussed under Ventilation/Perfusion Imbalance.

Hemoglobin deficiency. Hemoglobin deficiency may be of two varieties, absolute or relative.

Absolute. Anemia, with a quantitative lack of circulating hemoglobin, can seriously impair the oxygen-carrying capacity of the blood, even in the presence of normal supply and adequate diffusion.

Relative. For adequate oxygenation not only must there be enough hemoglobin, but it must be capable of transporting oxygen because abnormal hemoglobin can produce clinically significant hypoxia. For example, carbon monoxide in a breathing mixture will combine with hemoglobin much faster than will the oxygen present, and it forms carboxyhemoglobin, which is incapable of carrying oxygen. It is this mechanism that makes carbon monoxide such a lethal agent. Another abnormal form of hemoglobin is methemoglobin, an oxidized (not oxygenated) form in which the iron is in the ferric instead of the normal ferrous state. The result of hereditary defects or the ingestion of certain drugs in toxic doses, methemoglobin, like carboxyhemoglobin, is unable to transport oxygen and is an important cause of hypoxia.

Ventilation/perfusion ratio imbalance. This cause of hypoxemia involves blood perfusing areas of the lung where ventilation is reduced or an excessive amount of blood for the amount of ventilation present. Because of the clinical importance of the problem, its principles and consequences are discussed in some detail later in this chapter.

Anatomic shunts. A shunt is a bypass, or a short circuit, and in a cardiopulmonary sense it consists of a direct communication between the arterial and venous circulations. The result of congenital defects, disease, or trauma, a shunt may consist of a local communication between a peripheral artery and a nearby vein, or a large defect in the septa separating the left and right chambers of the heart. The latter type is the most clinically important; it is common in congenital heart disease and is described in Chapter 7.

Physiologic shunts. When blood flow in the lung passes alveoli that have no ventilation, the result is similar to that described for anatomic shunts. That is, deoxygenated blood mixes with arterialized blood, much like a right-to-left shunt. This can also be considered the extreme end of a low ventilation/perfusion ratio. This cause of hypoxemia is difficult to treat and does not respond well to simple oxygen administration methods. More discussion of this "venous admixture" problem is presented under Ventilation/Perfusion Imbalance in this chapter.

The problems discussed so far are common causes of hypoxemia. Of course all of these may also cause tissue hypoxia as well, especially if the hypoxemia is severe and cannot be compensated for by an adequate increase in cardic output to deliver oxygen. Also some problems, such as the following two, can cause tissue hypoxia even when there is an adequate amount of oxygen in the arterial blood.

Circulatory failure. Should the systemic circulation lose its thrust, there will be reduced tissue cell perfusion with resulting hypoxia. This may also be of two types, generalized or local.

Generalized. In the presence of generalized circulatory failure, as in shock or with a failing heart, oxygen deprivation will be widespread because of the decreased cardiac output.

Local. Venous or arterial obstruction can interfere with local circulation, causing tissue hypoxia of the affected area.

Histotoxins. Chemical substances that interfere with the enzyme systems of body cells responsible for oxygen use can produce lethal cellular hypoxia, in the presence of adequate oxygen supply. Cyanide poisoning is one of the best known clinical examples of this category.

Acute hypoxia

Acute hypoxia is caused by a rapid reduction of available oxygen, as from asphyxia, airway obstruction, blockage of alveoli by the fluid of edema or infectious exudate, abrupt cardiorespiratory failure, and acute hemorrhage. Some patients, depending on the cause, may exhibit hypoventilation and others, hyperventilation to the point of "air hunger," a seemingly insatiable attempt to breathe more and more air. In the latter, hyperpnea is usually present, and the increased ventilatory volume blows off excess carbon dioxide, dropping the blood level significantly and elevating blood pH. Both arterial oxygen tensions and saturation are low. If the degree of hypoxia is less than critical, the mental state it produces has been likened to that of alcoholic intoxication.[4] Headache is a frequent complaint, and often mental confusion occurs. However, in the early stages of oxygen deprivation, mental stimulation may be strikingly evident, the subject reacting in a euphoric and sometimes hilarious manner. This is followed by a state of depression and drowsiness. Muscle weakness ensues, accompanied by lack of coordination, and as the hypoxia progresses, serious loss of discrimination and judgment occurs.[5] With a more sudden hypoxia, there may be an acute abrupt loss of consciousness; this is not common except in those instances when the subject finds him- or herself suddenly in an airless environment, such as a gas-filled compartment.

The most critical target organ of hypoxia is the central nervous system, and with a few exceptions, survival of acute hypoxia depends on its effect on the brain. One of the early responses of the brain is vasodilation and an increased cerebral blood flow. However, because nerve tissue is so vulnerable to oxygen lack, a few minutes of severe hypoxia may produce irreversible damage to brain cells, and prolongation of lesser degrees can lead to death or permanent damage. Comas of days' or weeks' duration are not uncommon; and the half-living vegetative existence of the not-quite dead brain may be the most tragic consequence of hypoxia.

Other organs are also affected by hypoxia. Although the healthy heart can tolerate hypoxia to a considerable degree, one slightly compromised by disease may suffer seriously. This is especially evident in the patient with subclinical cardiac disorders (not quite to the symptom-producing stage), such as early or mild coronary artery narrowing or early heart failure. Functioning with a minimum reserve, such hearts, when perfused with hypoxic blood, will be adversely affected. Myocardial fibers, with a high oxygen demand, may weaken or die, or the cardiac rhythm may be seriously disturbed. Patients with known or suspected heart disease, especially those in the middle and older age groups, must be watched very closely, from the cardiac point of view; electrocardiographic changes are frequent indications of impending or actual myocardial hypoxia. Kidney cells also require constant and adequate oxygenation, and hypoxia can precipitate renal failure, interfering with the ability of the kidney to maintain normal electrolyte and water balance and to eliminate waste products efficiently. Finally, the carbon dioxide transport mechanism is less effective with hypoxia, since oxyhemoglobin is needed to displace carbon dioxide in the lung.

The depth of hypoxia that the body can tolerate and still survive is a matter of considerable interest. There are so many obvious modifying variables, such as the state of the circulation (especially the cerebral), the general body cellular health, the total metabolism, and the intensity of therapy, that there is no clear-cut lower limit of oxygenation. A guiding rule of thumb for some time has held that an arterial PO_2 below 20 mm Hg is probably incompatible with life[6]; yet experience has shown values as low as 9 mm Hg followed by recovery. The modern therapy of respiratory failure has most likely reduced the hypoxic threshold of viability. A more practical guide that the therapist may encounter is the so-called *rule of three*, which describes, as at least temporarily acceptable as minimal oxygenation, an arterial oxygen tension that is three times the value of the inspired oxygen concentration. Such a gimmick has no scientific basis, since it employs unlike terms of measurement. It is simply an expression of clinical observation that tells us the oxygen uptake and transport are probably holding their own if the PaO_2 follows the rule or are decompensating if it does not.

We make special mention of a common sign of hypoxia, *cyanosis*, present in both acute and chronic hypoxia although not invariably in either. Cyanosis is a blue or gray-blue imparted to skin, mucous membranes, and nail beds in the presence of hypoxia. Evaluation of the degree of cyanosis, or even its presence, depends on the perception of the examiner, modified by such factors as the ambient lighting, the color of the environment, and especially the skin color of the subject. In dark-skinned patients, cyanosis may be detected only in nail beds or mucous membranes. Thus, although failure to see cyanosis does not rule out hypoxia, its presence is a strong positive sign of hypoxia.

Cyanosis is related to the degree of oxygen *unsaturation of capillary blood* perfusing body surfaces, and generally it requires the presence of about 5 g/dl of unsaturated hemoglobin to be detected. Obviously, the greater the concentration of unsaturated hemoglobin, the deeper will be the cyanosis, since it is the reduced hemoglobin that gives to blood its bluish red "venous" appearance. Normally, capillary blood contains about *2.5 g of reduced hemoglobin per deciliter of blood,* a value derived as follows: Since capillary blood represents blood continuously giving up oxygen as it passes from the arterial to the venous end of the capillary, its unsaturated hemoglobin content may be considered the *average* of the unsaturation of the arterial blood entering the capillary and the venous blood leaving. At a normal oxygen saturation of 97%, 15 g/dl of arterial hemoglobin has 3% unsaturated hemoglobin, or 0.45 g/dl. Venous blood 70% saturated has 30% unsaturated hemoglobin, or 4.5 g/dl. The average capillary unsaturation would thus equal:

$$\frac{0.45 + 4.5}{2} = 2.5\% \text{ of unsaturated hemoglobin}^{[1]}$$

Assuming a hemoglobin concentration of 15 g/dl and an a-v oxygen saturation difference of 24% (corresponding to an a-v oxygen content difference of 5 vol%, as described earlier), we can calculate that an arterial oxygen saturation of 79% will produce a mean capillary unsaturation of 5 g/dl (Appendix 11). Hypoxia below this level, which the oxygen dissociation curve shows to be the equivalent of about 45 mm Hg partial pressure of oxygen, will probably produce visible cyanosis. However, since cyanosis depends on a specific concentration of unsaturated capillary hemoglobin, in anemia, with its reduced quantity of available hemoglobin, there may not be enough unsaturated hemoglobin to produce cyanosis until the arterial saturation drops well below 80%. Conversely, polycythemia, with its increased supply of hemoglobin, may show cyanosis even though there is adequate circulating oxygen.

Chronic hypoxia   If the onset of hypoxia is slowly progressive, the body may adjust to it without any acute reactions. Diseases most likely to cause chronic hypoxia include gradually destructive or fibrotic lung diseases, congenital or acquired heart diseases, and chronic blood loss. In general, a persistent state of chronic hypoxia simulates a condition of persistent mental and physical fatigue. Mental responses may become sluggish and acuity diminished, and patients frequently complain of inability to perform physical tasks with the same ease as formerly. As a rule, however, chronic hypoxia itself is not a common cause of disability; rather it is the underlying disease responsible for the hypoxia. Often, relief of the hypoxia only, with oxygen breathing, will have little effect on disability. In many patients with whom the respiratory therapist will have contact, the physical effort to maintain normal oxygen and carbon dioxide levels is the real cause of disability. Just as in acute hypoxia, if the oxygen lack is severe enough chronically, cyanosis will be present.

People who are born at high altitudes and who continue to live for several years at those altitudes must physiologically adjust from the prenatal period to an environment with a lower oxygen tension than that which exists at sea level. Inhabitants of mountainous areas, especially those of the South American Andes and the U.S. Rocky Mountains, have been extensively studied over many years, up to and including the present, to determine how the body adjusts to hypobaric conditions. Many people live normal and active lives at partial pressures of oxygen in the same range as that found in patients at atmosphere who are suffering from hypoxia as a result of disease. It is obvious that altitude residents must be endowed with some type of adaptation to their "hypoxic" environment; and although many of the details of their physiologic responses, cardiac as well as pulmonary, are still under investigation, a few pertinent facts have been established. These people have a larger "red cell mass" than do natives of lowlands. This means that the total mass (or volume) of all their circulating erythrocytes is greater than that of the average human population, generally accomplished by an increased number of such cells. In addition, altitude dwellers have significantly larger lung volumes. In a general way it may be safe to assume that mountain life has certain rigors not found at sea level, if for no other reason than the nature of the terrain itself and the fact that the economy of such areas has often been agrarian. The survival of generations in such an environment attests to the efficiency of natural adaptation. Indeed, extensive studies have failed to show any ill effects in the indigenous populations, as long as they remain at altitude. Apparently, however, if altitude dwellers leave their original environment for the lowlands for a certain period of time, they often lose their natural adaptation; and a return to low ambient oxygen tensions puts them at the same disadvantage as is experienced by any other transient from sea level. For the individual with a normal cardiorespiratory system, a period of several days may be required to acclimatize to the reduced oxygen partial pressure, during which time the individual may experience weakness and lassitude, headaches, and a marked impairment of his or her usual physical performance.

In a sense, the pulmonary hypoxic patient (with low arterial oxygen tension) is in a situation much like that of the altitude dweller or visitor, with the important difference that he or she has a defective respiratory mechanism. Nevertheless, chronic hypoxia is accompanied by an attempt on the part of the body to accommodate to the limited amount of oxygen that is able to reach the arterial blood. Hypoxia stimulates the bone marrow to increase its production of erythrocytes (an action called *hematopoiesis*) so that, as in the altitude dweller, there is an increase in the number of circulating red cells or, more specifically, an increase in the red cell mass. This state is referred to as *secondary polycythemia,* meaning a more than normal number of red cells secondary to the underlying pulmonary disease. As may be expected, there is also a condition called primary polycythemia, or polycythemia vera, entirely unrelated to cardiopulmonary dysfunction. In secondary polycythemia no increase in the other cellular blood components occurs. The presence of polycythemia is always suspected in a chronically hypoxic patient, but its actual identification may not be apparent. In many patients it may be readily detected by examination of the blood and by noting an increase in the *hematocrit,* which is the ratio between the volume of cells (mostly red cells, of course) and plasma, in a centrifuged sample of blood that has been treated with an anticoagulant. Normally, this does not exceed about 45%, but in polycythemia it may be nearly double. The hemoglobin content is similarly elevated from its usual upper limit of 15 g/dl to perhaps 20 g/dl, and measurement of the circulating erythrocytes will often show an excess above the normal high of around 5 million per cubic millimeter of blood.

It has been demonstrated, however, that such simple measures do not always reflect the hypoxic hematopoiesis responsible for polycythemia.[7] There is usually an associated increase in plasma volume; and if this is of sufficient degree, those measurements that relate red cell numbers or hemoglobin content to blood volume may appear erroneously normal. The most definitive diagnostic technique is an actual measurement of circulating red cell mass, using procedures that employ the dilution of dye by the blood, or the "tagging" of red cells by radioactive substances, which permits evaluation of both the total circulating blood volume and the erythrocyte mass. It is believed that polycythemia is common in patients with chronic lung disease and, if such tests are performed, many who would not otherwise be detected will be revealed.

Enough patients show elevated hematocrits and hemoglobin contents to warrant a few remarks about the clinical significance of such findings. With a sufficient increase in the ratio of red cells to blood fluid, viscosity of the blood can be expected to rise, constituting a matter of concern in the management of this condition.[8] At least in principle, the retarding effect on blood velocity and ease of flow of increasing viscosity may outweigh the advantages of the additional oxygen-carrying capacity of the enlarged red cell mass, and cellular distribution of oxygen may be impaired by a slowing of or interference with perfusion of body cells. It has been suggested that viscosity is not physiologically significant until the hematocrit reaches 55% to 60%.[9] Still there is justified fear that the sluggish circulation of polycythemia may cause intravascular thromboses, especially in vessels that may already be damaged by sclerosis or narrowing from other causes, because slowly moving blood clots more readily than does swiftly moving blood.

The patient with overt polycythemia is usually cyanotic, despite an actual increase in the volume of oxygen carried by the blood. This is because the cyanosis depends on the amount of circulating unsaturated hemoglobin, not saturated, and the patient with a greater than normal number of red cells can have a corresponding increase in the amount of hemoglobin that is unsaturated as well as saturated. Patients often complain of headache, fullness in the head, nasal stuffiness, lethargy, difficulty in taking a deep breath, and epistaxis (nosebleed). The small vessels of the sclera (the white of the eye) may be seen as grossly congested from an increased blood volume. Finally, the increased volume of circulating blood, especially if associated with significant viscosity, places an abnormal work load on the heart to overcome the resistance to flow. The less muscular right ventricle is especially affected; it becomes strained, enlarges in an attempt to sustain its increased load, and eventually fails. This produces the so-called *cor pulmonale*, "pulmonary heart," right-sided heart disease secondary to pulmonary disease.

The respiratory therapist will commonly encounter a physical sign in patients called *clubbing*. Although this condition is not exclusively associated with hypoxia, because of its frequency in this state, it is believed to be pertinent to the discussion here. Clubbing is one state of a more generalized process that affects bones and joints known as hypertrophic osteoarthropathy.[10,11] The essential lesion of osteoarthropathy is a chronic inflammatory process with thickening of periosteum, especially of the long bones, accompanied by the deposition of new bone. By x-ray examination the bones are seen to be thickened, giving rise to the term *hypertrophic*. Joints may also be affected with swelling and inflammation. In a well-developed case many bones and joints may be affected with pain and disabling limitation of motion. Since the changes in the joints and long bones may frequently be detected by x-ray examination only and since lesser degrees are more frequently encountered in patients seen by the respiratory therapist, we describe in greater detail that aspect of the process known as clubbing.

Clubbing may occur as an early stage of hypertrophic osteoarthropathy, or it may be found without subsequent long bone changes. It is manifested by a bulbous swelling of the terminal phalanges of the fingers and toes, which become enlarged and rounded, often but not always cyanotic. There is an increase in all diameters of the tips of the extremities, giving them a "drumstick" appearance. In contrast to the process found in long bones, pain is seldom a symptom of clubbing, although the soft tissue swelling at the ends of the digits may be considerable. A characteristic feature of clubbing is the contour of the nail, which becomes rounded both longitudinally and transversely. Curvature of the nail is not in itself necessarily a sign of disease and often is only a variation of the normal. In clubbing, however, the distortion of the nail is accompanied by a loss of the cuticular angle, the angle at the junction of the skin and nail as viewed from the side of the finger. This is shown in Fig. 8-1, illustrating a normal flat nail, a normal curved nail, and early and late clubbing. The marked cuticular angle in both normal nails is evident but is absent in clubbing. As the clubbing progresses from mild to severe, the degrees of curvature gradually increase. The first indication of imminent clubbing, before

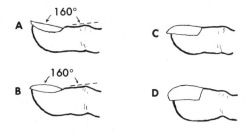

Fig. 8-1   Clubbing is characterized by marked curvature of the nail, a loss of the cuticular angle, an increase in the angle the surface of the nail makes with the terminal phalanx above the normal of 160 degrees, and a bulbous soft tissue swelling of the terminal phalanx. **A** and **B** show the contours of normal straight and curved nails; **C** and **D** represent increasing degrees of clubbing.

significant rounding is evident, is loss of the cuticular angle, associated with a "floating" nail base. This latter is characterized by a sponginess palpated under the base of the nail, which allows the nail to be moved up and down with compression.

Despite the frequency with which clubbing is seen, the specific cause of clubbing, or the full osteoarthropathy, is unknown. It has been speculated that some or many of the following are responsible: chronic infection, unspecified toxins, capillary stasis from increased venous back pressure, arterial hypoxia, and local hypoxia. There is some disturbance in the circulation of the terminal portions of the digits, manifested by an increased blood flow. This has been demonstrated, through microphotography of a nail bed, as an increase in the width of the capillaries.[12] This sign is an extremely important clinical one, even though it does not always indicate hypoxia, or even pulmonary disease. In adults approximately 75% to 85% of clubbing is caused by pulmonary disease (lung tumors, bronchiectasis, fibrosis, empyema); 10% to 15% to cardiac disease (congenital right-to-left shunt, subacute bacterial endocarditis); 10% to liver or gastrointestinal disease (cirrhosis, chronic diarrhea conditions); 5% to miscellaneous causes (heredity, tumors of the thyroid or pharynx, aneurysms of large branches of the aorta). In children, clubbing is predominantly found with cystic fibrosis, bronchiectasis, empyema, and congenital heart disease.[13]

In summary, clubbing suggests disease, first, of the respiratory tract, second, of the heart, and third, of the liver or gastrointestinal tract. The appearance of clubbing may antedate the x-ray signs of carcinoma of the lung by as many as 48 months. Finally, in many instances successful treatment of the underlying disease results in the resolution of the clubbing and a return of the digits to normal.

Treatment of hypoxia

The obvious need in hypoxia is oxygen to preserve the life of body cells, but the details of its administration are discussed elsewhere. It should be emphasized, however, that the objective of therapy is to restore arterial oxygen tension to normal, not to overload the blood with high pressures, except in very specific and limited circumstances. While hypoxia is being relieved, every effort must be made to correct the underlying pathologic conditions responsible for the hypoxia, for only when the latter is accomplished can we feel that the patient is improved. The therapist will see many patients in whom disease has left permanent lung damage of such a degree that sustained normal oxygenation is impossible to achieve, and the management of such patients will strain the ingenuity of physician and therapist alike. Again, when hypoxia is associated with hypercapnia in the presence of an unresponsive respiratory center and the chemoreceptor hypoxic drive is active, ventilation must be supported mechanically during the administration of oxygen to prevent fatal apnea.

Details of oxygen administration for treatment of hypoxia are found in Chapters 12 and 14. Basically, normal levels of arterial oxygenation can be achieved by simple oxygen therapy techniques when hypoxemia is caused by reduced alveolar oxygen, diffusion defects, and moderately low ventilation/perfusion ratios. These problems are generally adequately treated with less than 50% oxygen.

When hypoxemia is caused by extremely low ventilation/perfusion ratios or physiologic shunting, even 100% oxygen may not adequately raise the arterial PO_2. Instead, techniques of positive pressure to the airway such as mechanical ventilation, positive end-expiratory pressure (PEEP), or continuous positive airway pressure (CPAP) may need to be used. These techniques aid in opening airways so that gas exchange can improve, even with lower oxygen concentrations (see Chapters 13 and 14).

Other causes of hypoxia are treated to correct the underlying problem while supplemental oxygen is administered. As an example, anemias are treated with blood transfusions, some anatomic shunts may be surgically corrected, and generalized circulatory failure may be treated with drugs that enhance cardiac output.

Where polycythemia is clinically significant, *phlebotomy* is often a useful procedure. Literally meaning "opening of a vein," phlebotomy entails the venous withdrawal of blood, in increments of about 300 ml, at intervals of 3 to 4 days. The objective of therapy is to lower the hematocrit to a maximum of about 50%, removing a segment of the red cell mass. Since blood water is restored by a shifting of the body fluids, the result is a reduction of blood viscosity. Some believe that the beneficial effects of phlebotomy are attributed to relief of the enlarged blood volume, not just to lowered viscosity. The clinical results are often very rewarding, as patients feel better both physically and mentally and the progress of cor pulmonale is retarded.[9] During an acute hospitalization, a patient may have several phlebotomies and then return as an outpatient for follow-up treatment as needed, usually with gradually decreasing frequency.

Airway obstruction	Obstruction of the airways is one of the most common causes of cardiopulmonary disability and is almost always an important factor in the disease of patients treated by the respiratory therapist except for those with nonpulmonary ventilatory problems. Obstruction may be transient and reversible, or it may be permanent. We considered the effects of airway resistance on the mechanics of ventilation earlier and now concern ourselves with a description of the physiologic and pathologic changes brought about by obstruction. For our purposes, we do not include gross obstruction, as from an inhaled foreign body or a large tumor, but rather classify the causes of obstruction as *mucosal edema, bronchial spasm, increased secretions,* and *bronchiolar collapse* (Figs. 8-2 and 8-3).
Mucosal edema	Edema is an increase in the amount of interstitial fluid that bathes the body cells; pathologic changes cause a shift of body water from the plasma to the

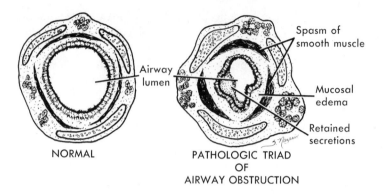

NORMAL

PATHOLOGIC TRIAD
OF
AIRWAY OBSTRUCTION

Fig. 8-2 Cross sections of airways comparing normal with obstruction caused by pathologic triad. Note narrowed airway lumen (opening) in obstructed airway.

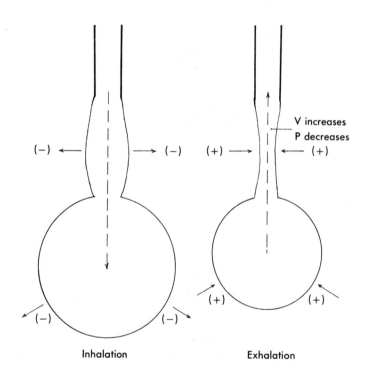

Inhalation

Exhalation

Fig. 8-3 A disease-weakened bronchiole is shown as thin walled and flaccid. Negative intrathoracic pressure inflates the alveolus with little difficulty. During exhalation, however, rising intrathoracic pressure compresses the diseased bronchiole as well as the alveolus, impeding airflow. In addition, the velocity (V) of air through the bronchiolar restriction reduces intraluminal pressure (P), encouraging further collapse and worsening the obstruction.

intercellular spaces, with resulting swelling of the affected area, which may be localized or extensive over larger areas of the body. The most common example of edema of the respiratory tract is the nasal swelling and inflammation (rhinitis) of the common cold, with the accompanying obstruction to breathing. This same reaction can be visualized in the lower portions of the respiratory passages. Severe edema of the larynx is well known as *croup,* and the same relative degree of airway narrowing can occur in the small bronchi and bronchioles.

Mucosal edema can be caused by:

1. Mechanical irritation or trauma to the respiratory mucosa, as from instrumentation, the presence of a foreign body, or the inhalation of caustic liquids or irritant fumes.
2. Infection, bacterial or viral, in which the reaction represents a body defense against the invading organisms.
3. Allergy to inhaled liquids or particulate matter, exemplified by the common allergic bronchial asthma.

In acute edema, respiratory mucosa becomes boggy soft, spongy, and waterlogged. There is usually an accompanying arteriolar and capillary congestion, which adds to the swelling. If of short duration, acute edema may be easily reversible following removal of its cause. However, if the edema is long lasting or frequently recurring, it may become *indurated,* giving to the tissue a permanent thickening and a firm, rather than soft, consistency. Such changes markedly interfere with mucosal function, especially through destruction of cilia, and the removal of the normal mucus blanket. Chronic respiratory infection aids in the perpetuation of such induration.

Bronchial spasm

Spasm may be defined as an involuntary excessive contraction of a muscle. Common examples are found in extremity muscle cramps, spasm of neck muscles after injury, and intestinal cramps. Bronchial spasm is produced by excessive and prolonged contraction of the involuntary muscle fibers in the walls of the bronchi and bronchioles. Such contraction can seriously reduce airway lumens and may be localized or general. The causes of bronchial spasm are the same as those of edema listed previously, but especially bronchial asthma, of which spasm is the major physiologic derangement.

Increased secretions

By *increased bronchial secretions* we mean an actual increase in *volume* of secretions produced, an increase in their *viscosity,* or both. Although such reactions may follow exposure of the respiratory mucosa to many irritants, infection is the most frequent offender, and the common cold is again a familiar example with its abundance of sputum.

Bronchial secretions are composed of many ingredients[14]: *mucus,* secreted by the goblet cells and mucous glands of the bronchial mucosa; *DNA* (deoxyribonucleic acid, as a protein salt) and *RNA* (ribonucleic acid, as a protein salt), released from nuclei and cytoplasm of disintegrating cells; and *plasma fluid* and *proteins,* including fibrinogen, escaping from pulmonary capillaries. The differentiation between normal and pathologic secretions depends on the relative concentrations of their components.

For purposes of discussion we can make a distinction between two broad types of sputum—mucoid and purulent. *Mucoid* secretions may be considered as a response by the airways to foreign matter invasion, infective or noninfective, in an attempt to remove the offending agent. One of the characteristics of a well-established chronic bronchitis is an actual increase in the number of mucous glands in the bronchial walls. The secretions so produced will consist of a high concentration of mucus, in respect to the other constituents.

Mucus contains mucoproteins, a combination of any of several proteins with substances known as mucopolysaccharides, and long-chain carbohydrate-containing compounds, and it is these mucoproteins that are responsible for the viscosity of the secretions. Thus, when stimulated to overproduction of sputum by some irritative or pathologic process, the airways will contain larger amounts of fluid of a greater than normal viscosity. It should be added that viscosity of normal secretions (normal relative concentrations of its components) can be raised to dangerous degrees simply by dehydration. This is considered again later with the subject of humidification.

Purulent secretions, on the other hand, are the result of invasion of the respiratory tract by pathogenic bacteria and the effect of such infection on the sputum. The natural inflammatory response to bacterial infection brings many leukocytes to the area, and they engage the organisms in destructive battle. The mucoid secretions, which are the first response, become grossly infiltrated with intact and fragmented bacteria, leukocytes, and tissue cells damaged by the process. Disruption of the cytoplasm and nuclei of the cells releases into the secretions a large amount of nucleoproteins, the DNA and RNA noted above. It is principally the DNA protein that gives to the secretions their purulent characteristics of viscosity to the point of tenacious stringiness and a yellow to green discoloration, in contrast to the colorless, clear or frothy, mucoid type. If the bronchial inflammation is acute, the sputum may have streaks of dark red or brown from extravasated blood. Finally, depending on the offending bacteria or the presence of secondary or mixed infection, putrefactive organisms will often distinguish purulent sputum with a disagreeable odor.

The usually effective mucus blanket with its escalator cleansing action becomes less effective as its viscosity and volume increase, and these factors interfere with ciliary action. Often much of the cilia is destroyed, removing a valuable protective mechanism from the respiratory tract. As viscosity increases, the ordinary cough mechanism is less able to remove the secretions, and these plug airways, seriously interfering with ventilation. Parts of the lung may become airless, a condition referred to as *atelectasis,* with potentially grave consequences.

Bronchiolar collapse

Usually associated with advanced bronchopulmonary disease, bronchiolar collapse is a clinically important form of small airway obstruction that, in many patients, becomes the most critical factor in ventilatory disability. The mechanism of its action is based on two components. First, there must be damage to the integrity of bronchiolar walls so that they are unable to maintain patency in the face of the second factor, a pressure gradient across the bronchiolar walls. The conditions predisposing to bronchiolar collapse are most frequently found in the destructive lung diseases such as emphysema, bronchiectasis, and cystic disease; and, by far, emphysema is the predominant influence.

The bronchioles, devoid of cartilaginous support, are essentially highly pliable soft-walled tubes that depend for their patency on surrounding structures. Encompassed by masses of alveoli whose septa are arranged in a radial fashion apparently attached to their walls, the lumens of the bronchioles are kept from collapsing by the weblike support of these air sacs. During normal exhalation the rising intrathoracic pressure is exerted on the bronchiolar walls, as on all other thoracic structures, and does slightly narrow them; but the intact surrounding alveoli prevent further collapse. Fig. 8-3 illustrates what happens in the presence of bronchopulmonary disease. With destruction of alveoli and the loss of their supportive septa, the bronchiolar walls are responsive to pressure changes between the intrabronchiolar lumens and the pleural space. During inhalation the increasingly negative intrathoracic pressure and the inflow of air are sufficient to dilate the bronchioles to full patency. During exhalation, however, the rising thoracic pressure, unopposed by alveolar septal countertraction, compresses the resilient bronchioles and narrows them to the point of interference with airflow. At the same time, as the exhaled air is being forced through the narrowing bronchioles, its velocity progressively increases. In keeping with the Bernoulli principle, with the increase in intraluminal velocity, there is a drop in intraluminal pressure, and the negative pressure gradient thus established across the bronchiole wall between the lumen and pleural space favors further narrowing. A vicious cycle is thereby set in motion that perpetuates the continuing airway collapse.[15]

The patients in whom this condition is clinically significant are usually those who already have expiratory difficulty from their underlying disease and must exert exceptionally great effort during exhalation. Thus, the element of bronchiolar collapse can contribute to a steadily worsening disability. In addition to its chronic influence on exhalation, bronchiolar collapse can produce an acute state referred to as *acute air trapping*. Frequently, without warning, a patient may suddenly find he or she is unable to complete a phase of exhalation already started. The chest is immobilized in a position of partial exhalation, and the patient is unable either to inhale or to empty the lungs further. He or she may struggle to move the chest and become severely cyanotic, especially in the face and neck. Such an episode may be triggered by an unnoticed early expiratory effort of greater force than usual; and as the sequence of events described previously comes into play after the movement of part of the exhaled air, a number of bronchioles completely collapse, trapping the remainder of the tidal volume. Although frightening to the point of panic to the patient and observers alike, these attacks are generally self-limiting. A series of sharp forceful lateral squeezes applied to both sides of the thorax will often supply spurts of air of sufficient pressure to overcome the collapse and empty the lungs. This technique is learned by many patients and especially by members of their families. To prevent acute trapping and to accomplish the maximum exhalation with the minimum of effort, patients either learn spontaneously or are taught the technique of "pursed-lip breathing." In the maneuver the patient slightly purses the lips while exhaling, deliberately prolonging exhalation and trying to maintain an even flow of air. The moderate obstruction he or she effects at the mouth builds up a back pressure in the airways, not enough to make exhalation difficult but enough to retard air velocity and reduce the transbronchiolar pressure gradient to prevent collapse.[16] It has also been suggested that pursed-lip breathing works predominantly by slowing the respiratory rate and increasing the tidal volume.[17]

Effect of obstruction on ventilation

Obstruction greatly increases the work of breathing because of the elevated resistance of smaller air passages and the retarding effect of air turbulence. Resistance to breathing may be more pronounced in one phase or the other of ventilation. For example, the laryngeal obstruction of childhood croup may necessitate such a strong inspiratory effort that there will be noticeable retraction of the sternum and epigastrium during inspiration, and the flow of air past the obstruction may produce a harsh sound known as a *stridor*. Most often, however, obstruction is a major problem in chronic bronchopulmonary diseases, and then exhalation is impeded. To a considerable degree the ventilatory muscles can overcome obstruction to inhalation, but the passive nature of normal exhalation is unable to deflate the lung to its resting position, and exhalation must employ muscular effort, at times very strenuous. The tremendous work involved in moving air against obstruction uses so much physical energy that it constitutes one of the major factors in the disability of chronic pulmonary diseases. Indeed, muscular fatigue may lead to ventilatory failure, hypercapnia, and respiratory acidosis.

Expiration time is usually prolonged beyond that of inhalation, and often contraction of the upper abdomen is evident during the latter part of exhalation. If bronchospasm is extensive or mobile secretions are present, characteristic breath sounds can be heard by the unaided ear or by the use of the stethoscope (auscultation) during exhalation. *Wheezes* are high-pitched squeaky noises produced by air passing with some velocity through passages narrowed by spasm or thick secretions. *Rhonchi* are coarser, lower pitched sounds caused by vibration of bronchial secretions in the airflow. *Rales* are fine bubbling or crackling sounds, usually noted during inhalation as air passes through fluid in the alveoli, and are not necessarily reflections of obstruction.

Treatment of obstruction

Details of treatment are considered elsewhere, but the general procedures include the following.

Aspiration (suctioning). Aspiration is the removal of secretions through the use of suctioning. It may be accomplished by means of *bronchoscopy*, the passage of a long, lighted tube, under direct vision, into the bronchi, allowing examination of these structures as well as extensive aspiration. Frequently employed is the insertion of a catheter into the main stem bronchi in patients in whom a *tracheostomy* tube has been placed just below the larynx, or in whom an *endotracheal* tube has been passed through the mouth and larynx into the upper trachea. Small catheters, passed through needles inserted between the tracheal rings just below the larynx, are occasionally used for aspiration of thin secretions. These procedures are described in more detail later.

Aerosols. The inhalation of very fine particles of liquids, in the form of a mist, is extensively used and includes the following:

1. Water—to thin secretions by increasing their water content.
2. Bronchodilators—agents that reduce bronchial spasm.
3. Decongestants—agents that reduce vascular congestion.
4. Liquefacients—agents that liquefy secretions by altering their physical or chemical characteristics.

Systemic liquefacients. Some medications, taken by mouth or vein, make bronchial secretions more liquid and easier to raise.

Postural drainage. Physical therapeutic techniques that use gravity in mobilizing secretions, by positioning the patient, are an important part of both short-term and long-term therapy.

Pulmonary distention	Pulmonary distention is a state of hyperinflation of the lung characterized by an increase in the functional residual capacity (FRC), and its two major causes are *airway obstruction* and *loss of lung elasticity*. As a rule, distention caused by obstructed airways is generally of a temporary and reversible nature, exemplified by an attack of acute bronchial asthma. In this condition, diffuse bronchial spasm is the outstanding feature, and during such an episode the FRC may be markedly increased. On subsidence and in the absnece of complications (especially bronchial infection), the resting throacic level returns to normal and the FRC is reduced. It is also probable that some distention may accompany acute episodes of obstructive bronchitis, but this is apt to be variable and evanescent.

From a practical, respiratory therapy point of view, *pulmonary distention* usually refers to the hyperinflation of pulmonary emphysema. Although we have not considered the clinical and pathologic nature of this disease in a specific discussion, we have mentioned it so many times that the student may already be forming a mental picture of its characteristics. There are many excellent descriptions of emphysema (often called obstructive emphysema, bronchitis-emphysema, and chronic obstructive lung disease) in any number of texts, and the student is encouraged to become very familiar with it, for it will probably be the most prevalent disease he or she will encounter. We note only a few of its details here as they pertain to distention.

Basically, emphysema is a destructive disease characterized by disruption of variable numbers of alveolar walls; the more disruption, the more severe is the disease. This destructive process converts the lung from an organ with a large number of uniform-sized air spaces into one with a smaller number of variable-sized spaces and fewer gas diffusion surfaces. A consequence of the resulting architectural change in the lung is a marked unevenness of airflow and air distribution and, most serious, a great loss of elastic fibers.

Until fairly recently, it was generally believed that destructive distention was a sequela of progressive or persistent airway obstruction. It was postulated that because of any of the common causes of bronchial and bronchiolar obstruction, the resistance to expiratory airflow developed an intraalveolar back pressure that eventually destroyed the alveolar walls. Somewhat oversimplified, it was like the rupture of a hyperinflated balloon. The continued expiratory resistance was then supposed to have trapped air in the enlarged air sacs. However, studies on normal individuals whose lungs are subjcted to very high intrapulmonary pressures from back pressure for long periods of time (e.g., wind instrument musicians) have failed to show any adverse effects on lung function and no signs of distention.[18] Refined pathologic techniques that permit better correlation between pathology and function have demonstrated that in many if not most instances the distention precedes and causes the airway obstruction so frequently seen with it. It is speculated that some factors not yet clearly defined (sometimes infectious?) destroy the alveolar walls, with loss of diffusing surface and elasticity. Bronchiolar collapse causes obstruction, which is worsened by an ensuing chronic bronchitis subsequent to failure of cough-clearance of the airways.[15,19] By this mechanism, following alveolar disruption the actual pulmonary distention is the result of loss of elasticity rather than of obstruction, since the thoracic expansile forces are now relatively unopposed.

Less well defined as a pathologic entity is the degenerative change that accompanies the aging process and that diminishes the tone of elastic tissue throughout the body. The loss of skin elasicity in older persons is a common observation, and apparently a similar phenomenon takes place in the lung. The increase in FRC often seen with advancing age is sometimes unwisely referred to as *senile emphysema*, although there is no concrete evidence that this constitutes a true disease.

Effect of distention on ventilation   The adverse effects of distention on ventilation can be described in the following three categories: reduced inspiratory capacity, low position of the diaphragm, and enlarged FRC.

Reduced inspiratory capacity. The elevated end-expiratory resting level of the thorax and the low, flat diaphragm (described next) produce the inspiratory position of the thorax. Thus at the resting level the lungs are already in a position of partial inspiration, since the lung-thorax relationship is unbalanced in the direction of the thoracic forces. The inspiratory capacity is encroached on, and increase in tidal volume in response to exertional needs is limited. (See Chapters 4 and 5.)

Low position of diaphragm. Increase in the FRC forces the chest into the inspiratory position as the lung-thorax resting level rises, and the overdistention of the lung depresses and flattens the contour of the diaphragmatic domes. In a low position, contraction of the diaphragm, even though feeble, instead of lowering itself, pulls in the costal margin and reduces the volume of the thorax during inhalation, rather than enlarging it. With loss of effective use of the diaphragm, reduction in intrathoracic pressure is dependent on contraction of the intercoastals and the accessory ventilatory muscles. The pull of the accessory muscles causes an upward and outward displacement of the sternum, an increase in the sternal angle (the junction of the manubrium and body of the sternum, at the level of the second rib), and eventually an increase in the anteroposterior diameter of the chest. This produces the *barrel-chest* deformity common to long-standing distention. The thoracic negative pressure, generated at a tremendous energy cost to the patient, also acts on the ineffective diaphragm, pulling it *upward* during inhalation, the so-called paradoxical ventilation. Thus, while the intercostals and accessories are working hard to enlarge the thorax, the rising diaphragm, sucked upward by their action, partially negates their efforts, and the net gain in intrathoracic volume is small in proportion to the physical effort expended. When inspiratory efforts are strenuous enough, not only is the diaphragm elevated during inhalation, but the abdominal wall is also retracted in a contrary manner. Exhalation, lacking the effective use of the abdominals, is a slow process, depending on inadequate passive recoil and expiratory action of the intercostals; and during exhalation, rising intrathoracic pressure drives down the diaphragm as the abdominal wall balloons outward. The clinical picture is one of a short, gasping inhalation, with extensive use of accessory muscles of ventilation and epigastric retraction, followed by a prolonged exhalation accompanied by varying degrees of epigastric protrusion. The presence of a barrel-chest defect, with or without paradoxical ventilation, signifies serious disruption of the normal lung-thoracic architecture, and the attentive therapist should always be on the watch for it.

Large functional residual capacity. The physiologic significance of an enlarged FRC can be appreciated only if the part it plays in ventilation is visualized clearly. Since the FRC is a substantial volume of air remaining in the lung at the end of a quiet exhalation, the next tidal volume of inhaled air must mix with it to reach the alveoli. In other words, air that is ventilating the alveoli with each breath is a mixture of air already in the lung and new air entering. The larger the residual air volume, the greater is the dilution of incoming tidal air. Since enlarged FRC is usually accompanied by airway obstruction, large and variable-sized air spaces, or both, an even distribution of tidal air to all alveoli is impossible. Thus *uneven distribution of inspired air* is characteristic of severe pulmonary distention and results in nonuniform alveolar ventilation, a hazard to gas exchange, since it interferes with the normal ventilation-perfusion balance described later.

An estimate of the evenness with which inspired air is distributed among the alveoli can be made in the cardiopulmonary laboratory (see Chapter 5). One technique involves the breathing of pure oxygen for a number of minutes, gradually washing out nitrogen remaining in the lung from previous air breathing. The exhaled air is monitored by an analyzer that measures the gradually decreasing concentration of nitrogen removed, and the time-concentration relationship is noted. In a lung disrupted by severe obstruction or especially in which variable sized air spaces empty in an irregular fashion, the relationship will be markedly abnormal. Another technique uses the inhalation of a known concentration of inert helium; by measurement of the time it takes for the lung air to reach equilibrium with the inhaled gas, the distribution characteristic of the lung can be determined.

Treatment of distention

The treatment of distention is nonspecific and is aimed to achieve the following.

Reduce obstruction. The methods employed to reduce obstruction are those described earlier, with emphasis on the use of aerosols and postural drainage.

Improve pulmonary air distribution. Closely related to the management of obstruction, treatment of distention employs the intermittent use of mechanical ventilators to assist air distribution by providing air under pressure. Aerosols to reduce obstruction, frequently delivered at the same time, help to maintain the integrity of the airways while ventilating alveoli that are otherwise poorly supplied with air.

Improve mechanics of ventilation. To help consolidate gains realized from the preceding two therapies, patients are retrained in the proper use of their ventilatory muscles through breathing exercises. Emphasis is placed on restoration of effective use of the diaphragm and on aiding the patient to limit reliance on the accessory muscles. This approach is incorporated into the long-term management of the patient, and its techniques become part of his or her daily activities.

Pulmonary restriction

Pulmonary restriction is defined as an interference with easy or adequate lung expansion and is often associated with a decrease in lung and thoracic compliance. There are many pathologic states that can restrict expansion of the lung, some of which are briefly described in the following four groups: thoracic, intrathoracic (nonpulmonary), pulmonary, and abdominal.

Thoracic causes. Some of the thoracic causes of restriction are the result of structural changes in the chest, others of reduced flexibility:

1. Kyphoscoliosis is an abnormal curvature of the spine that, when it affects the dorsal segment, distorts the thoracic cage by compressing one side or the other. In general, it is produced by an imbalance between the bilateral skeletal muscle groups, weakness of one group allowing unopposed traction by the other, with eventual tilting and rotation of the spine and chest cage. Poliomyelitis is a frequent offender, as are developmental defects of childhood and adolescence from causes as yet un-

known. The disfigured thorax may imprison portions of the lung, preventing normal expansion.

2. Destructive bone diseases of the spine and thorax, such as tuberculosis and osteoporosis, may produce restrictive distortion not classified as kyphoscoliosis.
3. Trauma, such as sternal and costal fractures, will cause severe, although usually temporary restriction.
4. Reduced thoracic flexibility can result from such diseases as arthritis, scleroderma, and fibromyositis.
5. Paralysis of ventilatory muscles, as in poliomyelitis and myasthenia gravis, although not reflecting a decrease in compliance, markedly interferes with lung expansion.

Intrathoracic (nonpulmonary) causes. Diseases within the chest often impede lung expansion because of the following:

1. Pleurisy limits ventilation by restrictive pain or by subsequent restrictive pleural thickening.
2. Fluid in the pleural cavity restricts pulmonary expansion by direct compression of the lung. Such fluid may be *serous* in character, from pleural inflammation of heart failure; *purulent,* from pleural infection or extension of a lung infection into the pleural space or from infected chest trauma; or *hemorrhagic,* from trauma or destructive lung disease.

Pulmonary causes. Most of the pulmonary causes of lung restriction can be put into one of two categories:

1. Fibrosis or scarring of the lung accounts for most of the restictive problems. It is a sequela of recurrent respiratory infections, often accompanying chronic bronchopulmonary disease such as emphysema, and follows such destructive diseases as tuberculosis, bronchiectasis, and many industrial or occupational diseases.
2. Intrapulmonary vascular congestion can significantly impair the compliance of the lung. Because of a failing heart, blood in the pulmonary circuit may back up, distending the vasculature of the lung with an increased blood volume. Since the total compliance of the lung depends on all stuctures in it, as the flexibility of the pulmonary vessels lessens with their congestion, the overall flexibility of the lung will be reduced. Mobility of the lung will be further impaired if the congestion is accompanied by pulmonary edema, with its increased fluid in the pulmonary intercellular spaces, and fluid in the alveoli.

Abdominal causes. Through immobilization of the diaphragm, abdominal pathologic conditions are a frequent cause of pulmonary restriction:

1. Abdominal splinting, a rigid contraction of the musculature of the abdominal wall, is usually an unconscious reaction to pain from intraabdominal disease or postoperative discomfort. Ventilation can be seriously impeded, and the combination of restriction and hypoventilation comprises a common respiratory complication of abdominal disease.
2. Abdominal distention results from excessive accumulation of gas or air

in the stomach or intestinal tract. This may be of such a degree that the abdominal wall is pushed outward into a rounded dome under great tension.

3. Abdominal fluid, referred to as *ascites,* usually the result of liver disease, heart failure, or some pathologic condition causing widespread peritoneal irritation, increases intraabdominal pressure to interfere with diaphragmatic descent.

Effect of restriction on ventilation

Restriction reduces the vital capacity and in severe instances may limit it nearly to the resting tidal volume. In this case, as with distention, there may be little or no inspiratory reserve volume to accommodate the needs of exertion. The FRC may be normal in the absence of associated distention, but despite this, the measured residual volume is often enlarged, since the rigidity of the lung, or the lack of muscular effort, reduces the size of the forced expiratory reserve volume. More often than not, other ventilatory disturbances accompany restriction, especially in patients with chronic bronchopulmonary disease.

Treatment of restriction

Some specific objectives of teatment are obvious, such as the removal of pleural or abdominal fluid, the removal of pleural adhesions, the repair of structural defects of the thorax, and the improvement of circulation. In many patients, however, such corrective causes are absent, and relief of the restrictive agent is not possible. In general, the treatment is that outlined for pulmonary distention. The more specific techniques of maintaining controlled mechanical ventilation of the restricted patient in respiratory failure are discussed separately in Chapter 14.

Ventilation/ perfusion imbalance

A disturbance in the ratio between ventilation and pulmonary perfusion is always secondary to some other disorder and is a condition that may be found with many types of diseases. In addition, this imbalance may also be the result of some of the disturbances already discussed in this chapter, but its clinical effects are so widespread and important that it deserves detailed consideration in any discussion of pathophysiology.

In terms of the body as a whole, with its myriad of individual cellular demands, the total exchange of oxygen for carbon dioxide is called the body *respiratory quotient* (RQ) and is expressed as the ratio of the quantity of carbon dioxide produced to oxygen consumed per unit of time, $\dot{V}CO_2/\dot{V}O_2$. Depending on the net metabolic needs of all parts of the body at a given moment, this ratio ranges from 0.7 to 1, with an average of 0.8. Because of biochemically limiting factors of metabolism, the RQ cannot exceed 1. Thus less carbon dioxide is produced by the body than oxygen is used, and to maintain necessary tissue gas exchange there must be a comparable exchange in the lung between alveoli and blood. For this the tidal flow of air into and out of the alveoli constitutes the pulmonary ventilation, and the pulmonary capillary blood flow, in direct contact with the alveolar walls, provides the perfusion of the lung. The relationship between the ventilation and perfusion is referred to as the *ventilation/perfusion ratio,* or the *respiratory exchange ratio* (R), symbolically designated as $\dot{V}_A/\dot{Q}_C$. It is the ratio between the minute flow of air into the alveoli and the minute flow of blood through the pulmonary capillaries. The R of the whole lung is the same as the RQ averaging 4:5, or 0.8.[20-22] This means that for every 4 ℓ of alveolar ventilation, there are 5 ℓ of pulmonary capillary blood flow.

A normal R in itself, however, is not adequate assurance of effective gas exchange, since it does not tell us how the ventilation and perfusion are distributed throughout the lung. Consider the hypothetical example of all the ventilation going to one lung and all the perfusion to the other. In this situation, although the total amount of ventilation and perfusion may be normal, and R equal to 0.8, gas exchange will be absent and survival impossible. It is important to grasp the concept of a whole host of respiratory exchange ratios scattered throughout the lungs, the so-called regional distribution of Rs. Each lobule of the lung might well have its own ratio, depending on the local balance ventilation and perfusion, but the overall lung R will be the same as the RQ. One can imagine generalized or localized disease or injury modifying both ventilation and perfusion so that the final functional effect on ventilation would depend on which was the more disturbed. Thus, when we attempt to classify the physiologic effects of disease as either ventilatory or circulatory imbalance of the ratio, we must recognize that either or both elements may be at fault.

Low $\dot{V}/\dot{Q}$. A ratio less than the normal body RQ of 0.8 results from a decrease in regional alveolar ventilation, physiologically producing what is known as a *venous admixture.* Through some pathologic process, variable numbers of alveoli are subjected to differing degrees of underventilation. If they remain fully perfused, the blood leaving them will not be normally saturated with oxygen and will be at least partially venous in nature as it combines with the mixed arterial blood leaving areas of normal R. Fig. 8-4 illustrates this mechanism with the complete obstruction of one alveolar unit.

The venous admixture is actually a *physiologic venous-arterial shunt,* although the term *admixture* is preferred in current terminology. It is a shunt because the effect, on mixed arterial oxygenation, of perfused blood denied its normal quota of oxygen is the same as that of blood bypassing the lung physically. It is termed *physiologic* because it is caused by a functional derangement of an organ that may have basically normal structure. We have already discussed how the natural human environment of ambient air at 1 atm pressure produces a small normal venous admixture because the distribution of ventilation throughout the lung is not even, and with any given breath some alveoli are incompletely ventilated. Thus the normal arterial oxygen saturation is about 97%. Fig. 8-5 diagrams the normal physiologic shunt, or venous admixture, showing the shunted blood as if it bypassed the lung.

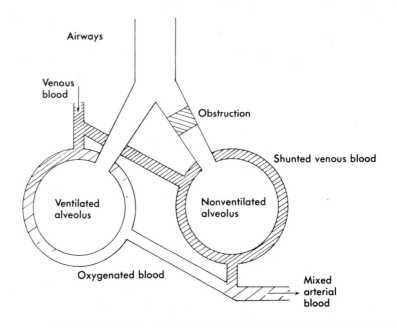

Fig. 8-4 *Venous admixture* is a term given to mixed arterial blood leaving the lung when it contains both fully oxygenated blood from normally ventilated alveoli and incompletely oxygenated "shunted venous blood" from poorly ventilated alveoli. In the sketch, ventilation to one alveolus is normal but is blocked to the other, and capillary shading represents a quantitative index of unsaturation. In the normal subject quietly breathing ambient air at 1 atm pressure, mixed arterial blood is approximately 97% saturated with oxygen.

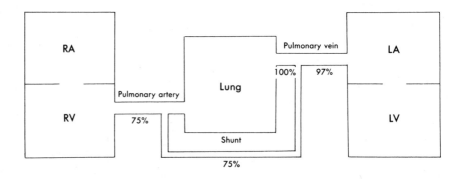

Fig. 8-5 The normal physiologic shunt, or venous admixture, during tidal ventilation of air at 1 atm pressure. Some venous blood is shown, with an oxygen saturation of 75%, as if it bypassed the lung as a result of perfusing scattered, nonventilated alveoli. The mixture of the shunted with the fully oxygenated blood gives arterial blood its usual saturation of about 97%.

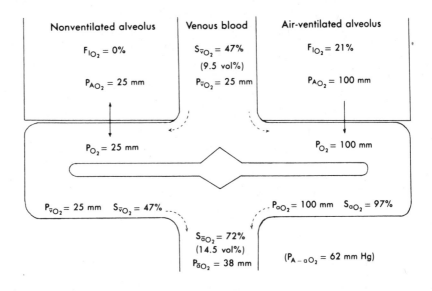

Nonventilated alveolus	Venous blood	Air-ventilated alveolus
$F_{IO_2} = 0\%$	$S_{\bar{v}O_2} = 47\%$	$F_{IO_2} = 21\%$
	(9.5 vol%)	
$P_{AO_2} = 25$ mm	$P_{\bar{v}O_2} = 25$ mm	$P_{AO_2} = 100$ mm

$P_{O_2} = 25$ mm $P_{O_2} = 100$ mm

$P_{\bar{v}O_2} = 25$ mm $S_{\bar{v}O_2} = 47\%$ $P_{aO_2} = 100$ mm $S_{aO_2} = 97\%$

$S_{\bar{a}O_2} = 72\%$
(14.5 vol%)
$P_{\bar{a}O_2} = 38$ mm $(P_{A-aO_2} = 62$ mm Hg)

Fig. 8-6 An alveolus with no ventilation and one with normal air ventilation, each being perfused by one half the venous blood entering the system. The data are based on a hemoglobin content of 15 g/dl and an a-v oxygen difference of 5 vol%. Arterialized blood leaving the ventilated alveolus combines with shunted (venous) blood leaving the nonventilated alveolus, giving the mixed arterial blood a saturation of 72% and a P_{O_2} of 38 mm Hg. There is thus an oxygen tension difference, or gradient, between the alveolar air and the mixed arterial blood of 62 mm Hg. This is called an A-a$_{O2}$ gradient, symbolized as P_{A-aO2}.

Discussing the effect of a venous admixture on blood oxygenation will serve the double purpose of acquainting the student with a useful technique of evaluating cardiopulmonary function and at the same time enabling the student to call upon some of the concepts of physiology that he or she has studied in an unavoidably isolated fashion so they can be put to practical use. Our purpose is to educate the respiratory therapist, not a professional postgraduate student, and although the detailed concepts of ventilation-perfusion relationships often tax the minds of the experienced physiologist, there is no reason why the therapist should not be stimulated to learn as much as possible about the patient he or she will be treating. We use two hypothetical situations, with a graphic illustration of each, to show the clinical effect of a significant venous admixture. In the interest of simplicity, we take some liberties with reality. First, the situations we create will be exaggerated for emphasis, and as shown in Figs. 8-6 and 8-7, the lung in question will consist of only two alveoli, each with its own perfusing capillary. One alveolus will be completely nonventilated and will resemble a closed space; the other will ventilate under differing conditions. Second, in considering blood oxygen content, we concern ourselves only with oxygen combined with hemoglobin, at 15 g/dl, ignoring the dissolved fraction. This facilitates calculation and, because of the minute quantities of dissolved gas at atmosphere, introduces little error. We further assume that as the venous

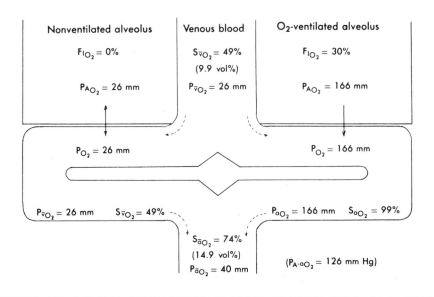

Fig. 8-7   This system is the same as that of Fig. 8-6, except that the functioning alveolus is ventilated with an inspired gas mixture containing 30% oxygen, resulting in a calculated $P_{A_{O_2}}$ of 166 mm Hg, and an A-a_{O_2} gradient of 126 mm Hg. Thus, as long as blood is being shunted, an increase in $F_{I_{O_2}}$ will lead to a disproportionately smaller increase in Pa_{O_2} and a widened A-a_{O_2} gradient.

blood enters our simple systems, its flow divides so that equal volumes perfuse each alveolus, and the arterial blood leaving is thus a mixture of equal parts from each alveolus. Finally, we assume that in each instance the a-v oxygen difference (respresenting oxygen given up to body cells) will remain steady at 5 vol%. To accomplish this, we have calculated values that allow the fully arterialized blood from the ventilated alveolus, when diluted with the shunted blood of the nonventilated alveolus, to have an oxygen content 5 vol% greater than it has when it returns to the lung as venous blood after perfusing body cells. All values are exceedingly lower than the normals to which the student has been exposed, but he or she must observe that these conditions represent what can be called a 50% shunt, in which half the circulating blood is denied oxygenation. Although they are grossly abnormal, there are clinical states that closely match them.

In Fig. 8-6, blood perfusing the air-ventilated alveolus, with its oxygen tension of 100 mm Hg, is fully oxygented and approaches the outflow tract with a P_{O_2} of 100 mm Hg and a saturation of 97%. On the other hand, blood perfusing the nonventilated alveolus picks up no oxygen. In fact, theoretically, there could be a diffusion of oxygen from the venous blood into the closed and oxygen-poor alveolus, maintaining a $P_{A_{O_2}}$ equal to the 25 mm Hg tension of the perfusing blood. This half of the blood volume thus reaches the outflow still as venous blood, with its P_{O_2} of 25 mm Hg and a saturation of 47%, and here the two streams unite and thoroughly mix. The oxygen content of the *mixed* arterial blood depends on the degree of saturation of each of its two components, since saturation is volumetrically related to hemoglobin content. In this instance the final saturation is the average of the values of the two halves, or 72%, and by the normal oxygen dissociation curve this represents a partial pressure of 38 mm Hg. Note that a saturation of 72%, in this very hypoxic arterial blood, is the equivalent of a combined oxygen content of 14.5 vol% (72% of 20.1 = 14.5). On this basis the oxygen content of the venous blood was established as 9.5 vol%, at a partial pressure of 25 mm Hg.

If this were a subject under study and we were to get a sample of exhaled alveolar air to measure its oxygen content, or if we calculated it according to the alveolar air equation, we would find a PA_{O_2} of about 100 mm Hg.* The nonventilating alveolus, of course, contributes nothing to alveolar sampling. The difference between the oxygen tensions in the alveoli and in sampled arterial blood constitutes a gradient, called an *alveolar-arterial oxygen tension gradient,* or more simply an $A\text{-}a_{O_2}$ gradient, symbolized as $PA\text{-}a_{O_2}$. Under normal conditions, with the small physiologic shunt usually present, the A-a gradient does not exceed 10 mm Hg while breathing room air. The gradient in our example is 62 mm Hg (100 − 38). A large gradient usually identifies a state of hypoxia as a result of some cause other than an inadequate alveolar supply of oxygen and generally resolves the diagnosis to a differential between a venous admixture and a diffusion defect. Although we have illustrated the manner in which a gradient can be caused by shunting, a block to diffusion of oxygen across the A-C membrane theoretically could just as well have been responsible. Let us now describe a procedure that will help to differentiate between an $A\text{-}a_{O_2}$ gradient resulting from a shunt and one from a diffusion defect.

Fig. 8-7 represents the same general arrangement as Fig. 8-6, but now the ventilating alveolus carries a 30% oxygen mixture instead of the 21% of air. An a-v oxygen difference of 5 vol% is still assumed for uniformity. With this breathing mixture the alveolar oxygen tension is calculated to be approximately 166 mm Hg, and the perfusing blood leaving the ventilated alveolus equilibrates at this tension. The arterial oxygen saturation corresponding to a partial pressure of 166 mm Hg is difficult to read with accuracy from the flat upper portion of the dissociation curve, but according to a table designed to overcome this problem, it is approximately 99%.[23] Employing the same technique as before in determining the characteristics of the mixed arterial blood leaving the lung, we find a final arterial oxygen saturation of 74% and an oxygen tension of 40mm Hg. If we now compare the alveolar and arterial oxygen partial pressures, we find an $A\text{-}a_{O_2}$ gradient of 126 mm Hg (166 − 40).

These two examples make it evident that as we increase the oxygen concentration in the breathing mixture and as long as some of the blood is consistently bypassing ventilated alveoli, we get a smaller proportionate increase in the oxygen content of the mixed arterial blood. This should be expected, and

*See Appendix 12 for an explanation of the alveolar air equation.

if the student examines the data carefully, he or she will see how the characteristics of the oxygen dissociation curve limit the value of increasing the oxygenation of the ventilated alveolus. We can thereby make the following generalization. If an A-a$_{O_2}$ gradient exists when room air is breathed and it is primarily caused by a shunt, the gradient will widen with increasing concentrations of oxygen in the breathing mixture. This holds true for the normal subject since the negligible gradient will also increase as he or she breathes oxygen-enriched air. Finally, whereas an A-a oxygen gradient is characteristically present with a lowered $\dot{V}/\dot{Q}$, an arterial alveolar PCO_2 gradient or difference is not. The greater diffusibility of carbon dioxide permits its easy escape through ventilated alveoli, aided by the often present hyperventilation accompanying hypoxia.

In contrast to venous admixture, the hypoxia caused by an impairment of oxygen diffusion is generally thought to be overcome by an elevation of the inspired oxygen concentration. With increasing alveolar oxygen partial pressure, enough additional oxygen molecules are diffused into the blood to bring the latter above the hypoxemic level, although at times breathing concentrations close to 100% may be necessary. Because of this, a subject with an A-a oxygen gradient from a diffusion defect will show a reduction in the gradient as an increased oxygen mixture is breathed, since the rise in blood gas tension will be proportionately higher than that of the alveoli (although, of course, the former can never exceed the latter). In both shunt and diffusion defects the hypoxia will worsen with exercise, and gradients will widen as the increased tissue use of oxygen lowers the venous gas content in the shunt and as the increased blood flow of exercise further reduces pulmonary gas exchange time of a diffusion defect.

The technique of subjecting a patient to two breathing mixtures with differing oxygen concentrations (often room air, and 30% to 40% oxygen) and calculating the two A-a gradients is termed a *double-gradient study*. This valuable diagnostic tool, although by no means foolproof, gives a dynamic perspective to cardiopulmonary function hampered by hypoxia. Fig. 8-8 is a nonquantitative sketch showing the double oxygen–gradient characteristics of the normal state, shunt, and diffusion defect. The PA-a$_{O_2}$, breathing air at 1 atm, in a given circumstance can be estimated by a simple equation.[24] With a normal mean PA_{O_2} of approximately 100 mm Hg and a mean PA_{CO_2} of 40 mm Hg, the sum of these two alveolar gases averages about 140 mm Hg. With such alveolar tensions it is believed that in the normal subject the sum of the arterial PO_2 and PCO_2 should be at least 120 mm Hg. We can say, then, that the alveolar-arterial PO_2 difference, if any, should be less than the difference between 140 mm Hg and the sum of the arterial gas tensions. This is expressed as

$$PA\text{-}a_{O_2} = 140 - (Pa_{O_2} + Pa_{CO_2})$$

which tells us that the gradient should not exceed 20 mm Hg and that higher values are abnormal.

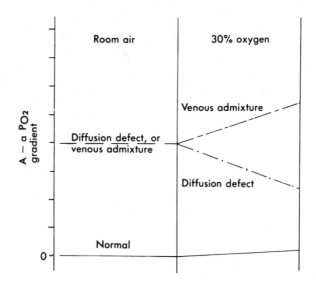

Fig. 8-8   Simplified schematic of differentiation between normal and abnormal *A-a P*o_2 *gradients,* the latter shown in nonspecific arbitrary units, using the double gradient technique. Normal lungs show no significant gradient with *room air* breathing but a slight one with *30% oxygen*. Both *diffusion defects* and *venous admixture* produce gradients with air, but the gradient (*not* the absolute alveolar and arterial tensions) with 30% oxygen decreases with diffusion defects and worsens with shunting.

If desired, a practical working bedside estimate of the A-a$_{O_2}$ gradient can be calculated for any known combination of FI_{O_2}, Pa$_{O_2}$, and Pa$_{CO_2}$. Sacrificing some accuracy in the interest of expediency, if we arbitrarily reduce the constant of 713 mm Hg in the air equation (which represents P$_B$ of 760 mm Hg minus saturated water vapor pressure of 47 mm Hg), to 700 mm Hg, and if the respiratory quotient R in the same equation is taken to be 1, then the difference between PA_{O_2} and Pa$_{O_2}$ will closely equal:

$$700(F_{I_{O_2}}) - (Pa_{CO_2} + Pa_{O_2})$$

We will look at a single-gradient procedure that permits the estimation of the degree of right-to-left shunt. The patient breathes *100% oxygen* for 15 to 20 minutes to ensure equilibration between alveoli and capillaries and to allow maximum washout of alveolar nitrogen. At this point a normal lung will contain but three alveolar gases, carbon dioxide, water vapor, and oxygen. The easy equilibration of carbon dioxide lets us substitute its measured tension in arterial blood for alveolar, and water vapor pressure is a constant. Therefore, theoretically at least, under conditions of perfect alveolar-arterial equilibration, the Pa$_{O_2}$ should equal the difference between atmospheric pressure and the sum of 47 plus arterial carbon dioxide pressure. This can be expressed as:

$$Pa_{O_2} = P_B - (47 + Pa_{CO_2})$$

Using normal values, this translates to a Pa_{O_2} of $760 - (47 + 40) = 673$ mm Hg. If measured arterial Po_2 is less than 673 mm Hg, the inference is made that venous blood is mixing with arterial. For practical purposes it can be assumed that a 5% *shunt* (5 parts venous blood to 95 parts arterial blood) is represented by every *100 mm Hg reduction in Pa_{O_2} below that claculated in the above equation*. Any difference between measured and calculated ideal Pa_{O_2} is included in the rewritten equation

(1) Percent shunt (100% O_2) $= \dfrac{P_B - (47 + Pa_{CO_2} + Pa_{O_2})}{20}$

or, in its usual applied form,

(2) Percent shunt (100% O_2) $= \dfrac{673 - Pa_{O_2}}{20}$

High $\dot{V}/\dot{Q}$. Regional elevations of the respiratory exchange ratio (R), which may reach 3 or more, result from the loss of adequate perfusion of ventilated alveoli; and when capillary flow to alveoli is reduced or absent, reduced or absent gas exchange occurs, even in the presence of normal or increased tidal alveolar airflow. As illustrated in Fig. 4-1, this constitutes *dead space ventilation*.

The basic effects of a highly localized elevated R are illustrated in Fig. 8-9, which shows two normally ventilated alveoli, one *(A)* with normal perfusion and the other *(B)* unperfused because of a block in its perfusing capillary. Because alveolus *B* is not perfused, it receives no carbon dioxide and its Pco_2 is 0. In the absence of carbon dioxide the gas of the alveolus consists of oxygen, nitrogen, and water vapor, and its oxygen partial pressure is approximately 150 mm Hg. With no component from the obstructed capillary, mixed arterial blood from the area has normal tensions of carbon dioxide and oxygen. The gas values of a mixed alveolar sample, however, are the averages of those of each alveolus, with a PA_{CO_2} of 20 mm Hg, and a PA_{O_2} of 125 mm Hg. Because of the perfusion defect, then, there are gas tension gradients present between the alveoli and arterial blood: an A-a oxygen gradient of 25 mm Hg and an a-A carbon dioxide gradient of 20 mm Hg. Again, this example is exaggerated, since one might expect to find a normal carbon dioxide gradient not in excess of 5 mm Hg, and a value of twice this would be considered highly significant. The only specific information that an elevated carbon dioxide gradient provides is to indicate that there is a general increase in pulmonary ventilation over pulmonary perfusion. This is dead space ventilation, but physiologically it means that there is a certain amount of work being invested in ventilation from which there is not a proportionate return in profitable blood gas exchange. The term *wasted ventilation* has been given to this uneconomical state.[21]

Clinically, this concept has a practical diagnostic application. Pulmonary embolism is a relatively common phenomenon and may express itself as a massive obstruction of a large branch of the pulmonary artery or as frequently

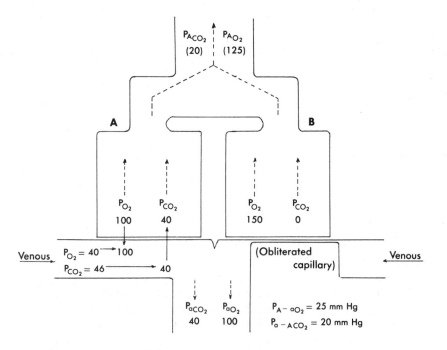

Fig. 8-9 Two normally air-ventilated alveoli are shown, one with full perfusion. **A,** The other without perfusion because of obstruction to (or destruction of) its capillary, **B.** Mixed arterial blood leaving the system has normal gas tensions, but sampled mixed alveolar air is high in oxygen and low in carbon dioxide. This produces an A-a_{O_2} gradient of 25 mm Hg and an a-A_{CO_2} difference of 20 mm Hg. The latter normally does not exceed 5 mm Hg, and higher values indicate ventilation of nonperfused alveoli, or dead space breathing.

recurring blockage of small arteries or arterioles. Within a few hours after the onset of such an episode, evidence of a high $\dot{V}/\dot{Q}$ may be noted. The terminal portion of the patient's tidal air, considered to be alveolar in quality, is analyzed for its carbon dioxide concentration and tension, while a sample of arterial blood is drawn for the same purpose. A significant difference between the carbon dioxide tensions of the two samples, indicating an elevated $\dot{V}/\dot{Q}$, is often helpful in complementing other data to support a diagnosis of embolism, although it obviously is not pathognomonic. The nature of the test has given it the familiar title of an *end-tidal CO$_2$ determination*.

In summary two statements can be made:

1. A low $\dot{V}/\dot{Q}$ produces a venous admixture, with hypoxia and an A-a oxygen tension gradient resulting from a drop in arterial oxygen tension but with little effect on the carbon dioxide.
2. A high $\dot{V}/\dot{Q}$ produces alveolar dead space ventilation, with little hypoxia but with an A-a oxygen gradient caused by an elevation of alveolar oxygen tension and an a-A carbon dioxide pressure difference.

These concepts are to be used to explain *local* events in the lung, not necessarily the lung as a whole. Also, in disease all degrees of both ratio imbalances may be present, with the final state of lung function dependent on the net resulting mixed pathophysiology.

References

1. Cherniack, R.M., Cherniack, L., and Naimark, A.: Respiration in health and disease, ed. 2, Philadelphia, 1972, W.B. Saunders Co.
2. Williams, M.H., Jr.: Clinical applications of cardiopulmonary physiology, New York, 1960, Harper & Row, Publishers, Inc.
3. Hypoxemia vs. hypoxia (editorial), N. Engl. J. Med. **274**:908, 1966.
4. Barcroft, J.: Anoxemia, Lancet **2**:485, 1920.
5. Van Liere, E.J., and Stickney, J.C.: Hypoxia, Chicago, 1963, University of Chicago Press.
6. Campbell, E.J.M.: The management of acute respiratory failure in chronic bronchitis and emphysema, Am. Rev. Respir. Dis. **96**: 626, 1967.
7. Shaw, D.B., and Simpson, T.: Polycythemia in emphysema, Q.J. Med. **30**:135, 1961.
8. Comroe, J.H., Jr.: Physiology of respiration, ed. 2, Chicago, 1974, Year Book Medical Publishers, Inc.
9. Filley, G.F.: Pulmonary insufficiency and respiratory failure, Philadelphia, 1967, Lea & Febiger.
10. Shulman, L.E.: Hypertrophic osteoarthropathy, Bull. Rheum. Dis. **7**:135, 1957.
11. Lipman, B.S., and Massie, E.: Signs and symptoms, Philadelphia, 1957, J.B. Lippincott Co.
12. Field, A.S., Jr., and Gray, F.D., Jr.: The width of the nail fold capillary stream in clubbing, Dis. Chest **41**:631, 1962.
13. Kenney, J. (Carney Hospital, Dorchester, Me.): Personal communication with D.F. Egan.
14. Tappan, V., and Zalar, V.: Pathophysiology of bronchial mucus, Ann. N.Y. Acad. Sci. **106**:722, 1963.
15. Pratt, P.C., and Klugh, G.A.: Chronic expiratory air-flow obstruction—cause or effect of centrilobular emphysema? Dis. Chest **52**:342, 1967.
16. Barach, A.L.: In Petty, T.L., editor: Chronic obstructive pulmonary disease, New York, 1978, Marcel Dekker, Inc.
17. Mueller, R.E., Petty, T.L., and Filley, G.F.: Ventilation and arterial blood gas changes induced by pursed lip breathing, J. Appl. Physiol. **28**:784, 1970.
18. Bouhuys, A.: Lung volumes and breathing patterns in wind instrument players, J. Appl. Physiol. **19**:967, 1964.
19. Colp, C., et al.: Diffuse emphysema as a result of non-obstructive interstitial pulmonary disease, Am. Rev. Respir. Dis. **96**:788, 1967.
20. Gray, F.D., Jr.: Ventilation-perfusion ratios in cardiopulmonary diseases, Conn. Med. **31**:338, 1967.
21. West, J.B.: Ventilation/blood flow and gas exchange, ed. 3, Oxford, England, 1977, Blackwell Scientific Publications.
22. West, J.B.: Pulmonary pathophysiology—the essentials, Baltimore, 1977, The Williams & Wilkins Co.
23. Dittmer, D.S., and Grebe, R.M., editors: Handbook of respiration, Philadelphia, 1958, W.B. Saunders Co.
24. Ayers, L.N.: A guide to the interpretation of pulmonary function tests, New York, 1974, Projects in Health, Inc.

Chapter 9   Elements of a systematic approach to reading the chest x-ray

RICHARD L. SHELDON and **RICHARD D. DUNBAR**

A. Airways	M. Mediastinum
B. Bones	N. Nodules
C. Cor	O. Overaeration
D. Diaphragm	P. Pleura
E. Esophagus	Q. "Quickly examine name plate"
F. Fissures	R. Respiration
G. Gastric bubble	S. Segments
H. Hila	T. Thoracic calcifications
I. Interstitium	U. Under perfusion
J. Junction lines	V. Volume
K. Kerley's lines	W. Women's breast shadows
L. Lobes	X. "X-tra" densities

To write a comprehensive discussion of chest radiology in one chapter is impossible. Whole lifetimes have been spent developing techniques, accumulating experience, and developing a sixth sense that would lead an experienced chest radiologist to identify an abnormal finding on a chest x-ray film. This chapter is not intended to make an expert radiologist of the student, but it is worthwhile for the student to recognize some of the basic areas of normality and abnormality.

All the abnormal chest findings cannot be covered in one brief chapter, so it is our intent to introduce a systematic approach to reading the chest x-ray film that will allow the student to develop a framework on which to hang information and experience while working in the exciting field of respiratory therapy. Before starting our systematic approach, we provide an explanation of the x-ray and how x-ray films are obtained.

X-rays are electromagnetic waves that radiate from a tube through which an electrical current has been passed. The tube is made of a cathode, which is attached to a low-voltage electron source (a transformer). The end of the cathode wire is inside the vacuum-sealed tube, and as the electrons flow through

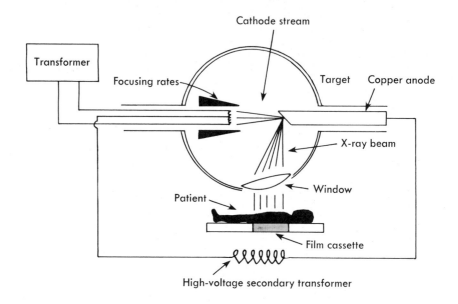

Fig. 9-1 The electrical current is generated by the transformer *(A)*, passes through the focusing plates *(B)*, and arrives at the cathode. The electrons are "boiled off," making a cathode stream *(C)*. They then strike the anode target *(D)* and are transformed into "x-rays" *(E)*. The x-rays leave the sealed vacuum x-ray tube through a window *(F)* and strike the patient *(G)*, pass through the patient, and cast a shadow on the film cassette *(H)* making an "x-ray picture."

the wire they are "boiled off," accelerate across a short gap, and strike a positively charged tungsten plate called the anode. The electrons coming off the cathode wire are focused so they hit a very small area on the anode. This area is called the "target" (Fig. 9-1).

On striking the target, physical changes occur, which result in the emission of "x"-rays. These x-rays are emitted in all directions, but because of the construction of the tube, only a few are allowed to escape through the window and are actually used. The rest are absorbed harmlessly into the wall of the x-ray machine.

X-rays are not reflected back like light rays but penetrate matter, and their ability to penetrate matter is dependent on the density of that matter. Very dense objects like bone will absorb (not allow penetration) more x-rays than air-filled objects like lung tissue. The four main objects shown in chest x-ray film are bone, air, soft tissue, and fat.

If a sheet of film is placed on the side of the patient opposite to where the x-ray tube is located, the x-rays passing through the patient will be absorbed by some objects and "cast a shadow" on the film. X-rays that pass through the low-density objects (air-filled), strike the film full force and turn it black. X-rays that strike bone are partially absorbed, and less darkening of the corresponding area on the x-ray film is seen. This area is relatively unchanged and is seen as white on the film.

The standard chest x-ray film is taken in two directions. First, with the patient standing upright with his or her back to the x-ray tube, the chest is pressed against a metal cassette containing the film, and the arms are positioned out of the way. The x-ray beam leaves the tube and first strikes the patient's back (posterior), moves through the chest, exits through the front (anterior), and then strikes the film. Since the beam moves posterior to anterior this is called a *P-A* view.

The patient is then turned sideways, and a *lateral* or side view is obtained. Thus two films are routinely taken, a P-A and lateral.

Other views are sometimes obtained when special problems are identified. If the patient is in an intensive care unit and cannot be moved, the film is placed in the bed, behind the patient's back, and the x-ray tube positioned in front. Since the x-rays are moving anterior to posterior, this is called an *A-P portable*. *Obliques* are done, left and right lateral decubitus, with the patient lying on the right or left side in order to see if free fluid (pleural effusion or blood) is present in the chest. Also, an *apical lordotic* is sometimes requested in order to look at the right middle lobe or the top (apical region) of the lung.

If an area of the lung consolidates because of pneumonia, tumor, obstruction, or collapse, it will show as a white patch on the film. Cavities will look like black holes. Diffuse patterns (interstitial markings) will be a fine, lacelike pattern in the lung tissue.

Some densities that appear on the film are normal, such as the heart and the lymph nodes. When they become abnormal they change shape, and by developing a clear understanding of what normal looks like, one can make an accurate diagnosis of the disease process by how the shape of the structure is altered.

One of the most important jobs the x-ray technician has is to make sure the patient is not rotated or turned. A very slight amount of rotation will so distort normal structures that they will start to appear falsely abnormal.

Now we take a step-by-step approach to chest x-ray films, thus forcing the student to concentrate on certain areas of the film rather than letting his or her eye scan it in a random manner. Many of the findings on chest x-ray films are subtle and require the ability to collect many pieces of information that may suggest where the abnormality can be found. Even though the student may be unable to identify what the abnormality is, attention can be directed to the fact that something is wrong with the film, and more expert help can be sought in delineating the precise nature of this problem.

We introduce here a systematic approach using the alphabet to make the student concentrate on specific areas of the film as suggested by the subsequent letters of the alphabet. This will make for a thorough inspection of the film.

NOTE: Throughout, the terms "right" or "left" always refer to the *patient's* right or left.

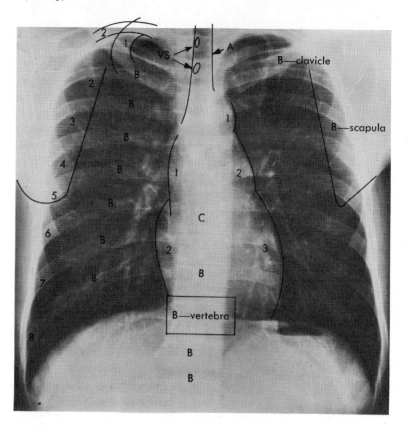

Fig. 9-2   *A,* Airways. Do the vertebral spinous processes seen end on *(VS)* go down the middle of the air column? In this case they do not. This patient is rotated slightly. *B,* Bones. Ribs numbered 1 through 8 on the right side where they swing anteriorly. Clavicles, scapula, and vertebrae are in the *B* category also. *C,* Cor. Cardiac shadow: *(right side) 1,* superior vena cava, *2,* right atrium; *(left side) 1,* aortic arch, *2,* pulmonary artery segment, *3,* left ventricle.

A. Airways (Figs. 9-2, 9-4 and 9-10)

Is the trachea midline? Do the vertebral spines go right through the middle of the tracheal air column? If not, the film has been rotated or the trachea may have been deviated to one side or the other because of fibrosis drawing it to one side, loss of volume in one lung drawing it to one side, or hyperinflation on one side forcing it to the opposite side.

Is the trachea the same width as the vertebral column? If not, tracheobronchomegaly, known as Mounier-Kuhn syndrome, may be present. This is a very rare disorder. Is the trachea buckling to the side opposite the aortic arch? This is a very common, normal finding. Are the larger bronchi, especially just distal to the main carina or at the openings to the lobes, tapering? This may suggest the presence of a bronchogenic carcinoma invading carinal lymph nodes, which in turn are compressing the main bronchi.

B. Bones
(Figs. 9-2 and
9-5)

The ribs should be equal distance apart. If the space between ribs is narrowed on one side more than on the other, this may suggest loss of muscle tone such as in a patient who has a paralysis involving that side of the chest. Notching of the ribs can be a significant finding that should be carefully examined. Notching of the superior aspect of the first rib bilaterally is suggestive of scleroderma or rheumatoid arthritis (Fig. 9-15). Inferior notching of the third through the ninth ribs suggests coarctation (narrowing) of the aorta.* Tetralogy of Fallot* may cause inferior rib notching on the left side only. The ribs can be inspected for cough fractures, which may be seen on the sixth through the ninth rib, usually the seventh in the posterior axillary line. Rib anomalies such as bifid ribs can be seen. These usually have no clinical significance. Pectus carinatum (pigeon breast) is associated with congenital atrial and ventricular septal defects or asthma from early childhood. The spine should also be inspected for such things as kyphoscoliosis, which, if severe enough, will result in loss of pulmonary volume and subsequently hypoventilation. Demineralization of the bones (washed out bones on the x-ray film) may be seen with steroid therapy, aging, renal disease, or other metabolic diseases.

C. Cor
(Figs. 9-2, 9-7,
9-9, 9-10, and
9-12)

The right heart border is composed of two bulges that should always be seen. If they are obliterated, it may represent pectus excavatum, as suggested in the previous section. The bulges will be blurred or absent in the presence of right middle lobe collapse, pneumothorax (Fig. 9-12), or pneumonia involving the portion of the lung that comes in contact with the heart. Loss of superior bulge may be seen with an abnormal aortic arch.

The left heart border is composed of three bulges, the most superior being the aorta, followed by the main pulmonary artery segment, and then the most inferior of the three, the left ventricle. Pneumonias located next to these bulges will obliterate the edges of the bulge; this can be helpful in identifying the presence of pneumonia. There are multiple congenital cardiac lesions that will be present as abnormal cardiac shapes, and they will not be dealt with in this chapter.

If the width of the heart is greater than one-half the distance across the lungs at the level of the diaphragms on the P-A projection, the cardiothoracic (C/T) ratio is increased, and the heart is considered enlarged, usually from congestive heart failure. Other heart problems can also cause the heart to enlarge.

*Congenital heart defects found in children.

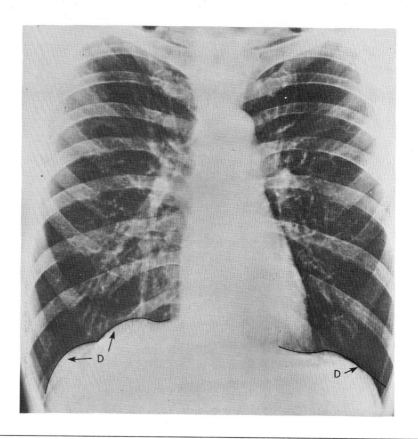

Fig. 9-3   *D,* Diaphragm. This example shows scalloping on the right, with the right side higher than the left. This is normal.

D. Diaphragm
(Figs. 9-3, 9-8,
9-11, and 9-15)

The right diaphragm is usually about one-half a rib interspace higher than the left. *Scalloping* can appear on the right side. This occurs in approximately 5% of all cases and is of no clinical significance (Fig. 9-3). One diaphragm may be elevated above the normal limits, in which case the following should be thought of: thoracic tumor with resultant paralysis of the phrenic nerve (Fig. 9-8); or old surgery to the chest, which will result in fibrosis; scarring of the pleura and subsequent entrapment of the diaphragm and elevation. Subphrenic abscess will usually result in the posterior portion of the right diaphragm being elevated. This can best be identified from a lateral view. Some rare causes of hemidiaphragm elevation include trauma (Erb's paralysis), stroke, tumor or infection in the neck or cervical spine, pneumonia, and radiation therapy.

An interesting anomaly of the diaphragm is the accessory diaphragm, usually on the right and associated with scimitar syndrome.* The accessory diaphragm is usually oriented upward and backward to the posterior wall and has a lower lobe between it and the true diaphragm.

*A congenital cardiac defect composed of both heart and lung malformations.

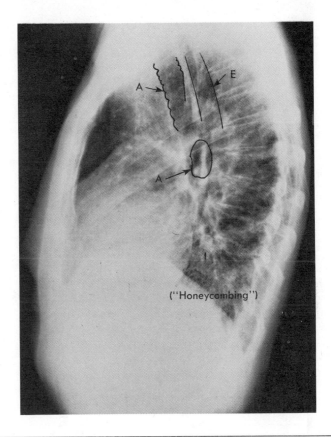

("Honeycombing")

Fig. 9-4 *A,* Airway. This is the lateral view of the trachea and the right and left main stem bronchi. *E,* Esophagus. Its proper position is behind the trachea. The vertical lines seen in this area are the scapulae on end. *I,* Interstitial markings are increased with a big esophagus. The increased markings are due in this case to scleroderma. Note the "honeycombed" appearance of the lung markings.

E. Esophagus (Fig. 9-4)   The esophagus will be located behind the trachea. An air fluid level would suggest certain diseases such as achalasia or stricture.

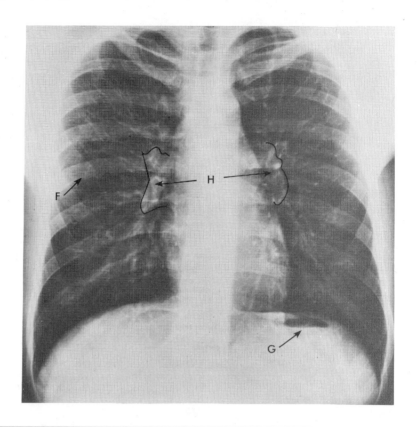

Fig. 9-5 *F,* The horizontal fissure line or "short" fissure is shown on the right. *G,* Gastric bubble. Note the thickness of the left diaphragm above it. This is normal. *H,* Hila. The left hilum is higher than the right. This is the proper relationship.

F. Fissures
(Figs. 9-5, 9-6,
9-8, and 9-9)

The fissure lines divide the lung into various lobes. The two long (major) fissures or the oblique fissures (one each for the right and left lungs) are best seen on the lateral view x-ray film. The inferior end of these fissures never runs into the anterior chest wall but ends in the diaphragm. Sometimes it is important to know which fissure is for the right lung and which is for the left. They usually run with the sixth rib, and on the lateral view the right fissure ends in the higher of the two diaphragms. The left fissure can be identified as the one that ends in the diaphragm that has a stomach bubble under it. If the stomach bubble is not well seen, this may cause some confusion. The heart will usually obliterate the anterior part of the left diaphragm.

The short fissure, also called the minor or horizontal fissure, is seen on the right. It is absent in approximately 20% of normal chest x-ray films. Approximately one half of the normal films show a short fissure, and it is rarely seen projecting all the way across the right lung (Figs. 9-5 and 9-6).

The azygos lobe (Fig. 9-11) is visible in about four tenths of 1% of normal chests. This fissure is very distinctive in its appearance. It is almost always seen on the right, but left azygos lobes caused by an accessory hemiazygos vein have been identified. The azygos lobe is evidence of a pleural reflection from the azygos vein, which has descended during the embryologic period into its proper resting position, bringing with it a piece of pleura that remains radiographically evident. It looks like an upside-down comma.

There is also a superior accessory lobe, which is found in about 5% of the normal films and is seen below the horizontal fissure on the right. It separates the superior segment of the right lower lobe from the rest of the lobe. Inferior accessory lobes also occur in about 5% of normal films, and it separates the medial basilar segment of the right lower lobe from the rest of the right lower lobe. It therefore runs obliquely from the right heart border. The left minor fissure occurs rarely and represents a separate minor fissure.

G. Gastric bubble (Fig. 9-5)

It is important to make sure that the gastric bubble, if present, is seen on the left. If it is found on the right, mislabeling of the chest x-ray film should be suspected, or the patient may have situs inversus. If the gastric bubble is absent, the possibility of achalasia should be considered. A bubble behind the heart could indicate the presence of a hiatal hernia. The top of the gastric bubble should be no more than 2 cm from the top of the dome of the diaphragm.

H. Hila (Figs. 9-5 and 9-6)

The displacement of this part of the chest anatomy constitutes the most important indirect sign of collapse of part of the lung. Ninety-seven percent of left hila are higher than right hila. The right is never higher than the left. The left should not be over 3 cm higher than the right. If any of these rules are violated, then the hilum is out of its proper position. This results from either hyperinflation of the lung on one side of the hilum pushing it in the opposite direction or collapse of an area of lung, which would pull the hilum in the direction of the collapse.

Enlargement of the hilar area is also an important finding. The hilar area can enlarge because of spreading cancer, infection somewhere in the lung, immunologic diseases, or sarcoid, to name a few. Enlarging left hila are hard to see; it is not as difficult to observe right hilar enlargement.

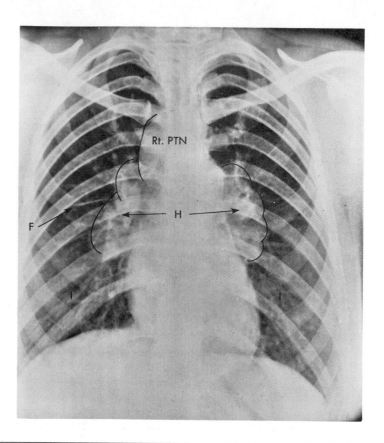

Fig. 9-6   *F,* Another example of a short fissure line. This horizontal fissure is a little thickened. *H,* Enlarged hila bilaterally and right paratracheal nodes *(Rt. PTN)* consistent with sarcoid. *I,* Note the diffuse, multidirectional lines in the lower portion of the lung. These lines are interstitial markings, and they are increased, consistent with interstitial disease. Sarcoidosis causes interstitial infiltrates and is the cause for the finding of hilar node enlargement and interstitial infiltrate in this patient.

I. Interstitium
(Figs. 9-6, 9-8,
9-9, and 9-15)

Interstitial infiltrates are separated classically into alveolar and interstitial patterns. If there is an interstitial infiltrate, its presence can be confirmed by looking at the anterior air space, the area behind the sternum and in front of the heart. This is best seen on the lateral film. If an interstitial infiltrate is seen in the lateral view in the anterior air space, this is good evidence that in fact the patient does have a true interstitial infiltrate. Breast shadows overlying the lower portions of the lung will accentuate normal lung findings, and the student should not be trapped into thinking that there is an abnormal interstitial pattern in female patients.

The alveolar pattern is caused by filling of the alveolus with water or near water density material such as pus, blood, or edema fluid. In the case of near drowning or congestive heart failure, the alveolar space fills up with water. With Goodpasture's disease or idiopathic pulmonary hemosiderosis, these spaces fill up with blood. In the case of pulmonary alveolar proteinosis, these spaces fill up with a proteinlike material. In the case of disquamative interstitial pneumonitis, these spaces fill up with cells. Sometimes this differential diagnosis can be narrowed if one has an idea of the type of material that the patient is coughing up.

J. Junction lines

Junction lines are vertical lines in the mediastinum seen only on the P-A projection. They include the right paraspinal line, left paraspinal line, right paraaortic line, left paraaortic line, posterior junctional line, anterior junctional line, right paratracheal line, and left paracardial line. These lines may be difficult to find, but if they are outlined or seen to bulge, this suggests a mass lesion displacing them.

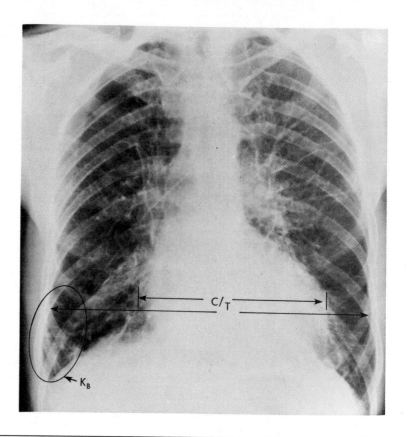

Fig. 9-7 K_B, Kerley B lines seen in their most common position. Note that the cardiothoracic ratio, which normally should be one half, is increased. This chest film is an excellent example of cardiogenic pulmonary edema.

K. Kerley's lines (Fig. 9-7)

Initially the Kerley B line was all that was observed, but now Kerley A and Kerley C lines have also been described. The Kerley B line is 1 mm thick and approximately 1 to 2 cm long and is found in the periphery of the lung, usually on the right at the base. It is a short, straight, horizontal line originating from the pleural surface. This is evidence of congestive heart failure. Kerley A lines are 1 mm thick and 2 to 4 cm long within the lung midway between the hila and pleura, oriented in many directions. The actual length of the Kerley C lines is controversial, but they have been reported to be associated with engorgement of the pleural lymphatics. These lines look like an interstitial infiltrate, mentioned previously under Interstitium. They have been called "everywhere lines."

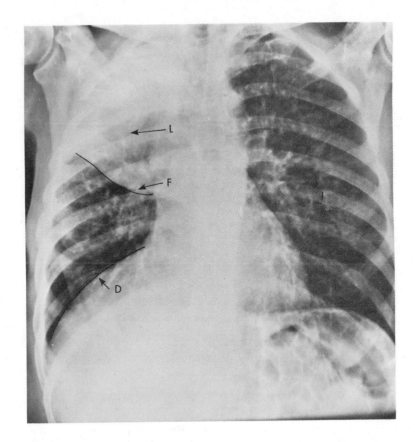

Fig. 9-8   *D,* The diaphragm is markedly elevated. Is the right phrenic nerve paralyzed? *F,* Fissure line. This horizontal fissure drifted up and is bulging. *L,* Lobe. This right upper lobe was full of tumor, which had blocked the bronchus. This resulted in collapse of the lobe. Forceful growth against the fissure line make it bulge, and growth of the tumor into the phrenic nerve caused paralysis of the right diaphragm. *I,* Interstitial marking. Another example of interstitial lines.

L. Lobes
(Fig. 9-8)

Collapse of a lobe is the result of obstruction of a bronchus either from an intrinsic mass, narrowing from tuberculosis, traumatic fracture of the bronchus, extrinsic pressure from the lymph nodes or cardiac enlargement, or mucous plugging. There are certain tumors that have been known to metastasize to the large bronchi and result in collapse. These include tumor from kidney, breast, and skin.

Cardiac enlargment as a result of certain disease states has been reported to be associated with obstruction. The left lower lobe bronchus can be compressed by a very large left atrium or left pulmonary artery.

Right middle lobe syndrome is a distinct clinical entity resulting from collapse of the right middle lobe. It is sometimes seen in persons with asthma and other allergic disorders. The signs of collapse of a lobe include displaced fis-

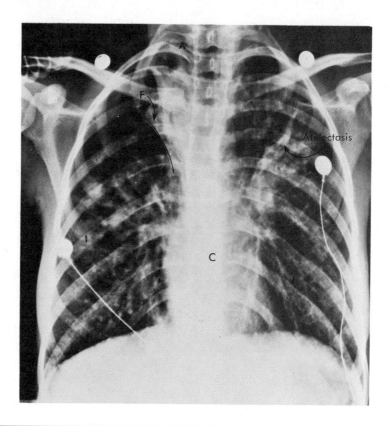

Fig. 9-9 *A,* Because of right upper lobe collapse the trachea is shifted to the right of the vertebral spines. *C,* The cardiac border on the left has been lost because of collapse of the lung on the left and because of several areas of atelectasis. *F,* The horizontal fissure line has been moved up and medially to the right. *I,* Interstitial markings are well seen. Several areas on the right upper-to-mid lung fields appear to be an alveolar infiltrate.

sure lines, loss of aeration, elevation of the diaphragm on the involved side, deviation of the trachea to the involved side, shifting of the heart to the right, narrowing of the trachea to the right, narrowing of the rib cage, compensatory overaeration, or hilar displacement.

It is helpful to know where each lobe goes when it collapses and how to find it. The right upper lobe is demonstrated by the horizontal fissure swinging up (Fig. 9-8) and with complete collapse swinging up to the right paratracheal mediastinum (Fig. 9-9). This is best seen on a P-A view. The left upper lobe moves anteriorly, and on P-A projection there is no sharp border to delineate the collapse. It is therefore best to see this form of collapse on a lateral film. The aortic knob can be obliterated.

The right middle lobe is seen best with a lateral or an apical lordotic view. On P-A projection the right heart border is obliterated when the right middle lobe collapses.

With collapse of the lingula, the left heart border is lost on the P-A projection, with displacement of the lower half of the left major fissure. This displacement is usually forward. The collapse of the right lower lobe results in downward posterior and medial displacement of the lung toward the spine. The right heart border is usually seen well. This collapse is best seen on P-A projection. The left lower lobe has the same direction of collapse as with the right lower lobe. The left heart border is seen well, but the "ivory heart" sign, as described by Dr. B. Felson,[1] may be seen. This constitutes loss of lung markings seen through the heart and results in a pure white heart shadow with no lung markings seen through it. This is best seen on the P-A projection.

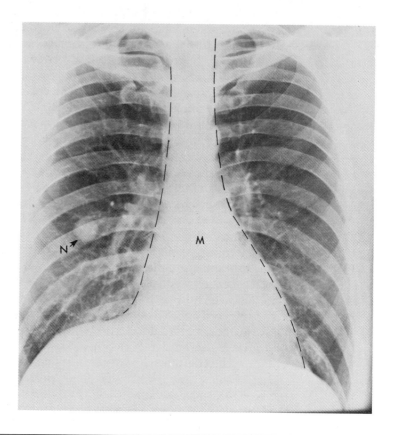

Fig. 9-10   *M,* Mediastinum is outlined with broken lines. *N,* Nodule with an area of calcium deposited in it—small white dot within the nodule at the 3 to 4 o'clock position. This means the nodule is benign; in this case it is a coccidiodomycosis scar.

**M. Mediastinum
(Fig. 9-10)**

The mediastinum is the part of the chest that is found between both lungs. It contains the heart, the great vessels, several very important nerves such as the vagus nerve and phrenic nerve (the nerve that controls the diaphragm), hilar nodes, and other soft tissue such as fat pads. It is classically described as having an anterior compartment, middle compartment, and posterior compartment. Several organs come to rest in each of these compartments, and enlargements or mass lesions found in these compartments give a clue as to the diagnosis of the disease entity.

Sometimes air gets into the mediastinum, which is called a *pneumomediastinum*. It can best be seen on the lateral view, but the subtle findings of a small line around the heart in the P-A view can be a tip-off that a pneumomediastinum has occurred.

N. Nodules
(Fig. 9-10)

Nodules can be of two types: benign, not indicating a serious clinical problem, or malignant, which is a much more serious diagnosis and prognosis. Nodules that are less than 1 cm are usually benign. Regardless of its size, a lesion that has calcium in it is most likely benign. If the nodule is 1 to 6 cm, it may well be malignant. Nodules in the 1 to 6 cm size are described as solitary coin lesions if they have clear areas of normal lung surrounding them.

If old films are available, whether or not a nodule is growing should be determined. Malignancy is highly likely if the lesion is enlarging. However, nonmalignant lesions can slowly enlarge, such as old scars from histoplasmosis.

Sometimes nodules can cavitate so that they have hollow centers. This occurs with squamous cell carcinomas. It also occurs with tuberculosis, coccidiomycosis, and Wegner's granulomatosis. Sometimes these cavities will become the home of a colony of fungus. The fungus will form itself into a ball and actually be able to roll around inside the cavity. This should suggest a method to diagnose fungous balls. If the patient is made to lie on his or her side, and a lateral decubitus film shows the density inside the cavity moving to a more dependent position because of gravity, the diagnosis is confirmed.

If possible, comparison should be made with old films to determine if the nodule is growing

O. Overaeration

A finding of overaeration on a chest x-ray film can be extremely subtle. The film should be checked for an area indicating more air in a part of the lung exceeding the aeration on the matching part of the opposite lung. This will be viewed as a much darker area on the film since air does not stop x-rays. Usually this will not have any distinct borders, so it will be a diffuse area of overaeration. It can be either an obstructed or nonobstructed area of the lung. Nonobstructed areas of overaeration usually suggest emphysematous blebs or bullae. Emphysema will present with overaeration.

The obstructive form of overaeration is usually secondary to an inhaled foreign body or tumor. Another cause of overaeration is a pneumatocele, an area of lung destruction following a staphylococcal pneumonia. It usually has a distinct border caused by a very thin wisp of tissue surrounding the area of overaeration. Another important clinical cause of overaeration is a tension pneumothorax. This occurs when rupture of the lung forces air into the pleural space, causing the lung to collapse. This will present with overaeration throughout the entire side of the involved lung.

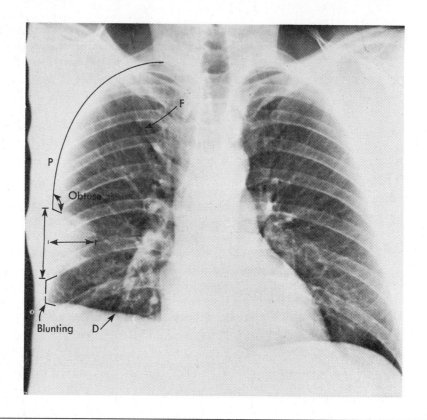

Fig. 9-11   *D,* Right diaphragm abnormally shaped. *F,* Fissured line showing an azygos lobe. Note the typical white, almost almond shape at the end of this fissure line. This is where the azygos vein came to rest. This is a normal, but uncommon, finding. *P,* Pleura with a typical pleural-based lesion showing an obtuse angle with the chest wall and vertical dimensions greater than horizontal. If it were reversed (acute angle with the chest wall and horizontal dimensions greater than vertical), then the lesion would be originating from lung tissue.

P. Pleura
(Figs. 9-11 and 9-12)

The student should run his or her eye all around the lung looking for thickening of the pleura, mass lesions, loss of markings in the lung sitting right next to the pleura, or blunting of the costophrenic (CP) angle. The CP angle is at the very bottom of the lung, where the diaphragm and chest wall meet. If there is any blunting of the sharp angle, formed by the diaphragm and lateral portion of the chest wall, this suggests the presence of fluid, called pleural effusion.

The thickening of the pleura at the apex of the lung field is caused by old tuberculosis in about half of the patients. There is no cause found for the thickening in the other half.

Very rare phrenic tumors called mesotheliomas are usually located along the lateral edge of the lung field.

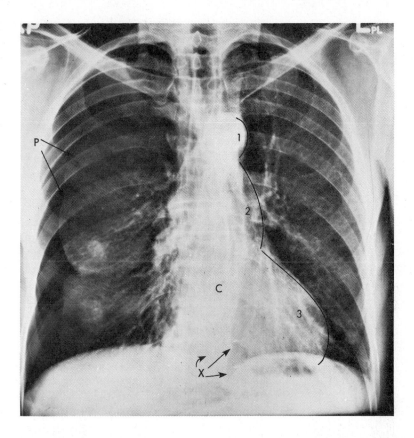

Fig. 9-12   *C,* Cardiac shadow shows the three bulges on the left, and bulge *1* and *2* are absent on the right. *P,* Pleural surface is displaced away from the chest wall, in this case because of a large pneumothorax. With the lung collapsing away from the chest wall, the right heart border has been obliterated. *X,* "X-tra" densities: surgical clips used to stop bleeding during surgery.

It should be determined whether the mass seen on the lung-pleural junction is actually arising from pleural tissue or whether it is arising from the lung itself. This will make a difference in treatment and clinical course depending on whether this lesion comes from the lung or from the pleura. There are two good rules of thumb to help. Pleural-based lesions tend to form an obtuse angle with the chest wall. In contrast a tumor originating from the lung forms an acute angle. Another important differentiation is that if the vertical dimension of the lesion is greater than the horizontal dimension, then the lesion is pleural based. If the opposite is true (Figs. 9-11 and 9-12), then the lesion is based in the lung.

If a pneumothorax occurs (Fig. 9-12), the pleural edges will become visible by looking through and between the ribs to see where the lung markings have pulled away from the chest wall. A thin line will be present just parallel to the chest wall. This can be easily missed if not carefully looked for.

Pleural effusions have some specific findings on chest x-ray films. One that has been mentioned is blunting of the CP angle (Fig. 9-11). However, one form of pleural effusion is called the subpulmonic effusion. This type of effusion will spare the CP angle because the fluid is tucked under the lung and is not free to migrate down to the most dependent corner that makes up the CP angle. If this does occur, the diaphragm will tend to be flattened and go straight out laterally toward the chest wall, almost reaching it, then sharply drop off into the CP angle.

Q. "Quickly examine name plate"	Since there does not seem to be a good Q relationship to chest x-ray film, this would be an excellent time for the student to quickly look at the name plate on the chest x-ray film and make sure that this film in fact belongs to the patient with whom the student is concerned.
R. Respiration	Respiration has effects on the chest film. The lung makes obvious shifts with inspiration and expiration. A great deal can be determined about the nerve supply to the diaphragm via the phrenic nerve by the *sniff test,* a form of rapid respiration. In addition, the heart size has been described as changing with respiration. Whether this actually happens is under some debate.
	If the chest x-ray film has been taken properly and inspiration has been deep enough, the diaphragm will have descended to the bottom of the sixth rib anteriorly or the tenth rib posteriorly. Anything less than that will misrepresent some of the markings that are used to evaluate the film.
	Inspiration or expiration films are taken to accentuate and clearly define the presence of a small pneumothorax.
S. Segments (Fig. 9-13)	It is sometimes important to find out which segment is involved with an infiltrative process. This requires understanding of the anatomy of the segments and which structures sit next to them. The *silhouette sign* as described by Dr. B. Felson[1] has been a very helpful technique used for identifying which segments are involved. The silhouette sign depends on the fact that an infiltrate will obscure the demarcating line of the structure it sits next to. We show some examples of this as we go through this section.
	There are ten segments on the right and eight on the left. Fig. 9-13 demonstrates where each of these areas can be found.

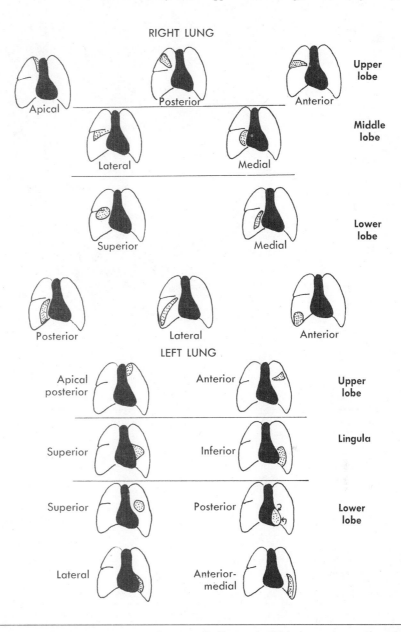

Fig. 9-13   The *dotted areas* show the approximate location of infiltrates should they occur in segments of the lung. Ten areas are shown for the right lung corresponding to the ten segments in the right, and eight areas are shown for the eight segments of the left lung.

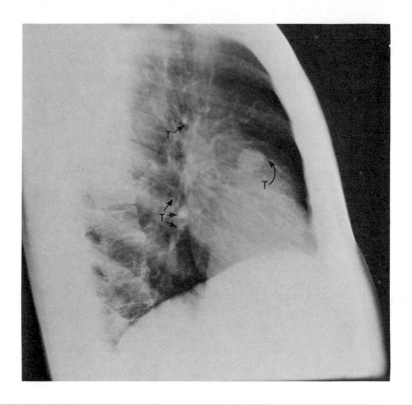

Fig. 9-14   *T*, Thoracic calcifications here represent old scars secondary to histoplasmosis.

T. Thoracic calcifications
(Figs. 9-14 and 9-16)

Areas of calcification within the lung are frequent and represent benign lesions the majority of the time. However, there are a few that need to be identified and discussed. *Eggshell* calcifications have been described to occur in the hilar lymph nodes in patients who have silicosis, sarcoidosis, and other granulomatous diseases. Calcifications of the pulmonary artery, much like the calcifications seen in the aorta, can imply severe pulmonary hypertension. The most common cause of calcifications seen in the lung are healed infections caused by histoplasmosis, coccidiomycosis, or tuberculosis. Also described are calcifications seen in patients who have had chickenpox, pneumonia, and paragonimiasis, a parasitic worm that will take up residence in the lung. Paragonimiasis is more commonly seen in patients who live in Asia.

The pneumoconioses, that is, silicosis, asbestosis, etc., present with calcifications not only within the lung and the hilar lymph nodes as noted above, but also with calcifications of the pleura.

A very rare, but interesting, lung disease has been called alveolar microlithiasis, a familial disease that presents with calcium phosphate deposits in the lung. With this disease the lung appears like a snowstorm because of the myriads of calcifications within the alveolar sacs and ducts. An interesting pleural sign has been described in this disease. It is called the "negative" pleural sign. It is a dark line running all the way around the outer border of both lungs. Lung tissue has been whited out because of the calcium phosphate deposits. The pleura, which does not absorb any of the calcium, appears as a very thin, dark line around the lung making the chest x-ray film look as though it were a negative from a photograph.

U. Under perfusion

Under perfusion involves loss of blood vessels in a portion of the lung. When this occurs in association with pulmonary embolism it is known as *Westermark's sign*. This is a very subtle finding and sometimes very difficult to spot. It is the loss of vessel markings past where a pulmonary embolism has impacted. This same finding can be associated with the malpositioning of a Swan-Ganz catheter so that the catheter itself becomes an embolic device and blocks the flow of blood from the tip on out.

Another important disease is MacLeod and Swyer-James syndrome. This is associated with loss of small peripheral vessels. There is no overinflation, and a normal to small hilum is associated with the syndrome. It is secondary to acute bronchopneumonia in infancy and may look like unilateral pulmonary agenesis.

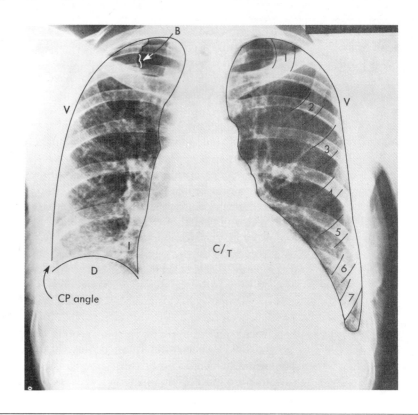

Fig. 9-15   *B,* Bone. The ribs on the left side are down by seven ribs anteriorly, so this is a good inspiration as far as the left side is concerned. The right side does not show as good an inspiration. Note the notching on the first rib on the right. *I,* Interstitial marking at both lung bases in this female patient show more "honeycombing." *V,* Volume. The right lung should be larger than the left. In this case the opposite is true and is therefore abnormal. *D,* Diaphragm. Why is the right diaphragm too high and the CP angle laterally is obsured? This is probably because of a pleural effusion. The *C/T* ratio is increased. The heart is therefore too large.

V. Volume
(Fig. 9-15)

In evaluating the lung volume it is important to know that the right lung represents 55% of the total of both lungs and therefore should appear larger than the left lung. A problem is suggested in a lung that disrupts this relationship.

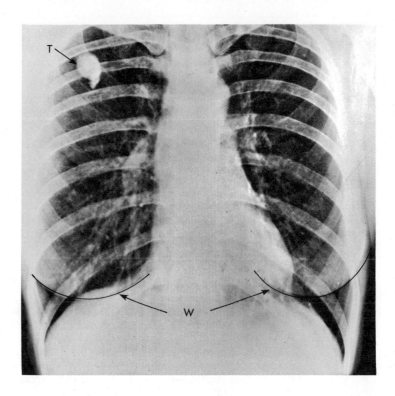

Fig. 9-16   *T,* Thoracic calcifications on this example are a result of old tuberculosis. *W,* Women's breast shadows. Note how the breast shadows accentuate the underlying tissue, making it appear as though there is an interstitial disease process present. As the lung tissue moves out beyond the breast shadow the increased interstitial pattern disappears.

W. Women's breast shadows (Fig. 9-16)

The difference in women's and men's anatomy must be taken into account in reading chest x-ray film. Women's breast shadows overlie the lower lung fields and will accentuate the lung markings behind them. This makes for an impression of increased interstial markings—a false impression. Absence of a breast shadow will make the chest film appear to be "overaerated" on the side where the breast is absent. It is a sign that the patient has undergone surgery to remove a breast, usually secondary to cancer.

Also, the nipples will appear as small coin lesions on chest x-ray films of women. Special techniques are used such as x-ray dense markers attached to the patient's nipples. The film is then retaken, and the film with the nipple markers is compared with the previous x-ray film to see if these "coin lesions" correspond to the area in question.

X. "X-tra" densities (Fig. 9-12)

"X-tra" densities, such as bullets, other foreign bodies within the chest well, and radioopaque dyes, can sometimes be seen. In Fig. 9-12, surgical clips used in a previous surgery to obtain control of bleeding can be observed.

• • •

Unfortunately there is no good way to finish this tour using Y and Z as a guide. If students remember the first 24 areas to examine specifically, they will have started down the long road leading to understanding and evaluating chest x-ray film.

Reference

1. Felson, B.: Chest roentgenology, Philadelphia, 1973, W.B. Saunders Co.

Bibliography

Felson, B., Weinstein, A.S., and Spitz, H.B.: Principles of chest roentgenology: a programmed text, Philadelphia, 1965, W.B. Saunders Co.

Fraser, R.G., and Pare, J.A.P.: Diagnosis of diseases of the chest, ed. 2, Philadelphia, vols. I to IV, 1977-1979, W.B. Saunders Co.

Lillington, G.A.: In Burton, G.G., Gee, G.N., and Hodgkin, J.E., editors: Respiratory care, Philadelphia, 1977, J.B. Lippincott Co.

Lillington, G.A., and Jamplis, R.W.: A diagnostic approach to chest diseases, ed. 2, Baltimore, 1976, The Williams & Wilkins Co.

Chapter 10   Humidity and aerosol therapy

We introduce the subjects involved in clinical respiratory therapy with a discussion of humidity and aerosols. This pairing was deliberately chosen because the use of water and drugs in the treatment of bronchopulmonary disease requires an understanding of the principles of water vapor and aerosols. From this point on in the text, our attention is directed primarily toward the patient's needs and how they are best served. During these forthcoming discussions we lean heavily on the physical and chemical fundamentals covered in the previous chapters.

In recent years the efficacy of certain respiratory therapy treatment modalities has been immersed in controversy. Certainly many of these modalities have been developed empirically.[1,2] Two conferences have been held to discuss the scientific basis for respiratory therapy; one concerned outpatients with stable chronic obstructive pulmonary disease,[1] and the other concerned inhospital patients of various types receiving respiratory therapy.[2] Both conferences found certain aspects of aerosol and humidity therapy to be lacking in hard scientific data to support their beneficial use, and they suggested various studies that still need to be conducted.[3] Our approach to these involved and complex modes of therapy is to present concepts and suggestions for practice based on available theoretic information, known physical principles, accepted "facts,"[2] and clinical experience.

Humidity concepts

Although humidity is introduced in Chapter 1, it is appropriate to briefly review certain concepts here and integrate them with clinical application in respiratory therapy. Humidity is water in its vapor form. It is the invisible,

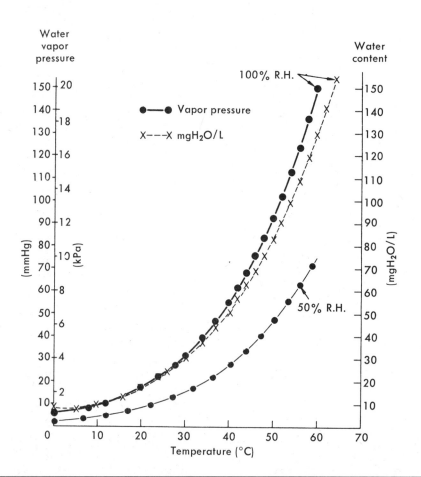

Fig. 10-1   Water vapor pressure (pH_2O) and absolute humidity (H_2O mg/ℓ) curves for gas which is fully saturated (RH = 100%) and gas which is half saturated (RH = 50%). (From Sykes, M.K., McNicol, M.W., and Campbell, E.J.M.: Respiratory failure, ed. 2, Oxford, England, 1976, Blackwell Scientific Publications.)

gaseous state of water, which exerts a temperature-dependent pressure. Humidity is sometimes referred to as "molecular water."

Absolute humidity is the actual amount of *water vapor* in a gas. It is usually expressed in terms of weight of water per unit volume of gas, such as milligrams per liter or grams per cubic meter. *Relative humidity* is a ratio of actual water vapor present in a gas to the capacity of the gas to hold the vapor at a given temperature. It is expressed as a percent and can be derived by the simple expression:

$$\%RH = \frac{\text{Content (absolute humidity)}}{\text{Capacity}} \times 100$$

The capacity of gas to hold water in its vapor state increases as temperature increases. Fig. 10-1 graphs this relationship.

When the content of humidity present is equal to the capacity for humidity, the RH is 100%, and the gas is considered *saturated*. If even slight cooling occurs with a saturated gas, condensation of water vapor occurs; i.e., the water will change state from vapor to liquid. This liquid formation occurs on whatever surface is available, such as sides of a container, walls of tubing or on suspended particles of liquid, or solid substances suspended in the air. The temperature at which water vapor condenses to water liquid is known as *dew point* and has considerable clinical importance, as discussed in other sections of this chapter.

When a gas is less than saturated with water vapor, the amount of humidity can be expressed in several ways. As an example, suppose a gas at 20°C has an absolute humidity level of 11 mg/ℓ, exerting a partial pressure of about 10.5 mm Hg. Fig. 10-1 shows that if that gas were holding its capacity of water vapor (i.e., saturated), it would have 18.5 mg/ℓ exerting about 17.5 mm Hg. The relative humidity percent can be calculated in the following manner.

Example 1: Using mg/ℓ values

$$\%RH = \frac{\text{Content}}{\text{Capacity}} \times 100$$

$$\%RH = \frac{11 \text{ mg/}\ell}{18.5 \text{ mg/}\ell} \times 100$$

$$\%RH = 0.6 \times 100 = 60$$

Example 2: Using mm Hg values

$$\%RH = \frac{\text{Content}}{\text{Capacity}} \times 100$$

$$\%RH = \frac{10.5 \text{ mm Hg}}{17.5 \text{ mm Hg}} \times 100$$

$$\%RH = 0.6 \times 100 = 60$$

Either set of figures shows us that the air has an RH of 60%; i.e., it has 60% of its capability for holding water in its vapor state.

The amount of water vapor in a given volume of gas is measured according

Table 10-1 Humidity deficit	Air temperature and relative humidity	Water vapor/gas (mg/ℓ)	Humidity deficit (mg/ℓ)
	37° C, saturated	44	0
	21° C, saturated	18	26
	21° C, 50% RH	9	35

to these principles of absolute and relative humidity. For evaluation of respiratory humidity the convenient term *percent body humidity* is sometimes used.[4] It refers to the amount of water vapor in a volume of gas as the percent of the water in gas saturated at body temperature. For example, air at 20°C, saturated with vapor, contains 18.5 mg of water per liter, whereas saturated air at body temperature contains 43.8 mg/ℓ. The room air could be said to have 42% body humidity.

Water vapor is used specifically to prevent or correct a "humidity deficit" in the respiratory tract (Table 10-1). Normally, the tracheobronchial tree can maintain saturation of inspired gas at body temperature by evaporation from the respiratory mucosa, most of which probably occurs proximal to the carina. Gas thus reaching the pulmonary tissue contains about 44 mg of water vapor per liter of gas. If the inspired gas contains less than this amount of water, its vapor pressure will be less than the 47 mm Hg of body humidity, and a vapor pressure gradient will be established between the inspired gas and the respiratory mucosa. Evaporation of body water from the mucosa brings the gas to full humidification. When the respiratory tract and the general body hydration are in good health, this humidifying mechanism works efficiently, but a humidity deficit of pathologic degree can be produced under two circumstances.

Breathing dry gas. The administration of therapeutic gases from a cylinder or central supply subjects the respiratory tract to large volumes of vapor-free gas. The normal humidification process may be inadequate to cope with this load and may have to draw on the water content of the entire mucosal surface. Such failure will be hastened or aggravated by an associated dehydration incidental to systemic disease. Depletion of mucosal moisture increases the viscosity of the mucus blanket of the tract and slows its escalator movement. At the same time ciliary action is adversely affected. Patients requiring gas therapy often have increased amounts of abnormal secretions, which tend to become dehydrated and less mobile.

Mucosal crusting. The secretions just noted, resulting from bronchopulmonary infection and irritation or systemic disease, can cover the mucosal surface with a dry and crusted coat. Impervious to the diffusion of moisture, it blocks the normal humidification process from the underlying mucosa. Further desiccation may be caused by the inhalation of therapeutic gases that are inadequately humidified.

Clinical humidity therapy

Clinical uses for molecular water, humidity, can be divided into two broad classes: first, to humidify dry, therapeutic gases to make them more comfortable to breathe, and second, to provide near body humidity levels of inspired gases for patients with artificial airways. Neither of these categories is concerned with physically adding *liquid* water to the respiratory tract per se. That clinical goal is discussed in the section on aerosol therapy in this chapter.

Humidifying therapeutic gases

By far the most common use for humidification in the modern hospital setting is the simple addition of water vapor to oxygen supplied from cylinders or a central supply to patients spontaneously breathing through their nose or mouth. Humidity is also often supplied to gases for anesthesics, to gases in the pulmonary function laboratory, or to therapeutic combination gases such as oxygen–carbon dioxide or helium-oxygen mixtures. Any of these medical gases supplied in cylinders or from a central supply is required to meet purity levels (see Chapter 12) such that no water vapor can be present. As we already mentioned, breathing these dry gases can cause undue stress on the respiratory tract of patients with respiratory disorders. Furthermore, just breathing these dry gases can cause discomfort.

The basic goal in this therapy is to provide at least a level of humidity that is similar to or exceeding that amount commonly found in room air. In modern, air-conditioned hospital rooms this is probably about 30% to 70% RH at room temperature, depending on the local climate and weather conditions. Common humidifiers currently used are generally capable of providing at least this level of moisture and often more.[5] Since patients using these simple systems are breathing through intact upper airways, the remainder of water vapor needed for body humidity is supplied in the usual fashion. This humidification of dry therapeutic gases adds little or no *extra* water vapor to the total inspired gases as compared to breathing room air, but rather it prevents these gases from adding to the normal humidity deficit.

Providing body humidity

Normally inspired air is warmed to nearly body temperature and is saturated with water vapor by the time it reaches about the level of the carina.[6,7] Heat and moisture are supplied by the respiratory mucosa of the upper airways. If an endotracheal tube or a tracheostomy tube is used, the upper airways are bypassed (see Chapter 14). It is well known that if inadequate humidification is supplied to inspired gases through these tubes, the patient's secretions will become thick, inspissated, and difficult to remove.[8-12] Because the upper airways are bypassed, the heat and water vapor needed for body humidity in the lung will have to be supplied by the lower airways or by artificial means.

To prevent this large humidity deficit from drying the patient's secretions, heated humidification systems are used.[5,12] These systems are capable of controlling the temperature and humidity levels of inspired air and providing saturated gases at or near the normal body temperature of 37°C. The primary goal here is to mimic the upper respiratory tract's ability to provide body humidity.

Some controversy exists in the literature concerning the optimum amount of humidity and temperature the inspired air should contain for patients with artificial airways. Traditionally, the recommendation has been to keep the air 100% saturated at 37°C in the same manner as the upper airway normally would.[5,9-11] However, some research in anesthesized animals and patients has presented conflicting data for mucus flow, pulmonary complications, and lung tissue and surfactant changes.[13-17] When all heat and moisture deficits are supplied artifically, some natural heat and water vapor losses from the respiratory tract are also stopped. The clinical significance of this is not well understood. However, since mucociliary clearance of secretions can be impaired by 50% to 75% body humidity[13] but is less affected by temperatures between 32° to 42°C with humidity levels of 33 mg/ℓ,[14] it seems reasonable that inspired gases for intubated patients be kept between 80% to 100% RH at temperatures between 32° to 37°C (90° to 99°F); at least, temperatures of inspired gases should be monitored closely (see Chapter 14). Our clinical experience agrees with others for the safe use of these guidelines.[8]

For patients having increased amounts of airway secretions, more than humidification of inspired air may be required. Since typical heated humidifiers have essentially no *liquid* water output, they cannot be used to *add* significant amounts of water to the patient's airways. Instead, aerosol generating devices that can deliver liquid to the respiratory tract are used to add fluid volume to retrained secretions.[10,18-20] This is discussed in more detail later in this chapter.

Humidifiers

Various types and brands of humidifiers have been described and evaluated elsewhere,[5,21,22] so our discussion here is limited to a general overview of the principles involved and to common type examples.

Several factors relate to the efficiency of any humidifier. Primarily, these factors are (1) the amount of the surface area exposure between the water and the gas to be humidified, (2) the time the gas and water are in contact, and (3) the temperature of both the water and the gas.

Surface area exposure. In order for effective evaporation of significant amounts of water to occur, the gas to be humidified must generally have a high level of interface area with the water. This can be accomplished several ways. The most common methods are dispersing the gas through the water as small bubbles or spraying the water as small droplets into the gas, or both.[5]

Time of contact between gas and water. In general, the longer a gas is in contact with humidifier's water, the greater the chance for that gas to be saturated with water vapor. In some humidifiers used for moisturizing therapeutic gases, the flow rate of the gas influences the level of humidity obtained,[22] indicating that perhaps the time of contact was not sufficient for saturation.

However, when a very high surface area is maintained or when temperature of the water is increased, saturation of the gas is reached very rapidly, and time of contact and the flow rate of the gas are much less important.[5,23]

Temperature of water and gas. The most important factor contributing to a humidifier's overall efficiency is temperature. Even humidifiers that have a relatively low surface area for exposure between water and gas can saturate the gas if the water is heated enough. Even when relatively high flow rates are used, if adequate heat is applied, high levels of humidity can result.[24] There is a loss of heat when evaporation occurs (see Chapter 1), and if the temperature of a gas is lowered, its ability to carry water vapor is also lowered (Fig. 10-1). Therefore, if a humidifier is not heated from some external source, as water vaporizes into the gas, heat is lost and the gas and the humidifier's water are cooled. This causes the level of humidity output to be somewhat limited to less than the potential for the room air since the gas leaving the humidifier is cooler than room air. This phenomenon is less significant in certain types of humidifiers, described next.

Pass-over humidifier

The pass-over humidifier is the simplest of all and depends on evaporation to supply humidity to air directed across its surface. Although its efficiency can be increased by heating either the water or the air, this type of humidifer has been replaced for the most part by the other humidifiers under discussion.

Bubble-diffusion humidifier

One of the oldest methods of humidifying oxygen or other gases consists of bubbling them through a reservoir of water, thus providing a large number of gas-to-liquid surfaces to enhance evaporation. Fig. 10-2 illustrates two commonly employed techniques. Gas enters the unit at *A* and passes through a tube immersed nearly to the bottom of a jar containing water. Sometimes the tube contains multiple perforations (*B*), through which the gas escapes as bubbles. The size of the bubbles is determined by the size of the openings and the gas flow rate. The relatively small amount of gas in each bubble, surrounded by a large amount of water, picks up water of evaporation to varying degrees of humidity and leaves the outflow port (*D*). Instead of the holes, the immersed oxygen tube may be fitted with a porous stonelike *diffusion head* (*C*) at its lower tip. This breaks the gas into much smaller bubbles than the perforated tube, thus increasing the total gas surface for evaporation of water among the much larger number of small bubbles.

These units are generally capable of supplying dry gases with 60% to 100% RH at their operating temperatures. As mentioned previously, the operating temperatures are generally cooler than room conditions, often by several degrees, because of the evaporative cooling effect. Since the humidified gases are usually carried to the patient by a small-diameter tube of 6 to 8 feet in length, some warming of these gases occurs before they are inspired by the patient. If no liquid water is available for evaporation in the tubing or gas stream, then the *relative humidity* of the gas will *drop* as its temperature rises towards room

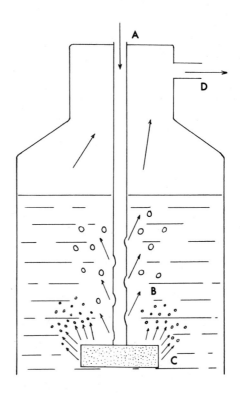

Fig. 10-2 The bubble-diffusion humidifier bubbles therapeutic gas, *A,* through a perforated tube, *B,* or a porous diffusion head, *C.* The larger the number of small bubbles, the greater the evaporation area to humidify the gas leaving outflow port, *D.*

temperature. Because of the evaporative cooling effect within the humidifer, even saturated gases leaving a bubble-diffusion humidifier generally can only supply about 35% to 40% body humidity.

Jet humidifier The jet humidifier increases the surface area for exposure of water to gas by breaking the water into small droplets, i.e., an aerosol. Although aerosols and aerosol therapy are discussed later in this chapter, because the jet humidifier uses similar principles, some discussion is appropriate here.

An *aerosol* can be defined as particles of liquid or solid suspended in a gas. For the jet humidifier a *water aerosol* is created so that a tremendous gas-water interface occurs. The purpose is solely to provide water vapor for the gas, however, and the particles are *not* intended for deposition in the patient's airways. An attempt is made to remove as many water particles as possible from the gas before it reaches the patient. *Baffling* the aerosol is an attempt to remove the particles from suspension, and some of the aerosol evaporates into the gas.

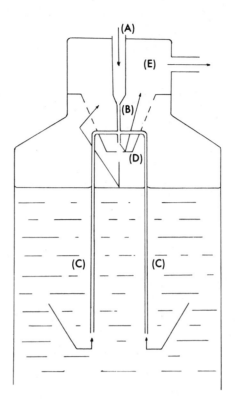

Fig. 10-3 Components of a jet humidifier. (See text for description.)

Fig. 10-3 depicts the jet principle employed in humidification. The power gas enters at *A,* passing through a restriction (*B*) into which twin capillary tubes (*C*) open. The venturi at *B* produces a foaming mixture of liquid and gas that meets a baffle (*D*) as it emerges from the jet orifice. The baffle may be a perforated plate against which some liquid particles impinge, fracture, and are reflected into the vapor chamber (*E*). Other particles penetrate the plate and are further baffled by the reservoir surface, which retains the larger ones; the remainder are screened once more as they enter the vapor chamber through the plate baffle. Baffled particles condense and return to the reservoir. The minute water particles that continue into the chamber evaporate into the gas to raise its vapor content, supplemented by water of evaporation from the reservoir surface. Gas issuing from the unit will thus have a maximum amount of water vapor and a minimum of liquid water particles.

Again, the temperature of the gas leaving the humidifier is several degrees cooler than the surrounding room air, and warming occurs as the gas travels to the patient. Some water particles do escape the humidifier's baffling system and are available to evaporate as the gas is warmed. Of the three types of

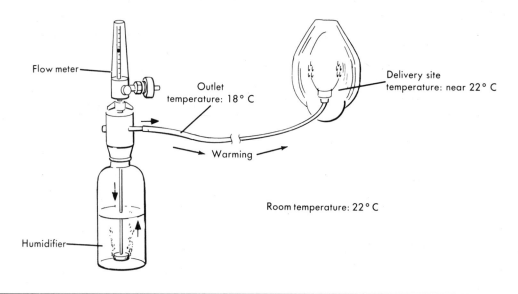

Fig. 10-4   Gases leaving outlet of the simple humidifier are cooler than room temperature due to evaporation. Warming toward room temperature occurs en route to patient delivery site.

humidifiers so far discussed, the jet humidifier has the greatest potential for water output when operated at or below room temperature.

Fig. 10-4 diagrams a typical setup using a simple humidifier for therapeutic gas administration and illustrates the effect of temperature differences between the humidifier and the delivery site.

Heated humidifier   When body humidity levels are needed, heat must be applied to the water of the humidifier or to the gas, or both. Typically, most heated humidifiers warm the reservoir or water. Some also maintain the heat of the warm, humid gases leaving the unit by using heating wires applied to the delivery tubing.[5] Heated humidifiers can be the pass-over or blow-by type, or a sophisticated bubble-diffusion style, sometimes referred to as a *cascade type,* or they can incorporate a water-absorbing material called a *wick.*[5] Because the surface area exposure is relatively high for the cascade type, high *relative* humidity can be achieved even without adding heat while the low surface area for the pass-over and wick types generally must have heat applied in order to raise the humidity levels, both absolute and relative. Therefore the pass-over and wick types are not recommended for use for high humidity output unless temperatures above room air are also applied.

The most common use for heated humidifiers is with mechanical ventilation systems, but they have also been used for patients with artificial airways who are spontaneously breathing.[5,24,25] As mentioned previously, the purpose of these devices is to replace the heating and humidification functions of the patient's upper airways, which have been bypassed by the artificial airway.

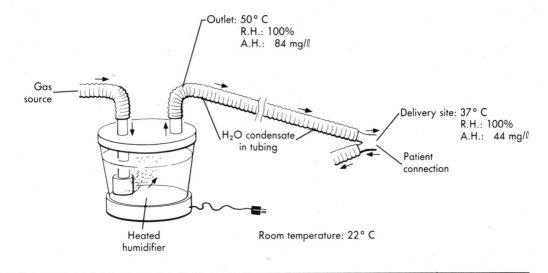

Outlet: 50° C
R.H.: 100%
A.H.: 84 mg/ℓ

Gas source

H₂O condensate in tubing

Delivery site: 37° C
R.H.: 100%
A.H.: 44 mg/ℓ

Patient connection

Heated humidifier

Room temperature: 22° C

Fig. 10-5   Gases leaving outlet of heated humidifier are hot and saturated with water vapor. As cooling occurs in tubing, vapor condenses and absolute humidity *(A.H.)* decreases while relative humidity *(R.H.)* remains 100% (saturated). Note that almost half the original water vapor is "lost" to condensate in this example.

These systems must be used so that they provide near body humidity levels at the point of delivery to the patient.

For these systems, tubing of about ³/₄ to 1 inch (2 to 2.5 cm) in diameter is used to deliver the warm, humid gases to the patients (Fig. 10-5). This "large-bore" tubing is used rather than the smaller diameter tubing of the other humidifiers discussed because significant *cooling* will occur between the heated humidifier and the patient. Since the gases leaving the humidifier are hot and generally saturated with water vapor, this cooling causes condensation of vapor to liquid state in the tubing. Small diameter tubing would very quickly occlude its lumen, so large-bore is used instead. Still this tubing will also fill with water and must therefore be drained periodically or water traps be used to collect the condensate. The magnitude of this cooling and condensation problem is illustrated in the following example.

In a typical hospital room, temperatures may be between 22° and 24°C. When gases near body temperature are delivered to the patient connection, temperature at the humidifier outlet may be 48° to 50°C. Because of a variety of factors involved, such as air-conditioning, air currents in the room, and insulation properties of the tubing, cooling occurs so that the gas temperature falls to near 37°C at the patient connection. By referring to the chart in Fig. 10-1, it can be seen that saturated air at 50°C holds about twice the water vapor that saturated air at near body temperature holds. During this cooling process then, about half of the original water vapor leaving the humidifier condenses or "rains out" into the delivery tubing as the capacity of the air for holding water in vapor state decreases (Fig. 10-5).

To express this example using humidity terminology, during the cooling of the hot saturated air, relative humidity *remains at 100%* while absolute humidity *decreases* as water vapor condenses to liquid. Of course the actual numbers in this example are used to illustrate the concept, and varying conditions will require different humidifier outlet temperatures, delivery temperatures, and amounts of condensation.

Heated wires placed around or inside the delivery tubing can decrease the gradient between the humidifier and the delivery site. This allows the humidifier to be operated at lower temperatures and tends to minimize the condensation in the tubing circuit.

Physical properties of aerosols

Therapists will better understand the clinical use of medical aerosols, as well as the important health effects of atmospheric contaminants, if they have a background knowledge of the nature of aerosols in general. An aerosol is defined as a suspension of very fine particles (particulate matter) of liquid or solid in a gas. In general, aerosol particles are considered to fall within the size range of 0.005μ to 50μ in diameter, but from a practical point of view only those are important that are less than 3μ in diameter, for at this mass size, gravity begins to lose its influence, a point of some importance, as we shall soon see.

Atmospheric aerosols can be considered to be either *natural* or *synthetic* and may consist of windblown dusts, bacteria, yeast, molds, water, dusts from explosions or earth-moving equipment, smoke, industrial wastes, and products of incomplete combustion of a large variety of commercial fuels, to list a few of the more prevalent. Another classification of atmospheric particulate matter, which is especially revealing in its relationship to disease production, is that which describes *neutral particles,* commonly referred to as dusts and "condensation nuclei." These are made up of hygroscopic substances (substances able to absorb water).[26] The neutral, dustlike particles range in size from 10^{-5} to 10^{-3} cm in diameter, have mostly a nuisance value, and are generally less harmful than the condensation nuclei. The latter are smaller, from 10^{-7} to 10^{-5} cm in diameter, and are composed mostly of chloride salts, sulfuric acid, phosphorus compounds, nitrogen oxides, and nitric acid. In the air such nuclei grow rapidly by the acquisition of water, as the RH exceeds 70%, and easily produce haze and fog. It should be apparent also that any hygroscopic aerosol might undergo the same change during inhalation into the moist environment of the respiratory tract. Finally, although we are not studying the atmosphere as such, it is relevant to note that condensation nuclei, often consisting of toxic or irritant trace gases, tend to form on the most minute speck of matter, giving stability to these otherwise vaporous substances so that they are able to enter the respiratory tract, with harmful effects.[27] Their participation in the damaging action of contaminated urban air and smothering smogs is a matter of record.

Aerosol terminology

Stability of an aerosol refers to its ability to remain in suspension for significant periods of time or to maintain its integrity as an aerosol. Such stability depends on a number of characteristics, including size and nature of the particulate matter, concentration of particles, ambient humidity, and the degree of mobility of the carrier gas. *Instability* is the reverse of the above—the propensity of a suspended particle to remove itself, or be removed, from suspension. From a therapeutic point of view it is apparent that the stability or instability of a given aerosol will bear directly on the aerosol's effectiveness and be a matter of considerable concern to the manufacturer. Although the size range of particulate matter is great, as the myriad particles intermingle, some will condense on others, some will coalesce to form larger masses (agglomerate), and other will vanish through instability. A large population of aerosols thus undergoes a process of "aging," whereby there is a gradual increase in the number of particles of optimum size and concentration for maximum stability, with a reduction in the range of sizes. This *ideal* state consists of particles from 0.2μ to 0.7μ in diameter, in concentrations of from 100 to 1000 particles per cubic centimeter of gas.[27] Fig. 10-6 is a graphic illustration of this phenomenon, showing the relationship among population, distribution of particulate diameters, and time.

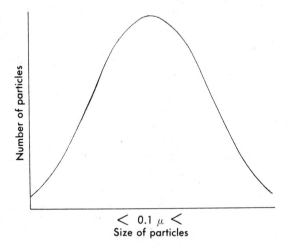

< 0.1 μ <
Size of particles

Fig. 10-6   Distribution curve of aerosol particle sizes. If a population of particles of many sizes is allowed to settle, the largest number will have diameters somewhere around 0.1μ, with decreasing frequency of sizes larger and smaller. (Modified from Lovejoy, F.W., and Morrow, P.E.: Anesthesiology **23:**460, 1962.)

Related to the characteristics of stability and instability and especially pertinent to the therapeutic use of aerosols are *penetration, deposition or retention, and clearance.* These terms describe the fate of particles once they have come into contact with the respiratory tract. *Penetration* refers to the maximum depth that suspended particles can be carried into the tract by the inhaled tidal air. *Deposition* is the result of an aerosol's eventual instability, permitting it to "fall out" on a nearby surface, whereas *retention* implies the deposition of a particle within the confines of a structure, such as the respiratory tract. Aerosol *clearance* is the opposite of retention and, depending on its specific use, may have two meanings. Most authors refer to aerosol clearance as the process of removal of particles once deposited in the respiratory tissues by one of several biologic mechanisms that are considered later. Occasionally the term implies the excretion of still-suspended particles in the exhaled air.

Penetration and deposition of aerosols

The location of the deposition of inhaled particles is of significance, for there is a considerable physiologic difference between particle contact with the relatively rugged and exposed nasal tissue and particle contact with the more secluded and reactive bronchial and alveolar cells. The latter areas are of more interest to us in the therapeutic use of aerosols. The depth of penetration of the respiratory tract increases as the particle size decreases. In fact, unless a particle is considerably less than 100μ in diameter, it will not even gain entrance. The nasal filtering process (deposition in the nose) is so effective that it will remove completely particles down to 5μ to 10μ in diameter, whereas sizes below 1μ can pass the upper tract and are retained in pulmonary tissue. We can make the generalization that the overall retention of particulate matter in the total respiratory tract is 100% for particles down to 5μ to 10μ in diameter, which are trapped in the nose, and about 25% for particles down to 0.25μ, which are deposited and retained along the rest of the tract. Deposition in the upper respiratory tract (conducting airways to the respiratory bronchioles) varies from 100% for large particles to no deposition for particles of 1μ, whereas deposition in the alveoli is 90% to 100% for sizes down to 1μ.[28] There are five major factors that influence aerosol penetration and deposition—*gravity, kinetic activity of gas molecules, inertial impaction, physical nature of the particle,* and the *ventilatory pattern.*

Gravity. The speed with which a particle will "settle" is a measure of its ease of deposition. The settling rate is related to the force exerted by gravity on the particle mass or the combination of density and size. The greater the mass of any body, the greater the influence of gravity on it. Suspended particles between 0.1μ and 70μ generally follow the prediction of Stoke's law of sedimentation.[29] In its entirety Stoke's law relates the velocity at which a small particle falls toward the earth with such physical factors as particle volume, density, acceleration of gravity, and viscous resistance of air. For our purposes, however, we can use it in a simplified proportionality and state that, within the previously stated size range, the settling velocity of a

	Particle	Density	Diameter	Velocity
Table 10-2 Gravity deposition	x	1	2	4
	y	1	4	16
	z	2	2	8

particle is proportional to the product of its density and the square of its diameter. Thus:

$$\text{Settling rate} \cong \text{Density} \times \text{Diameter}^2$$

Table 10-2 compares the relative velocities with which the three hypothetical particles will deposit under the influence of gavity. Particle x, with a density of 1 unit and a diameter of 2 units, will settle with a velocity of 4 units. Particle y, of the same density but with twice the diameter, will settle four times as fast; whereas particle z, with the same diameter but twice the density, will settle twice as fast.

Kinetic activity of gas molecules. This interesting force of particle deposition is effective on sizes 0.1μ or smaller. Because of their minute size, such aerosols are almost molecular in character and, as such, are subject to some of the physical activities attributed to gas molecules. They present the phenomenon of *brownian movement* under the influence of the kinetic activity of the molecules of their carrier gas. The suspended particles are under constant bombardment from the gas molecules and are thus impelled into high-speed random movements for very short distances. *The smaller the particles, the greater their velocities.*

This transferred activity and mobility causes many of the particles to come into contact with nearby surfaces, and it is referred to as *diffusion* of the aerosol. The resulting surface impaction is called *diffusion deposition*. How much of the suspended material will deposit is a function of its *diffusion coefficient,* defined as the volume of particles that can diffuse a distance of 1μ over an area of 1 cm^2 at a pressure of 1 atm and is inversely proportional to particle size. Whether a given particle will deposit or what fraction of a given volume of suspended particles will fall out is determined by the distance of the particles from the nearest suitable surface. The probability of deposition is related to time as well as to diffusibility and distance, and the average distance that the force of diffusion will move a minute particle is expressed by the following proportionality:

$$\text{Average distance traveled} \cong \sqrt{\text{Diffusion coefficient} \times \text{Time}}$$

We are not interested in quantitative values for such physical phenomena, but we should be aware that they play an important role in the efficiency of aerosol therapy, and we should recognize that consideration of these many factors in the design of aerosol generators can mean the difference between

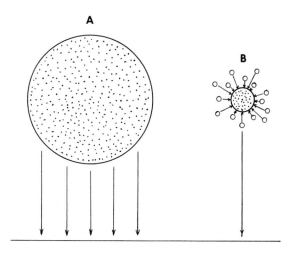

Fig. 10-7   The mass of the larger aerosol particle, **A,** makes it susceptible to the settling force of gravity. The smaller particle, **B,** is more affected by the bombardment of surrounding carrier gas molecules, eventually impinging on a nearby surface; this is called diffusion deposition.

good and indifferent equipment. Fig. 10-7 illustrates gravity and diffusion deposition.

Inertial impaction. A particle being carried in an airstream tends to continue on a straight course when the stream undergoes a sudden change in direction,[30] as shown by the large particles in Fig. 10-8. This divergence of the particle's path from that of the airstream is referred to as a "sideways slip." Because it occurs at angulations in the conducting channel, such a slip can precipitate a particle on a nearby surface. Whether a particle will deposit in such a manner depends partly on its location within the airstream, the probability increasing with the particle's proximity to the periphery of the stream. Whether it will deposit also depends on the force of inertia, which opposes any change in direction of a moving particle, being great enough to free the particle from others in the stream. To do this, inertia must overcome the resistance of air friction so that another probability of deposition depends on the net effect of the two forces of inertia and friction. In summary, then, inertial precipitation of aerosol particles of uniform density is related to particle velocity and size.

Physical nature of particles. Of the many physical and chemical characteristics of minute matter, probably the most important in terms of deposition and retention is its hygroscopic nature, noted previously. Initially small, a particle may absorb relatively large amounts of water from ambient air, especially in transit through the respiratory tract, and increase many times its diameter. This, of course, will alter its original probable point of impact.

The solubility and chemical nature of particles, especially those in a heter-

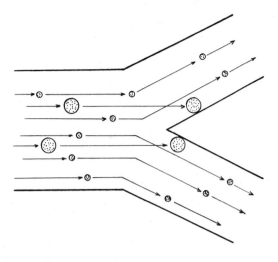

Fig. 10-8 Inertial impaction of large aerosol particles, whose masses tend to maintain their motion in straight lines. As airway direction changes, the particles deposit on nearby walls. Smaller particles are carried around corners by the airstream and fall out less readily.

ogeneous atmospheric mixture, may play an important role. Very small particles may dissolve in or chemically react with aerosolized water or other solvents of a larger size and thus eventually deposit at levels different from those dictated by their original sizes.

Finally, particle contour can influence deposition. Although we speak of aerosol particles as though they all had regular diameters like the spheroids of liquid particulates, some hard and brittle substances produce particles with many angulations and irregular plane surfaces. Such particles may follow transit and deposition paths considerably different from those predicted on the basis of physical laws we have been discussing. We might note here that our application of aerosol principles in the treatment of disease is somewhat simplified in that most therapeutic aerosols currently in use are liquids, and the aberrations that might be attributed to solid particles concern us less.

Ventilatory pattern. In general, deposition and retention of aerosol particles is directly related to inhaled volume and inversely related to respiratory rate.[18] This generalization, however, is not applicable to sizes less than 1μ in diameter. The character of air movement on particle behavior is significant down to the level of the terminal bronchiole, but air in the alveolar sacs is almost stagnant. Thus depth and frequency of ventilation have little influence on the deposition of particles once they have reached the alveolar level.[31, 32] The nature of ventilation higher in the tract does help to determine the volume of particles reaching alveoli and thus exerts an indirect influence. Deposition of particles is increased with both increasing tidal volume and decreasing frequency, and the effects of both are additive. Shallow breathing carries a reduced volume of aerosols per tidal volume, and a rapid breathing rate reduces the time available to the particles to settle.

If penetration and deposition are the objectives as in aerosol therapy, the ideal ventilatory pattern appears to consist of slow, moderately deep breathing, with breath holding at end-inspiration.[18] This facilitates the introduction into the respiratory tract of a significant volume of particles and allows adequate time for the smallest to enter the alveoli by diffusion and to settle by diffusion. This is a practical point that the therapist will have to keep in mind while supervising and teaching patients the techniques of effective aerosol therapy.

Like many aerosol therapy principles, disagreement and conflicting data persist concerning the optimum ventilatory pattern for maximum penetration and retention of mists.[33] Exercise during aerosol breathing appears to increase aerosol deposition, apparently related to the increase in minute ventilation rather than tidal volume.[33] Such exercise is often impractical or impossible for acutely ill patients. It is believed that for patients with poor distribution of inspired air, increased tidal volume may improve the distribution of aerosol and air to areas that usually receive low ventilation.[18]

Clearance of aerosols

We now concern ourselves with the removal of particles from the respiratory tract by means other than the exhaled air and discuss clearance of the upper and lower segments of the tract separately. The mechanism for cleansing the upper tract is referred to as the *ciliary mucus transport,* and there are several mechanisms to service the pulmonary areas.

Ciliary mucus clearance. We assume that the student already knows the anatomic structure of the airways and the pulmonary lobules. Of critical importance to the subject under discussion is the nature of the mucosal lining of the respiratory tract. We recall that the mucosa is characterized by the presence of microscopic hairlike structures called cilia that extend from the beginning of the trachea through all the ramifications of the airways to the level of the terminal bronchioles. Approximately 3μ to 4μ long, the cilia are in constant wavelike motion called "beating," which goes on at a rate of some 1000 to 1300 strokes per minute. The unique function of the cilia is made possible by more rapid upward strokes than downward recovery strokes. As the cilia wave cephalad (in the direction of the head), they propel an overlying thin layer of fluid called mucus.

Respiratory mucus is a thin clear substance, produced by specialized cells (*goblet cells*) throughout the tract to the respiratory bronchioles, and is on the average 5μ thick.[34, 35] Its function is to entrap foreign particles and, with the aid of the cilia, to remove them from the tract. Lying like a blanket over the cilia, the mucous layer is carried cephalad in an escalator fashion by the ciliary action at rates up to 13.5 mm/min. The mucus, with its captive particles, is brought into the trachea and then into the lower pharynx by a normal and almost imperceptible "throat clearing" action to be either expectorated or swallowed, depending on its volume.

The system is extremely efficient as long as both cilia and mucus are healthy. Should a pathologic process increase the depth of the mucous layer, its upward propulsion will gradually slow, becoming ineffective when the thickness of the fluid approaches four to five times the height of the cilia. Similarly, function will be impaired after damage to or destruction of the cilia. Airway obstruction from the prolific thick secretions accompanying bronchial irritation or infection can be self-perpetuating, as the increase in the secretory load retards its own removal.

Pulmonary tissue clearance. Particles in the lobular lung units can be removed by several routes. Some may be considered "functionally" removed in situ through encapsulation and immobilization by a deposit of fibrous tissue, remaining for the duration of the subject's life. It is not surprising that enough such reactions throughout wide areas of the lung might in themselves eventually present a problem. Other solid aerosols are picked up by wandering scavenger cells called *phagocytes,* whose mobility permits them to gather at sites of foreign matter deposition. After engulfing the particles within their own protoplasm, the phagocytes can transport them into the ciliary-mucous escalator for removal as described or into the interstitial lymphatics for incarceration in regional lymph nodes. Depending on solubility, some particles may dissolve in tissue fluid and diffuse into the general circulation to be disposed of by the body's metabolic processes.

Summary

Let us summarize the relation between particle size and deposition in the respiratory tract and point out that although much of the research done on inhaled particulate matter has used nontherapeutic solid particles, the results give us a practical insight into the expected behavior of the liquid aerosols that we will have occasion to use. It is generally agreed that there is a particle size of *minimum* deposition, around 0.4μ in diameter, and that above and below this size the incidence of deposition somewhere in the tract increases. The highest probability for pulmonary deposition is attributed to particles in the 1μ to 2μ range (gravity settling) and below 0.2μ (diffusion precipitation); the lowest probability is found with particles 0.25μ to 0.50μ, for which the effects of both gravity and diffusion are minimal.[36, 37] These data are summarized in Table 10-3.

As an aside from our specific topic of aerosol clearance, these mechanisms

Table 10-3 Particle size and site of deposition	Particle size (μ)	Deposition in respiratory tract
	100	Do not enter tract
	100-5	Trapped in nose
	5-2	Deposited somewhere proximal to alveoli
	2-1	Can enter alveoli, with 95% to 100% retention of those down to 1 μ
	1-0.25	Stable, with minimal settling
	0.25	Increasing alveolar deposition

are of great clinical importance in protecting the body from diseases caused by the inhalation of such pathogenic aerosols as bacteria and the toxic condensation nuclei described earlier. The ability of the respiratory tract to rid itself of foreign particles can be seriously hampered by such factors as smoke inhalation, exposure to cold air, ingestion of alcohol, and lack of adequate sleep.

The student should understand that in the preceding discussion of the properties of aerosols, many generalizations and assumptions are included that may or may not be valid.[33] The current great interest in aerosols has produced many changes in investigative techniques, making it difficult to correlate data from one source to another. These differences in technique account for much of the variance found in the literature, especially pertaining to effective particle sizes[33, 38] and to the degree of penetration by aerosols.[39] Nevertheless, we have reviewed the most widely accepted behavioral characteristics of aerosols as they apply to clinical medicine, and we can only be alert to new developments in this interesting field.

Clinical uses of aerosol therapy

Certainly aerosol therapy is being questioned, and much is still to be known about it.[3,33] In general, aerosol therapy is used with the following objectives in mind: *to provide humidification of the respiratory tract, to serve as an adjunct for mobilization of bronchial secretions for easier removal,* and *to provide relief from bronchospasm and respiratory mucosal edema.* The last has been well established, and potent drugs used for aerosolization for these purposes are described in Chapter 11. However, some brief comments concerning aerosol bronchodilator therapy are made here, and the remainder of this section is devoted to the other two general objectives.

While it is generally accepted that aerosolization of potent bronchodilator drugs provides relaxation of respiratory tract smooth muscle by local effect on these airways with minimum systemic side effects,[3,18-20,33,38] several problems are of concern. The dosage of drugs that are delivered to the airways by the aerosol route is often difficult to estimate.[3,33,40] A tremendous number of factors are involved, some of which we have already discussed. Many of the variables are not easily controlled, and much is yet unknown. Individual patients may not adhere to the prescribed routine, either underutilizing or overutilizing the drug. The dosage required for the desired effect may change significantly for a patient during acute exacerbations of airway obstruction and infection. Still, objective pulmonary function data can be dramatically improved by inhalation of these bronchoactive drugs. Thus their use is widespread, with generally good results (see Chapter 11).

Humidification of the respiratory tract

Aerosolized water serves a double function. Its principal duty is to deliver liquid water, in minute particle form, to the mucosal surface. The water that "rains out" in the airways is intended to dilute thick secretions or moisten dry crusts for easier removal by cough or aspiration. In addition to this local effect of physical water particles contacting the airway surfaces, aerosols provide an important source of moisture for humidifying the inspired carrier gas. As the gas enters the warmth of the body and its vapor capacity increases, suspended water particles evaporate into the gas, raising its vapor tension to that of body humidity. Humidification can be increased by heating the water to be aerosolized so that it reaches the respiratory tract with no humidity deficit, not only increasing the inhaled water content but also sparing the respiratory tract its duty of humidifying air.

Often heated water aerosol is used as a convenient substitute for a heated humidifier, described earlier. Again, for patients with artificial airways that bypass the upper airways, the primary aim is to at least supply near body humidity levels to the inspired gases. By using aerosol, potential for adding liquid water to the airways does exist. It seems reasonable that at least these water droplets aid in keeping the artificial airway cleared by not allowing respiratory secretions to become dried or crusted. Of course any secretions entering such a tube must be removed by coughing or suctioning (see Chapter 14) to avoiding occluding it.

Whether or not humidification of the *lower* respiratory tract by aerosolization is of real and measurable benefit for patients with respiratory disease, breathing through intact upper airways is yet to be proved.[1,3,33] Its usefulness in providing adequate humidification for patients with artificial airways is well accepted. The choice between using a heated humidifier or a heated water aerosol for this purpose is sometimes made when airway secretions are a problem, and the aerosol is used in hopes of gaining potential benefit from the available liquid. Reference is made again to this maneuver when equipment is discussed.

Warmed water aerosols are also often used for their soothing effect on inflamed tissues of the upper airway of patients immediately following removal of an artificial airway (extubation), following fiberoptic bronchoscopy, and in the treatment of inflammatory obstruction of laryngitis or croup (laryngotracheobronchitis).[20,41,60-62]

Aerosols for aiding in mobilization of secretions

Patients with acute and chronic respiratory diseases are often given various types of aerosol therapy in hopes of aiding the evacuation of the increased amounts or viscosity of airway secretions.[20] These aerosols may contain pharmacologically active mucolytic agents with or without other drugs, or they may consist of solutions thought to have little pharmacologic action, that is, *bland aerosols*. The actions and uses of mucolytic agents are described in Chapter 11. Let it suffice to say here that use of mucolytic aerosols is still debated, and their real role, if any, when they are given by inhalation is not settled.[3]

Bland aerosols are generally considered to be of water, hypotonic, normotonic, and some hypertonic saline solutions, propylene glycol, and detergents.[18,20,41] They are considered bland because they are believed to be soothing or nonirritating and lacking strong chemically or physically active ingredients. Review of the literature for use of bland aerosols recently failed to find substantial objective evidence of enhanced respiratory or mucociliary function.[41] However, subjective observation of improved efficiency of cough and ease of expectoration following aerosol inhalation infers that this form of therapy can be a useful *adjunct* to other forms of bronchial hygiene.[10,20,42,43] Lack of hard evidence of inhalation of bland aerosol to cause consistant and measurable improvements in respiratory and mucociliary function may only attest to the inadequacy of available testing methods and measurements. It was recently recommended that new experimental approaches be developed for further evaluation.[3]

When administration of bland aerosol appears to be indicated to ease the removal of secretions, several practical factors should be kept in mind. While it may be difficult if not impossible to systematically assess the absolute significance of each separately in a controlled study, the following suggestions are meant to provide optimum conditions for maximum benefit. Since only a portion of the inhaled aerosol is retained, large-volume, high-density mists have been recommended, using heated aerosols or ultrasonically produced mists.[20] Both of these methods produce more aerosol than conventional cool aerosol devices. Aerosol is best administered by a mouthpiece system, with the patient's head and tongue positioned to minimize obstruction to flow. If a mask is used, the patient should be instructed in proper mouth breathing. In either case, slow moderately deep breaths are recommended. Occasional sighlike breaths near inspiratory capacity may help open closed or poorly ventilated areas and aid in the subsequent distribution of mist.

The duration of therapy may vary because of individual need and tolerance. Generally if significant amounts of liquid are to be deposited, treatments may need to be from 30 to 60 minutes several times per day to virtually continuously for severe cases.[20,43] To minimize or prevent an increase in airway resistance produced by inhalation of high-density aerosols, bronchodilator drugs should be considered before bland mist therapy.[20,44]

The patient's ability to clear mobilized secretions should always be considered and monitored. Bland aerosols should be considered adjunct therapy, and other methods that help evacuation of secretions, such as proper coughing techniques and postural drainage (see Chapter 15), should also be used.

There is one special use of bland aerosol therapy that deserves individual attention because of its widespread use and importance—the induction of sputum specimens for laboratory examinations. Such examinations are done for two general reasons. First, specimens are prepared by skilled technicians called cytotechnologists and are carefully examined under the microscope for the presence of malignant cells in suspected cases of cancer of the respiratory tract. Often, if such disease is in communication with the airway, cells from the surface of the tumor will desquamate, mix with bronchial secretions, and be expectorated. Although the absence of malignant cells in this test, called a *cytologic* sputum examination, does not eliminate the possibility of cancer, their presence is strong evidence of the existence of cancer somewhere in the bronchi or lungs and necessitates a careful search for its location or for some other explanation for the abnormal cells. Second, a *bacteriologic* sputum examination attempts to determine the presence or absence of bacteria in the secretions and to identify those present. Initially the specimen is smeared on a glass slide, stained with a dye, and microscopically examined for organisms. This often gives a good idea of the general type of microbe present and permits the start of therapy. The rest of the specimen is mixed with several kinds of culture media (nutrients that promote bacterial growth) and incubated from a few hours to several days or weeks to allow maximum growth. Examination of the culture allows specific identification of the bacteria.

Most of the patients treated by the respiratory therapist will have little trouble providing sputum specimens for analysis, and no special procedures will be required. However, patients with suspected malignancy or nonacute tuberculosis may have very scanty sputum or none at all, and to obtain specimens from them may be critical. For these patients techniques are available to procure an *induced sputum* specimen, so called because agents are used by inhalation to promote an increased flow of bronchial secretion and to stimulate a cough. As indicated earlier, bronchial secretions will respond to almost any inhaled irritant, and for induction many have been tried, including 10% sodium chloride, dornase, acetylcysteine, sterile distilled water aerosols, and sulfur dioxide gas.[45] The last, although effective, has been found too irritating and is not generally recommended, and the mucolytics and proteolytics have little value in the absence of secretions. The salt-and-water aerosols, when delivered by standard aerosolization, are preheated to 140° to 185° F by any suitable means, but usually by an immersion heating unit in the aerosol generator.[46] This "superheated" aerosol is well saturated with humidity as the patient inhales it, and it also contains large numbers of particles for deposition throughout the bronchial tree.

The distilled water particles condense on the bronchial mucosa and mix with and increase the volume of the normal thin layer of mucus present. The abundance of fine particles also has an irritant effect, stimulating a cough that expectorates the diluted secretions. Sodium chloride aerosols have the same effect, and one additional: because a 10% concentration is more saline than the average body fluids (approximately 0.9%), this aerosol is hypertonic, and as it contacts the bronchial wall, its osmolarity draws fluid from the mucosal layer into the bronchial lumen, increasing the volume of secretions available for expectoration. With both fluid aerosols the stimulated cough causes the secretions thus moved to carry with them loose or superficial cells from the mucosal surface as well as any available bacteria close to the bronchial lumen. Cells and bacteria, which the subject would be unable to produce by voluntary cough, can thereby be examined.

When the technique of sputum induction became accepted, it was customary to use a 20% solution of propylene glycol as the saline solvent because of the stabilizing properties attributed to this agent. It was believed that the inclusion of propylene in the mixture ensured the penetration and deposition of a maximum number of particles in the respiratory tract. However, further experience demonstrated that propylene glycol itself had an inhibiting effect on the causative organism of tuberculosis *(Myobacterium tuberculosis),* destroying it or preventing its growth in culture.[45] This was a serious handicap, since the recovery of tubercle bacilli is an important function of sputum induction. From a practical point of view of the overall use of this technique, since it is diagnostic and the condition of the subject to be examined is therefore not known, it is advisable to omit propylene glycol from induced sputum mixtures and to use simply 10% sodium chloride in water.

Some hospitals have found ultrasonic aerosol generators, which are described later, to be most effective in inducing cough. Using distilled water at room temperature, these generators produce finely uniform particles that stimulate a heavy cough, usually after only a few breaths. As yet there are no available data comparing the relative amounts of secretions produced by ultrasonic aerosols as against the standard heated hypertonic saline aerosols. Precautions should be taken to protect medical personnel from possible contamination, especially when they are obtaining specimens suspected of containing tubercle bacilli. The use of a specially ventilated hooded table has been suggested and appears to be as practical a method as any.[47]

The usefulness of this procedure is widely recognized. For many years it was a common practice to aspirate the stomach through a long tube swallowed by the patient and to examine the gastric secretions for tubercle bacilli that the patient had inadvertently swallowed after unnoticed small coughs. Although not a difficult procedure, it was a nuisance and has been replaced by the much more convenient induced cough, which most investigators find to have a far greater bacterial yield.[48,49] It has proved to be a great boon to cancer detection, at times eliminating diagnostic procedures that are much more hazardous.[50,51] In addition to its diagnostic value, sputum induction often affords excellent symptomatic relief of airway obstruction by removing inspissated mucus, and not infrequently this technique of heated supersaturated aerosolization is used for its therapeutic benefit.

The duration of exposure to the aerosol, for diagnosis or therapy, can be varied to suit each individual. The patient is instructed to inhale the aerosol through the mouth in an easy and comfortable manner, resting as often as necessary, and at most the session should not exceed 15 minutes. Samples of sputum should be collected over the ensuing 30 minutes, and care should be taken not to collect saliva but only secretions that obviously arise from the depths of the airways. Sterile containers should be available for all specimens. If sputum is to be examined for malignant cells, it *must* be free of foreign particles. This is best accomplished by having hospitalized patients wash their teeth and thoroughly rinse their mouths before collection, and outpatients at least to rinse. As a maximum precaution against contamination, it is helpful to collect as many cytologic specimens as possible before breakfast; sputum yields are usually most abundant at that time.

Aerosol generators

This section is not intended to be a technical manual, describing the details of specific equipment or comparing the characteristics of competitive products, for such information is available through the commercial brochures and specification tables provided by all manufacturers. We discuss principles involved in the design and operation of aerosol and humidity generators so that therapists will recognize and understand the features of any piece of equipment with which they will have to work.

Instruments used to generate aerosols are called *nebulizers* (from "nebula," meaning a cloud or mist), as compared to those that increase water vapor content, *humidifiers*. There is a considerable overlap between the two in function and in application. They sometimes differ only in degree or in the use to which they are put. It may be generalized, however, that nebulizers are designed to deliver a maximum number of particles of desired size, of pharmaceuticals or water, for penetration and deposition in the respiratory tract, and that humidifiers are designed to deliver a maximum amount of water vapor with a minimum of particulate water. Some humidifiers produce varying amounts of aerosolized water, but the prime difference between them and nebulizers is the tremendous volume of particles of the latter. This difference may be a consideration when possible spread of infection is of concern. Bacteria, in general, are of the same size as aerosol particles and can thus attach themselves to the particles for transport directly into the lungs. In contrast, the absence of water mass of humidity provides bacteria with no mobile nuclei to carry them. Humidifiers therefore pose less of a threat of bacterial contamination to the patient than do nebulizers. Moistening the inspired gas with a humidifier rather than a nebulizer will at least deny bacteria easy access to the respiratory tract.

Nebulizers, like humidifiers, are available for use with water at room temperature or, by the inclusion of heating devices, with water at elevated temperatures. By raising the water temperature far above that of the body (up to 60°C), some humidifiers can add enough vapor to the inspired gas so that despite the drop in temperature in transit from instrument to patient, when gas enters the body it will be at or near body humidity. Some nebulizers, when used to deliver liquid water to the respiratory tract, employ the same principle so the carrier gas will have its quota of vapor and will not "steal" it from the suspended particles intended for deposition.[52]

Gas-powered (pneumatic) nebulizers

General description. Although the jet instruments can be used for both aerosol generation and humidification, for the sake of simplicity we will refer to them as nebulizers and differentiate between their specific uses when indicated. The jet nebulizer is the most versatile of this group of instruments and enjoys the most widespread usage. It is simple, can function without moving parts, and is based on the Bernoulli effect as illustrated in the simplified sketch of Fig. 10-9. Although jet nebulizers assume many shapes and sizes, they all have the fundamental features shown in the illustration. A source of gas pres-

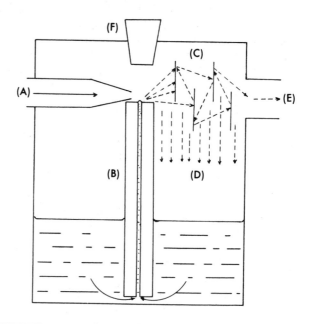

Fig. 10-9   Principle of jet nebulization. (See text for explanation.) (Modified from Egan, D.F.: Conn. Med. 31:353, 1967.)

sure must be provided that may be a simple hand-operated rubber bulb, a motorized compressor, or tanked gas. The gas enters the nebulizer chamber through a restricted orifice, providing a jet stream of high velocity *(A)*. The jet is directed across the end of a fine capillary tube *(B)*, the other end of which is immersed in the solution to be nebulized. The high velocity of the gas produces a local drop in pressure immediately adjacent to the capillary tube opening, and because the reservoir surface is subjected to atmospheric pressure, liquid is forced up the capillary *(solid arrows)*. As it reaches the top of the tube, the liquid is continuously blown off by the gas jets as small particles and thrown against one or more barriers called baffles *(C)*. Again, these baffles can be of many shapes such as small spheres, rods, or plates, or the configuration of the nebulizer chamber may function as a baffle. Here the particles are further fragmented, and many coalesce into masses too large to transport; these return to the reservoir as a condensate *(D)*. The outflow gas to the patient *(E)* contains aerosol particles of the desired therapeutic size. Many chambers provide an optional opening for the introduction of air into the gas-particle mixture *(F)*. When opened, the jet gas draws room air into the chamber (termed *air entrainment*), providing an increased flow through the nebulizer to the patient, increasing the rate of nebulization of the reservoir, and thus administering more liquid per unit of time. The need for such an additional source of gas varies with the instrument and its specific use, a matter to which we refer later. However, it must be remembered that chang-

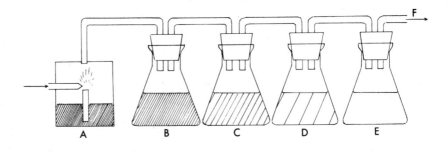

Fig. 10-10   Demonstration of the principle of liquid filtration in the production of microaerosols. Shading of the liquid represents the concentration of dye. (See text for further explanation.)

ing the physical environment of a nebulization chamber may alter the character of the aerosol output, especially in terms of the effect of the turbulence of higher flows on particle stability. These are influences that can be determined by carefully controlled measurements of equipment performance under various conditions.

Liquid filtration nebulizers.[53] Nebulizers of this type are reportedly able to produce aerosol particles consistently less than 0.5μ in diameter, the so-called microaerosols, or submicronic particles. Technically, they are classified according to a "D" series, such as D.10, etc., up to D.37, depending on size, particular structure, and other specifications. The basic feature of these nebulizers is the use of the nebulized solution as the baffling system of the units. The principle depends on the observation that if a mass of aerosolized liquid particles of heterogeneous sizes is brought into contact with successive volumes of the liquid, particles of increasingly smaller size will be removed from the aerosol until only completely stable, very small particles remain in suspension. Fig. 10-10 demonstrates this in the simplest fashion. Container A represents a typical air jet, nebulizing a dye-colored solution, whereas containers B to E are a variable number of glass flasks containing, initially, volumes of the uncolored solvent used to prepare the nebulizing solution. The flasks are connected in series so that the total output of the nebulizer will pass through each one in succession. In operation the solvent in each flask becomes increasingly colored, until one flask will show none. Thus relatively large numbers of large particles are trapped by the solvent in flask A, deeply staining the fluid, but by the time the aerosol issues from the last flask (at F), the particles are of such a uniformly small and stable size that none are baffled.

The use of this "scrubbing" process for the removal of unwanted large liquid particles in commercial nebulizers is modified according to the need of space economy and is illustrated in Fig. 10-11. A heterogeneous aerosol is generated by an air jet immersed in solution at A and passes upward through a series of constrictions (B). Turbulent flow removes from the stream all but the smallest and most stable particles, condensing them so that they return to

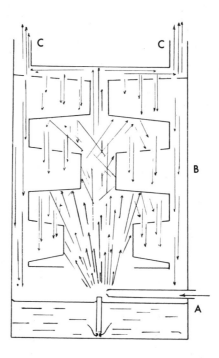

Fig. 10-11   Use of liquid filtration in an aerosol generator. Turbulent flow through the constrictions removes all but the smallest particles. (See text for description.)

the reservoir. Those particles leaving the ports *(C)*, in order to have escaped the scrubbing turbulence, are submicronic in size.

Inert gas-powered (metered dose) nebulizers. Popular because of their compactness and ease of operation, nebulizers with a self-contained power supply are in widespread use. They are made of a small vial containing the solution (or powder) to be nebulized and a physiologically inert gas under pressure as a propellant. With the supplied mouthpiece in place, a slight squeeze releases a small valve allowing the gas to nebulize the medication and deliver it in self-limited premeasured doses.

There is an unresolved controversy as to just how inert are the propellant gases of these units (and household commercial aerosols, as well.)[54-58] The gases are of a chemical group known as fluorocarbons, with many members, but of which Freon 11 is one of the most widely used. Animal experiments suggest that fluorocarbons may cause cardiac arrhythmias and death if inhaled in the presence of hypoxemia, and rhythm disturbances in humans have been reported. It is speculated that instances of sudden or unexpected deaths in asthmatic patients may be a result of fluorocarbon-induced cardiac arrest. This view is by no means unanimous, and some investigators question the evidence on which the claims of propellant hazards are based. Much of the dispute centers on the validity of projecting experimental animal data to humans and on the duration of fluorocarbon blood and tissue levels following inhalation. Despite the unsettled question of safety, gas-powered aerosol units are very popular, and as long as they continue to be used, patients should be instructed in their proper use and advised strongly to keep exposure to a minimum.

For the purpose of discussing the clinical use of jet nebulizers, we can arbitrarily divide them into two classes—intermittent nebulizers and reservoir nebulizers—although it will be obvious that there is no clear-cut line of demarcation between the two.

Intermittent medication nebulizers. This group comprises the relatively small instruments with a capacity of about 5 ml used for limited periods of time on an intermittent basis, mostly for the administration of pharmaceutic aerosols rather than water or humidity. The prototype is the so-called hand nebulizer, which combines a simple glass or plastic air jet powered by a hand-operated rubber squeeze bulb and is especially suited to the short-term administration of sympathomimetic bronchodilators (Chapter 11), for which it was originally designed. The therapist should be acquainted with the energy required to operate a hand bulb so that he or she appreciates the difficulty experienced by a patient attempting to use such a nebulizer for a long period of time. Most units of this type have air ports that permit two velocities of airflow and nebulization. In general, the slower rate without air entrainment is satisfactory, but the option permits adjusting therapy to individual needs. Simple though the instrument is, proper technique in its usage is essential for good results. All patients should be instructed in the nebulizer's use, with a demonstration by the therapist, and should not be permitted to rely only on the manufacturer's directions.

Two major points should be emphasized. First, the patient should be instructed to open the mouth widely so that the lips and teeth will not obstruct the aerosol flow, then hold the nebulizer so that its delivery port is directed toward the mouth but is about 1 inch away from the lips. This allows the aerosol to be entrained in the inspiratory airflow, but if the nebulizer tube is inserted into the mouth and the lips are tightly pursed about it, much of the aerosol will be deposited in the mouth. Second, the patient should be taught to inhale as slowly and deeply as possible and to deliver the first charge of aerosol just after starting an inhalation. The therapist will observe that many patients release the aerosol at, or even before, the start of inhalation, depositing much of it outside the respiratory tract. Depending on the length of inhalation, two or three aerosol doses may be delivered in one breath. At end-inspiration the breath should be held for 2 or 3 seconds to allow maximum aerosol distribution and deposition.

For the administration of mucolytic, proteolytic, or antibiotic aerosols (Chapter 11), or for longer therapy with dilute bronchodilators, the small-volume nebulizers can be adapted to a power source. A small compressor is most practical, since it does not need the pressure regulator or flow meter of tanked gas and is safe for home use. For treatments that may last up to 30 or

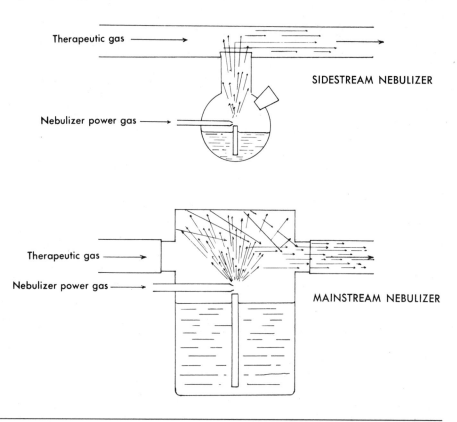

Therapeutic gas ⟶

SIDESTREAM NEBULIZER

Nebulizer power gas ⟶

Therapeutic gas ⟶

Nebulizer power gas ⟶

MAINSTREAM NEBULIZER

Fig. 10-12 Diagrammatic comparison of sidestream and mainstream nebulizers. The aerosol of the sidestream unit is considerably diluted by the large volume of dry therapeutic gas and provides limited humidity. It is used primarily to administer medication. The entire therapeutic gas flow passes through the mainstream nebulizer chamber and is able to pick up significant moisture. The effectiveness of this nebulizer can be increased by heating the fluid reservoir.

60 minutes, the use of an aerosol mask is advisable. Not only is the patient spared the nuisance and fatigue of holding a nebulizer to his or her face, but the design of such a mask holds a mass of aerosol particles about the mouth as a reservoir from which the patient can inhale. Since nebulization during the exhalation is wasteful of medication, a simple Y-connector can be inserted in the tubing from the pump to the nebulizer, with the stem of the Y connected to the pump and one of the arms to the nebulizer. The other arm, left free, can be obstructed by the finger during inhalation to permit nebulization and can be released during exhalation to shunt the airflow away from the nebulizer. Although the same general pattern of slow deep breathing is advised for prolonged therapy, as was described earlier, the patient should be warned about overbreathing to the point of discomfort from either the effort involved or possible hypocapnia.

One of the virtues of a skilled respiratory therapist is versatility. With knowledge of equipment and the objectives of therapy, he or she is able to choose the right instrument, or combination of instruments, to accomplish these objectives. The therapist will frequently be called on to use imagination and ingenuity in setting up equipment to suit the needs of patients with special problems. Because of the great variety and numbers of jet nebulizers, it would be impractical as well as needless to attempt to describe the idiosyncrasies of each, but we mention a few operational principles common to all which the therapist should bear in mind. To begin with, the relationship between the output of the jet nebulizer and the main flow of gas being humidified is important, and it may be described in one of two ways, *sidestream* nebulization or *mainstream* nebulization.[4,5,18] In sidestream nebulization the aerosol is discharged into the therapeutic gas flow between the delivery instrument and the patient, as shown in Fig. 10-12. The nebulizer has its own separate gas power supply, which is smaller than the therapeutic gas flow, and when the aerosol mixes with the greater volume of dry gas in the patient delivery tube, it is too diluted to raise the humidity of the gas to maximum. The sidestream method is mostly used with mechanical ventilators of the inspiratory positive-pressure type, or in hand-held, compressor-driven nebulizers. Although it is limited in the humidity it contributes, the moisture is usually sufficient for short-term therapy. Primarily, it is an effective way of administering medication during a treatment, and most of the pharmaceutic agents described in Chapter 11 can be given by this route.

In mainstream nebulization the entire gas flow to the patient passes through the chamber of the nebulizer. These units may be either small medication nebulizers or larger reservoir nebulizers (described next). When they are used inline with flow from a ventilator or from room air during spontaneous breathing, the extra flow passing through increases the aerosol output and humidity levels.[18,59] Some small nebulizers available can be used in either a sidestream or mainstream fashion.[5] Generally the sidestream method should produce fine, "dry" aerosol of small droplet size and would help optimize conditions for delivering bronchodilator drugs toward smaller airways. Using the same nebulizer but in a mainstream fashion, more aerosol leaves the unit, increasing volume output.[59] In this case drugs benefiting from increased volume deposition such as mucolytics or local anesthetics may be optimally given by this mainstream aerosol.

Reservoir nebulizers. As the name implies, reservoir nebulizers have a large capacity for the solution to be nebulized and are intended for prolonged intermittent or continuous use. Thus they are predominantly used for aerosolized water or humidity therapy, although occasionally for more active agents such as mucolytics or detergents. The most commonly used devices of this type generally incorporate an air entrainment system, making them function in a mainstream fashion. Often driven by oxygen to the jet, these units can generally entrain enough room air to dilute the oxygen to various levels. Common reusable reservoir nebulizers can reduce the 100% oxygen driving the jet to near 40% oxygen by entrainment and mixing of room air. Newer disposable units can produce an oxygen mixture of near 30%.

This air entrainment increases both aerosol and total gas flow output from these reservoir nebulizers but not necessarily in similar proportions. While aerosol output may increase by 1.5 to 2 times by adding air entrainment, total flow output may increase 4 to 8 times, depending on the amount of air entrainment available. Therefore, while total aerosol output increases with air entrainment, the concentration or density of the aerosol (milliliters of aerosol per liter of gas) decreases. Dilution of oxygen or jet gas in these nebulizers functions on principles further described in Chapter 12.

Temperature considerations. We already know how temperature affects humidity conditions from previous discussions of humidifiers, and these principles also apply to nebulizers. Some reservoir entrainment nebulizers can be heated to provide temperature control of the delivered mist.[5] Heating the water to be aerosolized raises gas temperature leaving the nebulizer and thereby increases the humidity carrying capacity (Fig. 10-1). This can increase the water output from the nebulizer a considerable amount by raising the absolute humidity. If the unit is not heated, cooling as a result of evaporation occurs, and absolute humidity is less.

It has been demonstrated that with unheated jet- or bubble-humidifying devices driven with oxygen, the reservoir water temperature drops significantly.[63] At flows of up to 12 ℓ/min, the temperature of the water may drop up to 13°C below its starting ambient temperature within 1 hour. Even the small-volume sidearm nebulizer shows a temperature drop of up to 5°C in 10 minutes.

The effects of temperature on aerosols after they have left the nebulizer are also significant. For instance, both small and reservoir nebulizers operated "cold" will produce aerosols at temperatures less than that of room air. As the aerosol travels to the patient some warming can occur, and this will allow more capacity for evaporation of water particles and an increase in absolute humidity. Relative humidity will remain near 100% as the temperature rises because of evaporation of water particles.

Table 10-4 Influence of tubing on vapor temperature*	**Distance from reservoir**		**Temperature in tube (°C)**
	cm	**ft**	
	30.5	1	48.5
	60.9	2	40.5
	91.4	3	37.0
	121.9	4	35.0
	152.4	5	34.5

From Wells, R.E., Jr., et al.: Humidification of oxygen during inhalation therapy, N. Engl. J. Med. **268**:644, 1963.

*Reservoir temperature = 53°C; tube length = 153 cm; internal diameter = 1.9 cm.

Heated reservoir nebulizers produce warm, humid aerosols that will cool as they travel through tubing toward the patient. As with heated humidifiers, this drop in temperature causes condensation of water vapor. The vapor will condense both on the walls of the tubing and on the aerosol particles, increasing their diameter and volume.

Table 10-4 illustrates the change in gas temperature at various distances from the heated reservoir using large-bore tubing.[63] Measurements were made at 1-foot intervals from the reservoir. Note that at a 1-foot distance the air was 48.5°C and that at only 3 feet it was normal body temperature of 37°C. Referring to the chart in Fig. 10-1 we again see that with this temperature drop, only half the original water vapor carried (assuming saturation) can be

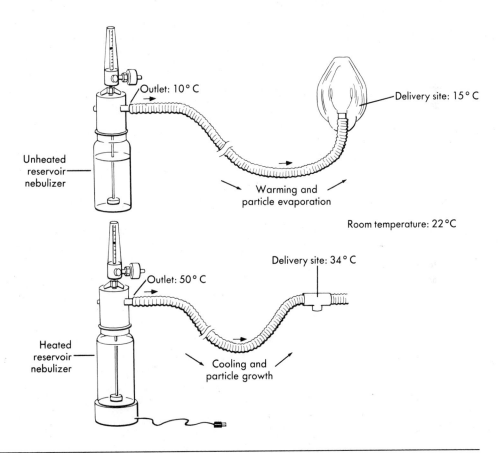

Fig. 10-13   Comparison of unheated versus heated reservoir nebulizers. Output from the unheated (cool) nebulizer is cooler than room temperature due to evaporation of aerosol in the nebulizer. As the aerosol warms on the way to the patient delivery site, further evaporation of particles occurs. Output from the heated nebulizer is hot and humid. Cooling occurs as the aerosol travels through tubing exposed to cooler room and water vapor condenses on aerosol particles, causing them to "grow" larger.

carried at 37°C. The condensation will cause the particles to increase their size, and some will fall out of the air stream. "Rain out" of water in the tubing will be increased, as compared to the same nebulizer used unheated.

It should also be noted in Table 10-4 that the drop in temperature from 1 to 2 feet is 8°C, while between 4 and 5 feet the drop in temperature is only 0.5°C. This illustrates that nearest the heated reservoir the temperature gradient from reservoir to room air is the greatest, causing the greatest heat lost. Fig. 10-13 illustrates the difference in heated and unheated reservoir nebulizers with respect to temperature effects and output.

Flow limitations. The jets used in gas-powered nebulizers are restricted orifices. Most nebulizers used in respiratory therapy operate with oxygen or compressed air from a source supplying up to 50 pounds per square inch (psi) of pressure. Because the jets are so small, there is an upper limit of flow for each nebulizer when operated at the maximum available pressure as a result of principles covered in previous chapters. Generally, common reservoir entrainment nebulizers are limited to 12 to 15 ℓ/min of gas through the jet alone when 50 psi is applied. If a small compressor is used with a less than 50 psi capability, the jet flows will be less. Some small intermittent medication nebulizers have very small jets and so may only provide 8 to 10 ℓ/min of flow. Therapists should know the maximum flow through the nebulizer jets they use for practical purposes. Total airflow from entrainment nebulizers is partly influenced by the jet flows. Certain systems such as oxygen hoods and tents require minimum flows that are greater than some nebulizers can provide (Chapter 12).

Hydro-Sphere nebulizer

To some degree the Hydro-Sphere is a modification of the jet nebulizer with same indications for its use. The basic difference between the two is the mechanism by which pressured gas is brought into contact with the liquid to be aerosolized. Instead of a capillary tube-jet complex, the Hydro-Sphere uses gravity flow over a glass sphere, as demonstrated in Fig. 10-14. A pumping mechanism (not shown) carries solution from the reservoir *(A)* through tube *(B)* to the top of a hollow glass sphere *(C)*. The solution is continuously and gently poured onto the upper pole of the sphere at *(D)*, where it distributes itself by gravity as a very thin film *(E)* over the spherical surface. The film is greatly exaggerated in the sketch for illustration purposes. A gas source, at pressures between 10 and 50 psi, enters the hollow sphere at *(F)*, pressurizing the interior of the sphere *(G)*, rupturing the overlying liquid film and dispersing it as small particles. An impactor baffle *(H)* removes the large droplets, permitting the outflow only of those within the therapeutic range. Excess, unnebulized fluid flows down the sphere and is directed by the sphere's tapered base back into the reservoir for recirculation *(I)*.

Among the virtues claimed for this aerosol generator are (1) the absence of moving parts minimizes maintenance; (2) 97% of its aerosol output is said to be within the 1μ to 10μ diameter range, and 50% below 5μ; (3) aerosol is delivered at a temperature of 6° to 10°F below ambient; and (4) there is an

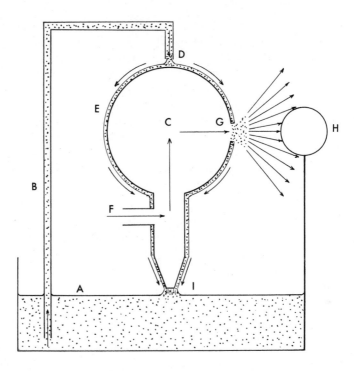

Fig. 10-14   Hydro-Sphere nebulizer. (See text for description.)

apparent consistent aerosol density over a wide range of airflows. Several published reports support the efficacy of the Hydro-Sphere's performance, and only the test of time is needed for final confirmation.[21,64,65]

Impeller nebulizer

With an impeller nebulizer, physical force of a rapidly rotating disc is used to break up water into fine particles and to emit it as a heavy mist. The disc, driven by an electric motor, sucks water from a reservoir and literally throws it through a meshed or slotted baffle. Of less uniform size than the particles from a well-constructed jet nebulizer, the aerosol does produce a grossly visible fog and affords the inspired air a good supply of water particles for evaporation, although, with the heterogeneous particle sizes, there tends to be more "rain out" about a patient enclosed in a tent. Because there is no need for a compressed gas source and the units are compact and easy to operate, the impeller nebulizer is popular for home use. It is available in a number of sizes and output capacities, some decorator styled for room size humidification.

Ultrasonic nebulizer

The ultrasonic nebulizer is a complex electronic instrument that has been adequately described elsewhere, and here we only briefly review its major features and applications.[66-68] An ultrasonic nebulizer consists of two compartments—a power chamber and a nebulizing chamber. The heart of the unit is a transducer, a device that is activated by one form of energy and relays it in another form. The transducer is ceramic and is classified as *piezoelectric* because it is able to change pressure *(piezo-)* energy into electric, and vice versa. Thus, when electrical energy is applied to a piezoelectric transducer, the latter responds by a rapidly oscillating change in shape, manifested by physical vibration, a form of pressure energy. Conversely, if the transducer is subjected to pressure, it will convert such energy to electrical.

In the ultrasonic nebulizer, alternating current is applied to the transducer, and electrical energy is transformed into vibrational energy at frequencies beyond the range of human hearing. Commercial units operate at frequencies of from 1.3 to 1.4 megacycles/sec. The rapid vibrations are carried through water (called a couplant) and are focused on a flexible diaphragm supporting the liquid to be nebulized, in the aerosol chamber. The diaphragm vibrates in sympathy and literally shakes the liquid into a mass of small particles. The transfer of energy is accompanied by the production of a small amount of heat, varying from 3° to 10°C above ambient. The aerosol particles can be carried to the patient by a small blower provided with the instrument, by oxygen as a carrier gas, or by the patient's own ventilation. Depending on the make and model of nebulizer, there are adjustments for variable aerosol concentrations, and up to 6 ml of water can be nebulized per minute. Because of the high aerosol output, heating is not necessary, and the therapy can be given at room temperature.

Fig. 10-15 demonstrates some of the important characteristics of ultrasonic nebulization. Each model is a rough representation of a nebulizer, showing the electrical input to the piezoelectric transducer at the bottom, the resulting vibrational wave transmission through a couplant liquid to a responsive diaphragm in the center, and the effect of diaphragm vibrations on the aerosol chamber liquid.[69] Vibrational frequency determines the response of the liquid surface to vertical oscillations. Fig. 10-15, *A,* shows that low-frequency energy, less than 0.8 megacycle/sec, produces surface waves, the crests of which break into droplets greater than 25μ in diameter, but no fine mist. As the frequency increases above 0.8 megacycle/sec, we see from Fig. 10-15, *B,* that the liquid surface is pushed up into a column, like a fountain, emitting fine particles from its base and coarser droplets from its top.

Let us now consider the influence of electrical power on aerosol production. At low power levels, such as 30 watts applied per square centimeter of liquid surface, the effect is pulsatile, and the high-frequency-generated column breaks discontinuously into a wide range of particle sizes. As power increases to about 50 watts/cm^2, with continued high frequency, pulsed fog emission becomes continuous, and as demonstrated in Fig. 10-15, *C,* there is a steady production of high-density mist of fine particles. The final control over particle size of aerosol delivered to the patient is a function of baffling, often by a

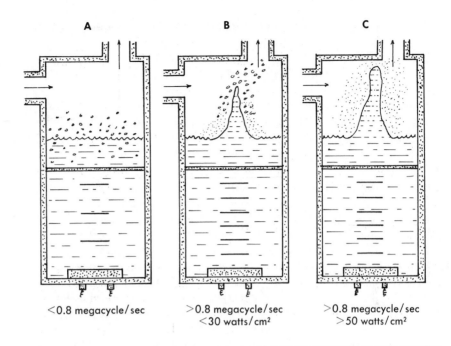

Fig. 10-15   Principles of aerosol production by ultrasonic nebulization. (See text for details.)

flow of air directed at the fountain. The higher the velocity of the impinging air stream, the smaller the emergent aerosol particles.

Clinical response testifies to the efficacy of ultrasonic nebulization and its ability to deposit water in the respiratory tract, but little specific information is available regarding mean particle size produced. On the one hand, it is asserted that measured mean values varied from 1μ to 10μ in diameter but with a narrow distribution range,[70] and on the other, it is claimed that the mass of particles falls within the 0.8μ to 1μ range with probable 80% deposition within the lung.[71] The lack of condensation of moisture on a piece of glass held in the aerosol steam indicates an effective stability of particle size.

In the process of determining the degree of humidity actually delivered to the respiratory tract, a revealing experiment was conducted on dogs.[71] Very small humidity transducers were introduced into the primary division of the bronchi and were attached to recorders responsive to the amount of water vapor with which the transducers were in contact. Calibrations were in arbitrary "humidity units," depending on the deflection of the recorder with known humidity. This permitted the comparison of the amount of moisture delivered to the airway with air-activated and ultrasonic nebulizers. Standard nebulizers increased bronchial vapor content an average of 0.18 units, whereas the ultrasonic achieved 0.71 and 4.03 units, on two volume settings. In addition, the duration of maintained humidity was longer with the ultrasonic than with the air-generated instruments.

With the large aerosol production of which the ultrasonic nebulizer is capable and the obvious penetration of water into the respiratory tract, the question of possible harm to the lung arose. Washing the lung with water or saline is known to disrupt its surface tension stability, presumably by the removal of pulmonary surfactant, and because it was important to know whether ultrasonic aerosolization posed the same risk, animal experimentations were carried out.[72,73] The lungs of dogs subjected to nebulization of isotonic saline and distilled water were examined, and no evidence of interference with surface tension stability was detected, even after 72 hours of aerosols. It was speculated that the small particle size and the total low fluid volume were not harmful, in this respect. On the other hand, after prolonged aerosol exposure all animals receiving saline mist, and a few of those on distilled water, showed microscopic pulmonary changes consistent with bronchopneumonia. The deposition of hypertonic saline, the result of water evaporating from normal saline, was felt to be responsible. It was concluded that continuous wetting of the lung with ultrasonic mist for long periods of time might be deleterious, although no time-limit safety guides were suggested.

In addition to its large aerosol volume, the ultrasonic nebulizer has other physical virtues. Of importance is the independence of the aerosol production from the flow of the breathing gas. Whereas the output of the jet nebulizer depends on the flow of its power gas, the ultrasonic nebulizer can dispense a steady particle volume regardless of the flow. This is an advantage when the nebulizer is incorporated into an oxygen therapy or mechanical ventilation procedure, since it will not materially disturb the therapeutic gas flow pattern. Because the only grossly moving part of the instrument is the small blower, operation is quiet and inoffensive. Parts are easily cleaned and sterilized, and the inflow can be filtered.

The clinical use of the ultrasonic nebulizer is extensive, but it is of prime value when the actual deposition of water in the respiratory tract is desired. The basic indication therefore is the liquefaction by dilution of bronchial secretions, and a secondary use is the maximum humidification of inhaled air. It is effective in stimulating cough for both therapeutic and diagnostic purposes, when its full output volume is held close to the mouth and slowly inhaled. Water aerosol is usually more irritating than saline for this purpose and is valuable in inducing a sputum specimen for laboratory examination, but it is seemingly equally useful in wetting thick bronchial secretions and stimulating expectoration. In general, the ability of the adult patient to cooperate with the techniques employing simpler and less expensive, heated or unheated, aerosol generators and humidifiers obviates the need for the ultrasonic instrument except for unusual circumstances. However, if mobilization of secretions by other methods is unsatisfactory, and it is thought that the problem can be corrected by an increase in the density of inhaled water particles, then an ultrasonic unit should be used. Unfortunately, there are no good data based on sound scientific principles that let us set up objective criteria for using aerosol therapy. Techniques employed in a specific instance generally depend on the personal experience and bias of the responsible attending physician. This is a branch of therapeutics desperately in need of practical basic and clinical research.

Ultrasonic nebulization has been used in all the usual pediatric diseases characterized by obstructive secretions and has also been used in the treatment of cystic fibrosis (cystic fibrosis of the pancreas, mucoviscidosis). Of unknown cause, cystic fibrosis is a complex hereditary disease involving several organ systems, characterized by a malfunction of mucus-secreting glands with the production of markedly viscid mucus. Early descriptions of the disease emphasized cystic destruction of the pancreas secondary to plugging of its excretory ducts by thick secretions and gave the disease its not quite accurate name. Because this disease is not uncommon, the student is encouraged to become familiar with its many clinical features, but we concern ourselves here with its pulmonary complications. Fatalities are usually a result of respiratory failure from pulmonary mucoviscidosis. Along with secretions elsewhere in the body, bronchial mucus is remarkably thick and tenacious, severely obstructing airways and leading to secondary bronchitis, bronchiectasis, emphysema, and repeated pulmonary infections. Although the total treatment program involves many aspects, none is more important than the constant effort to maintain airway patency. To this end the prolonged inhalation of aerosolized water has long been standard therapy, either on an intermittent basis when secretions develop acutely or on a regular regimen of a prescribed number of daily hours in a mist tent. In these situations ultrasonic nebulization as a valuable tool has been debated.[43,62]

The deposition of water in the respiratory tract may be able to thin secretions by dilution and to facilitate their removal by the natural cough mechanism, by vigorous postural drainage, and occasionally by aspiration. For prolonged nebulization there is no universal agreement as to the relative values of water (preferably sterile) or isotonic saline. Some believe that water is safer because the immature kidney of infants and small children has difficulty in excreting the added sodium load of saline, retention of which might seriously disturb water and electrolyte balance.[74] Others prefer normal saline because of the irritating effects of such a large volume of water particles.[75] During "normal" or nonacute phases of cystic fibrosis, as a prophylactic measure many patients are placed in a mist tent during the sleeping hours, a technique employed as part of home care that often reduces the number of hospitalizations for acute obstruction.

Although water and saline are the two most frequently used media in the ultrasonic nebulizer, there is increasing interest in the use of other substances with pharmacologic action. There has been concern about using substances with pharmacologic action because of the fear that the vibrational energy of ultrasonic nebulization might degrade or disrupt the structure of chemical substances and either destroy their specific action or produce harmful by-products.[74] However, studies of the complex relationships between high-frequency vibrations and mist production have resolved this apprehension. The power, or energy, applied to the target surface of an ultrasonic aerosol generator, and measured in watts per square centimeter rather than the sonic frequency, determines both fog output and the degree of particle damage. It has been shown that instruments with an acoustic power output of less than 20 watts/cm^2 and an aerosol production less than 2 ml/min will not degrade substances aerosolized. These are known as *drug nebulizers* and can safely dispense pharmaceuticals. Power outputs greater than 50 watts/cm^2 required to generate flows exceeding 2 ml/min are apt to disrupt the chemical structure of aerosolized particles. Such instruments produce large volumes of particles and are used as *fog nebulizers*.[76]

Another major limitation to drug nebulization is viscosity, and in general, liquids with viscosities greater than 10 centipoises are difficult to aerosolize. There still are no dependable guidelines for ultrasonic nebulization, but to date at least water, normal saline, saline propylene glycol, acetylcysteine, and some antibiotics have been so aerosolized. We have no way of knowing, however, whether or not the use of jet nebulization might have been just as effective.

Let us summarize ultrasonic nebulization with the following statements: (1) it is effective in producing a large volume of high-density mist; (2) sonic frequencies above 0.8 megacycle/sec prepare the necessary column or fountain of the liquid to be nebulized, while 20 to 50 watts/cm^2 power input to the transducer determines the volume of fog output; (3) delivered aerosol particle size is controlled by baffling; (4) solutes may be degraded by power levels of 50 watts/cm^2 needed for high-volume fog production but not by power at or below 20 watts/cm^2; (5) solutions with viscosities above 10 centipoises are difficult to nebulize with ultrasound.

Considerations for aerosol therapy	While aerosol therapy can be a clinically valuable tool when properly applied, certain hazards and considerations are associated with its use.

Medication side effects. Many of the drugs aerosolized for inhalation are extremely potent with considerable potential for producing undesired side effects along with their therapeutic benefit. Chapter 11 discusses various drugs commonly used and specific side effects, but some general statements are made here.

It is generally accepted that bronchodilator drugs given by aerosol inhalation can diminish the systemic side effects while giving maximum benefit compared to intravenous or oral administration of the same drug. This effect is probably enhanced when nebulizers producing small particles are used in a fashion that optimizes conditions of airway deposition, such as using the nebulizer as a sidestream unit, using dilute solutions over 10 to 20 minutes, and using the proper ventilatory pattern while the patient is in a relaxed, upright position.

In general, bronchodilators may cause cardiovascular effects, muscle tremors and nervousness. Other drugs such as mucolytics can cause bronchospasm. These effects should be monitored for by the therapist.

Increased airway resistance. It has been shown that ultrasonically produced, high-density bland aerosols can increase airway resistance, especially in patients with respiratory disease.[44] Administration of bronchodilators before high-density mist therapy can help prevent this problem. Heated aerosols given to the same subjects did not produce the same increase in airway resistance, but high-density cool aerosols from gas-powered nebulizers were not tested.[44] The chance of causing bronchospasm with wheezing and dyspnea should always be considered while giving large-volume aerosol therapy. Monitoring patients for these problems includes listening to breath sounds before, during, and after therapy, observation of the patient's breathing pattern and overall appearance, and most essentially, communicating with the patient during therapy.

It is well known that common mucolytics such as acetylcysteine can produce significant bronchospasms in sensitive persons. Therefore it is generally recommended that a bronchodilator drug also be used to prevent or minimize this occurrence.[40,42]

Evacuation of mobilized secretions. Care should always be taken to ensure that patients are capable of clearing secretions once they are loose and being mobilized following aerosol therapy. Proper coughing techniques, controlled deep breathing, and/or postural drainage and percussion should accompany aerosol therapy to promote secretion evacuation from the bronchial tree (see Chapter 15). For those patients unable to clear secretions adequately, airway suctioning or fiberoptic bronchoscopy is indicated.

Infection control. All aerosol-creating devices have the potential for spraying bacteria-laden mist into the patient's respiratory tract. Bacterial contamination of medical aerosols is well known and can be minimized by conscientious cleaning and disinfecting procedures.[77] Usually the contaminating organisms are gram-negative bacilli, commonly *Pseudomonas aeruginosa*. Various procedures have been recommended for reducing contamination and infection for respiratory therapy equipment.[12,77] Frequent changing (e.g., every 12 to 24 hours) and disinfection of equipment are essential. Precautions should also be taken to avoid cross contamination between patients.

Drug reconcentration. Before closing the subject of aerosol therapy, note should be made of a hazard of potential clinical importance. During the baffling and recycling of solutions undergoing nebulization, as droplets are continuously returned to the fluid reservoir, there has been observed a gradual increase in the concentration of the solution yet to be nebulized. The risk of drug toxicity is evident, as the patient is subjected to increasingly higher concentrations during the course of therapy. It was at first believed that this phe-

Table 10-5
Drug reconcentration
during ultrasonic
nebulization

Aerosolization time (minutes)	Percent acetylcysteine	
	Ambient air	Humiditied air
0	20.5	20.5
5	21.7	20.4
10	23.0	20.2
15	26.4	20.1
20	29.0	20.2
25	32.8	20.6
30	40.1	20.5

Modified from Glick, R.V.: Drug reconcentration in aerosol generators, Inhal. Ther. **15**:179, 1970.

nomenon was primarily a characteristic of jet nebulizers, but an excellent study has demonstrated that *drug reconcentration* is a function of both jet and ultrasonic nebulizers.[78]

One of the drugs used was acetylcysteine, and when subjected to 30 minutes of ultrasonic nebulization using ambient air as the carrier gas, concentrations of the drug rose from 20.5% to 40.1%. The experiment then demonstrated that when control of temperature and humidity ensured full water vapor saturation of the carrier gas, reconcentration did not occur. Table 10-5 vividly illustrates the effect of this humidification. The conclusion drawn was that in the presence of a humidity deficit of the carrier gas, the greater ease of evaporation of water-solvent molecules than of the heavier drug solute progressively raised the concentration of the shrinking residual solution.

In summary, with the widespread indications for aerosol therapy and the increasing variety of equipment appearing on the market, the respiratory therapist who has supervisory responsibility is faced with a difficult test of judgment. The medical director of a department of respiratory therapy and the hospital administrator will often rely on the therapist's recommendations as to type and quality of equipment to be purchased and the therapist must weigh the therapeutic value of each proposed addition to the inventory against its expected use and cost. The therapist's objective will be to provide the maximum service to a heterogeneous hospital patient population, within the limits of his or her budget, and he or she will have to consider the initial cost of new equipment, the service required to maintain it in workable condition, and the probability that all members of the department will not use it with the same degree of efficiency and uniformity. The decision may be a compromise between what the therapist would like to have and what is practical. He or she will find from experience that it is generally unwise to disburse a large fraction of the budget for the purchase of a few expensive items which, although desirable, may be essential for only a few patients when the same expenditure could provide more less sophisticated items that would be satisfactory for many. Again, this underscores the need for a competent therapist to understand fully the merits of his or her equipment and the general therapeutic needs of the hospital's patients.

References

1. Pierce, A.K., and Saltzman, H.A., chairmen: Conference on the scientific basis for respiratory therapy, Am. Rev. Resp. Dis. **110**(2):1, 1974.
2. Pierce, A.K.: Scientific basis of in-hospital respiratory therapy, Am. Rev. Respir. Dis. **122**(2):1, 1980.
3. Brain, J.: Aerosol and humidity therapy, Am. Rev. Respir. Dis. **122**(2):17, 1980.
4. Cushing, I.E., and Miller, W.F.: Considerations in humidification by nebulization, Dis. Chest **34**:388, 1958.
5. McPherson, S.P.: Respiratory therapy equipment, ed. 2, St. Louis, 1981, The C.V. Mosby Co.
6. Inglestent, S.: Studies on the conditioning of air in the respiratory tract, Acta Otolaryngoi. [Suppl.] (Stockh.) 131, 1956.
7. Sara, C.: The management of patients with a tracheostomy, Med. J. Aust. **1**:99, 1965.
8. Sykes, M.K., McNicol, M.W., and Campbell, E.J.M.: Respiratory failure, ed. 2, Oxford, England, 1976, Blackwell Scientific Publications.
9. Bendixen, H.H., et al.: Respiratory care, St. Louis, 1965, The C.V. Mosby Co.
10. Shapiro, B.A., Harrison, R.A., and Trout, C.A.: Clinical applications of respiratory care, ed. 2, Chicago, 1979, Year Book Medical Publishers, Inc.
11. Petty, T.L.: Intensive and rehabilitative respiratory care, ed. 2, Philadelphia, 1974, Lea & Febiger.
12. Burton, G.G., Gee, G.N., and Hodgkin, J.E., editors: Respiratory care, a guide to clinical practice, Philadelphia, 1977, J.B. Lippincott Co.
13. Forbes, A.R.: Humidification and mucus flow in the intubated trachea, Br. J. Anaesth. **45**:874, 1973.
14. Forbes, A.R.: Temperature, humidity and mucus flow in the intubated trachea, Br. J. Anaesth. **46**:29, 1974.
15. Chalon, Jr., et al.: Humidity and the anesthestized patient, Anesthesiology **50**:195, 1979.
16. Chalon, Jr., Loew, D.A.Y., and Malebranche, J.: Effects of dry anesthetic gases on tracheobronchial ciliated epithelium, Anesthesiology **36**:338, 1972.
17. Tsuda, T., et al.: Optimum humidification of air administered to a tracheostomy in dogs, Br. J. Anaesth. **49**:965, 1977.
18. Cushing, I.E., and Miller, W.F.: In Safar, P., editor: Respiratory therapy, Philadelphia, 1965, F.A. Davis Co.
19. Miller, W.F.: Fundamental principles of aerosol therapy, Respir. Care **17**:295, 1972.
20. Miller, W.F.: Aerosol therapy in acute and chronic respiratory disease, Arch. Intern. Med. **131**:148, 1973.
21. Klein, E.F., et al.: Performance characteristics of conventional and prototype humidifiers and nebulizers, Chest **64**:690, 1973.
22. Dolan, G.K., and Zawadski, J.J.: Performance characteristics of low-flow humidifiers, Respir. Care **21**:393, 1976.
23. Hemholz, H.F., and Saposnick, A.B.: In Burton, G.G., Gee, G.N., and Hodgkin, J.E., editors: Respiratory care, a guide to clinical practice, Philadelphia, 1977, J.B. Lippincott Co.
24. Poulton, T.J., and Downs, J.B.: Humidification of rapidly flowing gas, Crit. Care Med. **9**:59, 1981.
25. Comer, P.B., et al.: Airway maintenance in patients with long-term endotracheal intubation, Crit. Care Med. **4**:211, 1976.
26. Neuberger, H.: Condensation nuclei: their significance in atmospheric pollution, Mechanical Engineering **70**:221, 1948.
27. Goetz, A.: The physicochemical behavior of submicron aerosols, Am. Rev. Respir. Dis. **83**:410, 1961.
28. Brown, J.H., et al.: The retention of particulate matter in the human lung, Am. J. Public Health **40**:450, 1960.
29. Lovejoy, F.W., Jr., and Morrow, P.E.: Aerosols, bronchodilators, and mucolytic agents, Anesthesiology **23**:460, 1962.
30. Hatch, T.F., and Gross, P.: Pulmonary deposition and retention of inhaled aerosols, New York, 1964, Academic Press, Inc.
31. Altshuler, B., et al.: Aerosol deposition in the human respiratory tract, Arch. Industr. Health **15**:293, 1957.
32. Dautrebande, L., et al.: Lung deposition of fine dust particles, Arch. Industr. Health **16**:179, 1957.
33. Brain, J.D., and Valberg, P.A.: Deposi-

tion of aerosol in the respiratory tract, state of the art, Am. Rev. Respir. Dis. **120:**1325, 1979.

34. Hayek, A.: Cellular structure and mucus activity in the bronchial tree and aleoli, Ciba Foundation Symposium on Pulmonary Structure and Function, Boston, 1962, Little, Brown & Co.

35. Hatch, T.F., and Gross, P.: Pulmonary deposition and retention of inhaled aerosols, New York, 1964, Academic Press, Inc.

36. Hatch, T.F.: Distribution and deposition of inhaled particles in the respiratory tract, Bacteriol. Rev. **25:**237, 1961.

37. Dautrebande, L.: Microaerosols, New York, 1962, Academic Press, Inc.

38. Mercer, T.T., et al.: Output characteristics of several commercial nebulizers, Ann. Allergy **23:**314, 1965.

39. Muir, D.C.F.: Distribution of aerosol particles in exhaled air, J. Appl. Physiol. **23:**210, 1967.

40. Ziment, I.: Respiratory pharmacology and therapeutics, Philadelphia, 1978, W.B. Saunders Co.

41. Wanner, A., and Rao, A.: Clinical indications for and effects of bland, mucolytic and antimicrobial aerosols, Am. Rev. Respir. Dis. **122**(2):79, 1980.

42. Miller, W.F., and Geumei, A.M.: In Petty, T.L., editor: Chronic obstructive pulmonary disease, New York 1978, Marcel Dekker.

43. Miller, W.F., Johnston, F.F., and Tarkoff, M.P.: Use of ultrasonic aerosols with ventilatory assistors, J. Asthma Res. **5:**335, 1968.

44. Cheney, F.W., and Butler, J.: The effects of ultrasonically produced aerosols on airway resistance in man, Anesthesiology **29:**1099, 1968.

45. Yue, W.Y., and Cohen, S.S.: Sputum induction by newer inhalation methods in patients with pulmonary tuberculosis, Dis. Chest **51:**611, 1967.

46. Cohen, B.M., and Crandall, C.: Physiologic benefits of "thermo-fog" as a bronchodilator vehicle: acute ventilation responses of 93 patients, Am. J. Med. Sci. **247:**57, 1964.

47. Tomashefshki, J.F., et al.: An environmental contamination control unit for use during aerosol administration, Am. Rev. Respir. Dis. **96:**1246, 1967.

48. Hensler, N., et al.: The use of hypertonic aerosol in production of sputum for diagnosis of tuberculosis, Dis. Chest **40:**639, 1961.

49. Lillehei, J.P.: Sputum induction with heated aerosol inhalations for the diagnosis of tuberculosis, Am. Rev. Respir. Dis. **84:**276, 1961.

50. Umiker, W.O.: A new vista in pulmonary cytology: aerosol induction of sputum, Dis. Chest **39:**512, 1961.

51. Johnson, J.R., et al.: Aerosol-induced sputum: an effective, inexpensive method for nebulization of a super-heated mixture of 40 percent propylene glycol in isotonic saline. Dis. Chest **42:**251, 1962.

52. Egan, D.F.: Humidity and water aerosol therapy, Conn. Med. **31:**353, 1967.

53. Dautrebande, L.: Microaerosols, New York, 1962, Academic Press, Inc.

54. Taylor, G.J., IV, and Harris, W.S.: Cardiac toxicity of aerosol propellants, J.A.M.A. **214:**81, 1970.

55. Silverglade, A.: Cardiac toxicity of aerosol propellants, J.A.M.A. **222:**827, 1972.

56. Harris, W.: Aerosol propellants are toxic to the heart, J.A.M.A. **223:**1508, 1973.

57. Chiov, W.L.: Aerosol propellants: cardiac toxicity and long biological half-life, J.A.M.A. **227:**658, 1974.

58. Silverglade, A.: Aerosol propellants, J.A.M.A. **231:**136, 1975.

59. Mercer, T.T., Goddard, R.F., and Flores, R.L.: Effect of auxiliary air flow on the output characteristics of compressed-air nebulizers, Ann. Allergy **27:**211, 1969.

60. Lough, M.D., Doershuk, C.F., and Stern, R.C.: Pediatric respiratory therapy, ed. 2, Chicago, 1979, Year Book Medical Publishers, Inc.

61. Shibel, E.M., and Moser, K.M.: Respiratory emergencies, St. Louis, 1977, The C.V. Mosby Company.

62. Tabachmik, E., and Levison, H.: Clinical application of aerosols in pediatrics, Am. Rev. Respir. Dis. **122**(2):97, 1980.

63. Wells, R.E., et al.: Humidification of oxygen during inhalational therapy, N. Engl. J. Med. **268:**644, 1963.

64. Litt, M., and Swift, D.F.: The Babington nebulizer: a new principle for generation

of therapeutic aerosols, Am. Rev. Respir. Dis. **105**:308, 1972.

65. Swift, D.L.: Generation and respiratory deposition of therapeutic aerosols, Am. Rev. Respir. Dis. **122**(2):71, 1980.

66. Andrews, A.H., Jr.: Ultrasonic aerosol generator, Presbyt. St. Luke Hosp. Med. Bull. **3**:155, 1964.

67. Proceedings of the First Conference on Clinical Application of the Ultrasonic Nebulizer, Somerset, Pa., 1966, DeVilbiss Co.

68. Abramson, H.A., editor: Proceedings of the Second Conference on Clinical Application of the ultrasonic nebulizer, J. Asthma. Res. **5**:213-379, 1968.

69. Boucher, R.M.G., and Kreuter, J.: Ultrasonic nebulization, Ann. Allergy **26**:591, 1968.

70. Gauthier, W.D.: Operational characteristics of the ultrasonic nebulizer, Proceedings of the First Conference on Clinical Application of the Ultrasonic Nebulizer, Somerset, Pa., 1966, DeVilbiss Co.

71. Stevens, H.R., and Albregt, H.B.: Assessment of ultrasonic nebulization, Anesthesiology **27**:648, 1966.

72. Modell, J.H., et al.: Effect of ultrasonic nebulized suspensions on pulmonary surfactant, Dis. Chest **50**:627, 1966.

73. Modell, J.H., et al.: Effect of chronic exposure to ultrasonic aerosols on the lungs, Anesthesiology **28**:680, 1967.

74. Allan, D.: Artificial humidification, Med. Sci. **17**:41, 1966.

75. Doershuk, C.F., and Matthews, L.W.: Cystic fibrosis, Postgrad. Med. **40**:550, 1966.

76. Boucher, R.G.M., and Kreuter, J.: Fundamentals of the ultrasonic atomization of medicated solutions, Ann. Allergy **26**:591, 1968.

77. Pierce, A.K., and Sanford, J.P.: Bacterial contamination of aerosols, Arch. Intern. Med. **131**:156, 1973.

78. Glick, R.V.: Drug reconcentration in aerosol generators, Inhal. Ther. **15**:179, 1970.

Chapter 11   Pharmacology for respiratory therapy

JAMES A. PETERS

Respiratory pharmacology concerns those drugs that affect the pulmonary system. If all body systems were to be genetically and environmentally allowed to produce their quota of enzymes and substances necessary to maintain body functions, then drugs prescribed by a physician would never be needed. However, with respiratory patients, drugs are sometimes necessary to help the body meet its needs either temporarily or permanently. Determining when they are necessary is a responsibility of the physician. Administering those prescribed drugs in an intelligent and safe manner is the responsibility of the respiratory therapist.

Respiratory drugs can be administered through various means, but of primary concern for the therapist are those drugs that are administered by inhalation. These drugs include bronchodilators, mucolytics, expectorants, steroids, oxygen, various therapeutic gas mixtures, and occasionally antibiotics. Additionally, a local anesthetic, such as xylocaine, may be injected subcutaneously before an arterial puncture or nebulized before bronchoscopy.[1]

The respiratory therapist must be concerned with respiratory and nonrespiratory drugs that are administered by the physician, nurse, or patient. These drugs can add their effects to those that have been given by inhalation and may result in responses that are different than expected. Respiratory drugs can prove life saving or life threatening—which of these it is depends largely on the therapist's understanding of pharmacology.

Basic pharmacology

A *drug* is a chemical substance that exerts a biologic effect.[2] Medically, a drug can be defined as a substance that is used for the treatment, diagnosis, or prevention of disease.[3] *Pharmacology* is the study of how drugs affect the body and how the body acts upon drugs. Specifically, pharmacology concerns six basic areas: (1) the chemical and physical properties of drugs, (2) the physiologic effects that drugs produce and where they produce these effects, (3) how drugs exert their effects or the "mechanism of action," (4) what the body does with drugs, i.e., the absorption, distribution, metabolism, and excretion of drugs, (5) dosages and routes of administration of drugs, and (6) side effects and toxicity.

The respiratory therapist should be familiar with these six areas for each of the drugs he or she is responsible for administering. This is necessary to ensure the safe use of the pharmacologic agents prescribed.

Basic concepts

Every drug has more than one effect, and any effect a drug produces that is other than the desired one can be termed a *side effect*. Thus, every drug has side effects. A "drug of choice" is that drug that best achieves the desired response with minimal side effects (Fig. 11-1). An example of a side effect is a respiratory drug that exerts effects on the heart, such as increasing heart rate. This is an undesired response since a drug that was given for the lung pro-

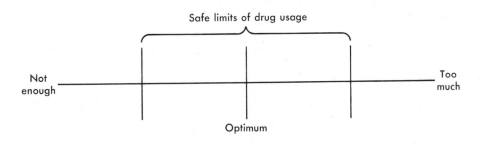

Fig. 11-1   The therapist must be familiar with the range of drug dose that produces therapeutic effect with minimal adverse effects.

duced an effect on the heart. Typically, the amount of drug (dose) that can be given a patient is limited by the side effects it produces, and many times these effects may be significant with less than the prescribed dose. Therefore, careful monitoring of the patient is essential.

It is as important to know when to discontinue the use of a drug as it is to know when to give one. Since no drug can cure disease or produce a new function for which there was previously no physiologic potential, a drug is limited to merely enhancing, modifying, or inhibiting an already existing function. This is only accomplished by producing undesired effects elsewhere. Thus, as soon as the body is capable of doing without the drug, and its use is discontinued, the better off the patient will be. As with the initiation of drug therapy, the modification or cessation of drug use should only occur as a result of a physician's order. However, the therapist's suggestions to the physician regarding drug regimen modification, based on observations of the patient's response to treatment, play an important part in overall patient care.

Drug safety and the response to drug therapy

The safe use of drugs requires awareness of many different factors, including the following:
1. Mode of action
2. Side effects
3. Toxicity
4. Range of common dosages
5. Rate and route of excretion
6. Individual differences in response
7. Interaction with other drugs or food
8. Contraindications

The administration of respiratory drugs may potentially be detrimental. Drugs that are inhaled increase the risk of contamination to the lungs, possibly resulting in infection. When preparing medications for delivery it is essential to observe proper techniques of cleaning and handling of the aerosolizing equipment.

The following list identifies what should constitute a proper prescription for respiratory drugs. The therapist should seek clarification from the physician if the order does not specify the necessary information.
1. Prescription should be complete with:
   a. Patient's name.
   b. Drug name.
   c. Dose.
   d. Frequency it is to be given.
   e. Duration of administration (for some aerosol treatments).
   f. Route of administration
   g. Signature of physician.
2. *Before administering the prescribed drug the therapist should double check:*
   a. Patient's chart for order.
   b. Patient's name band.

    c. Medication labels.

    d. Dates on medication.

    e. Dosage.

    f. Charted response to previous drug administration.

When administering the medication, nothing should be taken for granted. Double check all the information. If an error is suspected or a question arises the therapist should not proceed until satisfied that all is proper.

Although there are "standard" dosages routinely prescribed for patients, drug administration is an individualized event. Very young and very old patients generally have a more difficult time with drugs because of the body's decreased ability to handle drugs at the extremes of age. *Accumulation* of the drug ensues, and the drug level begins to build up in the body, resulting in adverse effects.

The *half-life* of a drug is an important concept. This simply refers to how rapidly a drug is broken down to an inactive form or excreted from the body. Specifically, half-life refers to how much time it takes the body to decrease a given concentration of a drug to half its initial level. A half-life is a constant for a given drug and helps determine how often a drug should be given so as to maintain a therapeutic level.

The half-life of a drug may be prolonged because of compromised liver function in the geriatric patient or in the infant because of lack of maturation of necessary enzyme systems, as well as in any patient with liver disease. The liver is responsible for most of the metabolism and transformation of drugs. The liver basically will convert a drug to a less active form and increase its solubility in water so that it can more readily be excreted by the kidneys. The kidneys are the major route of excretion for most drugs, and any compromise in their function can lead to toxic drug levels. The acid-base status of the body, which is regulated by the lungs and the kidneys, plays a role since drug excretion and drug activity are affected by pH. Clearly, the respiratory patient who has altered acid-base status and compromised respiratory and cardiac function, who is receiving a combination of various drugs, and who may be receiving continuous mechanical ventilation (which further compromises internal organ perfusion) is a prime candidate for poor handling of administered drugs.

The weight, and more specifically, the percent body fat, as well as the size of a person, will influence the response to a given dose of a drug. A person with more body fat has greater storage sites for fat-soluble drugs, and the larger a person is, the more potential there is for fluid volume diluting a given dose to a level that is less than effective. However, the size and amount of fat are less of a concern with drugs that are topically applied, such as those administered directly to the lungs by inhalation of aerosol.

Repeated use of a specific drug may result in a decreased response to the same dose. This is referred to as *tolerance* and is seen occasionally in asthmatic patients who have become "trigger happy" with their aerosol cartridge inhalers. This is corrected by educating the patient as well as giving a combination of different drugs that work by different mechanisms, thus minimizing the build up of tolerance to a specific drug.

Another factor that can alter the expected response to a given drug is the concomitant use of other drugs. Since the average patient receives about 10 different drugs while in the hospital, the potential for undesired interactions resulting in adverse effects are very real.[4] It is difficult to predict what effect various drugs will have when combined together, hence the danger of multiple drug usage. Drug interactions can result in *additive effects,* which is when one drug interacts with another and the resultant effect is the sum of the individual effects. *Potentiation* could also result, which is greater than an additive effect.[5] Many times this is referred to as *synergism,* which is simply two drugs working together in some fashion, the effect of which could be additive or multiplicative. Additional factors that affect the response a patient has may be the time of administration, the pathologic state of the patient, genetic factors, and psychologic factors.[6] When a drug is given may influence the drug effect, since many body processes vary in a cyclic manner throughout the day. There may be times at which a drug has greater effect than at other times. The pathologic condition of the patient is important in that certain body systems such as the liver or kidneys may not allow deactivation or excretion of the drugs as expected, thus possibly leading to cumulation. Furthermore, uneven distribution of gas within the lungs may not allow aerosolized drugs to reach the desired target sites at concentrations necessary to produce noticeable effects. Genetically, a person may lack certain enzymes that a particular drug requires to exert its effect. Last, the psychologic state of the patient can play an important part in the effectiveness of the drug. Belief that a drug will work typically results in a better therapeutic outcome. The therapist's attitude and confidence are of definite effect, and he or she may make the difference between a good or marginal response to the drug therapy given.

Receptor theory of drug action

Drugs are thought to produce their effects either by acting discretely at some specific *receptor* site or by acting diffusely at many tissues, the response being dependent on the degree of saturation. *Saturation-dependent* (or nonreceptor) drugs include alcohol, hypnotics, anesthetics, and mucus-diluting agents such as water and saline. However, the majority of drugs act at receptor sites. A receptor is a special location where specific molecules on cells form reversible bonds with a specific drug. Receptor-drug interaction has been likened to a lock and key, as illustrated in Fig. 11-2. Receptors are very specific as to what drugs will bond there. The shape, the size, and the polarity of the drug molecule have to be within the range of the receptor's specifications or no drug effect will occur. *Affinity* is the tendency a drug has to combine with a receptor.[5] If a drug has affinity and produces an effect, it is termed an *agonist.* A *partial agonist* is a drug that has affinity but cannot produce the full effect. In contrast to this, an *antagonist* is a drug that has affinity but produces no effect. An antagonist is capable of blocking any effect that an agonist would produce if the antagonist gets to the receptor first. This would be anal-

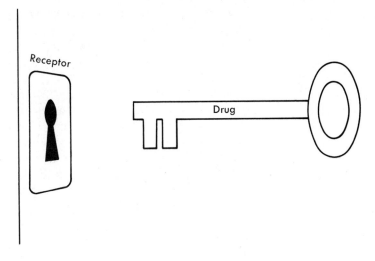

Fig. 11-2   Receptor-drug interactions are analogous to a lock and key. Only a drug with the right properties will activate or "fit" the receptor, thus resulting in a response.

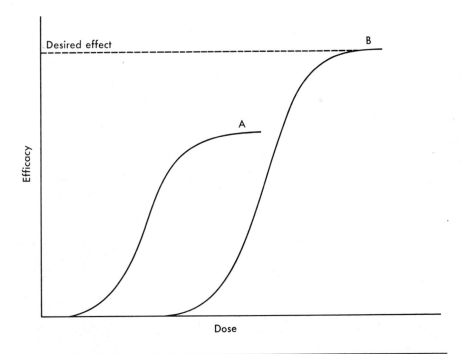

Fig. 11-3   Drug *A* is more potent but less effective than drug *B*. In this example drug *A* will never achieve the effect that drug *B* does.

ogous to putting a toothpick in a lock, thus not allowing the key to work. The toothpick fits inside the lock but is not able to open it. An antagonist can be *competitive* (forms reversible bond with receptor) or *noncompetitive* (forms irreversible bond), depending on the type of chemical bonds formed between the receptor and the drug.

It is well recognized that some drugs work better than others. The ability of a drug to exert an effect is known as the drug's *efficacy*. How large a drug dose is required to produce a given effect determines the *potency*. Fig. 11-3 illustrates the relationship of dosage and efficacy. The dosage is plotted on the horizontal axis and the drug effect on the vertical. Note that there is a maximum effect that can be attained by drug *A* or *B*, i.e., increasing the dose beyond a given point produces no change in efficacy. In this example, drug *A* is clearly able to achieve an effect at a low dose; therefore, it is more potent. However, it is not able to elicit the desired effect. Drug B, although not as potent (i.e., it requires a larger dose), achieves the desired effect. Our goal is to use those drugs that produce the desired effect. Potency is a minor consideration.

Pathologic triad and treatment

The primary purpose of respiratory pharmacology is to relieve the *pathologic triad—bronchospasm, retained secretions,* and *mucosal edema* of the airway (Fig. 11-4). The agents used to reduce these symptoms can be called the *treatment triad.* These consist of bronchodilators, mucokinetic agents, and decongestants. The pathologic triad and treatment are outlined below:

Pathologic condition	*Treatment*
1. Bronchoconstriction	Bronchodilator (e.g., isoproterenol, isoetharine)
2. Airway edema	Decongestant (e.g., phenylephrine)
3. Retained secretions	Hydration (e.g., water); mucolytics (e.g., acetylcysteine)

Bronchodilators increase the lumen of the airways by relaxing the spasm of the bronchial muscle, which is triggered by disease or irritation. *Mucokinetic*

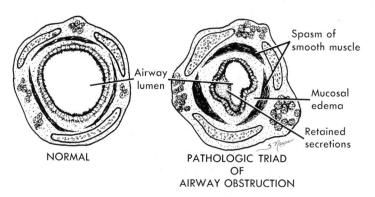

Fig. 11-4   Cross sections of bronchioles comparing normal with obstruction caused by pathologic triad. Note narrowed airway lumen (opening) in obstructed airway.

agents are used to loosen and mobilize secretions. The action is by simply diluting the mucus by direct application of liquid agents, by stimulating serous secretion within the airways and thus allowing a more liquid mucus that is easier to expectorate, or by chemical breakdown of secretion components. *Decongestants* (agents that relieve congestion) function in one of two ways. Most cause a contraction of the muscle fibers of the arterioles and small arteries, thereby reducing blood flow to the affected area and lowering the hydrostatic pressure that permits fluid to move into the tissues. Others interfere with the natural defense mechanism that stimulates increased blood flow to an injured area and are called "antiinflammatory" in action.

Bronchodilators and mucokinetic agents are discussed in detail later in this chapter. The decongestants are most often combined with bronchodilators for aerosol therapy either as a separate drug mixed with it or simply as a secondary action of the bronchodilator agent itself. Decongestants are discussed as applicable.

Autonomic-active bronchodilators

The autonomic-active group of bronchodilators is clinically the most widely useful and contains the largest variety of drugs of the three categories. Bronchodilators whose actions either simulate or interfere with tissue stimulation by the autonomic nervous system have been effectively used for many years. Although our major interest in their physiologic actions is limited to the single function of bronchial dilation, because of their extensive use and potency, it is essential that we understand their total effects. This necessitates a review of the autonomic division of the nervous system.

Autonomic nervous system

The nervous system and the endocrine system are the body's internal communication network. The nervous system is capable of rapid response and discrete control, while the endocrine system is slower and typically more diffuse in its response. Both systems help regulate the body's internal environment; this process of regulation is referred to as *homeostasis*. Both systems are similar in that pharmacologic agents can interact with them at receptor sites and thereby modify function at selected tissue locations.

Looking closer at the nervous system we can classify it into several major divisions, as follows:

A. Central nervous system
B. Peripheral nervous system
   1. Afferent system
   2. Efferent system
     (a) Somatic nervous system
     (b) Autonomic nervous system
       (1) Sympathetic nervous system
       (2) Parasympathetic nervous system

The *central nervous system* (CNS) consists of the brain and spinal cord, and the *peripheral nervous system* consists of those nerve pathways that are outside of the CNS. These pathways can be functionally divided into the *afferent pathways*—those that conduct information to CNS—and the *efferent pathways*—those that conduct information away from the CNS. The *somatic* and the *autonomic nervous systems* are subdivisions of the efferent system. The somatic nervous system, which is under conscious control, conducts impulses from the CNS to the skeletal muscles. The autonomic nervous system, in contrast, functions beyond the level of our conscious control, although biofeedback techniques can bring some conscious control to some of its functions. The autonomic system derives its name from the fact that it performs its many duties, minute by minute, whether we are awake or asleep, in an *automatic* fashion. Among other things, the autonomic nerves govern the activities of the cardiac muscle, the smooth or involuntary muscles of all body systems (such as smooth muscles in the lungs that regulate airway caliber), the digestive and genitourinary systems, the sweat glands, and certain endocrine glands. Functioning of the autonomic nerve system is vital for maintaining homeostasis.

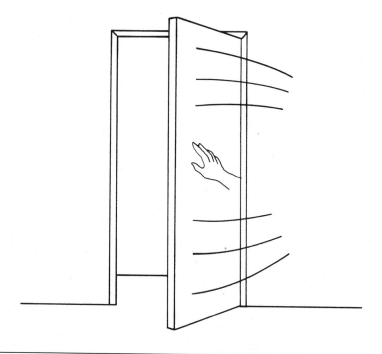

Fig. 11-5   Force applied to only one side of a door allows it to close but with no ability to open the door or regulate the speed at which it shuts. By applying a force on the opposite side of the door at the same time, one can exercise control over the door. Dual innervation by the sympathetic and parasympathetic nervous systems, which have opposite effects on the effector organs, allows for more precise control.

The autonomic division is itself divided into two competitive subdivisions, *sympathetic* and *parasympathetic,* and most of the structures listed above are innervated (supplied with nerves) by both. With organs innervated by two opposing systems, precise control is possible (Fig. 11-5). For a schematic diagram of autonomic organization refer to Fig. 11-6. Sympathetic fibers arise in the thoracic and lumbar spinal cord segments and travel uninterrupted until they reach a *ganglion,* which is simply a relay point where many interconnections (synapses) are possible. The preganglionic sympathetic fibers are short and terminate at ganglia, whereas postganglionic fibers are long and terminate at the *effector organs* (those organs or tissues that are affected by those nerves). The ratio of preganglionic to postganglionic fibers is from 1:11 to 1:17. Therefore, an impulse coming in on a preganglionic fiber results in impulses on many postganglionic fibers, producing an effect at many different locations. In addition, at the adrenal gland, epinephrine is released into the blood and is carried by the circulation. Thus, stimulation of the sympathetic system

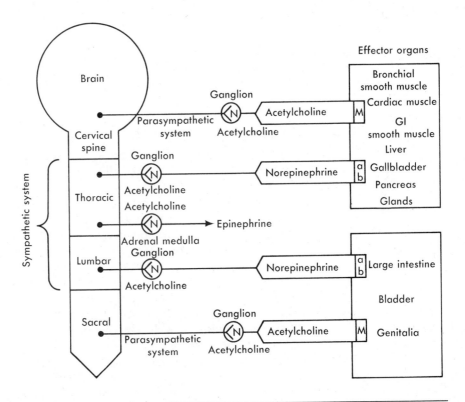

Fig. 11-6   Sympathetic and parasympathetic nervous system innervation. Note that there is dual innervation to effector organs. *Acetylcholine* is the transmitter at all ganglia and at parasympathetic sites. Their receptors are labeled *N* for nicotinic and *M* for musarinic. The transmitters for the *sympathetic system* at the *effector organs* are labeled *a* and *b* for alpha and beta respectively (see text).

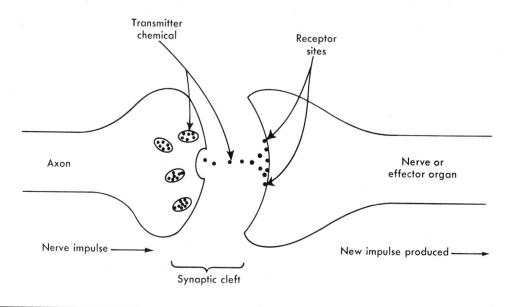

Fig. 11-7   The *nerve impulse* releases a chemical transmitter that flows across the *synaptic cleft* at the ganglion and effector organ. The chemical transmitter attaches to a receptor and initiates a new electrical impulse. Drugs can attach to the receptor sites, producing a response that is similar to the natural chemical transmitter released from the axon terminal.

results in a diffuse response throughout the body. The parasympathetic fibers originate from the brain and the sacral spinal cord segment and travel without synapsing until they reach the ganglia, which are located near the effector organs. The preganglionic fibers are long, and the postganglionic fibers are short; their ratio is about 1:2, resulting in a more discrete response.

The locations where the nerve fibers synapse, such as at the ganglia or at the effector organ (neuroeffector junction), are special sites where the nerve impulse is passed along only by a chemical *transmitter* or *mediator* (Fig. 11-7). It is at these locations that drugs exert their effects. The chemical transmitter is released when a nerve impulse arrives and depolarizes the membrane that contains the transmitter. The transmitter is then "transmitted" or flows across the synaptic cleft, where it combines with the receptors of other nerve fibers as in a ganglion or with receptors of the effector organ. When the receptors are activated by the right chemical transmitter the membrane depolarizes and produces a new impulse or results in a response at the effector organ.

For a drug to have the desired effect it must be similar to the chemical transmitter at the ganglia or effector organ we want to influence. The nature of the chemical transmitter and its receptor identifies the type of nerve and its response.

The chemical transmitter at all ganglia, both sympathetic and parasympathetic systems, is acetylcholine. At the effector organ the sympathetic fibers release *norepinephrine,* whereas the parasympathetic fibers release *acetylcholine* just as at the ganglia. As long as the chemical transmitter is present it will exert its influence. Since nerve stimulation does not lead to permanent effects, something must happen to the transmitter very soon after it is released. In fact, there are specific enzymes that destroy the transmitters as soon as they have exerted their effect. Norepinephrine (as well as epinephrine) is dealt with in several ways: (1) reabsorbed back into the axon terminal that secreted it, (2) deactivated by catechol-o-methyl transferase (COMT) enzyme, or (3) deactivated by monoamine oxidase (MAO) enzyme. The parasympathetic transmitter, acetylcholine, is deactivated by acetylcholinesterase enzyme. The removal or deactivation of the transmitter makes it possible for the receptor sites to be stimulated again and again.

The receptors for these chemical transmitters are very specific. The ganglia receptors are called *nicotinic receptors,* named after the drug nicotine, which was found to exert a stimulating effect here. (Nicotinic receptors are also found at skeletal muscles in the somatic nervous system.) The receptors at the parasympathetic effector site are called *muscarinic receptors,* named after the muscarine drug (poison) from mushrooms, which was found to exert its stimulating effects here. It is interesting to note that acetylcholine is the transmitter that works at both of these locations, but the receptors are slightly different. This can be understood with our lock and key illustration (Fig. 11-2). In this case, the lock (receptors) are slightly different, but the key (acetylcholine) is a master key that can "unlock" both nicotinic and muscarinic "locks." However, we have drugs that selectively work only at one site or the other, thus allowing us to achieve a specific effect. Table 11-1 summarizes the effects seen when nicotinic and muscarinic receptors are stimulated.

The sympathetic system receptors at the effector sites are of two basic types, *alpha* and *beta,* and their characteristic effects are shown in Table 11-2. Beta receptors can be differentiated into two groups according to their abilities to (1) hydrolyze fatty acids, (2) stimulate the heart, (3) dilate bronchi, and (4) relax arterioles. Some beta stimulators primarily produce lysis of fatty acids and cardiac stimulation, while others produce bronchodilation and arteriole relaxation. Receptors that, when stimulated, affect primarily the heart are called *beta$_1$ receptors,* and those that primarily dilate bronchi are called *beta$_2$ receptors.* Drugs that primarily stimulate beta$_2$ receptors are the desired drugs to use for bronchodilation since fewer side effects accompany their use.

Alpha-receptor stimulation in the cardiopulmonary system results in vasoconstriction, slight bronchoconstriction, and a reflexive decrease in heart rate. Various other effects are listed in Table 11-2. Alpha-stimulating drugs have been used in respiratory therapy for decreasing congestion in the airway mucosa and are also used as nasal decongestants.

Broadly speaking, the effects of each subdivision of the autonomic nervous system on a given receptor organ are antagonistic to the other; inactivity of one allows the action of the other to dominate the organ response. Each thus exerts a constant action against the other, like two forces maintaining a steady

Table 11-1
Effects of nicotinic and muscarinic stimulation on various organ systems

Organ system	Nicotine effects	Muscarinic effects
Autonomic ganglia	Stimulated	—
Airways in lung	*	Constriction
Heart rate	*	Decreased
Blood pressure	*	Decreased
Blood vessels	*	Dilation
Gastrointestinal		
Tone	Increased	Increased
Motility	Increased	Increased
Sphincters	—	Relaxed
Salivary gland secretions	First increase, then decrease	Increase
Sweat glands		Increase
Bronchial gland secretions		Increase
Eye	—	Pupil constriction; decreased accommodation
Skeletal muscle	Stimulated	—

Modified from Bergersen, B.S.: Pharmacology in nursing, ed. 14, St. Louis, 1979, The C.V. Mosby Co.
*Stimulation of nicotinic receptors at ganglia produces both sympathetic and parasympathetic effects. If muscarinic effects are blocked with atropine, then nicotinic stimulation results in sympatheticlike results.

Table 11-2
Alpha- and beta-receptor effects in the cardiopulmonary system and elsewhere

	Alpha	Beta$_1$	Beta$_2$
Cardiopulmonary	Vasoconstriction	—	Vasodilation
	Slight bronchoconstriction	—	Bronchodilation
	Decrease in heart rate (reflex)	Increase in heart rate	—
	—	Increase in heart contraction	—
	Enhancement of histamine release		Inhibition of histamine release
Other effects	Constriction of GI sphincters	Lypolysis	Skeletal muscle tremor
	Contraction of ureters	Relaxation of GI system	
	Dilation of pupils	Relaxation of uterus	
	Contraction of pilomotor muscles		
	Hepatic glycogenolysis		
	Contraction of uterus		

pull on each end of a rope. This action is called *tone,* and it establishes a balance of influence on receptor function, ensuring fine control over function and rapid response. Generally, the sympathetic division is designed to protect the integrity and maintain the safety of the organism, which involves the expenditure of energy. The parasympathetic division, on the other hand, is less kinetic in its objectives and is more concerned with conservation and restoration of function. Table 11-3 summarizes the sympathetic and parasympathetic autonomic systems and their differences.

Table 11-3
Differentiation
between sympathetic
and parasympathetic
systems

	Sympathetic nervous system	Parasympathetic nervous system
Origin	Thoracolumbar	Craniosacral
Preganglionic fibers	Short	Long
Postganglionic fibers	Long, with many branches	Short, with few branches
Transmitter at ganglia	Acetylcholine	Acetylcholine
Receptor at ganglia	Nicotinic	Nicotinic
Transmitter at effector organ	Norepinephrine (acetylcholine at sweat glands, blood vessels of skeletal muscles)	Acetylcholine
Receptor at effector organ	Alpha, beta	Muscarinic
Major effect	Fight or flight	Feed or breed

We can begin to compact this information for practical use in our special area of interest by introducing some new terms that describe these opposing autonomic divisions. *Adrenergic* nerves act through the release of norepinephrine (or epinephrine) and derive their name from the fact that the medulla of the adrenal gland releases adrenaline or epinephrine; therefore drugs that act like adrenaline are known as adrenergic. Since these drugs mediate the effects of the sympathetic nervous system they are also frequently called *sympathomimetic* drugs, or drugs that mimic the sympathetic system. One other synonym for these drugs is *catecholamine*. This name is derived from the plant *Mimosa catechu*, which has a chemical agent with a ring structure that is called a catechol. Drugs that resemble the chemical structure from this catechu plant and have an amino group are called catecholamines.[7] Epinephrine and norepinephrine have this same basic structure so they are often referred to as catecholamines.

Cholinergic nerves release and produce their effects via acetylcholine. Drugs that have acetylcholine-like effects are called cholinergic. Since acetylcholine is the mediator in the parasympathetic nervous system, drugs with its effects can be called *parasympathomimetic* drugs.

Drugs that block the above effects can be referred to as *adrenergic-blockers* or *cholinergic-blockers* (or *anti*cholinergic). The above terms are simply broad classifications of autonomic drugs.

Therapists will encounter more specific drug names, and to minimize confusion, Table 11-4 lists the nomenclature of pharmacologic agents. Most frequently, the *generic name* or the *trademark* or *brand name* will be used. In this text the generic name will be used, and if the brand name is mentioned it will be in parentheses following the generic name.

To summarize the preceding concepts and provide a working model that can help us visualize the functioning of the sympathetic and parasympathetic systems in regards to respiratory drugs, refer to Fig. 11-8. Beta$_2$-adrenergic

Table 11-4 Naming of drugs	Name	Explanation	Example
	Chemical name	Name based on chemical structure	1-(3,5-dihydroxyphenyl)-2-isopropylaminoethanol
	Generic name	Common name; may reflect chemical name	Metaproterenol, orciprenaline
	Official name	The name that is used in an official drug publication; may be the same as generic name	Alupent, Metaprel

Modified from Ziment, I.: Respiratory pharmacology and therapeutics, Philadelphia, 1978, W.B. Saunders Co.

drugs bind to the receptor, *adenylate cyclase*, which is an enzyme that initiates the conversion of *adenosine triphosphate* (ATP) to *cyclic adenosine monophosphate* (cAMP). The level or concentration of cAMP is important in mediating the effect of the drug that is bound to the receptor. cAMP exerts its effects through various enzyme systems (*kinases*), which results in the primary effect, bronchial relaxation. The level of cAMP is a result of the stimulation of the receptor adenylate cyclase and the breakdown of cAMP to 5′ AMP by the enzyme *phosphodiesterase*. Stimulation of the alpha receptor also results in *decreased* levels of cAMP. Any drugs that can promote an increased cAMP level will result in bronchial relaxation, and any drugs that decrease cAMP promote bronchial constriction. As can be seen, a beta$_2$-adrenergic drug can increase cAMP levels as well as any drug that will block the action of phosphodiesterase, which would result in maintenance of cAMP levels. The action at the cholinergic receptor is very similar, only the nucleotides are different. In this case, *guanosine triphosphate* (GTP) is converted to *cyclic guanosine monophosphate* (cGMP). As these levels increase, the result is an increasing bronchial constriction. As may be seen, the bronchial smooth muscle tone is a function of the amount of cAMP and cGMP present at any given time. The level of cAMP and cGMP is a result of the sympathetic and parasympathetic nervous system activities as well as the action of any drugs that may be present.

At the letters in Fig. 11-8, drugs can block the action of drugs that stimulate. At *A,* phentolamine is a drug that blocks alpha-stimulation effects. Propanolol is a beta blocker and acts at *B,* whereas xanthines, such as theophylline, block phosphodiesterase at *C,* not allowing it to deactivate cAMP. At *D,* an anticholinergic drug, atropine (which is a competetive antagonist at muscarinic receptors), blocks cholinergic stimulation.

Adrenergic bronchodilators

Adrenergic bronchodilators are the most commonly used type of bronchodilators. Some preparations of these drugs are administered orally, others by inhalation, and some are effective given either route. As we begin, we will refer to several figures and tables. It is important to be familiar with these before studying the individual drugs. The general mechanism of action of these drugs has been summarized in Fig. 11-8. The major effects that these

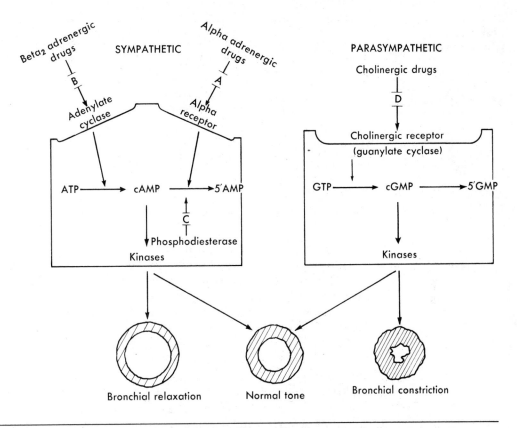

Fig. 11-8   Model of drug mechanism of action for adrenergic and cholinergic drugs. Note that drugs act at specific receptor sites, which then influences *cAMP* or *cGMP* levels. The amount of cAMP to cGMP determines the outcome on the bronchial smooth muscle. At *A*, *B*, *C*, and *D*, blocking agents can inhibit the function of the specific enzyme system.

drugs produce on the body have been summarized in Table 11-2, and a quantitative estimation of these effects for the commonly used adrenergic bronchodilators are listed in Table 11-5. This table can be referred to as the drugs are discussed.

It is important to note the commonly experienced side effects with adrenergic bronchodilators, and these are summarized below.

Side effect	*Cause*
Increased heart rate	Beta$_1$ stimulation
Arrythmias, palpitation	Beta$_1$ stimulation
Skeletal muscle tremor	Beta$_2$ stimulation
Anxiety, nervousness, insomnia, nausea	Beta$_2$ CNS stimulation
Decreased Pa$_{O_2}$ (occasional)	Beta$_2$ vasodilation in lung producing altered $\dot{V}/\dot{Q}$ match-up

Table 11-5
Receptor site stimulation, relative strength, and duration of action of some adrenergic drugs

	Alpha	Beta$_1$	Beta$_2$	Duration of action
Epinephrine (Adrenalin)	3+	4+	3+	Short
Racemic epinephrine (micronefrin, Vaponefrin)	2+	3+	2+	Short
Ephedrine	2+	3+	3+	Long
Isoproterenol (Isuprel, Isoprenaline, Aludrine, Norisodrine)		4+	4+	Short
Isoetharine (Dilabron)		1+	3+	Medium
Metaproterenol (Metaprel, Alupent)		2+	2+	Long
Terbutaline (Bricanyl, Brethine)		1+	3+	Long
Solbutamol (Ventolin, Albuterol)		1+	4+	Long
Fenoterol		1+	4+	Long

Key: short, $^1/_2$ to 2 hours; medium, 2 to 4 hours; long, 4 to 6 hours (1+, minor effect; 4+, strong effect).

All patients will experience one or more of these side effects while using adrenergic bronchodilators. Some patients will be more sensitive to adverse effects than others, and the dose that is necessary to achieve adequate bronchodilation may result in excessive side effects. Thus termination of treatment occurs before therapeutic effects are achieved. Careful monitoring of respiratory patients is always essential, especially for those patients who are receiving heart medication or using other adrenergic drugs. Proper monitoring by a respiratory therapist, while administering an aerosolized bronchodilator, minimally includes the following: obtain pulse and respiratory rate before, during, and after the treatment; measure tidal volume during treatment; auscultate lung fields before and after treatment; and observe for excessive hand tremor, patient fatigue, or other undesired responses. A treatment should be terminated if pulse rate becomes excessive (increases more than 20 beats/min) or should not even be started if a patient is experiencing tachycardia. Respiratory rate is usually controllable by the patient and simply requires educating the patient during the treatment to breathe in a manner that is slow, relaxed, and of proper volume to ensure maximum therapeutic effect. All of the above monitored parameters should be charted, as well as any other patient response to the treatment. There are many individual variations that may modify these general recommendations, and specific problems or questions should be discussed with the patient's physician.

At least some of the adrenergic bronchodilators perform the additional valuable role of increasing the transport of airway mucus. Studies following the parenteral use of the beta stimulant, terbutaline, showed up to 110% of average tracheal mucous velocity in patients with chronic obstructive airway disease.[8] There was no apparent increase in flow in normal subjects. It is thus possible that the effectiveness of catecholamines in the treatment of obstructive disease is a result of the dual action of bronchodilation and increased mucus transport. Although the mechanism for the latter is not apparent, it may account for instances of subjective evidence of increased mucus removal even though tests of airway patency show no improvement.

Additionally, it has been observed that beta$_2$-adrenergic compounds, specifically fenoterol, could induce a decrease in lung recoil pressure that is dose related.[9] Possibly, this could result in a decrease in work of breathing for some patients. This effect is of short duration (30 minutes) and appears to be more closely related to the action of the drug that was absorbed into the circulation through the bronchial mucosa and exerted its effects, via the circulation, to the parenchyma of the lung. It is well recognized that many of the effects of bronchodilators—especially side effects and possibly some bronchodilator effects—occur as a result of the aerosolized drug being absorbed into the circulation. Studies indicate that only about 10% of the aerosolized drug actually deposits in the lung, the remainder either being exhaled or deposited in the mouth or oropharynx and swallowed.[10] Thus plasma levels of the drug may be responsible for some of the drug action via absorption in the gastrointestinal tract, if not metabolized, or via bronchial absorption.[11,12]

Epinephrine. Epinephrine is the standard against which most sympathomimetics are judged. Epinephrine is a potent drug, and since it stimulates all three adrenergic receptors, its use carries with it the risk of serious unwanted side effects. It performs important functions in regulating the body's metabolism and maintaining a state of alertness to cope with the environment. The therapist sees this drug used frequently in the hospital for its effect on the circulation and to combat allergic reactions, for which purposes it is administered by injection under the skin, into muscle, or into superficial veins. It is almost completely inactivated in the stomach; thus oral use is not feasible. However, it has been used parenterally for many years for the relief of acute bronchial asthma.

Epinephrine is one of the most powerful bronchodilators and decongestants, whether given by injection or by aerosol. Indeed, its action by aerosol is both topical (local, by application to a surface) and systemic (distributed to many parts of the body), since the small particles act by direct contact with the bronchial mucosa and are also absorbed into the circulation by way of the pulmonary blood flow. Thus inhalation generally affords quicker response than does subcutaneous or intramuscular injection, although not exceeding the intravenous route.

There are two major hazards to aerosolized epinephrine. First, the unwanted side effects may be a danger as well as a nuisance, and the effect on the cardiovascular system may outweigh its benefits. This is especially true in elderly patients or in those with known heart or vascular disease. Second, repeated use of epinephrine often leads to a condition of "fastness," in which there is a progressively decreasing response to the drug and dangerously larger doses are required for therapeutic effect. A patient exhibiting this phenomenon is considered to be epinephrine-fast. Less commonly seen is a third complication apparently attributable to any of the sympathomimetic compounds by which the symptoms of acute bronchial asthma are made worse by these aerosols. It is believed that this adverse effect is a result of the development of an allergy to some of the metabolic end products of the drugs.[13]

If epinephrine is to be used as a bronchodilator-decongestant aerosol, nothing stronger than a 1% aqueous solution (1:100) should be considered safe. Two effective inhalations from 30 to 60 seconds apart are sufficient, and treatments should be spaced at least 4 hours apart. Because of the development of safer preparations, some of which are described later in this chapter, the use of epinephrine aerosol has rapidly declined in recent years.

Racemic epinephrine. This drug is a mixture of two isomers (chemical formula is identical but atoms arranged differently) of epinephrine. It is a little less potent in its effects than epinephrine and therefore exerts fewer side effects, yet can achieve reasonable bronchodilations. It serves the purpose of relaxing bronchial smooth muscle and decreasing mucosal congestant by its alpha action. It has been recommended for laryngotracheobronchitis[14] and may be of value in recently extubated patients because of its decongestant action. The use of racemic epinephrine has shown to be effective for the acute signs of croup.[15]

Ephedrine. Although ephedrine is not used as an aerosol, its close similarity to the action of epinephrine and its frequency of use warrants its mention at this time. Ephedrine is an alkaloid (nitrogen-containing organic compound with physiologic action) derived from a plant, with a less intense but longer lasting bronchodilating effect than epinephrine. Unlike epinephrine, it is a strong cerebral stimulant. A major advantage of ephedrine is its oral effectiveness, and most commonly it is used in conjunction with other bronchodilators, expectorants, or sedatives. Excessive use, as by patient self-administration, can cause serious mental excitation.

Isoproterenol. A powerful beta stimulator with negligible alpha effects, isoproterenol has enjoyed wide use as an aerosol bronchodilator. Although much more selective in its effects than are epinephrine and ephedrine, its role as a bronchodilator is somewhat limited by its stimulation of $beta_1$ receptors. Cardiac output increase may reduce the ventilation/perfusion ratio by raising pulmonary perfusion more than bronchodilatation improves ventilation, and thus worsen hypoxia. Further, the risk of cardiac arrhythmias is increased by $beta_1$ stimulation in the presence of hypoxia.[16] However, clinical experience with it is extensive enough that it can still be used effectively as an inhalant, with a wide range of safety. A major advantage of this aerosol is its somewhat better bronchodilating effect than that of epinephrine, with nearly complete absence of vasopressor action. In contrast to epinephrine, isoproterenol produces vasodilation and thus has negligible decongestant value. It tends to lower diastolic and not systolic blood pressure but may encourage a sinus tachycardia. Its symptomatic side effects are infrequent, tend to be mild, and include nausea, excitement, tremors, and rapid heart action.[17]

Although available in aqueous concentrations of 1:100 and 1:200, for routine aerosol use the *1:200 strength is recommended*. For intermittent short-term therapy, as in self-administration, two to four well-spaced inhalations at 4-hour intervals is a conservative program, although the general safety of the drug allows for considerable flexibility according to clinical need. Since all aerosols are, in a sense, foreign bodies, overuse of them often causes severe pharyngeal and laryngeal irritation, further aggravating the very condition being treated. Warning of this possibility should be included in instructions given to all patients who are to treat themselves. For prolonged bronchodilation, especially as administered with mechanical ventilators, the isoproterenol should be further diluted to concentrations of 1:400 or 1:600.

l-Norepinephrine; levarterenol. The major sympathetic nerve stimulus mediator, when administered therapeutically, is very limited in its action and, although not a bronchodilator, is included here for completeness. Levarterenol is exclusively an alpha-receptor stimulant, with its primary effector the cardiovascular system. Given intravenously, its only clinical use is the support of blood pressure in certain types of shock.

Isoetharine. Isoetharine is a commonly used bronchodilator with a bronchodilating effect that is somewhat less than that of isoproterenol. The cardiovascular side effects of isoetharine have also been noted to be less intense.[18] It is claimed to be mostly a $beta_2$ stimulator, with clinically insignificant $beta_1$ activity. In one test of cardiovascular responses to a strong exposure to the drug, intravenous administration of isoetharine to anesthetized patients caused a decrease in systolic and diastolic blood pressures ($beta_2$ effect) and an increase in heart rate ($beta_1$ effect) but no arrhythmias.[19] Isoetharine can be administered orally as well as by aerosol, and it is reportedly more effective in conditions characterized by diffuse bronchospasm, as in bronchial asthma, than in those with obstructing secretions, as chronic bronchitis.[20]

Solbutamol. Clinical experience with solbutamol has been obtained for some time in Europe, and recently solbutamol has been introduced into the United States. Clinical response to the drug is excellent, resulting in significant bronchodilation with fewer side effects than isoproterenol.[21,22] Nebulized solbutamol appears to take longer to achieve bronchodilation but has a longer lasting effect because of its slower rate of metabolism.[23] A major asset is its effectiveness, whether given by mouth, intravenously, or in aerosol form. However, for many conditions the administration of the aerosolized drug appears to offer fewer side effects, and there are some indications that better results are achieved by this route in acute asthma.[24] This drug will prove to be a valuable therapeutic aid in the treatment of bronchospasm.

Metaproterenol. A derivative of isoproterenol, metaproterenol has many of the same effects.[25,26] It can be taken orally or inhaled as an aerosolized powder from a pressurized cartridge, or a liquid form can be nebulized. It has $beta_1$ side effects when given by inhalation and comparable $beta_2$ effects when compared with isoproterenol but with significantly increased duration of action.

Terbutaline. Terbutaline is used primarily as an orally administered bronchodilator and is a very specific beta$_2$ adrenergic with minimal beta$_1$ effects. It is comparable to metaproterenol but with slightly better bronchodilation and longer duration of action.[27]

Fenoterol. Fenoterol is not yet available for general clinical use in the United States. Studies indicate that it is an effective beta$_2$ stimulant, whether given orally or by inhalation. Its duration of effect appears to be very persistant (about 8 hours) and is accompanied by minimal beta$_1$ effects. However, a recent study using aerosolized fenoterol versus terbutaline reported a better overall clinical effect for terbutaline.[28] More clinical studies will determine its overall usefulness.

It should be emphasized that adverse effects, or at least failure to achieve or sustain benefit, are commonly seen with most of the adrenergics now in use. Such results may not always be caused by stimulation of unwanted effector sites but are often the result of local airway mucosal irritation or the blockade of beta receptors by accumulated adrenergic metabolites.[29] Isoproterenol is especially susceptible to the latter reaction, particularly if used too frequently or over too long a period of time. Metabolic products of the breakdown of isoproterenol can accumulate faster than enzymatic degradation can destroy them. Some of the metabolites block the beta receptor from bronchodilator action, and further administration of isoproterenol increases bronchospasm. Also, the student will find that there is a wide variety of adrenergic bronchodilators commercially available that differ chemically from one another, and many are combined with other agents for supposed multiple effect.[30]

It is not our purpose to comment on the relative virtues of these varied compounds, but the respiratory therapist may have occasion to note the presence of propylene glycol in many preparations, and its function should be explained at this time. Propylene glycol is a fairly simple organic compound, related to glycerin but less irritating, that is frequently used as a vehicle or solvent for active substances to be administered by intramuscular injection and is itself completely inert physiologically. In liquids designed for aerosol use, advantage is taken of another characteristic of propylene glycol: It is hygroscopic, and through its ability to absorb water, it supposedly will minimize shrinkage of aerosol particles by evaporation as the particles enter the warmth of the respiratory tract. However, the probability is just as great that aerosol size may so increase through hygroscopic growth that penetration will be hampered, and it is sometimes suspected that aerosol particles may become so stable that they exert no therapeutic effect in the respiratory tract and are exhaled intact.

Anticholinergic bronchodilators

Atropine is an alkaloid found in the plants *Atropa belladonna* and *Datura stramonium,* and it has been used for many years in the treatment of airway disease. Inhalation of the smoke of stramonium leaves was a favorite remedy for asthma, but the increased use of adrenergic drugs gradually displaced atropine therapy until, at present, little reference to it can be found in modern treatment regimens. Yet, because we frequently encounter patients who are resistant to the common drugs, we should at least keep it in mind as a potential agent.

Related to other drugs such as scopolamine and hyoscyamine, atropine blocks the effect of parasympathetic stimuli by increasing the threshold of response of effector cells to acetylcholine. It thereby depresses the reactions of structures supplied by the parasympathetic division, and its action generally resembles stimulation of adrenergic receptors, since these are freed of competing and counteracting cholinergic stimulus. The most extensive of the cranial nerves are the paired vagus nerves, large conveyors of parasympathetic fibers. Coursing from the brain, the vagi pass through the neck, supplying all the organs in the thorax, and continue into the abdomen, where they innervate the digestive system and other abdominal viscera. Thus in our area of interest, the action of atropine inhibits vagal stimulation of the heart and respiratory tract, elevating blood pressure and cardiac rate and dilating bronchi by paralyzing the terminals of the vagal parasympathetic nerve endings. In addition, atropine is believed to have action in the central nervous system, stimulating the cerebral respiratory center to generate rapid, deep breathing.[31]

Relative to the patient with airway obstruction, the two most important actions of atropine can be summarized as follows:

1. *Reduction of secretions.* Atropine inhibits secretions of nose, mouth, pharynx, and bronchi and, by reducing their fluid volumes, increases their viscosities. This property made atropine and related derivatives popular in compounds prescribed to relieve symptoms of the common cold and in preoperative medication to reduce the mucus-producing stimulus of anesthetics and airway instrumentation. However, this effect of atropine poses a potential threat to the patient already handicapped by thick bronchial exudates and subjects him or her to the risk of serious aggravation of the obstruction. This hazard has probably been the major impediment to the continued use of atropine in respiratory problems.

2. *Bronchodilation.* By blocking cholinergic constricting influences on bronchial muscle, atropine potentiates beta-adrenergic dilation and widens the airways. Because there is no evidence that acetylcholine plays an active role in generating bronchospasms, atropine is a less effective dilator than either epinephrine or isoproterenol in therapeutic doses, yet the beneficial effect of atropine on bronchoconstriction has been well demonstrated in airways that were subjected to dust inhalation and protected by the drug parenterally administered.[32] Aerosol studies have employed 1% and 0.2% concentrations of atropine in equal parts of propylene glycol and water.[33] It has been emphasized that the medication must be microaerosolized, with mean particle diameters from 0.03μ to 0.05μ. This avoids potential toxic effects from the powerful drug by ensuring maximum deposition in the alveoli and minimizing absorption from the upper tract. Through the use of very small particle size, total dosage of the alkaloid is kept within safe limits, but microaerosolization to such a controlled degree can be achieved only with specialized equipment (see

Chapter 10). With the proper administration of atropine aerosol, airway resistance can be significantly reduced in normal subjects as well as in obstructed patients. Bronchi are also protected against the induced bronchospasm of inhaled irritants such as carbachol and aluminum dust. It was also found that results were equally satisfactory with the 0.2% as with the 1% solution. It has been suggested that atropine in small amounts be added to sympathomimetic mixtures, and one study demonstrated that an aerosol of isoproterenol and atropine methonitrate gave better bronchodilation than either alone, combining the rapid onset and short duration of isoproterenol with the slower but more prolonged effect of atropine.[34]

Currently undergoing study in Europe and the United States, and not yet available for clinical use, is a derivative of atropine, *N*-isopropyl nortropine, for experimental use designated as Sch 1000.[35,36] Administered as an aerosol in doses of 10 to 20 μg, it produces bronchodilation about as effectively as does isoproterenol. Onset of its action is three to six times as long as isoproterenol's, but its duration is four times greater. The major effect of Sch 1000 seems to be in large rather than peripheral airways, and apparently no subjective drying of oral or ocular secretions has been noted. Finally, bronchodilation is better in patients with chronic bronchitis than with asthma, an observation consistent with the theory that bronchitics are more sensitive to vagal activity than are asthmatics. It is to be hoped that Sch 1000 soon becomes clinically available, giving us an effective alternative bronchodilator to the many adrenergics that now dominate the market.

Xanthines

There is a group of vegetable organic compounds called the xanthines, of which the three most important are *caffeine, theophylline,* and *theobromine.* We are all familiar with caffeine as the important ingredient of coffee, tea, cola drinks, and cocoa, but the xanthine group as a whole has some specific physiologic actions that make them valuable as pharmacologics. Although the degree to which these three react varies, in general their activities include the following: CNS stimulation, respiratory stimulation, smooth muscle relaxation, diuresis (increased production of urine), coronary artery dilation, cardiac stimulation, and skeletal muscle stimulation. It is evident that there is a great potential for the medical use of these substances. Frequently used in the past for cardiac stimulation (caffeine) and diuresis (theobromine), for the most part they have been replaced by more effective agents, with the exception of theophylline. This agent, used plain or compounded as theophylline ethylenediamine (aminophylline), still plays an important role in therapeutics. It is useful in certain types and stages of congestive heart failure and is especially valuable in correcting Cheyne-Stokes' ventilation. It has more recently received attention from its ability to decrease the frequency of apneic episodes in premature infants.[37,38,39]

The value of theophylline can be appreciated from reviewing Fig. 11-8. Its action is to *maintain* cAMP levels by inhibiting phosphodiesterase (rather than increasing cAMP as with adrenergics), thus promoting bronchial smooth muscle relaxation. This allows a patient to alter medications between beta$_2$ adrenergics and xanthines and decrease the chances of developing tolerance to adrenergics as well as minimizing adverse effects that may be seen by excessive use of only one agent.

The therapist sees aminophylline frequently used for patients with diffuse bronchospasm and in cases of intractable bronchial asthma, especially when there is refractoriness to the sympathomimetics. Acute exacerbations of bronchospasm are commonly treated with intravenous administration of aminophylline. Intramuscular and rectal routes are sometimes used, but these are less effective. For overall treatment of patients prone to bronchospasm, oral theophylline or its derivatives are frequently part of the drug regimen along with adrenergic agents. The desire is to maintain therapeutic levels of theophylline in the plasma, which is around 10 to 20 mcg/ml of serum. However, the therapeutic dose is very close to the toxic dose, and adverse effects are more likely. Many physicians periodically monitor serum theophylline levels on their patients in order to more accurately adjust for maximum effectiveness with minimal side effects.[40] The most common side effects are anorexia, nausea, and vomiting. Cardiovascular effects such as tachycardia, palpitations, and arrhythmias as well as CNS effects of nervousness, insomnia, and tremulousness may be seen. Variables that affect the half-life of the drug and therefore alter the dose or frequency of administration of theophylline are listed below.*

Situations requiring increased dosage	*Increase†*
1. Cigarette smoking	25-75%
2. Exposure to smog or hydrocarbons	10-25%
3. High caffeine intake	10-20%
4. Barbiturate or phenytoin use	10-15%
5. High-protein diet	10-15%
6. Suboptimal blood levels	—
7. Patients known to have high tolerance to theophylline	—
8. Children 2 month to 16 years	—

Situations requiring decreased dosage	*Decrease†*
1. Hepatic congestion or insufficiency	20-50%
2. Marked obesity	20-50%
3. Overt heart failure	20-30%
4. Marked hypoxemia	10-25%
5. Febrile illness	10-20%
6. Antibiotic use of erythromycin, troleandomycin, lincomycin, or clindamycin	10-20%
7. Cimetidine use	10-20%
8. Patients exhibiting toxic symptoms	—

*Modified from information supplied by Irwin Ziment, M.D. Used by permission.
†Approximate guidelines for dosage adjustments. Serum levels provide more accurate guidance.

Patients who smoke cigarettes have a shorter half-life of theophylline and therefore require greater frequency of administeration.[41] It has also been reported that certain upper-respiratory-tract viral infections can increase the half-life of theophylline in a significant manner.[42]

As an aerosol, aminophylline has not enjoyed as widespread usage as the sympathomimetic agents, although the effectiveness of this technique has been recognized for many years.[43] The intravenous preparation is used for aerosolization, by any convenient method available. Continuous nebulization has been used until relief is obtained, often requiring as much as 0.5 to 0.7 g of aminophylline. Intermittent therapy, with positive pressure or an aerosol mask, alone or in conjunction with sympathomimetics, is also effective in bronchial asthma. Because of the relatively small amounts of the drug absorbed, side effects of aerosol administration are very rare.[44,45] It seems practical to consider aerosolized aminophylline in those patients with diffuse bronchospasm who no longer respond to safe doses of sympathomimetics, for the speed of action and economy of the latter still justify their consideration as first-line drugs.

Adrenocortico-steroids

Adrenocorticosteroids have assumed a position of great importance in the therapy of almost all branches of medicine. Again, although we are interested in a relatively limited aspect of their use at present, some general background knowledge of them is essential because the therapist will encounter them throughout his or her patient care experience. For the sake of convenience, we use the commonly employed abbreviated expression "steroid," with the understanding that we mean adrenocorticosteroid. We must understand also that, like many familiar terms, it is not really correct, for steroids comprise a large group of organic compounds, many of which have other physiologic properties than those in which we are interested. The steroids that concern us are potent hormones secreted by the *cortex* (outer layer) of the adrenal glands, as opposed to the sympathomimetic products of the adrenal medulla, already described. There are some five general groups of complex organic compounds produced in the adrenal cortex, of which the only one of importance to our present needs is the *glucocorticoids*. The name of this group derives from its involvement in carbohydrate metabolism, and its two most clinically useful members are *cortisol* and *cortisone*. Many commercial preparations and modifications of these two are available, with variable potencies and supposed specific responses.

The adrenal steroids exert a tremendous influence on the body physiology, touching all organ systems. They have been referred to as "stress hormones" because they are secreted in excessive amounts when the body is put under stress, and severe trauma or prolonged grave illness may cause a depletion of their supply. In a complex way the steroids give support to the body to aid it through a crisis, and if they are acutely depleted or if their production is interrupted by abrupt destruction of the adrenals, the body functions deteriorate rapidly. On the other hand, a slow, chronic increase of cortical function does not produce a catastrophic picture but rather a multiplicity of signs and symptoms described as *Cushing's syndrome*. A patient beginning to show evidence of excessive steroid action is often referred to as "Cushinoid." We describe some of the more common and important effects of hyperadrenalism to illustrate the wide range of steroid action. The glucocorticoids have the following effects.[46-48]

Formation of glucose from body protein. When excessive, the formation of glucose from body protein can raise the blood sugar level high enough to produce "steroid diabetes" or to activate a latent, subclinical true diabetes. There can be associated protein loss with muscle wasting and weakness.

Depletion of bone calcium. Through a process of resorption, calcium is removed from bone, so thinning is consistency that fractures are frequent. This state of the bone is called *osteoporosis*.

Increase in fat production. Excessive amounts of fat are produced, also from body protein, and are characteristically deposited in the subcutaneous tissues of the head and trunk. This results in a rounding of the facial contour, referred to as *moon face,* and an accumulation of fat at the base of the neck and upper back, called *buffalo hump*. These are two of the most prominent visible signs of a Cushinoid state.

Impairment of immunologic response. Steroids inactivate circulating antibodies and thus can protect the body against the harmful effects of severe allergies. By the same token, however, this function lowers the body's resistance to infection, a point of significance in the therapeutic use of steroids.

Reduction of inflammatory response. Steroids decrease the local vascular congestion and cellular infiltration that is the natural response to injury or infection. In addition, the deposition of fibrous tissue as part of the reparative process is inhibited. Of use in controlling the adverse effects of inflammation, this function also facilitates the spread of infection, since it interferes with the usual process of localization. This is a serious threat to the patient with quiescent tuberculosis.

Elevation of blood pressure. Steroids, through the mediation of certain electrolytes and other hormones, elevate the blood pressure. Of therapeutic significance, in state of shock, when the cardiovascular system no longer responds to sympathomimetics, steroids often aid the vasoconstrictors to regain their pressor effects on the arterioles.

To complete the review of steroid action, mention should be made of the pituitary gland. The adrenal cortex is directly controlled by the anterior division of the pituitary gland, through a pituitary hormone called *adrenocorticotropic hormone*. The name itself describes a substance that stimulates (*-tropic*) the adrenal cortex and, not surprisingly, is almost always referred to as "ACTH." Administration of ACTH can be expected to elicit the same response as cortisol and cortisone, by stimulating the adrenal production of these substances. This presupposes that the adrenal cortex is in a functioning state, able to respond. Because the adrenals are likely to slacken in their activity during the therapeutic administration of steroids (the body is receiving adequate hormone from its outside source), there is risk of adrenal atrophy with prolonged loss of function. Under such circumstances, ACTH may be given for periods of time to stimulate the adrenals to function and to prevent their atrophy.

For the most part, in the treatment of respiratory diseases, steroids are administered orally and by inhalation. They are used for their potent antiinflammatory and antifibrogenic effects already mentioned, as well as for their ability to inhibit production and release of histamine (histamine produces bronchospasm) and to make $beta_2$ receptors more responsive to $beta_2$ adrenergics.[43,44] Thus, steroids not only help decrease the frequency of acute bronchospasm but also increase the effectiveness of adrenergic bronchodilators, especially in conditions where some tolerance has developed to them. Steroids are of particular value in the treatment of persons with asthma and with resistant allergies of the respiratory tract. The therapist will witness dramatic responses to steroid therapy, but because of the diffuse action of the drug, various undesired effects can frequently accompany its use. Unlike the other respiratory agents, which typically exert their side effects during or soon after the treatment, steroid side effects are typically those that are of insidious onset and develop over a period of time (days to months).

One fairly common side effect is a fungal infection, candidiasis, of the oropharynx or larynx, which can occur with the aerosol administration of steroids.[45] Using the proper dosage can greatly minimize this complication,[45] as well as having patients rinse their mouth out after treatments. Fortunately, for some of the more recently introduced steroids, candidiasis may be the only real side effect, since systemic absorption from the lung is minimal. Among the many steroids that have been aerosolized, the following deserve special mention.

Dexamethasone sodium phosphate

Dexamethasone is available in a gas-propelled pressurized capsule and can be used alone or mixed with isoproterenol. The consensus of its users is that this steroid is therapeutically active and effective throughout the entire respiratory tract from the nose to the bronchioles in the treatment of nasal allergies, allergic asthma, and some chronic obstructive states.[49,50] However, with no doubt concerning its local effects, dexamethasone has been found to have definite systemic effects, readily detected by special urinary excretion tests. The systemic side effects have limited the use of aerosolized dexamethasone in the lungs in favor of some newer products to be mentioned.

Triamcinolone acetonide

The steroid triamcinolone is a poorly soluble compound with good local and negligible systemic effects, which can be aerosolized for respiratory tract action. It is packaged as a suspension for intramuscular, intraarticular, or intrabursal injection but not intravenous. One dilution that is especially useful for our purposes contains 40 mg/ml of steroid in 1-, 5-, and 10-ml vials.

Starting aerosolization with a 10-mg dosage can be titrated for each patient by clinical response and serum cortisol levels. The majority of patients who are dependent on oral steroids can achieve a therapeutic effect with minimal side effects by using aerosolized triamcinolone.[51,52]

Beclomethasone dipropionate

After several years of use in Europe, the inhalant steroid beclomethasone became available in the United States in mid-1976. This drug is a significant step forward in the treatment of patients with bronchospasm. It is indicated in patients over 6 years of age with intrinsic, extrinsic, or mixed asthma who need chronic steroid therapy.

Studies show that in asthmatic patients, symptoms decrease in about 80% of the cases concomitant with an improvement in pulmonary function. This occurs without the systemic side effects of oral steroids,[53-55] although candidiasis may occur in a few. Most patients who have been dependent on oral steroids can switch to beclomethasone aerosol and maintain control of the asthmatic symptoms.[56-58] However, during acute exacerbation, oral steroids may be needed in previously steroid-dependent patients,[59] as well as in patients with pulmonary infiltration with eosinophilia.[60]

Beclomethasone has been reported to be of value in cases of perennial rhinitis to minimize the symptoms that develop in people susceptible to various antigens such as pollen.[61-63]

Overall, the use of beclomethasone appears to be an effective aerosolized steroid with minimal adverse effects that is of great therapeutic value to many patients.

No matter what steroid is aerosolized, the determination of the actual dose of steroid aerosol to be administered is a matter of professional judgment and is the responsibility of the attending physician. By and large, since steroid aerosols are usually packaged in self-administered gas-propelled units, the physician gives directions for use directly to the patient. However, should the therapist be assigned to oversee the patient's treatment program, he or she should make certain that the physician gives specific orders. Whereas this should be the practice for any treatment, there are many instances in which established routines can be used, allowing the therapist some flexibility to adjust techniques to individual needs. The great potency of the steroids and the possibility of adverse reactions mitigate against their administration with anything less than specific instructions for each patient. The many variables that influence the efficiency of aerosol treatment, such as function of the nebulizer, depth of ventilation, and ventilatory rate, make it impossible to predict the systemic absorption of the drug. The physician must "play it by ear," judging total dosage necessary by clinical response.

Cromolyn sodium

Cromolyn sodium is often part of a treatment program for asthma, used cooperatively with bronchodilators. It is a powder packaged in 20-mg dosages in capsules, effective only as an aerosol with a special inhaling device that punctures the capsule, releasing the powdered drug for transport to the lung during inhalation.

Cromolyn apparently interferes with the release of mediators that result from contact, in allergic persons, between allergen (substance to which an individual is allergic) and antibody (a protein mobilized by the body to inactivate allergen). Such mediators as histamine and SRS-A (slow-reacting substance of anaphylaxis) can cause severe bronchospasm, and although their exact roles are not known, they are thought to participate in initiating or propagating asthmatic attacks. Cromolyn is also able to provide good protection against nonallergenic challenges. Possible action is on cholinergic or irritant receptors in addition to inhibition of mast cell degranulation.[64] It must be emphasized very strongly that cromolyn is only of value in preventing or moderating asthmatic attacks and is completely ineffective once bronchospasm is established. It has made two important contributions to asthma management. The regular use of cromolyn inhalations during remission of symptoms may reduce the frequency and severity of attacks and lessen the amount of adrenocorticosteroids previously needed to control symptoms.[65-67]

Cromolyn has demonstrated clinical effectiveness and an ability to allow reversal of histologic changes that occur with perennial rhinitis,[68-70] as well as being effective in exercise-induced asthma.

Although not effective on everyone, cromolyn should be tried on any patient suffering frequent bronchospasm because of its great efficacy on many patients and minimal side effects.

Prostaglandins

New products are constantly being evaluated for safe and effective treatment of obstruction. Currently of interest, although yet in the investigative stage, is a bronchodilator of an entirely different type. A group of biologics called *prostaglandins* is found chiefly in seminal plasma but also in other organs. There are six primary prostaglandins, designated PGE_1, PGE_2, PGE_3, PGF_{1a}, PGF_{2a}, and PGF_{3a}, and they elicit many and varied responses from several organ systems. Because of the experimental nature of prostaglandins, a detailed description of their actions is unjustified in this text, and the interested student can find many good references in the literature.[71-74] Both PGE_1 and PGE_2 produce bronchodilation, while PGF_{2a} contricts bronchial smooth muscle. Aerosolized PGE_1 has been shown to decrease airway resistance in asthmatic patients to a greater degree than isoproterenol, and PGE_2 has an additive effect to beta-adrenergic stimulation. Approaching the problems from a different direction, bronchodilation can also be achieved experimentally by the action of a substance known as polyphloretin phosphate, which inhibits the constrictor effect of PGF_{2a}. It is expected that the future will show the prostaglandins revealing previously unknown mechanisms in the production of bronchospasm and at the same time increasing our arsenal against airway obstruction.

Mucokinetic drugs

Mucokinetics is concerned with the movement of mucus in the respiratory system. The continual movement of the mucus blanket ensures the clearing from the lung particulate matter that has deposited there during the respiratory cycle. There are two major components to the mucus clearing system: the mucus blanket and the cilia. Fig. 11-9 is a schematic of the anatomy of the important aspects of the mucokinetic system. The mucus blanket is composed of a mucopolysaccharide gel layer that "floats" on top of the more watery sol layer. The composition of the mucus blanket is a balance between the production of the goblet cells and the bronchial glands. The goblet cells produce primarily the gel layer and are stimulated to increase their production because

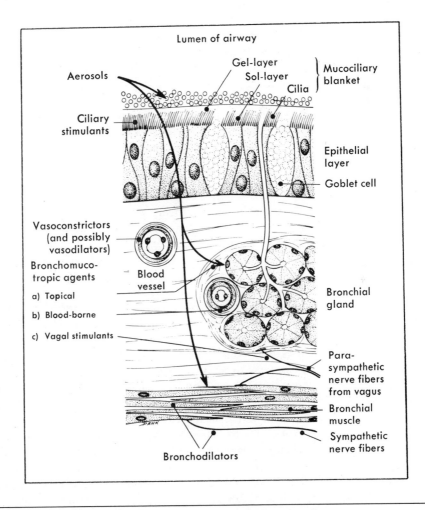

Fig. 11-9   Schematic of anatomy showing important components of mucokinetic system. (From Ziment, I.: Secretions of the respiratory tract: physiology and pharmacology, New York, 1976, Projects in Health, Inc.)

of irritants that are breathed in as particulate or gaseous form, or because of infections within the respiratory tract. The bronchial glands are primarily stimulated by the vagus nerve (part of the parasympathetic system) and probably produce most of the sol layer. The bronchial glands are affected either by agents that are taken orally and then act directly on the bronchial glands via the circulation or by stimulation of the vagus nerve. The vagus nerve at the bronchial glands can be stimulated by cholinergic drugs, higher brain centers, or agents that irritate the stomach via a vagal reflex pathway.

The cilia, primarily responsible for moving the mucus, beat in a coordinated manner: On their forward stroke they straighten up, making contact with the gel layer, propelling it toward the upper airways; on the return stroke they bend and reposition themselves without touching the gel layer. The action is analogous to rowing a row boat, where the oar contacts the water on the forward stroke and is lifted out of the water on the return. For the cilia to function properly they must be beating in the sol layer where they meet minimal resistance to their rapid "flickering" (beating) of about a 1000 times per minute.

Mucokinesis, then, depends on the proper composition of the gel and sol layers as well as optimum functioning of the cilia. Impairment of either of these systems may necessitate coughing, postural drainage, application of specific aerosols, use of oral mucokinetic agents, or possibly direct suctioning of the airways.

Diluting agents

Water. Of all the agents used to modify the character of respiratory tract secretions, rendering them more fluid for easier removal, none is more important than water. Water can be aerosolized or vaporized or can be taken enterally. Generous consumption of water is necessary for optimum functioning of the respiratory system as well as the body in general. Water is one of the few agents that has no side effects unless taken in ridiculus quantities. Only in those patients with congestive heart failure or excessive fluid retention is water restriction considered. Water is the first and most important agent to be considered when patients have difficulty mobilizing bronchial secretions. The aerosolization and vaporization of water is discussed in Chapter 10.

Saline. Saline (NaCl) is one of the most commonly used aerosols—either alone or with bronchodilators. Normal saline (0.9% NaCl) is considered physiologic since its osmolarity approximates that of tissues, and therefore it is considered a bland aerosol. Normal saline can be nebulized for diluting the mucus and enhancing clearance, or it can be instilled directly into the airway to increase the effectiveness of suctioning. Saline solutions and even water when used alone in an aerosol form can precipitate brochospasm, and the use of a bronchodilator may be necessary at times. Half-normal saline (0.45% NaCl) is also used for mucosal hydration, and it is thought preferable by some because of the composition of the droplet on termination in the respiratory tract. As an aerosol particle of half-normal saline travels down the respiratory tract the fluid contained in it has a chance to evaporate. The consequence is that as water leaves, the concentration of saline increases, thus achieving close to normal saline on arrival. Half-normal saline is often preferred with ultrasonic nebulization since the small particles can face significant evaporation.

Hypertonic saline (1% to 15% NaCl) is used for sputum induction since it has several effects that promote sputum production. First, its increased osmolarity is thought to result in increased movement of fluid into the mucosal blanket (bronchorrhea), and second, the irritation promotes coughing, which helps mobilize secretions. Since absorption of saline from the lungs into the circulation does occur, frequent use of the hypertonic saline in sodium-restricted patients is contraindicated.

The remainder of the aerosols that we discuss can be classified under mucolytics. Some mucolytics are most effective against sputum that is predominantly mucoid, and some with proteolytic properties work best on purulent sputum with its high protein content. Some products are claimed to be of equal value against both.

Mucolytics   Although mucolysis means the disruption of the long chains of organic compounds that constitute mucoid sputum, fragmenting them into smaller more mobile molecules, we include wetting agents here for convenience. These substances do not break molecular bonds and thus are better referred to as "mucoevacuants" than mucolytics, but through their surface-active effects they lessen the integrity of secretions and aid in their separation from airway walls.

Wetting agents (detergents). The commercially trademarked product Alevaire contains 0.125% aqueous solution of the wetting agent tyloxapol (Superinone), 2% sodium bicarbonate, and 5% glycerine for stability. Sodium bicarbonate in this concentration has itself mucolytic properties, since some of the polysaccharides will separate in a sufficiently alkaline medium. In vitro studies of the action of tyloxapol on homogenized specimens of sputum demonstrated its surfactant action. The sputum, with a measured surface tension of 52 dynes/cm, was not altered in the addition of water, but when subjected to the action of tyloxapol, the surface tension dropped 20%.[75] It was concluded that a second major function of the wetting agent took place at the wet surface interface between the respiratory mucosa and the mucoid layer, breaking the adherence of the mucus to the bronchial wall. This allowed the mucoid layer to be separated and then removed by cough.

Tyloxapol has been used for several years, and although the mechanical effect of its detergent on mucoid specimens in the laboratory is unquestioned, there is not a uniform opinion as to its value in clinical application. Many believe that it is effective in removing secretions from both sinuses and bronchi and that it can be used continuously for long periods of time for its humidifying effects as well as for mucoevacuation.[76, 77] In the treatment of acute infections of the respiratory tract, tyloxapol has been found to increase the effectiveness of simultaneously administered antibiotics.[78] Other users feel strongly that the value of tyloxapol lies in the humidifying effects of its water-glycerin solvent and that the wetting agent does not influence viscosity or amount of sputum or clinical improvement.[79] It has been suggested that histologic changes in the lung as membrane damage and interstitial infiltration, sometimes seen in postmortem examination of patients succumbing to ventilatory failure.

The therapeutic use of wetting agents might be summarized by saying that they do have a limited effect on bronchial secretions, and by rendering these secretions less viscid, they will supplement the efforts of an existing effective cough mechanism. They are physiologically nontoxic and, when employed as a vehicle for other active substances, enhance the latter's probability of contact with respiratory tissue. However, detergents have little value against frankly purulent sputum.

Acetylcysteine. In the search for agents other than detergents effective in breaking the mucoproteins responsible of the viscosity of sputum in chronic respiratory diseases, the action of the naturally occurring amino acid, L-cysteine, was studied. Although it was found to be a potent mucolytic, it had irritating properties that could be minimized by modifying the acid into an acetyl form, as it is now employed. The chemical reaction between acetylcysteine (N-acetyl-L-cysteine, Mucomyst) and bronchial mucus has been extensively studied,[80] and basically it consists of a disruption of chemical bonds holding together segments of the long-chain mucoproteins by the direct action of specific groups of the amino acid. It is thus a true mucolytic and reduces the viscosity of mucoid sputum in direct proportion to its concentration. Some claim is made for a liquefying action on purulent sputum, but since acetylcysteine has no specificity for the ribonucleic acids characteristic of purulency, such action is probably indirect and mediated through associated mucoid components.

Some studies have indicated that mucolysis is as effective with a 10% as with a 20% concentration, and whereas the stronger preparation tends to induce bronchospasm in some patients, the lesser strength is a negligible hazard.[81] Other studies have found both 10% and 20% to be harmless, neither producing significant bronchospasm.[82] One can now obtain acetylcysteine and isoproterenol in a premixed solution. This combination can help minimize the bronchospasm that occurs in susceptible patients.

The possibility of damage to alveolar surfactant has been of concern with the inhalation of microaerosols of any kind and especially with one of potent lytic qualities. Examination of both human and animal lung tissue after use of 10% acetylcysteine aerosol showed no change in surface activity.[83] Serious complications are rare. A burning sensation in the upper passages is occasionally reported, and nausea may be experienced. Some patients complain of the rotten-egg odor, but most become adjusted to it quickly and appear to ignore it.

In general, the clinical response to this aerosol for the removal of mucoid secretions has been favorable, with indications for its use covering a wide range, from the cystic fibrosis of childhood (in which it seems to have scored considerable success), through the suppurative lung diseases, to the chronic bronchitis-emphysema of late adulthood.[84, 85] Nevertheless, a small minority have felt that acetylcysteine, though effective in vitro, has not shown any benefit in patients and is of no clinical value.[86]

A practical point to note is the chemical reactivity between acetylcysteine and certain component parts of nebulization equipment, especailly iron, copper, and rubber. To avoid the loss of potency of such reactions, parts coming in contact with the amino acid (liquid or aerosol) should be made of glass, plastic, aluminum, chromed metal, silver, or stainless steel.

There is no critical dosage schedule for administering acetylcysteine aerosol; it is used according to individual needs. However, when using the premixed acetylcysteine and isoproterenol solution one must limit the frequency of administration with respect to the isoproterenol. It can be administered by hand nebulizer, pump, or aerosol mask and in positive-pressure breathing devices, but the drug iteslf should not be put in a heated nebulizer. In addition to the aerosol route, acetylcysteine is often effectively used by direct instillation, especially to facilitate bronchial aspiration through tracheostomy or endotracheal tubes.

Ethyl alcohol. As a matter of convenience, ethyl alcohol (ethanol) is included with the mucolytics, though not without some justification, for it is used to modify surface tension of pulmonary fluids. More often, however, it is referred to as an antifoaming agent. Its action is not directed primarily to abnormal mucoid substances but rather to the thinner but equally hazardous edema fluid that frequently obstructs bronchioles and alveoli. Aerosolized alcohol performs a valuable service in the treatment of acute pulmonary edema, but when the acute episode subsides its use should be discontinued because of the irritating effects that alcohol has on the respiratory mucosa.

Acute pulmonary edema is characterized by the accumulation in the alveoli and bronchioles of a thin watery fluid, often containing some blood. There is enough protein in edema fluid to produce froth as air passes through it with tidal ventilation. A relatively small volume of fluid can thus be increased to a much larger volume of massed bubbles that severely obstruct the small airways and alveoli. This foamy edema fluid seriously compromises the alveolar ventilation/perfusion ratio and in a sense drowns the patient in his or her own water.

The function of aerosolized alcohol is to mix with the edema fluid, where its ability to reduce the mass of suffocating frothy foam had been observed long before the advent of current respiratory therapy techniques.[87] Delivered by the force of inspiratory positive-pressure breathing instruments, alcohol aerosolized by oxygen has become part of the standard treatment of acute pulmonary edema. Frothy fluid is converted to a liquid state that not only occupies less bronchiolar and alveolar space, with relief of obstruction, but is more readily removed by the cough mechanism and the perfusing pulmonary circulation. Despite the observed benefit of this therapy, there is no uniform agreement on, or clear-cut explanation of, the exact mechanism by which alcohol disperses pulmonary foam. Most authorities attribute the action to a modification of edema fluid surface tension that decreases the stability of bubbles, but they differ as to what direction this change takes.

Concentrations between 25% and 50% are suitable for therapeutic effect, without undue risk of local airway irritation. Although absorption does occur in the alveoli, the actual amounts of alcohol in the bloodstream at any one time are well within the limits of sobriety. Alcohol can be given by any standard aerosol generator by way of an aerosol mask or by positive pressure.

The effects of alcohol on the respiratory system are not limited to the aerosol form. Ingested alcohol can inhibit ciliary function and macrophage activity and may induce bronchospasm in some patients.[88] Studies show a definite relationship between obstructive lung disease and chronic alcohol consumption.[89,90]

Sodium bicarbonate. Reference was made to the mucolytic effect of this common household commodity, baking soda, in the preceding discussion of the action of tyloxapol. Large mucoid molecular chains tend to break as the pH of their environment rises, and local bronchial alkalinity can reach a pH of 8.3 without untoward irritation or damage.[91] Indeed, the treatment of acutely obstructive episodes of cystic fibrosis often includes, along with other modalities, the deliberate production of systemic alkalosis by the intravenous and oral administration of bicarbonate to make full use of its mucolytic properties. Although this regimen is less necessary with the availability of more potent mucolytics such as acetylcysteine and proteolytics (discussed next), sodium bicarbonate aerosol still has a place not only with this disease but also with chronic states of the adult. It is not uncommon to encounter patients in whom mucolysis from the usually effective agents lessens, and for such patients it is occasionally beneficial to switch to aerosolized 2% sodium bicarbonate to see whether mucus flow can be stimulated. For home use a teaspoonful of the soda in a cup of sterile water makes a readily available solution.

Proteolytics. As the name indicates, members of this group lyse the protein material found in purulent sputum. Although there is only one commercial preparation, for all practical purposes, enjoying widespread use, a brief description of the development of this therapy is felt to be pertinent here.

Trypsin. Because the effectiveness of mucolytics decreases with increasing purulency of bronchial secretions, the early efforts to find an adjuvant agent centered on trypsin, a proteinase (enzyme active against protein) of the pancreas. Trypsin plays an important role in the natural digestion of ingested protein, but it is most effective on protein that is already partially digested. It also acts on respiratory and intestinal mucin and on fibrin. The use of trypsin as an aerosol demonstrated its effectiveness in cleansing the upper airways of proteinaceous accumulations, apparently without damage to living cells or impairment of ciliary function. Some early investigators were disappointed with its results, feeling that it sometimes worsened the obstruction. Hoarseness was a frequent and troublesome complication, attributed to too high concentrations of the drug or too rapid administration.[92-94] Aerosolized trypsin was used for several years and, in my opinion, produced fairly satisfactory results, superior to other products then available. There were a few febrile reactions noted, and because of the real or imagined risk of an allergic reaction it was common to include an antihistamine in the treatment program. The effectiveness of a proteolytic aerosol was enough to prompt further search for better products, and trypsin has now been replaced by dornase.

Dornase. Dornase (pancreatic dornase, pancreatic deoxyribonuclease, Dornavac) is not a digestant in the same manner as trypsin, although it, too, is an important natural proteolytic. It is more specific in its action than is trypsin, since it depolymerizes (breaks long chains into smaller ones) deoxyribonucleic acid (DNA).[95] Therapeutically, this is most important, since it has been determined that from 30% to 70% of the solid matter of purulent secretions is composed of DNA.[96] The principal source of dornase is beef pancrease, but dornase is also produced by the pathogenic bacterium hemolytic *Streptococcus*. Indeed, the filtrate of a culture of hemolytic *Streptococcus* contains two active enzymes, streptococcal fibrinolysin (streptokinase) and streptococcal deoxyribonuclease (streptodornase). We might infer from its name that streptokinase acts mostly on fibrous tissue and as such is not particularly relevant to our present needs. A combination of these two enzymes is commercially prepared as Varidase, and although it is rather widely used for local application and intracavitary instillation, it has had limited use as an aerosol.[97,98]

Clinically, dornase has been indicated in any bronchopulmonary condition in which the accumulation of purulent sputum interferes with ventilation or with the resolution of an infection. It was thus of use in pneumonia, pulmonary abscess, bronchiectasis, cystic fibrosis, and especially in an acute respiratory infection superimposed on chronic lung disease.[99] As might be expected, some believe that enzyme aerosols have no useful role in clinical medicine.[100] However, others believe it to be one of the most valuable of available aerosols for *specific* use.[101] It is effective only against infected sputum, and indications for its use can be determined by visual examination of the sputum for color and consistency. For predominantly mucoid secretions it is of little value. No significant side reactions have been noted, and the only common patient complaint is posttreatment burning of the mouth, easily prevented by a vigorous mouthwash immediately following therapy. Inhalation of 100,000 units two to three times daily for no more than 4 consecutive days is generally sufficient. More prolonged use in one sequence is inadvisable because of the possible appearance of an inhibiting antideoxyribonuclease, which inactivates proteolytic action.[102] Formal approval of dornase by the FDA for clinical use was withdrawn in 1977 because of insufficient evidence to support its effectiveness.

Administration of antibiotics   When it became apparent that a new effective route was available for the administration of drugs, interest soon developed in the use of this new route in treating respiratory tract infections, especially such localized bronchopulmonary diseases as lung abscess, necrotizing pneumonia, and bronchiectasis, which were especially resistant to conventional therapy. In the mid-1940s sulfonamides were aerosolized, but the advent of penicillin and subsequent antibiotics stimulated extensive use of aerosols and the accumulation of a significant background of experience.[103-108]

The rationale for aerosol therapy was based on the speculation that even with adequate blood levels of systemically administered antibiotics, the diffusion of the drug from blood into infected tissue for its direct antibacterial action was blocked by tissue reaction to the infection. In localized lesions, especially, it was believed that the presence of thick bronchial and alveolar exudates composed a formidable diffusion barrier. Also, it was thought probable that interstitial edema and fibrosis of the diseased area were additional factors in preventing therapeutic antibiotic tissue levels. These observations were borne out by the frequent observation of active microbial growth in sputum while intensive systemic therapy was being administered.

The ideal antibiotic for aerosol use has effective topical action and is poorly absorbed. Further, it is necessary that the infection being treated is accessible from the respiratory tract surface. From a practical point of view it can be generalized that aerosolized antibiotics play their greatest role in the treatment of stubborn gram-negative respiratory tract infections, where the nature of the infection and the frequently accompanying airway obstruction require long-term therapy. Large doses of effective antibiotics can be used, self-administered at home if desired, with minimal hazard of untoward reactions. In the interest of economy, antibiotics should be aerosolized during inhalation only, using either a simple pump or gas-powered hand nebulizer or an ultrasonic nebulizer. Table 11-6 lists those antibiotics that have been found suitable for aerosolization, with suggested doses for their use.

The reported results make it apparent that there is no magic cure in the technique of aerosolization and that although some patients respond dramat-

Table 11-6
Antibiotics for aerosol use

Antibiotic	Aerosol dose
Carbenicillin	1-3 g
Neomycin*	50-400 mg
Bacitracin*	5000-200,000 units
Streptomycin	750-1000 mg
Chloramphenicol	200-400 mg
Kanamycin*	100-400 mg
Colymycin-M	25-150 mg
Polymyxin*	10-50 mg
Gentamicin*	40-120 mg
Amphotericin*	5-20 mg
Mycostatin*	100,000-400,000 units

From Miller, W.F.: Fundamental principles of aerosol therapy, Respir. Care 17:295, 1972.
*Poor or nonabsorbed in aerosol state.

ically, others show little or no benefit.[109,110] In view of the modifying factors listed previously and with variability of bacterial susceptibility encountered in systemic therapy, this is not surprising. However, the efficacy of aerosolized antibiotics can be significantly increased by using a technique that deserves special mention.[111] The same exudates and secretions that impair drug diffusion from blood to tissue are able to interfere with the action of aerosolized particles, and they are probably responsible for many instances of therapeutic failure. The prior or concomitant use of bronchodilators will aid penetration of antibiotic particles but will not bring them into bacterial contact in the presence of thick secretions. Often, extensive therapy with heated water aerosol and chest physical therapy are essential to clear the airways for penetration and deposition of antibiotic aerosols. If a secretion's barrier still blocks contact of antibiotic with the infected area, the antibiotic may be combined with pancreatic dornase. The latter reduces viscosity of purulent sputum and, while so doing, exposes the infecting organism to the action of the inhaled antibiotic.

In summary, we can say that, for the most part, aerosolized antibiotics are not intended to supplant the systemic but rather to supplement them in treating diseases characterized by copious purulent sputum. The respiratory therapy reduces the amount of secretions and clears it of bacterial growth, but we must remember that the risk of distant spread of infection to other parts of the body can best be controlled by maintaining therapeutic blood levels by systemic antibiotics. Of special interest to the therapist is the frequent appearance of *Pseudomonas aeruginosa (Bacillus pyocyaneus)* in the respiratory tract of patients suffering from chronic respiratory disease or who have been receiving treatment from poorly maintained respiratory therapy equipment, especially patients who have been tracheotomized and require frequent tracheobronchial suctioning. A potentially serious infection, it is notoriously resistant to systemic therapy, even by those drugs which sensitivity tests would indicate to be effective. The most encouraging results appear to follow the combined therapy of pancreatic dornase and gentamicin, which, because systemic absorption from the aerosol is so slight, can be used safely.

References

1. Hodgkin, J.E., Johnson, L., and Lopez, B.: An improved method for aerosolizing anesthetic for flexible bronchoscopy, Resp. Care **21**:134-137, 1976.
2. Goodman, L.S., and Gilman, A.: The pharmacological basis of therapeutics, ed. 4, New York, 1970, The MacMillan Co.
3. Meyers, F.H., Jawetz, E., and Goldfien, A.: Review of Medical pharmacology, ed. 5, Los Altos, Calif., 1976, Lange Medical Publications.
4. Issellbacher, K.J., et al.: Harrison's principles of internal medicine, ed. 9, New York, 1980, McGraw-Hill Book Co.
5. Goth, A.: Medical pharmacology, ed. 9, St. Louis, 1978, The C.V. Mosby Co.
6. Bergersen, B.S.: Pharmacology in nursing, ed. 14, St. Louis, 1979, The C.V. Mosby Co.
7. Harper, H.A., Rodwell, V.W., and Mayes, P.A.: Review of physiological chemistry, ed. 16, Los Altos, Calif., 1977, Lange Medical Publications.
8. Santa Cruz, R., et al.: Tracheal mucus velocity in normal man and patients

with obstructive lung disease: effects of terbutaline, Am. Rev. Respir. Dis. **109**:458, 1974.

9. DeTroyer, A., Yernault, J.C., and Rodenstein, D.: Influence of beta-2 agonist aerosols on pressure-volume characteristics of the lungs, Am. Rev. Respir. Dis. **118**:987, 1978.

10. Ziment, I: Why are they saying bad things about IPPB? Respir. Care **18**: 677-689, 1973.

11. Davies, D.S.: In Junod, A.E., and De Haller, R., editors: Lung metabolism, New York, 1975, Academic Press, Inc.

12. Blackwell, E.W., et al.: Metabolism of isoprenaline after aerosol and direct intrabronchial administration in man and dog, Br. J. Pharmacol. **50**:587, 1974.

13. Keighley, J.F.: Iatrogenic asthma associated with adrenergic aerosols, Ann. Intern. Med. **65**:985, 1966.

14. Singer, O.P., and Wilson, W.J.: Laryngotracheobronchitis: 2 years' experience with racemic epinephrine, Can. Med. Assoc. J. **115**:132-134, 1976.

15. Wesley, C.R., Cotton, E.K., and Brooks, J.G.: Nebulized racemic epinephrine by IPPB for the treatment of croup: a double-blind study, Am. J. Dis. Child **132**(5):484-487, 1978.

16. Sympathomimetic bronchodilators (editorial), Lancet **1**:535, 1971.

17. Sollman, R.: A manual of pharmacology, Philadelphia, 1957, W.B. Saunders Co.

18. Lands, A.M., et al.: The pharmacologic actions of the bronchodilator drug isoetharine, J. Am. Pharm. Assoc. **47**:744, 1958.

19. Shulman, M., et al.: Cardiovascular effects of isoetharine administered to surgical patients during cyclopropane anesthesia, Br. J. Anaesth. **42**:439, 1970.

20. El-Shaboury, A.H.: Controlled study of a new inhalant in asthma and bronchitis, Br. Med. J. **5416**:1037, 1964.

21. Kelman, G.R., et al.: Cardiovascular effects of solbutamol, Nature **221**:1251, 1969.

22. Owen, J.A.: A bronchodilator well-known in Europe, Hosp. Formulary, Aug. 1975, pp. 386-388.

23. Snider, G.L., and Laguanda, R.: Albuterol and isoproterenol aerosols. A controlled study of duration of effect in asthmatic patients, J.A.M.A. **221**:682-685, 1972.

24. Bloomfield, P., et al.: Comparison of solbutamol given intravenously and by intermittent positive-pressure breathing in life-threatening asthma, Br. Med. J. **1**(6167):848-850, 1979.

25. McEvoy, J.D.S., Vall-spinosa, A., and Paterson, J.W.: Assessment of orciprenaline and isoproterenol infusions in asthmatic patients, Am. Rev. Respir. Dis. **108**:490-500, 1973.

26. Sobol, B.J., and Reed, A.: The rapidity of Alupent and isoproterenol, Ann. Allergy **32**:137-141, 1974.

27. Brogden, R.N., Speight, T.M., and Avery G.S.: Terbutaline: a preliminary report of its pharmacological properties and therapeutic efficacy in asthma, Drugs **6**:324-332, 1973.

28. Trembath P.N., et al.: Comparison of four weeks' treatment with fenoterol and terbutaline aerosols in adult asthmatics. A double-blind crossover study, J. Allergy Clin. Immunol. **63**(6):345-400, 1979.

29. Eisenstadt, W.S., and Nichols, S.S.: Adverse effects of adrenergic aerosols in bronchial asthma, Ann. Allergy **27**:283, 1969.

30. Cohen, A.A., and Hale, F.C.: Comparative effects of isoproterenol aerosols on airway resistance in obstructive pulmonary disease, Am. J. Med. Sci. **249**:309, 1965.

31. Davison, F.R.: Handbook of materia medica, toxicology, and pharmacology, St. Louis, 1949, The C.V. Mosby Co.

32. Nadel, J.A., and Widdecombe, J.G.: Mechanism of bronchoconstriction with dust inhalation, Clin. Res. **10**:91, 1962.

33. Dautreband, L., et al. : Effects of atropine microaerosols on airway resistance in man, Arch. Int. Pharmacodyn. **139**:198, 1962.

34. Chamberlain, D.A., et al.: Atropine methonitrate and isoprenaline in bronchial asthma, Lancet **2**:1019, 1962.

35. Storms, W.W., et al.: Aerosol Sch 1000, Am. Rev. Respir. Dis. **111**:419, 1975.

36. Gross, N.J.: Sch 1000: a new anticholinergic bronchodilator, Am. Rev. Respir. Dis. **112**:823, 1975.

37. Gerhardt, T., McCarthy, J., and Banca-

lari, E.: Aminophylline therapy for idiopathic apnea in premature infants: effects on lung function, Pediatrics **62**(5):801-804, 1978.

38. Brazier, J.L., Renaud, H., Ribon, B., and Salle, B.L.: Plasma xanthine levels in low birthweight infants treated or not treated with theophylline, Arch. Dis. Child. **54**(3):194-199, 1979.

39. Aranda, J.V., and Turmen, T.: Methylxanthines in apnea of prematurity, Clin. Perinatol. **6**(1):87-108, 1979.

40. Iwainsky, H, and Sehrt, I.: Theophylline therapy—foundations and possibilities, Z. Erkr. Atmungsorgane **152**(1):21-36, 1979.

41. Powell, J.R., et al.: The influence of cigarette smoking and sex on theophylline disposition, Am. Rev. Respir. Dis. **116**:17-23, 1977.

42. Chang, K.C., Bell, T.D., Laver, B.A., and Chai, H.: Altered theophylline pharmacokinetics during acute respiratory viral illness, Lancet **1**(8074):1132-1133, 1978.

43. Aviado, D.M., and Carrillo, L.R.: Antiasthmatic adtion of corticosteroids: a review of the literature on their mechanism of action, J. Clin. Pharmacol. **10**:3-11, 1970.

44. Ellul-Micallef, R., and Fenech, F.F.: Effect of intravenous prednisolone in asthmatics with diminshed adrenergic responsiveness, Lancet **2**:1269-1270, 1975.

45. McAllen, M.K., Kochanowski, S.J., and Shaw, K.M.: Steroid aerosols in asthma: an assessment of betamethasone valerate and 12-month study of patients on maintence treatment, Br. Med. J. **1**:171-175, 1974.

46. Forsham, P.H.: The adrenal gland, Clin. Symp. **15**:3, 1963.

47. Kleiner, I.S., and Orten, J.M.: Biochemistry, ed. 7, St. Louis, 1966, The C.V. Mosby Co.

48. Williams, R.H., editor: Textbook of endocrinology, Philadelphia, 1962, W.B. Saunders Co.

49. Norman, P.S., et al.: Adrenal function during the use of dexamethasone aerosols in the treatment of ragweed hay fever, J. Allerg. **40**:57, 1967.

50. Fisch, B.R., and Grater, W.C.: Dexamethasone aerosol in respiratory tract disease, J. New Drugs **2**:298, 1962.

51. Golub, J.R.: Long-term triamcinolone acetonide aerosol treatment in adult patients with chronic bronchial asthma, Ann. Allergy **44**(3):131-137, 1980.

52. Chervinsky, P., and Petraco, A.J.: Incidence or oral candidiasis during therapy with triamcinolone acetonide aerosol, Ann. Allergy **43**(2):80-83, 1974.

53. Clark, T.J.: Corticosteroid treatment of asthma, Schweiz. Med. Wochenschr. **110**(6):215-218, 1980.

54. Chambers, W.B., and Malfitan, V.A. Beclomethasone dipropionate aerosol in the treatment of asthma in steroid-independent children, J. Int. Med. Res. **7**(5):415-422, 1979.

55. Datau, G., and Rochiccioli, P.: Corticotropic testing during long-term beclomethasone dipropionate treatment in asthmatic children, Poumon Coeur **34**(4):247-453, 1978.

56. Richards, W., et al.: Steroid-dependent asthma treated with inhaled beclomethasone dipropionate in children, Ann. Allergy **41**(5):274-277, 1978.

57. Imbeau, S.A.: Aerosol beclomethasone treatment of chronic severe asthma. A one-year experience, J.A.M.A. **240**(12):1260-1262, 1978.

58. Kass, I., Vijayachandra Nair, S., and Patil, K.D.: Beclomethasone dipropionate aerosol in the treatment of steroid-dependent asthmatic patients. An assessment of 18 months of therapy, Chest **71**(6):703-707, 1977.

59. Lee-Hong, E., and Collins-Williams, C.: The long-term use of beclomethasone dipropionate for the control of severe asthma in children, Ann. Allergy **38**(4):242-244, 1977.

60. Hudgel, D.W., and Spector, S.L.: Pulmonary infiltration with eosinophila. Recurrence in an asthmatic patient treated with beclomethasone dipropionate, Chest **72**(3):359-360, 1977.

61. Neuman, I., and Toshner, D.: Beclomethasone dipropionate in pediatric perennial extrinsic rhinitis, Ann. Allergy **40**(5):346-348, 1978.

62. Brown, H.M., Storey G., and Jackson, F.A.: Beclomethasone dipropionate aerosol in treatment of perennial and

seasonal rhinitis: a review of five years' experience, Br. J. Clin. Pharmacol. **3**:283S-286S, 1977.

63. Girard, J.P., Cuevas, M. and Heimlich, E.M.: A placebo controlled double-blind trial of beclomethasone dipropionate in the treatment of allergic rhinitis, Allergol. Immunopathol. **6**(2):109-116, 1978.

64. Woenne, R., Kattan, M., and Levison, H.: Sodium cromoglycate–induced changes in the dose-response curve of inhaled methacholine and histamine in asthmatic children, Am. Rev. Respir. Dis. **119**(6):927-932, 1979.

65. Mathison, D.A., et al.: Cromolyn treatment of asthma, J.A.M.A. **216**:1454, 1971.

66. Smith, J.M.: Prolonged use of disodium cromoglycate in children and young persons—ten years experience, Schweiz. Med. Wochenschr. **110**(6):183-184, 1980.

67. Turner-Warwick, M.: Clinical practice with regard to management of the adult asthmatic with cromoglycate, Schweiz. Med. Wochenschr. **110**(6):181-183, 1980.

68. Liern Caballero, M., Alberola Carbonell, C., and Climent P'erez, J.L.: Clinical and histological study to assess changes in the nasal mucosa in patients with chronic perennial rhinitis comparing sodium cromoglycate and placebo, Scand. J. Respir. Dis. **59**(3):160-166, 1978.

69. Goodman, M.L., and Irwin, J.W.: Disodium cromoglycate in anaphylaxis and pollinosis, Ann. Allergy **40**(3):177-180, 1978.

70. Frostad, A.B.: The treatment of seasonal allergic rhinitis with a 2% aqueous solution of sodium cromoglycate delivered by a metered dose nasal spray, Clin. Allergy **7**(4):347-353, 1977.

71. Nikano, J.: Prostaglandins and the circulation, Mod. Concepts Cardiovasc. Dis. **40**:49, 1971.

72. Parker, C.W., and Snider, D.E.: Prostaglandins in asthma, Ann. Intern. Med. **78**:963, 1973.

73. Katz, R.L., and G.J.: Prostaglandins—basic and clinical considerations, Anesthsiology **40**:471, 1974.

74. Said, S.I., et al.: Pulmonary alveolar hypoxia release of prostoglandins and other humoral mediators, Science **185**:1180, 1974.

75. Tainter, M.L., et al.: Alevaire as a mucolytic agent, N. Engl. J. Med. **253**:764, 1955.

76. Miller, J.B., et al.: Alevaire inhalations for eliminating secretions in asthma, sinusitis, and bronchiectasis of adults, Ann. Allergy **12**:611, 1954.

77. Sadove, M.S., and Miller, C.E.: Postoperative aerosol therapy, J.A.M.A. **156**:759, 1954.

78. Denton, R.: Continuous nebulization therapy, Pediatr. Clin. North Am. **1**:625, 1954.

79. Palmer, K.N.V.: The effect of an aerosol detergent in chronic bronchitis, Lancet **272-1**:611, 1957.

80. Sheffner, A.L.: The mucolytic activity, mechanisms of action, and metabolism of acetylcysteine, Pharmacotherapy **1**:47, 1964.

81. Hirsch, S.R., and Kory, R.C.: An evaluation of the effect of nebulized N-acetylcysteine on sputum consistency, J. Allerg. **39**:265, 1967.

82. Moser, K.M., and Rhodes, P.G.: Acute effects of aerosolized acetylcysteine upon spirometeric measurements in subjects with and without obstructive pulmonary disease, Dis. Chest **49**:370, 1966.

83. Thomas, P.A., and Treasure, R.I.: Effect of N-acetyl-L-cysteine on pulmonary surface activity, Am. Rev. Respir. Dis. **94**:175, 1966.

84. Webb, W.R.: New mucolytic agents for sputum liquefaction, Postgrad. Med. **36**:449, 1964.

85. Mucolytic agent, Br. Med. J. **2**:603, 1966.

86. Anderson, G.: A clinical trial of a mucolytic agent—acetylcysteine—in chronic bronchitis, Br. J. Dis. Chest **60**:101, 1966.

87. Luisada, A.A., et al.: Alcohol vapor by inhalation in the treatment of acute pulmonary edema, Circulation **5**:363, 1952.

88. Geppert E.F., and Boushey, H.A.: An investigation of the mechanism of ethanol-induced bronchoconstriction, Am. Rev. Respir. Dis. **118**:135-139, 1978.

89. Emirgil, C., and Sobol, B.: Pulmonary

function in former alcoholics, Chest **72**:45-51, 1977.

90. Heinemann, H.O.: Alcohol and the lung, Am. J. Med. **63**:81-85, 1977.

91. Tainter, M.L., et al.: Alevaire as a mucolytic agent, N. Engl. J. Med. **253**:764, 1955.

92. Limber, C.R., et al.: Enzymatic lysis of respiratory secretions by aerosol trypsin, J.A.M.A. **149**:816, 1952.

93. Unger, L., and Unger, A.H.: Trypsin inhalations in respiratory conditions with thick sputum, J.A.M.A. **152**:1109, 1953.

94. Prince, H.E., et al.: Aerosol trypsin in the treatment of asthma, Ann. Allergy **12**:25, 1954.

95. Salomon, A., et al.: Aerosols of pancreatic dornase in bronchopulmonary disease, Ann. Allergy **12**:71, 1954.

96. Sherry, S., et al.: Presence and significance of deoxyribose nucleotide in purulent exudate, Proc. Soc. Exp. Biol. Med. **68**:179, 1948.

97. Meunster, J.J., et al.: Treatment of unresolved pneumonia with streptokinase and streptodornase, Am. J. Med. **12**:367, 1952.

98. Craven, J.F.: Treatment of obstructive atelectasis by aerosol administration of proteolytic enzymes, J. Pediatr. **42**:228, 1953.

99. Clifton, E.E.: Pancreatic dornase aerosol in pulmonary, endotracheal, and endobronchial disease, Chest **30**:1, 1956.

100. Lyons, H.A.: Use of therapeutic aerosols, Am. J. Cardiol. **12**:461, 1963.

101. Egan, D.F.: Fundamentals of respiratory therapy, ed. 3, St. Louis, 1977, The C.V. Mosby Co.

102. Miller, W.F.: In Kagan, B.M., editor: Antimicrobial therapy, Philadelphia, 1970, W.B. Saunders Co.

103. Olsen, Am.: Streptomycin aerosol in the treatment of chronic bronchiectasis: preliminary report, Proc. Staff Meet. Mayo Clin. **21**:53, 1946.

104. Garthwaite, B., and Barach, A.L.: Penicillin aerosol therapy in bronchiectasis, lung abscess, and chronic bronchitis, Am. J. Med. **3**:261, 1947.

105. Eastlake, C., Jr.: Aerosol therapy in sinusitis, bronchiectasis, and lung abscess, Bull. N.Y. Acad. Med. **26**:423, 1950.

106. Christie, H.E., et al.: Aerosol therapy for lung abscess, Can. Med. Assoc. J. **62**:478, 1950.

107. Melica, A., et al.: Oxytetracycline inhalation in the treatment of acute and chronic bronchial infection, G. Clin. Med. **47**:416, 1962.

108. Naumov, G.P.: Pathologic changes in upper respiratory passages and lungs following use of antibiotic electroaerosols, Fed. Proc. **25**:654, 1966.

109. Pines, A., et al.: Gentamicin and colistin in chronic purulent bronchial infections, Br. Med. J. **2**:543, 1967.

110. Bilodeau, M., et al.: Studies of absorption of kanamycin by aerosol, Ann. N.Y. Acad. Sci. **132**:870, 1966.

111. Spier, R., et al.: Aerosolized pancreatic dornase and antibiotics in pulmonary infection, J.A.M.A. **178**:878, 1961.

Chapter 12   Gas therapy

Medical gases

The administration of therapeutic gases is a very important function of the respiratory therapist. Indeed, it is from the humble beginning of the "oxygen service" of the average general hospital that the present skilled technology of respiratory therapy evolved, and even though the therapist has now assumed a host of duties and responsibilities, gas therapy is the foundation of the therapist's work. We have covered many aspects of gases—something of their behavior and characteristics, the mechanics of introducing them into the body through ventilation, and the activities of some of them as they participate in body functions. In this chapter we consider the packaging and distrubution of compressed therapy gases and the clinical equipment and techniques for using them to treat patients. We call on some previously discussed principles as we describe both the gaseous and liquid forms of gases.

Much of the data in this section of the chapter are drawn from two sources with which all respiratory therapists should be familiar, the codes of the National Fire Protection Association[1] and pamphlets of the Compressed Gas Association, Inc., especially those that describe the common medical gases and the many important safety measures for which the therapist must be held responsible.[2] In addition, the student will find useful information in the many good brochures and other publications of the manufacturers of gases and gas equipment.

Agencies

Many agencies are involved in the control of manufacturing and the safe use of medical gases and devices employed in pulmonary medicine. A general outline of these agencies is presented below, with the knowledge that more detailed information is available in other sources.[3-7] The areas of responsibility covered by various agencies is being redefined continually to meet the demands of ever-changing technology. The agencies discussed in this chapter can be divided into two general groups: regulating and recommending.

Regulating agencies. Regulating agencies are federal, state, and local bodies that have the legal right to regulate, and the regulations often use standards prepared by the many recommending bodies. An example of a regulating agency would be a local county government that has adopted the standards for the storage of bulk oxygen as established by the National Fire Protection Association.

Recommending agencies. Recommending agencies are usually made up of individuals involved in some aspect of technology. An example would be the Compressed Gas Association, which is made up of equipment, container, and valve manufacturers and distributors and others involved in compressed and liquified gases.[7]

Clinicians involved in respiratory therapy can provide input to recommending bodies through their representative of a body, and most recommending bodies are looking for input from knowledgeable individuals. An example of a recommending body into which a clinician could provide input would be the Z-79 Committee of the American National Standards Institute.

Some of the major regulating and recommending agencies that are involved in respiratory therapy are listed here. These agencies may also be interested in other areas of technology.

Regulating bodies

1. Interstate Commerce Commission (ICC): The commission that regulated the construction, transport, and testing of compressed gas cylinders from 1948 to 1970.
2. Department of Transportation (DOT): The department of the federal government given for the responsibility in 1970 for compressed gas cylinders, which were previously regulated by the ICC.
3. Department of Health and Human Services (HHS): This department of the federal government was formerly called the Department of Health, Education and Welfare (HEW). HHS has created many agencies that are involved in health delivery. As an example, the Food and Drug Administration (FDA) is an agency that requires a certain level of purity for medical gases.

Recommending bodies

1. Compressed Gas Association (CGA): The CGA is made up of individuals involved in the compressed gas industry. It has created standards and safety systems for compressed gas systems.
2. National Fire Protection Association (NFPA): The NFPA is an agency involved in improved methods of fire protection and prevention, including creating standards for the storage of flammable and oxydizing gases.
3. International Standards Organization (ISO): The ISO is the international agency for standardization covering most areas of technology.

4. Food and Drug Administration (FDA): The FDA is an agency of HHS and requires a certain level of purity for medical gases.

4. American National Standards Institute (ANSI): ANSI is a private, nonprofit organization that coordinates the voluntary developments of national standards in the United States and represents U.S. interests in the area of international standardization.

5. Bureau of Medical Devices (BMD): The BMD is an agency of the FDA and was formed in 1976 to classify, provide standards for, and regulate medical devices.[1]

5. Z-79 Committee: Z-79 is a committee of ANSI and is the American National Standards Committee on standards for anesthetic equipment. It has produced a series of standards for anesthesia and ventilatory devices. These devices include anesthesia machines, reservoir bags, tracheal tubes and their connectors and adaptors, humidifiers, nebulizers, and other oxygen-related equipment.

6. Occupational Safety and Health Agency (OSHA): OSHA is an agency of the federal Department of Labor and is responsible for occupational safety.

6. Association for the Advancement of Medical Instrumentation (AAMI): AAMI is a nonprofit organization involved in education and standards relating to biomedical engineering.

Pressures for compressed gases

As noted in Chapter 1, the commercial gas industry and the various fields of related engineering use the English system of measurement almost exclusively, and the student must become familiar with the necessary units when considering the packaging of gases; however, we must move back into the metric system when discussing their application to the patient. Before we attempt to discuss the matter at hand, there is one variation of measurement we have not had occasion to use in the past but which is essential in considering gas therapy. Pressure in the English system is expressed as pounds per square inch and, in the parlance of commercial gases, is abbreviated *psi*. However, it is often necessary to be more specific and to denote whether a given pressure includes that of the atmosphere or is in excess of atmospheric. This need arises because of the use of calibrated gauges to measure and record pressures. A pressure gauge, which usually consists of a numbered circular dial with a centrally pivoted needle indicator, registers zero pressure under atmospheric conditions. In other words, at zero gauge pressure there is already 1 atm of pressure (14.7 psi) active, and any deviation above zero by the gauge indicates pressure above atmospheric. Therefore the recorded pressure is referred to as *pounds per square inch, gauge* (psig). Less commonly used in ordinary gas therapy, but widely used in hyperbaric medicine, is the concept of absolute pressure. This means that actual total pressure of a gas, including that exerted by the atmosphere, and is called *pounds per square inch, absolute* (psia). The student can remember that psia is always 1 atm, or 14.7 lb/in^2, greater than psig. Thus 14.7 psig = 29.4 psia; 371.2 psig = 385.9 psia. For completeness it should be noted that hyperbaric terminology frequently employs units of atmospheres and refers to so many atmospheres, gauge (atg), or atmospheres,

Table 12-1 Therapy and anesthetic gases	Limited therapy, laboratory gases	Therapy gases	Anesthetics
	Carbon dioxide (CO$_2$) Helium (He) Nitrogen (N$_2$)	Air Helium-oxygen (He/O$_2$) Oxygen (O$_2$) Oxygen–carbon dixide (O$_2$/CO$_2$) Oxygen-nitrogen (O$_2$/N$_2$)	Cyclopropane (CH$_2$)$_3$ Ethylene (C$_2$H$_4$) Nitrous oxide (N$_2$O)

absolute (ata), with the same relationship described for pounds per square inch. By common usage, in compressed gas data, gauge pressure is implied unless otherwise specified, and psi and psig are used interchangeably, although the latter is more correct.

Cylinder gases   Of all the many gases that are compressed into cylinders for distribution, we are interested in the few that are called medical gases. Even of these, we discuss in detail only some because a few are used mainly in the laboratory and others are anesthetics, which are not in the province of the respiratory therapist. Initially, we include in our discussion the groups of gases listed in Table 12-1. These, prepared and packaged for medical use, give us a wide scope to discuss techniques involved and characteristics of compressed gases; then our clinical discussions are limited to the therapy gases.

From a safety point of view, compressed gases are classified as nonflammable (will not burn), nonflammable but will support combustion, and flammable (will burn readily). The above gases can be grouped according to their flammability as follows:

Nonflammable: nitrogen, carbon dioxide, helium
Support combustion: oxygen, nitrous oxide, air, oxygen-nitrogen, oxygen–carbon dioxide, helium-oxygen
Flammable: cyclopropane, ethylene

Gas cylinders. The containers used to hold and ship compressed or liquid medical gases are high-pressure units, carefully controlled in their specifications by regulations, both federal and industrial. They are made of seamless steel, finely tempered and nonreactive with their gaseous or liquid contents, and are classified as type 3A or 3AA cylinders. We compare various pressures used in medical gas cylinders; but regardless of the cylinder pressure, all tanks used for therapy have valves that in clinical use are fitted with devices to reduce the pressure going to the patient to a "working pressure," typically 50 psig. The valves also have safety releases that will give way before the cylinders burst should exposure to sudden heat dangerously elevate the gas pressure.

Medical gas cylinders are marked by metal stampings on their shoulders that are supposed to supply specific information (Fig. 12-1). The letters ICC (Interstate Commerce Commission) on cylinders manufactured before 1967 or DOT (Department of Transportation) on cylinders new since then are

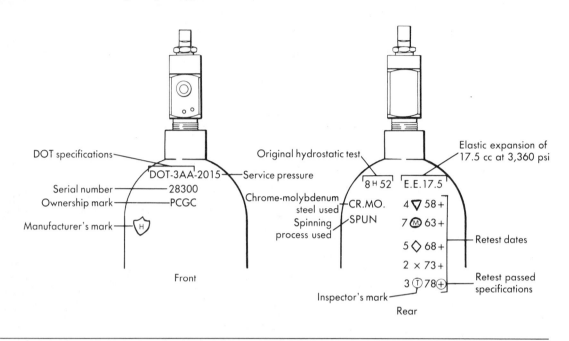

Fig. 12-1   Typical markings for cylinders containing medical gases. Front and back views are for illustration purposes only; exact location and order of markings is variable.

followed by the designation of the cylinder as a 3A or 3AA type and then by the maximum working pressure of the cylinder in pounds per square inch. This is the filling pressure of the tank, which can generally be exceeded by 10%. For example, a frequently encountered cylinder has a marked pressure of 2015 psi but is usually filled to about 2200 psi. Below these data the letter size of the cylinder is marked (E, G, etc.) followed by the serial number of the cylinder. A third line of stampings includes the initials of the company that owns the cylinder, and on fourth line a mark identifies the inspecting authority. On the opposite surface of the tank there is another set of stampings, the first line of which indicates the method by which the cylinder was manufactured, often noted as "Spun Cr-Mo," indicating the use of chrome-molybdenum. Below are a series of symbols that include the identification of the manufacturer of the cylinder, the data of its original safety test, dates of all subsequent tests as prescribed by regulation, and frequently the notation "E.E.," followed by a number that indicates the cubic centimeter elastic expansion of the cylinder under test conditions. In addition to these permanent marks, all tanks should have securely attached to them labels clearly identifying the contents and their concentrations, and some will tell the liters or cubic feet measurement of the gas.

Cylinders are given a letter designation according to size. Following is a list of most of the common sizes, in inches of diameter and height including

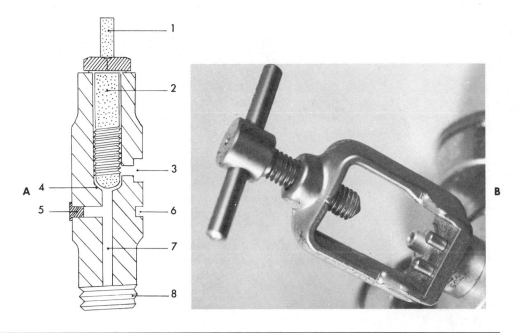

Fig. 12-2   **A,** Diagrammatic sectional sketch of a small cylinder valve. **B,** Photograph of the yoke connector used with small cylinders. (See text for description.)

valve, with an asterisk indicating the relatively few with which the respiratory therapist can expect to have frequent contact:

A	B	D*	E*	F	M	G*	H&K*
3×10	$3^{1}/_{2} \times 16$	$4^{1}/_{4} \times 20$	$4^{1}/_{4} \times 30$	$5^{1}/_{2} \times 55$	$7^{1}/_{8} \times 46$	$8^{1}/_{2} \times 55$	9×55

Sizes A through E are referred to as "small cylinders" and are used most often for anesthetic gases and portable emergency oxygen supply. These small tanks differ from the larger ones in the mechanism by which they attach to the appliances they serve. They employ a connector called a *yoke,* whereas the large cylinders (F to H&K) have a threaded outlet from their valves to which a nut attaches a pressure reducer. Fig. 12-2 illustrates the general structure of the cylinder valves and the yoke used with small cylinders. *A* represents a small cylinder valve, but the principle of the large valves is similar. *1* is the stem on which a handgrip is placed when in use; *2* is the valve plunger with its threaded lower end; *3* is the outlet of the valve, a recess in the small valves but a projecting threaded nipple in the large ones; *4* is the valve seat; *5* is an emergency pressure release; *6* is one of a pair of borings in the valve body of the small cylinders only, part of the Pin-Index Safety System; described later; *7* is the gas channel into the valve; and *8* is the threaded connection between the valve and the cylinder. *B* is an illustration of a yoke connector for the A to E cylinders that fits about the cylinder valve, showing the aperture that is slipped about the valve; a screw that holds the yoke firmly onto the valve; the small receiving nipple that fits snugly into the gas outlet *(3, in A);* and the pins of the Index System just noted.

As an aid to the easy identification of medical gases, Table 12-2 lists the color code for the size E cylinders, specially those intended for use on anesthesia machines, that has been adopted by the Bureau of Standards of the U.S. Department of Commerce.

It is strongly emphasized that the color of a cylinder is to be used only as a rough guide, and the therapist *must always check* the cylinder contents by *carefully reading its label.* Many of the larger cylinders employ essentially the same color scale, but there is enough variation among the many tanks the therapist may have occasion to handle to make the color identification unreliable. It is hoped that soon there will be a fully uniform international color marking system.

Every 5 to 10 years compressed gas cylinders must be subjected to a safety inspection and testing as specified in DOT regulations. Under compression

	Gas	Color
Table 12-2 Color code for size E gas cylinders	Oxygen	Green
	Carbon dioxide	Gray
	Nitrous oxide	Light blue
	Cyclopropane	Orange
	Helium	Brown
	Ethylene	Red
	Carbon dioxide and oxygen	Gray and green
	Helium and oxygen	Brown and green
	Air	Yellow

	Liters	Cubic feet	Gallons
Table 12-3 Gas volumes conversion factors	28.316	1	7.481
	1	0.03531	0.2642
	3.785	0.1337	1

	Gas	Physical state	psig	Gas	Physical state	psig
Table 12-4 Pressure ranges of medical gases	Air	G	1800	CO_2	L	825
	O_2	G	1800-2200	He	G	1650-2000
	O_2/N_2	G	1800-2200	$(CH_2)_3$	L	75
	O_2/CO_2	G	1500-2200	N_2O	L	745
	He/O_2	G	1650-2000	C_2H_4	G	1250
	N_2	G	1800-2200			

such factors as leaks, cylinder expansion, and wall stress are determined, and the cylinders are inspected internally and cleaned. The date of each such testing is stamped on the cylinder shoulder.

Because of the many ways of expressing gas volume measurements, it is helpful to be able to convert from one to the other by the use of the factors in Table 12-3.

Because of the different filling pressures of gases, volumes of different gases in the same size cylinder will vary. For example, a G cylinder contains about 187 cubic feet of oxygen but only about 147 cubic feet of helium. Table 12-4 gives an idea of the approximate filling pressure ranges of medical gases, depending on the types of cylinders used, calibrated at 70°F.

Filling (charging) cylinders. We differentiate here between gases and liquid gases.

Gases. The general rule is that gas cylinders will be filled at a temperature of 70°F to the pressure specified for a given cylinder, as stamped on its shoulder. However, certain gases, including oxygen, helium, helium-oxygen, and oxygen–carbon dioxide, may be filled to 10% in excess of the stated pressure. Thus a cylinder certified for 2015 psi may be filled to a pressure of 2217 psi and is generally referred to as a 2200 pound tank.

Liquid gases. For those gases that are packaged in liquid form, a limiting "filling density" determines how much may be put in each cylinder. The filling density is the ratio between the weight of liquid gas put in a cylinder and the weight of water that the cylinder can contain. Thus the carbon dioxide filling density of 68% means that the weight of the liquid gas allowable to charge a cylinder is equal to 68% of the weight of water that the cylinder has the capacity to hold. The filling densities of cyclopropane and nitrous oxide are 55% and 68%, respectively.

Cylinder pressures for liquid gases are considerably lower than those for vaporous gases, and the critical temperatures of the three liquid gases under consideration are all above average room temperature (carbon dioxide = 88° F; cyclopropane = 256°F; nitrous oxide = 98°F). Because liquid gas does not fill the entire volume of a given cylinder, the space above the liquid surface contains vapor of the gas in equilibrium with the liquid, and the measured pressure in the cylinder is the pressure of the *vapor* at any given temperature. Thus, although the pressure of a tank of carbon dioxide at its critical temperature of 88°F would be 1071 psig (critical pressure) and would rise with continued elevation of temperature, at room temperature of 70°F it is only about 825 psig. Similarly, the pressure of cyclopropane at its critical temperature of 256°F is 797 psig but is only 75 psig at room temperature. To compare vapor gas cylinders with liquid gas, we can say that the pressure in the former represents the force required to squeeze into a cylinder a given volume of gas; whereas in the latter it is the vapor pressure of the gas over the surface of a given weight of liquid poured into the closed container. The liquid gas pressure is dependent on the temperature and is the result of the filling of the cylinder, not the cause.

Measuring cylinder contents

Gas cylinders. The volume of gas in a cylinder is directly related to the cylinder pressure at a constant temperature. If a tank is full at 2200 psig, it will be but half full as usage drops the pressure to 1100 psig. The usual method of monitoring the depletion of cylinder contents is by the use of gauges. If greater accuracy is needed, weighing the cylinder when the weight of the empty cylinder and the density of the gas are known is more precise.

Liquid gas cylinders. Since the pressure in a liquid gas cylinder is that of the gas vapor in balance with the liquid at a given temperature, it gives no indication of how much liquid remains in the cylinder at any one time. As long as there is liquid in the cylinder, the vapor pressure and thus the recorded gauge pressure will remain unchanged even though gas is being drawn off. When the liquid is finally gone and the cylinder contains only vapor, then the pressure will fall in proportion to the reduction in the remaining gas volume until the tank is empty. Thus gauge pressure is of use in monitoring cylinder

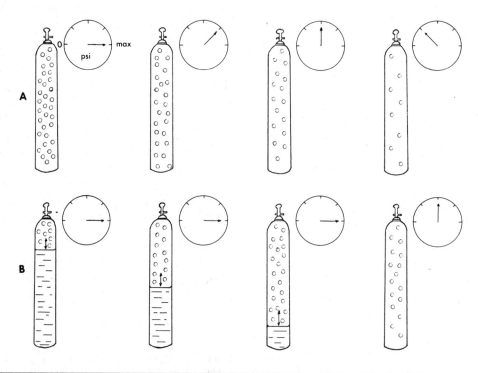

Fig. 12-3   The content of a gas-filled cylinder, **A,** is directly proportional to the gas pressure. As gas is withdrawn, for example, a pressure drop of 50% indicates a loss of 50% of the contained gas. In a liquid-gas cylinder, **B,** gauge pressure measures only the vapor pressure of gas in equilibrium with the liquid phase, and this remains constant at a given temperature as long as liquid is present. Only when all the liquid phase has vaporized, as the cylinder nears depletion, does the gauge pressure drop proportionately to the terminal volume of remaining gas.

contents only terminally; if contents must be determined, the cylinder must be weighed. Fig. 12-3 compares the pressure behavior of gas and liquid gas cylinders. Of course, the vapor pressure of liquid gas cylinders will vary with the temperature of their contents. Whereas carbon dioxide has a cylinder pressure of 838 psig at 70°F, at 60°F it has a cylinder pressure of only 733 psig. Then, as the temperature rises and approaches the critical point, more liquid will vaporize in the cylinder with an accompanying rise in pressure. Should a tank of carbon dioxide warm up to 88°F, the entire liquid contents will convert to gas; and if the temperature does not drop, as the gas is withdrawn, the cylinder gauge pressure will fall proportionately. Ethylene, on the other hand, is a gas at room temperature but with a relatively high critical temperature of 49°F; should it cool below this value, it will liquefy and its gauge pressure will stabilize as long as liquid remains in the cylinder.

Estimating duration of cylinder flow. When we set up a therapeutic procedure that uses cylinder vapor gas and that is expected to cover an extended period of time, it is a matter of both safety and convenience to be able to predict the approximate time to prepare for the replacement of the cylinder. Although this cannot be done with unerring accuracy because of the possibility of irregular flow, a practical rough estimate can be made on the basis of the average anticipated gas flows, the cylinder size, and the cylinder pressure at the start of therapy. Factors that can be used to convert these data into a time estimate can be calculated from the information on commonly used gases and cylinder sizes in Table 12-5.

Here is an example of the cumbersome combination of both the English and metric systems of measurement. Commercial gas cylinder calibrations and values are often recorded in the English system; but once a therapeutic gas leaves the cylinder pressure reducing gauge, it is subject to the medical custom of using metric measurements. In essence, we wish to determine the length of time a given number of liters of gas per minute will flow from a source of a given cubic footage of gas under a measurable pressure in psig. We now know that at a given temperature the cylinder gas volume will decrease in proportion to the drop in gauge pressure; therefore each reduction in pounds per square inch or pressure represents a specific volume of gas loss from the cylinder. This factor, relating pressure drop to gas volume, is calculated as follows:

$$\frac{\text{Cubic feet of gas in full cylinder} \times \text{Factor to convert from cubic feet to liters}}{\text{Pressure of full cylinder in psig}}$$

For example, an oxygen G cylinder contains about 187 cubic feet of gas under a filling pressure of 2200 psig. Therefore the volume of gas leaving the cylinder for every psig drop in pressure would be $(187 \times 28.3) \div 2200 = 2.41$ liters per psig (ℓ/psig).

Factors, so calculated for the gases and cylinders listed above, are shown in Table 12-6.

The principle employing the use of these factors is based on the relation-

Table 12-5
Pressures and volumes of commonly used cylinders

Gas	Full cylinder pressure	Liters/Cubic feet of gas			
		D	E	G	H&K
O_2	2200	360/12.7	623/22	5300/187	6900/244
O_2/CO_2	1800	360/12.7	623/22	5300/187	6900/244
He/O_2	2200	306/10.8	501/17.7	4250/150	5500/194
O_2/N_2	2200			5300/187	6900/244
Air	2200			5300/187	6900/244

Table 12-6
Factors to calculate duration of cylinder flow in minutes

Gas	Cylinder size			
	D	E	G	H&K
O_2, O_2/N_2, air	0.16	0.28	2.41	3.14
O_2/CO_2	0.20	0.35	2.94	3.84
He/O_2	0.14	0.23	1.93	2.50

ship that tells us: liter loss in cylinder volume per drop in each pound per square inch of cylinder pressure, multiplied by the observed cylinder gauge pressure and divided by the liter per minute gas flow delivered to the patient, equals the number of minutes the gas will flow until the cylinder is empty. Thus:

$$\text{Duration of flow in minutes} = \frac{\text{Gauge pressure in psi} \times \text{Factor}}{\text{Liter flow}}$$

As an example, let us estimate the duration of a G cylinder of oxygen with a gauge pressure of 800 psi if we use a flow of 8 ℓ/min. Referring to Table 12-6, we find the oxygen G cylinder factor of 2.41 and set up the simple fraction:

$$\frac{800 \times 2.41}{8} = 241 \text{ minutes, or approximately 4 hours}$$

Bulk oxygen

Because of the tremendous volume of oxygen used in the average general hospital, a separate discussion of special large bulk storage systems is warranted. Bulk oxygen storage consists of any system capable of accommodating more than 12,000 cubic feet of the gas ready for use or more than 25,000 cubic feet including unconnected reserves. Such systems may be located out of doors or in a special building set aside for the purpose. Strict regulations for locating and maintaining bulk oxygen systems have been established by the NFPA, subject to further control by local community fire and building codes. The supervision and maintenance of bulk oxygen units are not always functions of the respiratory therapist but often are responsibilities of oxygen service companies and hospital departments of engineering and maintenance. Nevertheless, the therapist should be acquainted with the systems, since they concern his or her most important therapeutic tool and because the therapist should be knowledgeable enough to be able to participate in dealing with emergency interruption of gas supply.

Bulk oxygen systems may provide either gaseous or liquid oxygen, and these are discussed separately below. Bulk oxygen is used as a "central supply," or "piped-in system," in which the gas is carried from its station to the hospital divisions by a system of pipes built into the walls of new construction or often added to the wall surfaces of older buildings. It is thus possible to have an oxygen outlet conveniently located by each patient's bed and any other area desired. The great values of such a centrally located oxygen supply should be obvious. There is almost no risk of a depletion of oxygen during therapy, and the inconvenience and hazard of transporting and storing individual tanks are obviated. Finally, pressure reduction of oxygen is accomplished at the central station, and the gas is piped to the clinical areas already reduced to the standard working pressure of 50 psig. This eliminates the need for pressure-reducing valves at the patient outlets and requires the use of only flow meters. As opposed to cylinder gas supply, a central system is referred to as a "low-pressure system."

Gaseous bulk oxygen. There are three general systems that employ large central supplies of the gas form of oxygen.

Standard cylinders. Large-sized standard cylinders can be banked together, usually pressurized at 2200 psig. Numbers of them can be tied together by a *manifold,* which, essentially, converts the individual units into one continuous supply. The manifold mechanism contains pressure-reduction valving and flow-control and alarm systems that warn of impending depletion or malfunction. As tanks empty, they are replaced by others. Sometimes packages of six or more tanks are manifolded together, each package replaced as needed.

Fixed cylinders. In contrast to the cylinders just described, fixed cylinders consist of large banks of up to 75 cylinders permanently fixed at a stationary site. When empty, they are refilled on location from a truck that contains liquid oxygen and converts the liquid to gas for pumping into the cylinders.

Trailer units. Mounted on trailers, tanks of a variety of sizes can be towed to the central area and connected to the distribution circuit. For heavy oxygen consumption, large trailers with up to 30 permanently attached long horizontal tubes are available. Replacement is a simple matter of switching trailers. Like the other tank systems, trailer gas is also at 2200 psig pressure.

Liquid bulk oxygen. An extremely economical method of transporting and storing oxygen, liquid gas systems are widely used where the demand justifies their installation. Although we have already discussed the liquid form of some medical gases packaged in standard cylinders, because of its physical characteristics, liquid oxygen deserves special consideration. The major physical difference between oxygen and those liquid gases noted previously is its very low critical temperature ($-181.1°F$) and boiling point ($-297.3°F$). The mechanisms for producing and maintaining the liquid state of oxygen are much more complex than are those for other medical liquid gases, but the practical returns justify the effort. Of prime importance is the fact that at its boiling point, 1 cubic foot of liquid oxygen is the equivalent of 860.6 cubic feet of gaseous oxygen at ambient temperature and pressure.

Brief reference has been made earlier to the method of producing liquid oxygen from the compression and cooling of air. To prevent the liquid from reverting to gas, the liquid must be kept below $-297°F$, both in transportation and storage. This is accomplished by keeping it in special containers, under a pressure not to exceed 250 psig. All such containers for liquid oxygen, whether trucks for transporting the substance or hospital supply stations, are constructed on the principle of a large thermos bottle with which we are all acquainted. They consist of inner and outer steel shells, separated by a vacuum, which effectively blocks the transfer of heat into the liquid. This evacuated space is filled with a noncombustible insulation, and the inner shell is silvered to aid in repelling heat. The containers are vented so that vaporized liquid oxygen can escape if warming occurs. It should be apparent that when liquid oxygen is kept below its boiling point, it can be exposed to atmospheric pressure, at least for short periods of time, without immediately vaporizing. Otherwise, transferring the material from supply truck to bulk container, for example, would be difficult. There are two types of containers for hospital use of liquid oxygen: the liquid oxygen cylinder and the permanent station.

Liquid oxygen cylinder. This unit is not necessarily classified as part of a bulk system because individual tanks of liquid gas can be used. These cylinders measure 58 inches high and 20 inches in diameter and hold the equivalent of 3000 cubic feet of gas at ambient temperature and pressure, matching the contents of more than 12 large gas cylinders. As with the gas tanks, the liquid cylinders can be banked by manifold to provide a space-saving supply of oxygen.

Fixed station. These units are cylindrical or spherical containers with ca-

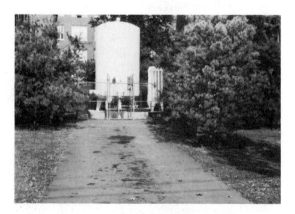

Fig. 12-4   Typical liquid oxygen storage facility in a hospital setting.

pacities up to a gaseous equivalent of 130,000 cubic feet. The liquid is converted to usable gas by a heating unit called a *vaporizer,* which may be heated by steam, hot air, electricity, or hot water. Elaborately controlled to ensure a steady, even conversion of liquid to gas according to need, these systems ensure an unlimited gas supply no matter what the peak demand load may be. They are refilled from service tank trucks according to schedules suited to each hospital. All liquid gas sources reduce their already low pressure to the 50 psig hospital line pressure. Fig. 12-4 illustrates a typical unit.

Safety indexed connector systems

With the tremendous number of compressed gases in current commercial, medical, and scientific use, one of the greatest risks in medical gas therapy is the inadvertent administration of a wrong gas to a patient. Certainly, care on the part of the medical attendant in reading labels or other identifying marks is the most important deterrent to such an accident. The human error, however, must always be considered a potential risk, and to compensate for this, specially designed connectors have been developed for compressed gas tanks and their accessories. The purpose of an indexed connector system is to make impossible certain connections between cylinders and delivery systems. When properly used, for example, a cylinder of any gas other than oxygen could not be functionally attached to any system for which only oxygen is specified. The importance of such a precaution for anesthetic gases is obvious. The systems commonly in use are briefly described here, but the therapist is encouraged to become familiar with their details as set forth in publications of the CGA. There are three basic indexed connector systems: the American Standard Compressed Gas Cylinder Outlet and Inlet Connections, the Diameter-Index Safety System (DISS), and the Pin-Index Safety System.

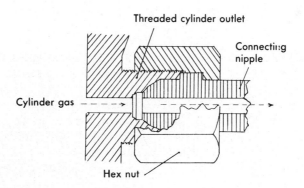

Fig. 12-5 This sketch illustrates the structure of a typical American Standard connection, such as might be used to attach a reducing valve to a large high-pressure cylinder. The hexagonal nut is held onto the nipple of the reducing valve by a circular collar, seen as a cross-sectional projection on the nipple. As the hex nut is tightened on the threaded cylinder outlet, the end of the nipple is snugly seated into the conical outlet. (Modified from CGA Pamphlet V-1, connection no. 540, Compressed Gas Association, Inc., New York.)

American Standard Compressed Gas Cylinder Valve Outlet and Inlet Connections. In the United States and Canada the specifications for threaded connections between compressed gas cylinders and their attached tubing have been standardized according to the type of gas concerned and are explained in detail in one of the publications of the CGA.[9] This system is confined to cylinders with threaded outlets from their valves and includes specifications for the mating nipples and hexagonal nuts by which an appliance (usually a pressure regulator) is attached to the valve. Fig. 12-5 illustrates a cutaway of a joined threaded outlet and nipple. The gas channel through the nipple of the regulator is aligned with the channel through the threaded outlet, and the two parts are secured by a wrench-tightened hexagonal nut that is held loosely on the nipple by a shoulder and flange mechanism.

The Standard system is based on varying dimensions of the cylinder outlet and nipple to limit the introduction of cylinders into a gas circuit specific to certain groups of gases. There are four fundamental divisions of the calibrated system: internal and external threads and right-handed and left-handed threads. Each division is further segmented by varying the number, pitch, and diameter of the threads. In general, left-handed threads are used for fuel gases, and right-handed threads are used for nonfuel. Most of the valve outlets have external threads, and their corresponding nipples internal threads. The threads of the Standard system are usually classified as NGO (National Gas Outlet), but a few are NGT (National Gas Taper). Each gas does not have its own specific connection, but 1 to 13 gases may share the same one since there are some 26 different connections for about 62 listed gases. The Standard system of classification is not binding on manufacturers, and the respiratory therapist must certainly read the specifications of cylinders supplied to his or her hospital so as to be completely familiar with any deviations from standard design.

In catalogues of cylinder gas dealers, the therapist will see the connection specifications listed for each type of cylinder and gas. A typical description is as follows for a large cylinder of oxygen:

CGA-540 × 0.903-14NGO-RH-Ext

This tells us that the connection for the threaded outlet of this cylinder is listed by the CGA as connection no. 540, that the outlet has a thread diameter of 0.903 inch, that there are 14 threads per inch of the NGO type, and that the threads are right handed and external.

Generally, respiratory therapists will use but one or two outlet connections, since most of the relatively small number of different gases they employ are grouped within a few connector sizes. They should be familiar with the classifications, however, since expanding instrumentation and scope of services may bring them into increasing contact with gases and tubing systems in the future.

Pin-Index Safety System (PISS). Pin-Indexing is incorporated in the specifications of the American Standard listing just described but as a special section applicable only to the flush valve outlets of the *small cylinders,* up to and including size E, which use a yoke connection. These valves do not have a threaded outlet but, rather, a recess in a flat face of the valve into which fits a nipple on the yoke to receive the gas (Fig. 12-2). The Pin-Index is intended for use on anesthesia machines or similar equipment, where fixed yokes are attached to internal gas circuitry, and is designed to prevent the wrong cylinder from being attached to a given yoke.

Two holes are drilled in the face of the valve, their exact position varying with the gas in the cylinder. There are two pins in corresponding positions on the yoke, and unless the pins and holes align perfectly, the yoke nipple will not seat in the recess of the valve. Six hole-pin combinations comprise the total system, but because of overlapping, adjacent holes cannot be used, and there are thus ten possible combinations, of which nine are now in use. Fig.

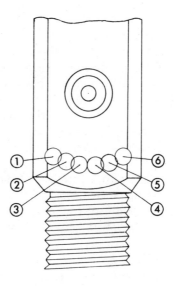

Fig. 12-6 Location of the Pin-Index Safety System holes in the cylinder valve face, various pairs of which constitute indices for different gases. (See text for the complete pairings.) (Modified from CGA Pamphlet V-1, Pin-Index Safety System, Compressed Gas Association, Inc., New York.)

Table 12-7
Pin-Indexed gases

Gas	Index hole position
O_2	2-5
O_2/CO_2 (CO_2 not over 7%)	2-6
He/O_2 (He not over 80%)	2-4
C_2H_4	1-3
N_2O	3-5
$(CH_2)_3$	3-6
He/O_2 (He over 80%)	4-6
O_2/CO_2 (CO_2 over 7%)	1-6
Air	1-5

12-6 is a composite illustration of the location of all six possible holes and the numbers by which they are indexed. Table 12-7 is based on CGA information and lists the gases now in Pin-Indexed cylinders, with their index positions.

Diameter-Index Safety System (DISS). As a sequential companion to the American Standard system just described, the DISS was established to prevent accidental interchanging among the removable threaded connectors used for medical gas—administering equipment at pressures of *200 psig or less* and is *not* part of a cylinder safety system directly. Specifically, DISS in respiratory therapy is used in effecting safe union between pressure regulators or flowmeters and any threaded connectors that are frequently engaged or disengaged in routine use. Such connections will also be used with therapy equipment and anesthesia apparatus. It should be noted that the standard removable threaded oxygen connector that has been in long use, 0.5625 inch in diameter, 18 threads per inch, has been given a DISS number (1240) and included in the system.

The system is designed as follows: Each connection consists of an externally threaded body and a mated nipple with hex nut, illustrated in Fig. 12-7. The body of the connector has two concentric borings, a primary bore, noted as *Bore 1,* and a counterbore, *Bore 2.* The accompanying nipple has two shoulders, identified as *1* and *2,* and a loose hex nut secured by a flange behind *Shoulder 2.* It can be seen that, as the two parts are joined, the corresponding shoulders and bores mate, and the union is held by the tightened hex nut. Indexing is achieved by varying the dimensions of the borings and shoulders; starting with a basic set of dimensions, bore 1 is increased and bore 2 decreased in increments of 0.012 inch. The nipple shoulders are changed accordingly. The final connection is a smooth-bored body and a nipple of regular diameter. There are 11 indexed connections, which accommodate 11 gases or

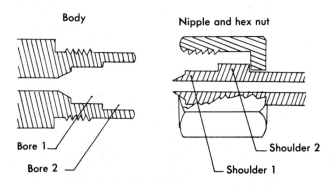

Fig. 12-7   Schematic illustration of components of a representative DISS connection. The two shoulders of the nipple allow the nipple to unite only with a body having corresponding borings. If the match is incorrect, the hex nut will not engage the body threads. (Modified from CGA Pamphlet V-5, DISS connection no. 1100, Compressed Gas Association, Inc., New York.)

gas mixtures, and Table 12-8 lists the DISS connection numbers with the gases assigned to each from data of the CGA.[9]

To illustrate the use of the DISS, let us imagine an equipment catalogue listing the specifications of a pressure regulator to be used on a cylinder of 100% carbon dioxide. The *inlet* (inlet of regulator, which mates with the threaded outlet of the cylinder) will require an American Standard connection designated as CGA-320. According to CGA data this will be a 0.825-inch

Table 12-8	Connection number	Gas	Connection number	Gas
DISS connection numbers and assigned gases	1020	Unassigned	1120	Unassigned
	1040	N_2O	1140	C_2H_4
	1060	He	1160	Air
		He/O_2 (O_2 <20%)	1180	He/O_2 (He 80% or less)
	1080	CO_2	1200	O_2/CO_2 (CO_2 7% or less)
		O_2/CO_2 (CO_2 >7%)	1220	Suction
	1100	$(CH_2)_3$	1240	O_2 (standard)

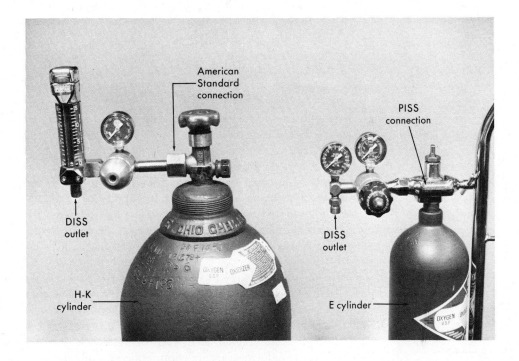

Fig. 12-8   Comparison of safety systems used for compressed gases. Note that the D.I.S.S. connections are for outlets having reduced pressures (less than 200 psig) while the American Standard connection is shown for a large cylinder and the P.I.S.S. connection is shown for a small cylinder.

14NGO-RH-Ext cylinder outlet for which there is a specific regulator nipple.[8] The *outlet* (of the regulator, to which a low-pressure line is attached to supply an appliance) will require a DISS connection CGA-1080.

Most of the time the therapist will use oxygen from a regulator, utilizing the standard removable connection designated as CGA-1240, which is not a DISS unit; but he or she will frequently have occasion to administer helium–oxygen mixtures and oxygen–carbon dioxide mixtures, both of which have DISS connections. To avoid the cumbersome stocking of a large variety of pressure regulators and to make economical use of those on hand, the therapist can use adapters to convert the outlets of the common oxygen regulators to suitable DISS dimensions for special gas use.

Fig. 12-8 illustrates the uses of and relationships between the three safety systems just described.

Quick-connect units for station outlets.[5] Another system that is also used to avoid connecting equipment to inappropriate gases is one used for station outlets. Various manufacturers active in producing station outlets have designed specially shaped connectors for each gas. These are commonly called "quick-connect" units because they allow for rapid connection or disconnection of equipment to and from the wall outlet. Because the connector for each gas has a distinct shape, its connector will not fit an outlet for another gas. Each manufacturer also has its own shape-coded system, which will not connect to other manufacturer outlets.

Regulating gas pressure and flow

Whatever the source of medical gas, a device is needed to regulate its pressure and flow as it is administered to a patient. A device that controls *both* pressure and flow is called a *regulator*. When gas pressure alone is controlled from a high to a lower pressure, the device used is called a *reducing valve*. A *flow meter* is a device that adjusts the flow of a gas, usually after the gas pressure is already controlled.

For cylinder gases such as oxygen or compressed air, the pressure leaving the cylinder must first be reduced to lower, more usable pressure. For respiratory therapy in the United States, this pressure is usually 50 psig and is commonly referred to as "working pressure." If cylinders are to feed a manifold system with individual station outlets as mentioned before, then a reducing valve is used to drop the cylinder's pressure to 50 psig first. Then flow meters or other devices can be used to properly adjust flow from these outlets.

When a cylinder is used to provide a gas for patient use without a manifold, both reducing valve and a flow meter are combined, forming a regulator. Since it is more common to use a regulator on cylinders than just reducing valve, we discuss here three types of regulators: preset, adjustable or Bourdon, and multiple-stage regulators. In each of these, the section that reduces the pressure is the reducing valve portion. Following the description of regulators for cylinders, we discuss flow meters used from a low-pressure, centrally supplied gas system and the concept of pressure compensation.

High-pressure cylinder gas regulators. There are three types of cylinder

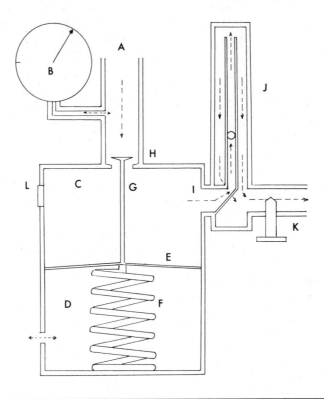

Fig. 12-9   Diagram of preset, high-pressure gas regulator. (See text for details.)

regulators, and though they function on the same basic principle, they deserve individual description.

Preset regulator. Fig. 12-9 shows a schematic illustration of the preset regulator. Attached to the cylinder outlet, high-pressure gas enters the regulators through *A*, with cylinder pressure (and thus contents) recorded on the pressure gauge *(B)*. The body of the regulator is divided into a pressure chamber *(C)* and an ambient pressure chamber *(D)* by a flexible diaphragm *(E)*. Attached to the diaphragm, in the atmospheric chamber, is a spring *(F)* fixed to the other side of the chamber. Also attached to the diaphragm, but in the pressure chamber, is a valve stem *(G)*, the other end of which controls the flow of gas through a valve *(H)*. Gas goes to the patient through the outflow *(I)*, passing through a Thorpe-tube flow meter *(J)*. The amount of gas released to the patient is regulated by the needle valve *(K)* and is read on a calibrated scale as liters per minute according to the height at which the ball is elevated in the Thorpetube flow meter. The pressure chamber is supplied with a safety vent *(L)* that prevents an accidental buildup of pressure beyond 200 psig (as an example) in the event of malfunction. This regulator is called *preset* because it is so constructed that the spring *F* will give if pressure on the diaphragm *E* exceeds 50 psig. When this happens, the valve stem *G* will be pulled back and the valve *H* will close, preventing further entry of gas into the regulator. As long as the needle valve *K* is open, allowing the escape of gas from the pressure chamber, the valve at *H* will remain open and permit gas flow. Thus a balance will be established so that the valve at *H* is open just enough to meet the demand of valve *K* and the automatic adjustment of the diaphragm-spring combination will prevent excessive pressures from building up in chamber *C*.

    Adjustable or Bourdon regulator. The adjustable regulator is one of the most commonly encountered regulators, differing from the preset type in two aspects, as shown in Fig. 12-10. The identifying feature of this regulator is the threaded hand control on its face *(K)*. This is attached to the end of the spring and allows displacement of the diaphragm. Whereas the valve *(H)* in the preset regulator is open until gas enters the pressure chamber and closes it by pressure against the diaphragm, in the adjustable regulator the valve *(H)*

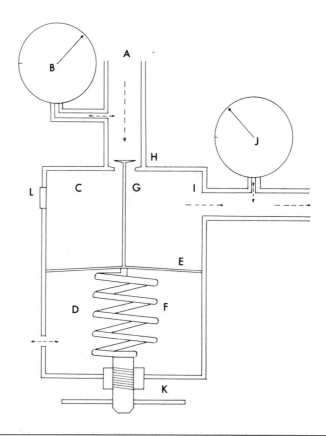

Fig. 12-10   Diagram of an adjustable, high-pressure gas regulator. (See text for details.)

is closed until the hand screw advances the whole mechanism and opens it to allow gas flow. The valve can thus be opened to permit a wide range of flows, and the pressures in chamber *C* will vary according to the relation between the amount of high-pressure gas entering and the amount leaving the regulator, but the spring will prevent the pressure from exceeding about 100 psig. In the preset one, pressure in the chamber is always 50 psig, but in the adjustable regulator it can be anything up to about 100 psig. A second characteristic of the adjustable regulator is the use of a Bourdon flow gauge *(J)* instead of a Thorpe. In reality, the Bourdon meter is a pressure gauge, like that at the regulator inflow *(B)*, and functions on the principle crudely schematicized in Fig. 12-11. The heart of the gauge is a curved, flexible, closed tube *(A)* that responds to the pressure of gas entering it by changing shape. The force of the gas tends to straighten the tube, causing its distal end to move as indicated by the arrow; and through a gear mechanism *(B)* this motion is transmitted to an indicating needle *(C)*. A numbered scale is calibrated by its manufacturer to read the needle movement either as pressure or liter flow, and gauges are constructed to varying degrees of sensitivity according to the ranges of pressure to which they are to be subjected. The Bourdon gauge is a low-pressure device (less than about 100 psig) that meters the gas leaving the regulator, with a scale that converts pressure to flow in liters per minute.[5]

By placing a fixed-size orifice at the outlet of the regulator (not shown in Fig. 12-10) the pressure against this orifice is proportional to flow. That is, each pressure pushing gases through the orifice will do so at a known rate. Therefore, while the gauge is actually *sensing* pressure, it can be calibrated to display a flow rate at each pressure available.

Multiple-stage regulator. As the name implies, this instrument accom-

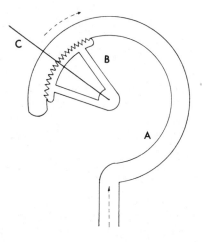

Fig. 12-11   Crude diagram of the principle of a gas-pressure gauge. (See text for description.)

plishes pressure reduction in two or three steps instead of one and is essentially one or two valves in one. Therapists may have occasion to use two-stage reducing valves, but rarely three. The first stage of high-pressure reduction is preset at the factory and lowers cylinder pressure to an intermediate level, e.g., 200 to 700 psig; in three-stage units the second stage lowers it to about half the first. The final stages, second or third as the case may be, therefore work off a lower pressure than does a single-stage valve and presumably are able to effect somewhat more precision and smoothness in flow control. A multiple-stage reducing valve may be provided with either Bourdon or a Thorpe-tube metering device. It is larger and more costly than a single stage and is indicated where minimal fluctuations in pressure and flow are critical factors. For routine hospital work the simpler single-stage regulators are satisfactory. The number of stages in a reducing valve can be easily determined by noting the number of safety vents present; there will be one for each pressure chamber.

Low-pressure gas regulators. It was emphasized earlier that one of the assets of a central gas supply system is the reduction of pressure at the central location so that the gas is at its working pressure when it reaches the outlets. This eliminates the need for pressure-reducing devices for patient administration and requires only a simple flow meter. The Thorpe-tube flow meter is used for this purpose, since it is calibrated to work off a pressure of 50 psig, as shown in Fig. 12-9. With outlets of a low pressure—oxygen or compressed-air system located by the patient's bed, therapy can be instituted in moments merely by plugging in a flow meter and adjusting its flow as desired.

Pressure compensation. The term *pressure compensation* refers to a design in the Thorpe-tube flow meter to prevent changes in gas pressure flowing through it from affecting its liter flow calibration. Although all standard manufacturers of these devices now supply them pressure compensated, the therapist should understand the importance of this and be on the alert for old equipment still in use that might not conform to present standards. Also, some other equipment such as ventilators do use uncompensated flow meters routinely.[5]

The problem of pressure compensation is the result of the effect of back pressure on a flow meter, when the gas outlet of the meter is connected with a therapeutic instrument. Practically all gas-administering equipment contains some restrictions in its circuits, and in some, such as jet aerosol generators, these restrictions are acute. When gas flow encounters a restriction, a back pressure is generated. At this point we might define back pressure as a pressure drop across a restriction, according to concepts considered in some detail earlier, when we learned of Bernoulli's principle and the relations among pressure, flow, and resistance. Therapeutically, we are interested in the delivered pressure distal to an obstruction, and if this is lower than the line pressure entering the restriction, we have a back pressure proximal to the restriction. Let now compare three flow-measuring devices, a Bourdon flow (pressure) gauge, an uncompensated flow meter (Thorpe-tube), and a compensated flow meter.

Bourdon gauge. As just described and illustrated in Figs. 12-10 and 12-11, the Bourdon gauge on the Bourdon regulator measures pressure and thus is not a flow meter. It measures the pressure of gas flowing from the pressure chamber of an adjustable reducing valve, and at the factory it is calibrated to indicate given flow volumes of gas at different pressures with its outflow *open to the atmosphere.* Thus the face of the valve shows supposed flows. In clinical use, however, the gauge output may be faced with the back pressure resistance of therapeutic appliances, and it would respond to this pressure, indicating a flow *higher* than the patient actually receives. Indeed, because the gauge records reducing valve chamber pressure, it will register (flow on its printed face) with the valve open and *the output completely blocked.* It should be remembered that the Bourdon gauge is in direct communication with a pressurized chamber, which may be either part of a reducing valve or the cavity of a gas cylinder. If outflow is blocked and the valve opened, the gauge and chamber will immediately equilibrate, and pressure will be recorded by the gauge. If the gauge is calibrated in units of flow, then flow will be indicated although no gas is moving.

Uncompensated flow meter. The uncompensated flow meter is also calibrated in liters per minute against the atmosphere, without restriction. Gas flow at 50 psig into the meter is controlled by a needle valve *proximal* to the meter, as shown in Fig. 12-12, *A.* The heart of the meter consists of a tapered transparent tube with a float, as shown much exaggerated in Fig. 12-13, with its diameter increasing from below upward. The float is suspended in the tube by the flow of gas past it, and its position is noted against an adjacent scale, which indicates the flow. Because the tube is part of the gas conduction system, the float cannot occlude it and must depend for its support partly on the Bernoulli effect. The space between the float and the inner surface of the tube constitutes a restriction, and the increased velocity of gas through this restriction produces a pressure drop immediately above the float.

In Fig. 12-13, pressure above the float (P_2) is less than that below it (P_1), and the float rises in the tube until its own weight equals the lifting force. When therapy equipment is attached distal to the meter, back pressure is generated in the atmosphere-equilibrated circuit, from the point of restriction in the equipment back through the flow tube to the needle valve, Fig. 12-12, *A.* As long as the back pressure does not exceed the source pressure of 50 psig, gas will continue to flow into the tube, but the back pressure does increase the pressure distal to the float $(P_2$ in Fig. 12-13). This reduces the pressure differential from P_1 to P_2, lessens the lift effect, and lets the float drop to a lower position. Therefore a flow meter that does not compensate for back pressure, when faced with a restriction, records *less* gas flow than the patient actually receives.

Compensated flow meter. In contrast to the preceding two instruments, the scale of the compensated flow meter is calibrated against a constant pressure of 50 psig instead of the atmosphere, and its major structural feature, shown in Fig. 12-12, *B,* is a flow control needle valve *distal* to the flow tube. Thus

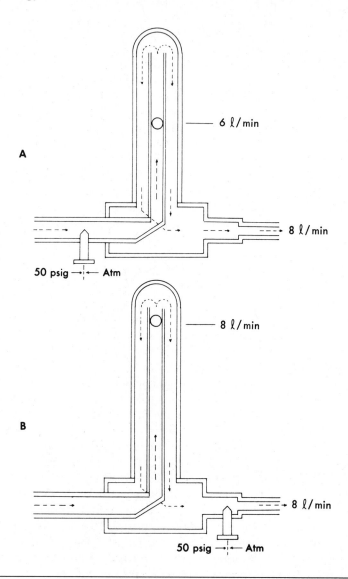

Fig. 12-12 Comparison of, **A,** pressure-uncompensated, and **B,** pressure-compensated flowmeters. In the former, the flow-control valve is proximal to the meter, and the gauge records less than the actual output. In the latter, location of the valve distal to the meter correlates the gauge reading with the output. (See text for detailed explanation.)

the entire meter, including the tube, to the needle valve is at a constant pressure of 50 psig, whereas in an uncompensated meter the 50 psig inlet pressure stops at the needle valve proximal to the tube. With a restriction distal to the meter, back pressure will develop in the atmosphere-equilibrated portion of the circuit, from the restriction back to the needle valve. However, as long as

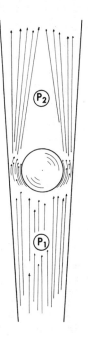

Fig. 12-13 The position of a flowmeter float depends upon a Bernoulli-generated pressure differential across it so that $P_1 > P_2$. Back pressure on the float increases P_2, reducing the differential and permitting the float to drop even though actual flow may be maintained.

the back pressure does not exceed 50 psig, it can have no effect in the tube and will not alter the flow kinetics, which are responsible for the lifting force on the float. Such a pressure-compensated flow meter, regardless of restrictions, will accurately record the flow to the patient and is the preferred instrument for clinical use.

Oxygen therapy	The mechanisms of oxygen uptake by the lungs and transport in the blood to the tissues are introduced in Chapter 6, and descriptions of hypoxia and hypoxemia are discussed in Chapter 8. With those concepts kept clearly in mind, we now describe oxygen used as a therapeutic gas.
Objectives for oxygen therapy	The primary objective for oxygen therapy ultimately is to provide sufficient amounts of oxygen to the tissues so that normal metabolism can occur and life can be maintained. From a clinical standpoint, however, simple inhalation of oxygen, usually at ambient pressure, is used to raise the level of oxygen in both alveolar air and in arterial blood so that adequate amounts of oxygen are available for delivery to the tissues.

The clinical objectives for oxygen therapy can be summarized in the following categories:

1. To reduce or correct arterial hypoxemia and tissue hypoxia.
2. To reduce or correct the need for physiologic compensatory mechanisms to hypoxemia.

The causes of arterial hypoxemia and tissue hypoxia are introduced in Chapter 8. Generally simple oxygen therapy methods can be used to correct hypoxemia when it is caused by hypoventilation, low ambient PO_2 of high altitude, diffusion defect, or moderate ventilation-perfusion imbalance. The hypoxemia caused by physiologic shunt is generally less responsive to simple oxygen therapy methods. With shunt fractions of about 25% or less, and common physiologic conditions, moderate to high concentrations of oxygen may maintain the PaO_2 above 60 mm Hg while shunt values above this may not provide an adequate PaO_2 even on 100% oxygen.[10]

We know from previous discussions that when blood oxygen levels decrease, the body attempts to compensate. A patient may have what appears to be an acceptable arterial oxygen content by arterial blood gas analysis, but in order to achieve that level the patient may be hyperventilating. When oxygen therapy is appropriately applied, this elevated work of breathing can be decreased. Similarly, a patient presenting with arterial hypoxemia may not have tissue hypoxia if the cardiac output is increased in order to compensate, such as with tachycardia. If oxygen therapy can adequately relieve the hypoxemia, the circulatory system will not need to be stressed. Therefore, both ventilatory work and circulatory work can be decreased by oxygen therapy.

Controlled oxygen therapy

Devices for oxygen administration are discussed later in this chapter, but it is appropriate to briefly discuss the concept of *controlled oxygen therapy* here. Because oxygen has both beneficial and detrimental effects it should be treated as a drug. As such, only the amount or "dose" required to obtain the appropriate response should be used. Depending on the device or system used, oxygen is generally ordered either in liters per minute or as a concentration of oxygen.[11-14] The concentration can be expressed as a percent, such as 30% oxygen, or as a fraction of inspired oxygen (FI_{O2}) such as 0.3.

Once an amount of oxygen desired is being administered, evaluation of therapy with arterial blood gases and clinical assessment are generally made. If the response to the oxygen used is not appropriate, then the amount being administered is adjusted and reevaluated. This dose-response approach is generally used in an attempt to use the least amount of oxygen to obtain the desired therapeutic effect. More about this principle is discussed throughout this chapter in sections under hazards in the use of oxygen and equipment techniques.

Characteristics of oxygen

Oxygen is a colorless, transparent, tasteless, and odorless gas occurring in nature as free molecular oxygen and as a component of a host of chemical compounds, both organic and inorganic. It comprises almost 50% of the weight of the earth's crust and occurs in all living matter as water and in combination with elements other than hydrogen. At 0°C and 1 atm pressure, oxygen has a density of 1.429 g/ℓ, compared with the density of air, 1.30 g/ℓ. It is only slightly soluble in water; at room temperature and 1 atm pressure 3.3 volumes of oxygen dissolve in 100 volumes of water. Nonetheless, this small amount is essential to aquatic life, both plant and animal.

Oxygen does not burn. However, it does support combustion, a matter of considerable importance to its widespread use in hospitals. A minute spark can become a large hot flame in an enriched oxygen environment, or a glowing ember can burst into open flame. The relationship between the burning intensity of a combustible substance and the amount of ambient oxygen is direct but not simple. Burning speed increases with an increase in the partial pressure of oxygen in the environment. Thus either an increase in concentration of oxygen at a fixed total pressure or an increase in total pressure of a constant gas concentration will augment the kinetics of combustion. However, burning speed will also increase if only oxygen concentrations are raised, and the partial pressure of the various oxygen percentages is kept constant by suitably lowering the total pressure.[15] These data demonstrate that both oxygen concentration and partial pressure influence rate of burning.

Another factor to consider in the relation between burning and the amount of oxygen is the self-perpetuating effect of combustion in oxygen. The reaction of oxygen with other elements is markedly enhanced at elevated temperatures, and once combustion starts in a high-oxygen atmosphere, the heat produced potentiates further combustion and is not wasted on the relatively inert nitrogen content of ordinary air.

Although oxygen can be produced by many chemical reactions and the electrolysis of water, as noted in Chapter 1, its main source is compressed air. Under the influence of tremendous pressure followed by the cooling effect of sudden expansion combined with heat exchangers, the components of air are converted to liquid.[6] Through the process of fractional distillation, as the liquefied air is allowed to heat slowly, nitrogen, with its boiling point of −195.8°C (−320.5°F), escapes first; then the trace gases of argon, krypton, and xenon are removed. Standards require that the final remaining oxygen have a purity of at least 99%, a value that is usually exceeded. The liquid oxygen is stored in special containers or converted to gas under high pressure in tanks.

Hazards in the use of oxygen

We have emphasized the importance of oxygen in the treatment of disease and have considered in some detail the seriousness of oxygen deprivation (Chapter 8), but it must not be thought to be a completely innocuous agent. The respiratory therapist must be familiar with all aspects of the physiologic action of oxygen, the harmful as well as the beneficial. He or she must be aware of those conditions in which oxygen is not indicated, when it may even be a threat to life, for such caution will make him or her a safe as well as effective therapist. Before discussing the equipment and techniques for administering oxygen, we consider some of the risks of its use and explore a bit its pathologic potential.

Ventilatory effects of oxygen

Oxygen-induced hypoventilation. This is not a new topic, for in the study of cardiopulmonary physiology earlier, we covered oxygen-induced hypoventilation superficially in discussions of ventilatory control and the role of the peripheral chemoreceptors. Here, we are interested not only in the specific academic relationship between oxygen and the ventilatory control mechanisms but also in the practical clinical use of oxygen in patients suffering from failure of these mechanisms.

For example, for the patient who is in ventilatory failure with its accompanying hypercapnia, we may usually assume that oxygen can be safely administered at concentrations slightly above ambient, at 1 atm pressure. Flows of 1 to 2 ℓ/min carry little risk and can be achieved by techniques to be discussed subsequently. Even so, the arterial carbon dioxide level may rise slightly but, after a period of perhaps 1 hour, will usually plateau at a level still within the bounds of safety. It has often been noted that if the oxygen administration is stopped, oxygen tension in arterial blood may fall below pretreatment levels.[16] In such a situation it is evident that intermittent use of the gas may be dangerous to the patient's respiratory equilibrium, and to ensure adequate oxygenation, oxygen should be given constantly with mechanical support of ventilation if necessary. This latter aspect is dealt with in detail in another chapter.[17] As a guide for the use of oxygen in patients with ventilatory failure, it has been suggested that an arterial oxygen tension of about 50 to 60 mm Hg will prevent immediate death from hypoxia while keeping the adverse effects of oxygen to a minimum.[18,19] This does not imply that such a level is therapeutically desirable as definitive therapy but that this tension will prevent rapid deterioration of the patient's state while other measures are being prepared.[20]

The effect of oxygen administration on ventilation is well documented in a study of several patients with chronic respiratory disease who were tested for their response to concentrations of oxygen in the 90% to 100% range.[19] When a normal subject breathes 100% oxygen, the chemoreceptors remain inactive, and because of the increased oxygen in the blood, there is less reduced hemoglobin available for carbon dioxide transportation and arterial P_{CO_2} tends to rise. To maintain a normal acid-base balance, the increased Pa_{CO_2} acting on the chemoreceptors, plus the irritating effect of the high concentration of oxygen on the respiratory mucosa, can produce a 5% to 20% increase in ventilation and correct the hypercapnia. In the presence of hypoxia, the arterial unsaturation stimulates the chemoreceptors, and if there is no airway obstruction to carbon dioxide excretion, the augmented ventilation may produce hypocapnia. This reaction is not uncommon in patients at high altitude, with venous-arterial shunts, and with diffussion defects. Of course, this sensitive response implies a normally functioning respiratory center. In contrast, when hypoxia exists with the hypercapnia of ventilatory failure, because the latter denotes an unresponsive respiratory center, oxygen administration suppresses the chemoreceptors and produces a hypoventilation that is not compensated.

It was observed that, on the average, when the arterial carbon dioxide tension was greater than 50 mm Hg, the risk of oxygen-induced hypoventilation increased, and this value seemed more significant than the pH level. This substantiates the observation, which the respiratory therapist will have frequent occasion to make, that the obstructed patient with hypoxia presents the greatest hypoventilation risk and that not far behind is the patient whose respiratory center is obtunded by sedation or narcosis.

This hazard of oxygen therapy does not militate against its use when indicated, for the relief of hypoxia is the most critical therapeutic need, and even for the most unresponsive patient there are methods of giving oxygen. It does mean, however, that the therapist assigned to administer oxygen must never assume such administration to be a "routine" procedure. The therapist should take time to become acquainted with the basic disease problem under treatment and be alert to potential danger. This point is important enough that we return to it again when we specifically discuss the management of ventilatory failure.

Atelectasis. The collapse of alveoli as the result of high concentrations of oxygen in the inhaled air is a result of the elimination of nitrogen from the lung and the effect of oxygen on pulmonary surfactant. We consider the first here and the second below. Normally, the most prevalent gas in the alveoli is nitrogen, the bulk of which comes from the inspired air, with a much smaller amount coming from the general body metabolism. Breathing pure oxygen depletes the circulating nitrogen within several minutes as each tidal air excursion washes it out of the alveoli, into which the gas has diffused from the blood. The patient who is excessively relaxed and ventilating at a minimal tidal level, especially if he or she has some degree of airway obstruction as from retained secretions, is liable to suffer ill consequences of 100% oxygen breathing. As the patient breathes the oxygen, should the easy tidal flow be impeded to and from a partially blocked alveolus or one somewhat hampered by a dependent location, the oxygen that gains access to the alveolus may diffuse into the pulmonary circulation faster than it can be replaced by ventilation. This results in a gradual shrinking of the alveolus and, when aided by other factors, may lead to complete collapse. In the alert patient this is not as great a risk, since the natural "sigh" mechanism periodically hyperinflates the lung, ventilating those alveoli that may be considered sluggish in their tidal exchange. However, the effect of this alveolar collapse following 100% oxygen breathing can result in an increase in physiologic shunt as demonstrated by West.[22]

It is of historical interest only that, in the past, the nitrogen-washout effect of 100% oxygen was used to relieve intestinal distention. Nitrogen is one of the major intestinal gases causing distention, especially postoperatively. Because of its diffusibility into the lungs, 100% oxygen was used to remove it from the blood, thereby creating a gradient that allowed the nitrogen to move from the bowel into the circulation, then to the lung, and out. It was shown that a given amount of nitrogen could be reduced 62% in 24 hours by this method, as against 10% by breathing room air. Breathing 95% oxygen for no longer than 10 hours was one recommended technique; and we can only wonder how often recovery may have been retarded by pulmonary complications, even though bowel distress may have been relieved.

Oxygen toxicity. Humans find themselves fully dependent for existence on a gas basically lethal to them, a fascinating biologic paradox. No substitute energy source for metabolic machinery has yet been found, and the poisonous gas remains a person's most indispensable need. The fact of aerobic survival is testimony to the effective defenses against the toxic actions of oxygen. We now review the important manifestations of oxygen toxicity. The classic description of oxygen toxicity in the lung, written by Lorrain Smith in 1897, accurately describes the congestion, inflammation, and edema that we have come to recognize as the problem in oxygen toxicity. As modes of delivery have increased, oxygen concentrations have improved, and our knowledge of how to prolong life especially in the intensive care area has improved, we have found that a major limiting factor has been oxygen toxicity to the lung.

More is not better in the case of oxygen administration. The lung is designed to handle an oxygen concentration of approximately 21% of inspired air. Increased concentrations above 21% can be adapted to up to a point, but after that, the lung damage can be devastating. What the safe point of oxygen percent is, for how long a period it can be breathed, and what techniques are most useful in "damage control" make up a very important area of knowledge for the respiratory therapist.

From the respiratory therapist's standpoint, oxygen toxicity is exclusively a pulmonary problem, but we must not forget that oxygen toxicity also involves central nervous system dysfunction. These dysfunctions are usually seen in hyperbaric chambers and include tremors, twitching, and convulsions. These problems are discussed later in this chapter.

It is generally accepted that 100% oxygen breathed continuously for 24 hours or more leads to pulmonary damage. But since there are such wide variations in human susceptibility, definite experimental support for this is lacking. Also it is important to note that astronauts have breathed 100% oxygen at one-third atmosphere for long periods of time with no ill effects. Thus many other factors besides oxygen concentrations are operative. Breathing oxygen in increased atmospheric conditions (hyperbaric chambers) greatly accelerates oxygen toxicity.[23-25] Twelve hours of 100% oxygen frequently result in the patient complaining of a cough and intestinal tightness and burning, with increasing dyspnea soon developing.

A review of the literature suggests that no significant damage occurs to the lung at F_{IO_2} up to 50% for extended periods of time.[26] To complicate this observation is the report of patients receiving low-flow oxygen therapy at home for 7 to 61 months whose lungs at autopsy showed evidence of oxygen toxicity.[27] However, it was concluded that the oxygen toxicity in this small group of patients did not contribute to an accelerated mortality.

Several pathologic changes are seen in autopsied lungs exposed to high oxygen concentrations for prolonged periods of time under certain clinical conditions. The Type II pneumocyte is relatively resistant to high $F_{I_{O_2}}$, but Type I is not. It may be killed early on, followed by destruction of basement membranes. An exudative phase follows. Capillary beds swell and in some cases may become obliterated.[26] Hyaline membranes and fibrosis follow.[26] The most useful index for following these changes is the vital capacity, which becomes progressively reduced as the damage progresses.[25] The changes then result in edema, congestion, atelectasis, and hemorrhage and potentially expose the patient to increased incidence of pneumonia.

Several situations will delay the development of oxygen toxicity. Occasionally patients with chronic lung disease such as a patient with chronic obstructive pulmonary disease (COPD) will be able to withstand prolonged oxygen exposure with no noticeable problems beyond what would be expected from a healthy person. This is in some way related to the concept of oxygen tolerance; that is, the lung is able to adapt to high levels of oxygen. Some lungs can do this better than others. Below are listed factors that modify the development of oxygen toxicity.*

Hasten onset or increase severity	*Delay onset or decrease severity*
Adrenocortical hormones	Acclimatization to hypoxia
Adrenocorticotropic hormone	Adrenergic blocking drugs
Carbon dioxide inhalation	Anesthesia
Convulsions	Antioxidants
Dexamethasone	Chlorpromazine
Dextroamphetamine	Gamma-aminobutyric acid
Disulfiram (ATA base)	Ganglionic blocking drugs
Epinephrine	Glutathione
Hyperthermia	Hypothermia
Insulin	Hypothyroidism
Norepinephrine	Immaturity
Paraquat	Intermittent exposure
Thyroid hormones	Reserpine
Vitamin E deficiency	Starvation
X-irradiation	Tris-aminomethane
	Vitamin E

Metabolic effects. This aspect of oxygen toxicity is complex and in some details very speculative, for it includes biologic responses to oxygen that may be apparent only to molecular scientists or theoretic biochemists. Much of the information comes from laboratory animal experiments, and one can question how much animal data can justifiably be projected to the human. Nevertheless, some of the reported work is convincing, and the implications that oxygen can adversely affect our basic life processes are so awesome that we cannot ignore them. As has been our custom with so many other topics, we simplify

*Modified from Clark, J.M.: The toxicity of oxygen, Am. Rev. Resp. Dis. **110**(2):40, 1974.

this discussion to highlight the few most important relationships between oxygen and cellular integrity.

It is believed that oxygen toxicity is mediated through the actions of chemical units known as *free radicals*. These are extremely reactive atoms or groups of atoms, which have half-lives in aqueous solution of 10^{-5} seconds or less and which carry at least one unpaired electron. They can exist "free" for only the merest moment and then must stabilize themselves by chemically combining with other atoms. Detailed consideration of the chemistry of free radicals is much too involved for us here, but we should be aware that three of them are believed to be involved in oxygen toxicity: the hydroxyl, perhydroxyl, and superoxide free radicals, of which the last is of the greatest interest to us.

We know that plus and minus superscripts denote ions. In contrast, a free radical is identified by a small dot representing the unpaired electron. Two of the radicals just noted are written with the dot, thus: hydroxyl radical = $OH\cdot$, and perhydroxyl radical = $HO_2\cdot$. The unpaired electron gives to superoxide an extra negative charge so that it is both an anion and a free radical. Theoretically, therefore, superoxide could be written $O_2^{\overline{\cdot}}$ showing its dual designation, but by custom it is symbolized as an ion, O_2^-, implying the presence of an unpaired electron and its free radical role.

As oxygen participates in cellular biochemical actions, it takes on electrons and is reduced, while its electron donors are oxidized. It is this intracellular reduction of oxygen that is responsible for producing the superoxide radical. In its electron structure, oxygen has two single, or unpaired, electrons in its outer orbit, and during reduction tends to accept electrons one at a time. This is called *univalent reduction,* and as a result there is a brief moment when one of the electrons is unpaired and the oxygen is a superoxide radical. Superoxide thus is referred to as an intermediate product of oxygen reduction. As metabolic reactions continue, superoxide is converted to another free radical, perhydroxyl, and this is turn reacts with additional superoxide to produce the powerful hydroxyl radical. We are not interested in the details of such reactions, and this sequence is noted only to emphasize the metabolic interactions that generate a continuous supply of these potent substances.

Inhibition of tissue cultures. It has been known that 100% oxygen at atmosphere is able to inhibit growth of living tissue cultures, apparently by interfering with the synthesis of DNA and RNA. It is now believed that free radicals are responsible for this action, possibly by blocking the metaphase stage of cellular mitotic reproduction or through mechanisms still undefined. If any substance can be considered the basic matter of life, in our present state of knowledge it is certainly the DNA-RNA complex. We can scarcely help but wonder at the circumstance of chemical reactants manufactured in the body from the gas on which we are so dependent that can imperil our own cellular survival. As yet there are no direct clinical implications of this action of free radicals.

Inactivation of enzymes. Free radicals are also able to inactivate some enzyme systems that regulate the efficiency of our metabolism. Especially vulnerable are those enzymes whose functions are dependent on sulfhydryl groups. These are highly reactive paired SH atoms present in many biologically active compounds, such as proteins, enzymes, and co-enzymes. In addition, the sulfhydryl group is needed to help maintain the exact state of cytoplasmic fluidity, referred to as the gel/sol relationship. Again, interference in these areas by free radicals puts at great risk some very critical and delicate metabolic mechanisms.

The evidence highly suggests that one of the major sites of injury caused by oxygen is the mitochondria—the little "power packets" inside each cell that use oxygen in the production of ATP. Mitochondrial activity is highly dependent on sulfhydryl enzymes, which are easily destroyed by oxygen.[29]

Damage to capillaries and pneumocytes. Specifically related to our sphere of interest are two targets of free radical activity in the lung—the pulmonary capillary endothelium and the Type I alveolar cell. Integrity of the capillary wall is damaged by toxic action of oxygen, allowing the escape of fluid from capillary into lung interstitium and parenchyma. We will see that this can present an acute and difficult clinical problem to manage. The alveoli are composed of two kinds of cells, called pneumocytes, and designated Types I and II. Type I pneumocytes are flat, elongated, membranous cells that cover most of the alveolar surface, while Type II cells are more cuboidal, contain many inclusion bodies (implying diverse cellular functions), and produce the important lipoprotein surfactant. The free radicals, and apparently especially superoxide, destroy Type I pneumocytes and threaten disruption of alveolar walls.

Morphologic effects. Our primary interest in oxygen toxicity is its varied clinical manifestations, and these are related to the pathology of the toxic reactions, the abnormal structural changes that occur in tissues and organs. We now review a half dozen examples of tissue responses to high tensions of oxygen.

Reduced mucociliary action. Feline experiments have shown that the rate of cephalad movement of minute particles deposited on the distal tracheal mucosa is markedly slowed in the presence of 100% oxygen.[30] If this unwelcome action of oxygen can be extrapolated to the human airway, serious clinical implications are obvious. It is of considerable interest, however, that administration of low concentrations of oxygen also slow mucus transport time. Apparently the system will not work if it is not fueled with sufficient oxygen and can be inactivated by too much.

Perhaps it is clinically important to note that the retarding action of high-tension oxygen can be prevented or reversed by parenteral or aerosol administration of epinephrine, isoproterenol, and adenosine triphosphate.

Interference with pulmonary surfactant. Further animal experiments have established that prolonged exposure to high oxygen concentrations can interfere with the function of pulmonary surfactant.[31] It has been postulated that the surfactant probably is not destroyed because it can still be demonstrated in extractions of affected lungs. More than likely the oxygen causes a redistribution of the surfactant, removing it from close contact with alveolar walls. The potential for this toxic reaction of oxygen to produce atelectasis is very evident, and when coupled with the risk of oxygen absorption from poorly communicating alveoli, subjects the patient to a double hazard.

Oxygen pneumonia. Prolonged exposure to inspired oxygen concentrations in excess of 50% can give the lung an x-ray picture identical to that of a diffuse bronchopneumonia.[32] Patchy infiltrates tend to be most prominent in the lower lung fields, but all areas may be involved. Pulmonary pathologic conditions includes alveolar wall edema and an intraalveolar exudate of large cells. Polymorphonuclear leukocytes, white blood cells that protect us against infection by destroying bacteria, are not prominent, and bacteria are few. As with any pneumonia, because of alveolar exudate, patients with oxygen toxicity pneumonia suffer increasing hypoxemia. If patient survival can be maintained while inspired oxygen concentrations are lowered, the pulmonary lesion may resolve.

Bronchopulmonary dysplasia. To some extent this pathologic state carries lung damage beyond the stage of the oxygen pneumonia just described and depicts the destructive healing that accompanies chronicity.[33] Two microscopic pathologic stages have been identified, defined by one study as exudative and proliferative.[34]

The following excellent description needs no amplification:

> The lungs in the *exudative phase* showed capillary congestion, an alveolar proteinaceous exudate, intra-alveolar hemorrhage, and a fibrinous exudate. Prominent "hyaline" membranes lined the alveolar walls, alveolar ducts, and respiratory bronchioles. Only a sparse chronic inflammatory component was present. The striking features of the lungs in the *proliferative phase* were marked alveolar and interlobular septal edema, fibroblastic proliferation with early fibrosis, prominent hyperplasia of the alveolar lining cells, and a variable component of the alterations characteristic of the exudative phase. It is our impression that these 2 categories are stages of a progressive deterioration, with the exudative phase representing an earlier change that progresses, if survival is sufficiently prolonged, to the proliferative or fibrotic phase.[35]

An additional tissue response sometimes accompanying the proliferative phase is referred to as *capillary tufting.*[35] From the thickened alveolar septa, proliferated (overgrown) pulmonary capillaries project as tufts or small masses into alveolar spaces. These capillary tufts probably resolve and disappear in surviving patients, but while present they are intraalveolar, space-occupying lesions that add to existing problems of ventilation and gas exchange.

Finally, the damaging effect of oxygen on the lungs tends to be less in patients with well-established lung disease than in those without intrinsic disease. The implication is that preexisting exudate, fibrosis, edema, and the like from chronic disease protects the pulmonary tissue from a direct assault by oxygen. The validity of this conclusion may need additional support.

Alveolar membrane formation. Alveolar membrane was referred to previously, but its clinical importance as one of the major manifestations of oxygen toxicity justifies a detailed description. To introduce the topic, we digress just a bit and describe a relevant pediatric disease.[36,37]

Many infants born prematurely suffer from a condition called *hyaline membrane disease,* or respiratory distress syndrome of the newborn (RDS).[36-38] The major defect in this disease is a severely noncompliant lung, placing a tremendous physical strain on the ventilatory mechanics of the underdeveloped child. Many of these patients succumb in their early postnatal life, and others may survive only after intensive mechanical ventilatory support. The alveoli of the victims are lined with a thin but definite membrane, which because of its clear, transparent homogeneity is referred to as a "hyaline membrane." Such a structure is a normal prenatal component of the lung, but one that disappears before birth, and premature birth often does not allow time for its natural disappearance. One of the more serious complications of high concentration–oxygen therapy is the appearance of a hyaline membrane, in adults as well as children.

As a demonstration of the ease with which a membrane can be formed, 75% of a group of guinea pigs exposed to 98% oxygen at atmosphere from 40 to 100 hours developed such a defect. Interestingly, if a subject survives despite this injury, there is apparently no residual damage. The hyaline membrane produced experimentally with high oxygen concentrations appears to be structurally identical with that which occurs in RDS and seems to be the result of injury to the alveolar duct and terminal bronchiole. If the experimental animal is given high doses of adrenocorticosteroids with the elevated oxygen concentration, it deteriorates rapidly and dies from fulminating pulmonary vascular damage. Human postmortem lung specimens demonstrated reactions similar to the experimental response if the patients had been treated with high oxygen concentrations. The membranes noted consisted of layers of fibrin on the alveolar walls, extending into the alveolar ducts and respiratory bronchioles. Many patients succumbing to oxygen toxicity not only had received oxygen concentrations in the 90% to 100% range but had also had this delivered by mechanical ventilators. However, little correlation exists between the pulmonary pathologic changes and the mechanical ventilation, per se, but there is close correlation with the oxygen therapy. As yet, no dependable safety limits have been determined for oxygen administration, but it is evident that both factors of gas concentration and duration of treatment are critical. There is some evidence that prolonged administration of oxygen concentrations above 70% will increase the risk of membranous toxicity and that levels above 90% are dangerous.

Retrolental fibroplasia (RLF). The term *retrolental* means "behind the lens" and refers to an ocular condition of premature infants associated with oxygen administration. The disease was established as a specific entity in the 1950s, when it was observed that some premature infants given oxygen therapy developed damage to the eyes that was severe enough to produce permanent blindness. The pathology is basically a fibrotic process behind the ocular lenses, which impairs light penetration to the retina. Apparently excessive blood oxygen levels produce retinal vasoconstriction, and if this is severe enough to persist after the cessation of oxygen therapy, permanent damage is likely.[38-41]

This risk poses a serious management problem, for the premature infant is often in great need of supplementary oxygen, and as in the infant with a lung expansion defect, sometimes large amounts of oxygen are necessary for survival. Experience and a cooperative study have demonstrated that if the concentration of inspired oxygen delivered to the small patient does not exceed 40%, the risk of retrolental fibroplasia is significantly reduced,[41] especially when therapy is of short duration. When long-term oxygen therapy (longer than 10 days) of 30% has been given to small premature infants, 10% of infants can have RLF.[38]

Most incubators, which provide the proper environment for premature infants, have devices that limit the oxygen concentration to 40%. However, more experience will be needed to determine more precisely the critical arterial oxygen tension level that is associated with oxygen damage to the eyes.[38,40] As a final note, it should be mentioned that oxygen-induced eye damage has not been considered an adult hazard, but in what might be the first such recorded incident, near total blindness was reported in a 32-year-old man. The apparent cause of visual loss was retinal arterial constriction following prolonged arterial oxygen tensions of 250 to 300 mm Hg.[42]

Defense against oxygen toxicity. An organism as complex as the human body doubtless has many mechanisms that prevent oxygen damage, but at the present the one attracting the most interest is the enzyme *superoxide dismutase* (SOD).[43-45] The lung is not only an exchange membrane for gases; it is also a metabolically active organ dealing with oxygen with enzymatically active compounds.

The "free radical therapy" of oxygen toxicity is simply stated as follows: The damage seen with oxygen toxicity is a result of the overproduction of oxygen free radicals. These compounds include hydrogen peroxide, superoxide radical, and singlet excited oxygen.[28] Oxygen free radicals are normally produced by cellular elements of the lung and detoxified rapidly by SOD. Other naturally occurring detoxifying agents include catalase, glutathione peroxidase, lipid membrane constituent, vitamin E, ascorbate, glutathione, cysteine, and cysteamine.[27] The one frequently attracting the most interest is SOD.

By definition, a dismutase is an enzyme able to effect simultaneous oxidation-reduction. SOD specifically catalyzes the following reaction

$$O_2^- + O_2^- + 2H^+ \rightarrow H_2O_2 + O_2$$

whereby dangerous superoxide is transformed into hydrogen peroxide and molecular oxygen. Hydrogen peroxide, in turn, is metabolized into water and more oxygen by enzymes, peroxidases and catalases.

Most experimental rats exposed to 100% oxygen die within 72 hours. However, if they are first exposed to 85% oxygen for a week, they can then survive 100% oxygen for a long time. This phenomenon is called *tolerance* to 100% oxygen, and while it is developing, lung content of SOD increases by about 50%. Apparently SOD production is stimulated by inhalation of moderately elevated oxygen concentrations, and the body subsequently can tolerate 100% oxygen, since SOD controls the levels of superoxide.

It has been established that while experimental oxygen tolerance is being generated and pulmonary SOD levels are rising, alveolar Type II pneumocytes increase in number up to 300%. This tremendous proliferation of alveolar cells is obviously related to the increasing SOD. It probably represents a high initial dismutase cell content, allowing cell survival in the face of high oxygen tension, or stimulation of increased SOD production by the pneumocytes. It thus seems that Type II alveolar cells are an important source of superoxide dismutase and the primary defense against pulmonary oxygen toxicity.

In concluding this section, it is only just to point out that the villain is not all bad. Scavenging granulocytes, comprising a major body defense against infection, manufacture and release superoxide and the other free radicals to kill invading bacteria.[46,47] The lethal potential of these substances is thus directed in chemical warfare against other threats to our survival.

Summary. There are important clinical implications in the available data concerning the scope and mechanisms of oxygen toxicity. We frequently encounter patients whose hypoxia demands oxygen therapy, often with mechanically assisted ventilation, but who show a progressive downhill course while increasing concentrations of oxygen are administered in a vain attempt to maintain adequate blood levels. Not only is alveolar-capillary diffusion impaired, but obstruction of small airways and alveoli by edema, hemorrhage, and capillary proliferation produces an increasing venous admixture, demonstrated in the laboratory by a widening alveolar-arterial oxygen tension gradient.[48] We appreciate that this can be the direct result of the topical action of high-concentration oxygen on the pulmonary tissue, with the creation of a chaotic disturbance of physiology as the lung is beset, simultaneously, with shunting and atelectasis. Because the relation between pure oxygen breathing and absorption atelectasis was recognized before the more deep-seated oxygen damage to the lung was known, it was frequently assumed that the morbidity and mortality of oxygen breathing was associated with atelectasis. On this basis, it has been suggested that prevention of lung injury might be accomplished by alternating periods of oxygen breathing with the breathing of air, permitting expansion of alveoli by the nitrogen content of the latter. Studies of this maneuver, however, have failed to substantiate its predicted virtue.[49]

We can summarize the topic of the danger of oxygen by emphasizing again, strongly, that when oxygen is needed, it must be given, even though we recognize its potential risk. After all, the patient might not suffer toxic reactions, since these are not predictable with any precision, but failure to supply oxygen may well cause irreversible tissue damage. Nevertheless, oxygen, like any potent medicine, should be used with reason and according to indications. If high concentrations of oxygen are necessary, the duration of administration should be kept to a minimum and reduced as soon as possible. In general, the objective of therapy is to administer oxygen sufficient to maintain arterial oxygen tension between 60 and 100 mm Hg, not 150 or 200 mm Hg. The exceptions are those circumstances in which delivery to the pulmonary blood is normal but the oxygen-carrying capacity of the hemoglobin is impaired. Anemia and carbon monoxide inhalation are two common clinical conditions needing high blood gas tensions to increase dissolved plasma oxygen, compensating for the deficient hemoglobin transport. Frequent arterial blood monitoring is a mandatory safety measure when concentrations above 50% are used. Also, the exact concentration of inspired oxygen should be measured, especially when the gas is used in mechanical ventilators, and if air-diluting mechanisms cannot be depended on to deliver desired concentrations, then premixed gases should be used. The safe and effective administration of oxygen to suit any individual need is one of the most important services that a knowledgeable and skilled respiratory therapist can offer, a service matched by few other technical members of the hospital health team.

Oxygen delivery equipment and techniques

The evolution of oxygen therapy since the turn of this century is interesting, with some devices such as the nasal catheter remaining basically unchanged while various masks, tents, and whole oxygen rooms developed and changed dramatically. In the interest of space we do not dwell on history here, but for the interested reader a recent review by Leigh is recommended.[50]

Nearly all of the devices described in this section that can be applied to the face of patients are disposable units usually intended for single-patient use. Where permanent, reusable devices are discussed, special mention of that fact is made.

Classification of oxygen therapy devices. Most commonly used oxygen therapy devices can be classified into one of two types: those that can provide a relatively controlled oxygen concentration when a variable breathing pattern occurs and those that cannot. Two sets of terminology have become popular in recent years in the United States and Great Britain.[14,51-55] One set uses the terms *high-flow* and *low-flow*,[51-53] while the other uses *fixed-performance* and *variable-performance*.[14,54,55]

Fixed-performance, or high-flow, devices can be defined as units that supply all the inspired gases at a preset $F_{I_{O_2}}$ and generally are not affected by changes in ventilatory pattern. Variable-performance, or low-flow, devices are defined as units that do not supply all the inspired gases so the patient inhales some room air along with the oxygen. As the patient's ventilatory pattern changes, different amounts of air are mixed with the constant flow of oxygen, and the inspired oxygen concentration varies.

For each of the following devices discussed we consider the factors that make them either fixed- or variable-performance devices as well as the oxygen concentrations they generally can deliver.

Variable performance devices

Nasal cannulas and catheters. We discuss these two similar items together, for their general principles of function are the same. Their proper designations are *nasal cannula* and *nasal catheter*.

The *nasal cannula* (Fig. 12-14, *A*) is a plastic appliance (formerly made of metal) consisting of two tips about $^1/_2$ inch long arising from an oxygen supply tube and inserting into the nostrils. It is held in place by looping over the ears and snugging under the chin like a lariat. The cannula has the advantages

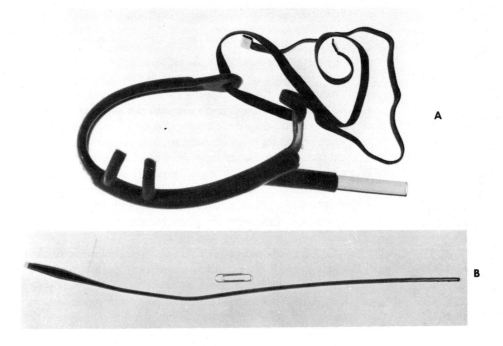

Fig. 12-14   **A,** Nasal oxygen cannula. **B,** Oropharyngeal catheter.

of ease of application, lightness of weight, economy, and disposability. It has the disadvantage of instability, being easily dislodged from a restless or unobservant patient. It is a common experience, while making medical rounds, to note open oxygen flow meters with cannulas so twisted out of place that the patients could not possibly get any significant therapy. It is also necessary to pay attention to the patient's comfort when instituting treatment, since excessive flows (variable among patients) can produce considerable pain in the frontal sinuses. Finally, such nasal pathologic conditions as a deviated septum, mucosal edema, mucous drainage, and polyps may interfere with adequate oxygen intake.

The *nasal catheter* is so named because it is placed through the nasal passage with its tip in the oropharynx (Fig. 12-14, *B*). Made of soft flexible rubber or plastic, the catheter has several holes in its terminal 1 inch. Success in catheter therapy depends on its proper insertion and maintenance, techniques with which every respiratory therapist should be familiar.

Before introduction, the distal one third to one half of the catheter is lubricated with a water-soluble lubricant. A low flow of oxygen is started to ensure patency of the tube and its apertures and continued during the insertion. The catheter is gently slid along the floor of either naris into the oropharynx until, in the cooperative patient, direct viewing into the mouth while the tongue is depressed shows the tip of the catheter just below the uvula. It is then retracted out of sight and fastened to the bridge of the nose with adhesive tape.

If direct vision is not possible, there are two "blind" procedures that can be used. The catheter can be placed on the side of the patient's face and the distance from the nose to the ear measured off; this length of the catheter is then inserted through the nose into the pharynx. Alternatively, with a moderate oxygen flow, the catheter can be introduced into the pharynx until the patient starts to gulp air and can then be retracted approximately 1 inch and fastened. Under no circumstances must force be used to advance the catheter through the nose, and if significant resistance is encountered, the opposite naris should be used. Nasal disorders as enumerated above may block passage of the tube, and attempts to ram it through will only produce mucosal edema and worsen the condition. There are patients in whom this therapy cannot be used.

Catheters should be removed and fresh ones inserted in the opposite nostril at least every 8 hours, since because they are foreign bodies in the nose, nasal secretions will cause them to adhere to the nasal mucosa if they are not changed periodically and their removal is a painful event. Generally, a well-placed catheter is not uncomfortable and allows at least a bit of bed mobility for the patient.

This therapy should be used with some caution in a deeply comatose patient with completely obtunded reflexes and in a patient who is elderly and debilitated, such as in a post-stroke state. With ineffective epiglottal reflexes or epiglottal paralysis, the administered oxygen stream may be directed down the esophagus and seriously distend the stomach. The risk of gastric rupture is real, and distention will further handicap ventilation that is already impaired. After inserting a catheter in such a patient, the therapist should observe and palpate the epigastrium for several minutes to see whether distention develops and, if present, the therapist should remove the catheter and employ some other technique. Finally, because oxygen is delivered as a blast in the pharynx, its desiccating effect on the respiratory tract must be prevented by adequate humidification. For this a good humidifier is safe and effective because it provides good water vaporization with a minimal amount of particulate water to deposit in and obstruct the oxygen tubing.

There has been considerable controversy over the relative merits and efficiency of the nasal cannula versus the nasal catheter. The issue has been clouded by failure of partisan advocates to apply uniform criteria in evaluating these appliances. Some have studied their performance in healthy subjects, others in patients; some have used the delivered oxygen concentration as a gauge, others have used arterial oxygen tension. Nevertheless, there seems to be enough available data to make at least some valid generalizations. With oxygen flows up to 6 ℓ/min, concentrations of near 40% can probably be achieved with a well-placed nasal cannula; with flows to 8 ℓ/min concentrations up to 50% can be delivered by a nasal catheter.[56] Because these oxygen flow rates are far below the typical peak inspiratory flow rates of spontaneously breathing adults,[10] room air is also inhaled, thus diluting the oxygen. Both of these devices are therefore variable-performance units. The actual $F_{I_{O_2}}$ achieved at any one oxygen flow can vary considerably from patient to patient and with breathing pattern changes in the same patients.[56-59]

In patients having a regular breathing pattern with relatively consistent rate and tidal volume, oxygen at low flows of 0.25 to 4 ℓ/min have been successfully used with cannulas to provide "controlled" oxygen therapy.[11,12,27] Under usual circumstances it is difficult to achieve consistently high $F_{I_{O_2}}$s with these devices unless the patient breathes shallowly[51] or is given sedation.[12] Both nasal cannula and nasal catheter are probably best used to provide relatively low concentrations of oxygen to stable patients with regular breathing patterns. Cannulas are often used for long-term therapy in adults,[12,27] and catheters can also be used for babies.[27,60]

It has been suggested that for the mouth-breathing patient a catheter is preferable to a cannula on the grounds that mouth breathing would dilute the nasal flow of oxygen below a therapeutic level. Some studies have shown that the eventual delivery of oxygen to the blood is not significantly different when either a cannula or catheter is used and whether the mouth is open or closed,[59,61] while other studies show tracheal concentration differences during similar conditions.[62] There is little doubt that the cannula is more comfortable or less of a nuisance than the catheter, but patient acceptance as a determinant must be weighed against the reliability of each technique. It might be practical to suggest that a cannula be considered for the cooperative and alert patient who can be depended on to keep the appliance in its proper position, and the catheter for the restless or less dependable patient.

Nasal mask. Brief mention will be made concerning a new version of an old idea,[50] the nasal mask. This device fits loosely over just the nose, and oxygen enters from tubing on either side. While comparative studies have not been done with this mask yet, it is reasonable to assume that the $F_{I_{O_2}}$s delivered will be similar to that of a nasal cannula. The primary advantage seems to be that the mask does not protrude into the nose, and some patients may find it more comfortable than the cannula. It can also be used for patients receiving long-term therapy who may desire to alternate with the cannula when the nares are sore from continued wearing of the cannula. If the level of oxygen received is critical for these patients, then arterial blood gases should be used to establish the proper flow for the nasal mask in the same manner as with the cannula.[11,12]

Masks. Oxygen masks are of many different types, varying in style of construction, materials, and specific purpose. Not too long ago most masks were of rubber, but now most are made of plastic and can be discarded after use, minimizing the risk of cross-contamination, work of sterilizing, and storage space. Although we discuss some critical differences among them, oxygen masks have some important common characteristics. The therapist will note variation in the use of masks, as with other pieces of equipment, among the hospitals with which he or she may have contact; but in general, we can say that the oxygen mask is used where oxygen is needed quickly and for relatively short periods of time. It is the emergency equipment of choice, and some type of a mask should be available wherever patients are being treated. A mask may be used for up to several hours, but other techniques are more appropriate for prolonged constant therapy.

Masks can be uncomfortable as a result of the frequent need for a tight seal between the unit and the patient's face, and the head strap or harness necessary to hold it in place adds to the discomfort. Masks are often quite hot, as they confine heat radiating from the face about the nose and mouth. The therapist must ever be aware of the risk of producing pressure necrosis of the skin when he or she attempts a tight fit of the mask to the face. Constant pressure of the edge of the mask over areas where little subcutaneous tissue separates skin from underlying bone, such as the bridge of the nose and the malar eminences of the cheeks, can readily interrupt cutaneous blood flow. Within a short time the skin may become devitalized, with the risk of permanent scarring. A snugly fitted mask should be removed frequently and dried, and the face should be dried and gently massaged over the pressure areas to stimulate circulation, then powdered to minimize the accumulation of moisture, which tends to soften the skin and to augment danger of pressure damage. An oxygen mask can be hazardous on a patient who is prone to vomit, for it can block the flow of vomitus and subject the patient to dangerous aspiration. Because of this risk of aspiration, and the possibility of airway obstruction by a flaccid tongue, a mask should never be strapped onto an unconscious patient. If mask therapy is indicated in such a patient, an oral airway should be inserted to prevent the tongue from retracting into the pharynx, and the oxygen mask should either be held in place by an attendant or loosely set on the face.

Finally, the therapist must recognize that by the nature of their construction, face masks add dead space to the patient's airway, which may be considerable with some appliances. The space under the mask, about the nose and mouth, is functionally an extension of anatomic dead space and, depending on the location of the exhalation ports, may cause a significant accumulation of carbon dioxide. Assuming a normally responsive respiratory center, the dead space of many masks produces an increased ventilation that may add to the patient's work of breathing, and in the patient with an obtunded center and hypercapnia, such dead space can be an added hazard.

Despite these shortcomings, however, oxygen masks have a wide use in therapy and are often lifesaving. In this section we describe some of the characteristics of the following four general types of masks: simple, rebreathing, partial rebreathing, and nonrebreathing.

Simple mask. The usual simple mask, shown in Fig. 12-15, is a disposable plastic unit with neither valves nor reservoir bag, exhaled air being vented

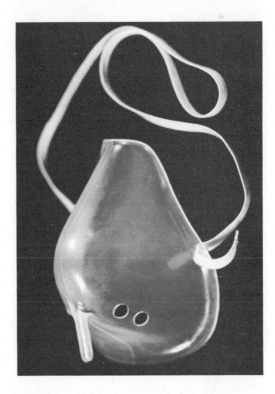

Fig. 12-15   Simple plastic mask with an oxygen inlet and exhalation holes (pediatric size shown).

through holes in its body. Generally, it is relatively loosely fitted without the capability of close molding to facial contours possible with more elaborate types. In the event of an interrupted oxygen supply, air is drawn in through the exhalation ports as well as around the edge of the mask. The mask dead space and its "reservoir effect" influence the relationship between oxygen flow and the resulting alveolar oxygen concentration.[63] A minimal flow is necessary to flush the dead space for removal of carbon dioxide, but beyond a given flow, since the oxygen supply is continuous throughout the ventilatory cycle, the reservoir or dead space is filled with oxygen at the end of exhalation.

The oxygen enrichment of inhaled air depends on the balance between the patient's ventilatory need and the oxygen supply during inhalation. The deeper the tidal volume or the greater the inspiratory flow of the patient, the more the oxygen will be diluted by supplementary air drawn in through the ports or around the mask since at any given instant the inspiratory flow may exceed many times the delivered oxygen flow. The more oxygen supplied during inhalation, the greater its alveolar concentration.

Because of its convenience and relative comfort, the simple mask has been widely used whenever moderate oxygen concentrations have been desired for short periods of time. This includes the postoperative recovery state, temporary therapy while awaiting definitive plans, and interim therapy while weaning a patient from continuous oxygen administration. The crudeness of a simple mask makes it impossible to predict exact amounts of oxygen going to the patient, but in general the delivered concentrations vary from 35% at gas flows of 6 to 10 ℓ/min.[56,59] It must be kept in mind that such values give no indication of the alveolar or arterial oxygen levels and are quite variable from patient to patient. Relatively high concentrations *can* be delivered by masks in an uncontrolled fashion to patients with slow, shallow breathing patterns, while only low concentrations may be delivered to tachypneic patients. Therefore, simple masks are often not a good choice for patients in acute ventilatory failure from chronic obstructive diseases nor for patients with acute restrictive disease (such as pulmonary edema) with a rapid breathing pattern and severe hypoxemia.

Rebreathing mask. The rebreathing mask is not used for clinical respiratory therapy and is only briefly described here. It consists of a mask tightly covering the mouth and nose, with an attached reservoir bag into which the breathing mixture flows and from which the patient inhales. The bag and mask are used in a closed system whereby the exhaled gas is circulated through a carbon dioxide absorber, and additional breathing gas is added to replace that metabolized by the patient. The chief use for a rebreathing circuit is the administration of anesthesia, since it prevents waste of anesthetic agents and permits the addition of desired amounts of oxygen to the breathing mixture.[4]

Partial rebreathing mask. Like the rebreathing mask, the partial rebreathing mask is a combined face mask and reservoir bag, but unlike the rebreathing mask, it is an open circuit without a carbon dioxide absorber. The purpose of the partial rebreathing mask is to conserve oxygen by a technique that, as the name implies, permits the patient to rebreathe some exhaled air. Fig. 12-16, *A*, schematically illustrates the basic parts and function of such an appliance. Source oxygen flows into the neck of the mask and during the inhalation phase passes directly into the mask proper, but during exhalation it enters the reservoir bag. Ideally, as the patient exhales, approximately the first third of the exhaled air is returned to fill the reservoir bag and to mix with source oxygen. This fraction of the exhaled volume essentially represents the pulmonary dead space, which contains mostly oxygen, and it is flushed into the bag to be reinhaled. As the bag distends with both source oxygen and exhaled air,

Fig. 12-16   Diagrammatic illustrations of the difference between, **A,** disposable partial rebreathing oxygen mask and, **B,** disposable nonrebreathing mask. In both, oxygen flows directly into the mask during inspiration and into the reservoir bag during exhalation. However, the early portion of exhaled air in **A** returns to the bag to be rebreathed with incoming oxygen in the next breath. Terminal air escapes through exhalation ports. In **B** all exhaled air is vented through a port in the mask, and a one-way valve between the bag and mask prevents rebreathing.

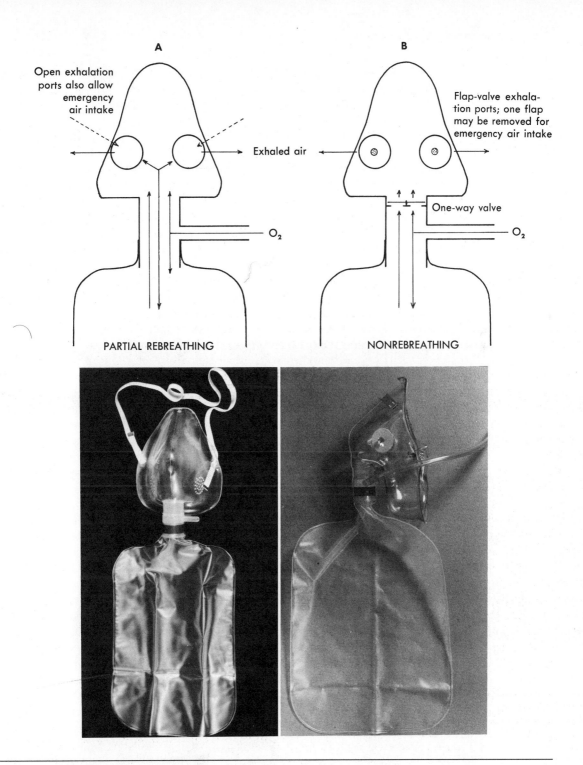

A

Open exhalation ports also allow emergency air intake

Exhaled air

O_2

PARTIAL REBREATHING

B

Flap-valve exhalation ports; one flap may be removed for emergency air intake

One-way valve

O_2

NONREBREATHING

Fig. 12-16 For legend see opposite page.

pressure in the system then directs the terminal two thirds of exhaled air, with its carbon dioxide load, out the exhalation ports. If the oxygen inflow is adjusted so that the bag does not collapse during inhalation and the rate is over 4 ℓ/min, the amount of carbon dioxide contaminating the reservoir is negligible.[64] The exhalation ports of many masks are only vents in the facepiece, and they also serve as emergency inlets for room air during each inspiration and in the event of a failure of source oxygen. With a well-fitted partial rebreathing mask, adjusted so that the patient's inhalation does not deflate the bag, inspired oxygen concentrations of from 35% to 60% can usually be achieved at delivered flows between 6 and 10 ℓ/min for disposable units and up to about 75% for rubber (BLB[50]) types.[59]

Disposable nonrebreathing mask. Also a mask and reservoir bag device, the name of the nonrebreathing mask indicates that there is no exhaled gas rebreathing. Fig. 12-16, *B,* depicts the essential differences between the partial and nonrebreathing masks. The one major characteristic of the nonrebreathing mask is a one-way valve placed between the bag and the mask. As in the partial rebreather, source oxygen flows either into the bag only (during exhalation) or into the mask and bag (during inhalation). However, the valve between bag and mask prevents exhaled air from returning to the bag and diverts it into the atmosphere through a flap valve in the facepiece. Somewhere, either in the neck or in the mask itself, flap- or spring-loaded valves permit the intake of room air should source oxygen fail or the patient's needs suddenly exceed the available oxygen flow. In some disposable units one of the exhalation ports does not have a one-way valve covering it, and it is therefore used as the safety inlet valve. This also allows room air to be inhaled through this port even when oxygen is attached, and dilution of the oxygen occurs.

A common misconception is to assume that the term *nonrebreathing mask* means that nearly 100% oxygen (or other source gas) will be administered. Particularly with typical disposable masks this has not been the case in our clinical experience as well as evidenced by a laboratory study.[56] This study found that a typical example of this mask delivered an average of 63% oxygen (range 57% to 70%) in healthy volunteers. Factors involved can be several. Most disposable masks do not fit snugly enough on most patients for the one-way valves to function adequately. Leaks around the mask are common, and room air enters during inspiration. As mentioned previously, some nonrebreathing masks have an open exhalation port that also is a source of room air dilution on inspiration. Because of these factors, common *disposable* nonrebreathing masks should generally be considered variable-performance devices. Well-fitting, usually reusable nonrebreathing masks are discussed under the next section.

Fixed-performance devices. As mentioned earlier, this category of devices includes systems that provide a relatively constant ("fixed") concentration of oxygen by supplying all the gases the patient requires during inspiration without further dilution of room air. We now discuss four systems that have been

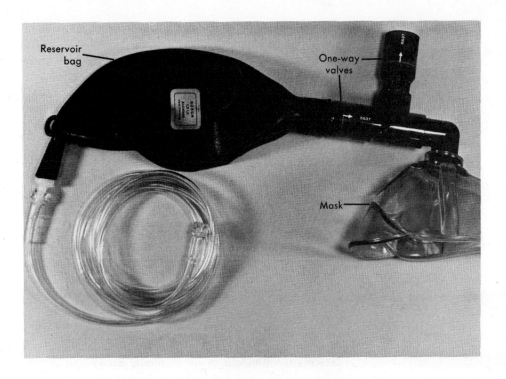

Fig. 12-17   Example of a permanent style, nonrebreathing oxygen system. One-way valves prevent both re-breathing and inhalation of room air while mask is held on patient's face.

used for this purpose: a well-fitted nonrebreathing system, air-entrainment masks, air-entrainment nebulizers, and oxygen blender systems.

Well-fitted nonrebreathing system. When a mask is used with this system it is similar in design to the disposable unit shown in Fig. 12-16, *B.* However, when a permanent anesthesia-style face mask is combined with dependable one-way valves and a 1- to 2-ℓ reservoir bag, 100% oxygen can be administered. This system can provide a snug fit when properly applied and avoid room air dilution at the mask site. Such systems can be built from equipment common to respiratory care or anesthesiology departments,[56] and they also are commercially available[5,50] (Fig. 12-17). Flows greater than the patients *total minute ventilation* are needed, and the reservoir bag should hold a volume greater than the patients typical *tidal volume* to ensure adequate fresh air delivery and prevent the bag from collapsing.

Because the patient inhales only the gas present in the bag, the nonrebreathing technique can be a most precise method of administering a specific gas concentration, but to be effective there must be no significant leakage about the face or elsewhere in the system. This type of apparatus can be used to deliver 100% oxygen, blended oxygen and air, or tanked gases of precise composition such as oxygen-nitrogen, helium-oxygen, and oxygen–carbon dioxide mixtures. Care must be taken to provide suitable humidification, and some reservoir bags have drain plugs for removal of accumulated moisture. Nonrebreathing systems can also be connected to patients with artificial airways when proper connections are used instead of a face mask. In this instance high-humidity conditions (Chapter 10) are needed, and the one-way valves chosen must be able to function with minimal resistance even when wet. If resistance to breathing is increased significantly with this system it will prove unsuitable for some patients for extended use.

Air-entrainment masks. In 1941, Barach and Eckman reported the use of an oxygen mask that provided controlled oxygen concentrations.[65,66] Oxygen was mixed by passing it through a jet and entraining specific amounts of room air. This device is often referred to as a "venturi" or "injector."[10,50] Barach's system provided relatively high concentrations of oxygen (above 40%) and controlled the amount of air mixed with oxygen by adjustable air-entrainment ports or orifices. The mixed gases were fed into a nonrebreathing mask with bag system and vented through a valved exhalation port on the mask.

In 1960, Campbell reported on an entrainment mask designed to provide a *low* oxygen concentration with high flow rates of air over the patient's face.[67] Fig. 12-18 is an example of a mask fashioned after Campbell's prototype and represents the function of other similar masks that are available. Because of the high airflows and low oxygen concentrations from these devices they have been referred to as *high airflow* with *oxygen enrichment* or *HAFOE* systems.[67,68] These masks by Campbell and later commercial units are often referred to as *venturi* masks, although this is not precisely correct.[5,69,70] These devices do not have an actual venturi tube in them (see Chapter 4). They do, however, use a jet (restricted orifice) through which oxygen flows at high velocities. Air is mixed or "entrained" at the jet site, and the higher the velocity of oxygen at the jet, the more air is entrained. Traditionally, this occurrence has been attributed in the medical literature to the Bernoulli effect. A recent article disclaimed this connection and explained instead that the mixing of the oxygen and air is caused by the forces of fluid viscosity and not pressure gradient per se.[70] Whether or not the decrease in pressure measured at the side of the jet occurs because of the high forward velocity alone or is created by the removal of air molecules as they adhere to the oxygen molecules by sheer force is a matter for gas physicists to discuss. The clinical considerations for these air-entrainment systems remain the same.

All entrainment masks have a common clinical goal: to provide a controlled oxygen concentration at flow rates sufficient to ensure that no further dilution of room air occurs during inspiration. In order for this to be accomplished, the total flow rate across the patient's face must exceed that patient's *peak inspiratory flow rate*.[10,14,70] Unlike the nonrebreathing mask described earlier, the entrainment mask of today has no reservoir for gases to be collecting during the patient's expiratory phase. Therefore, the mask must provide flow

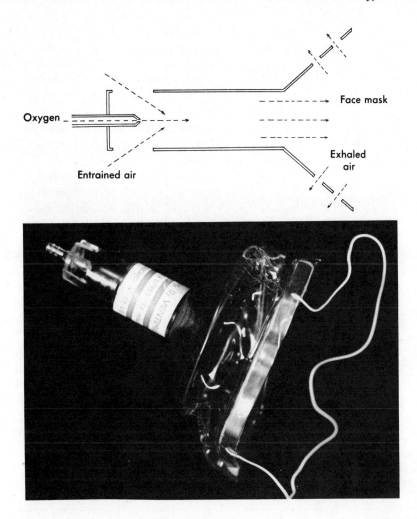

Fig. 12-18   Entrained air mixes with oxygen, which is supplied through the jet of an entrainment mask. Construction design maintains a constant air/oxygen ratio, ensuring a fixed concentration of inhaled oxygen over a wide range of oxygen flows.

rates that can meet instantaneous needs during each inspiration. During quiet breathing, a common peak inspiratory flow rate is probably less than 30 ℓ/min, but this can easily be doubled or tripled during times of stress or hyperventilation. A general clinical guide that has been suggested is to provide at least 40 ℓ/min of total flow[14] for resting patients and more if needed for tachypneic patients.

Peak inspiratory flow during spontaneous breathing is not easily measured at the patient's bedside without elaborate equipment such as a pneumotachygraph. (This resting *inspiratory* maneuver should not be confused with the peak *expiratory* flow rate during a forced maneuver described in Chapter 5.) Some correlation between peak inspiratory flow rate and exhaled minute volume has been shown by Nunn to exist for normal or anesthetized patients.[10] In general if a measured minute volume is multiplied by a factor of 4 to 6, an *estimate* of the peak inspiratory flow can be obtained. The exhaled minute volume is easily measured at the bedside using commonly available equipment.[5] However, no studies have been done to support this relationship in chronically or acutely ill patients of various types, and so this must be thought of only as a clinical guide.

Oxygen concentrations and total flows from entrainment devices are primarily determined by (1) the oxygen flow to the jet, (2) the air-to-oxygen ratio of the device, and (3) the amount of resistance encountered in the system.[69,70]

Most manufacturers list a single or narrow range of oxygen flow for the jet of their entrainment device for each concentration desired, and users appear to be reluctant to deviate from these flows. Several studies have shown that the oxygen concentrations are generally consistent, remaining within 1% to 2% oxygen when flows of 2 to 15 ℓ/min are used to drive the jet.[69,71,72] Some individual exceptions do exist, and up to a 6% oxygen change has been measured under changing jet flows.[72] The clinicians using these devices should become familiar with the brand of masks they use and measure the oxygen concentration entering the mask under different conditions. Once the desired concentration is established, the $F_{I_{O_2}}$ the patient actually receives will be primarily a function of the total flow available and the patient's peak inspiratory flow rate.[73]

The air-to-pure oxygen ratio is a mathematic relationship for each oxygen concentration. Common oxygen percentages and their *approximate* air-to-oxygen ratios are listed in Table 12-9.

Table 12-9 Approximate air-to-oxygen ratios for oxygen concentrations in common use	% Oxygen	Approximate air-to-oxygen ratio*	Total ratio parts†
	100	0:1	1
	80	0.3:1	1.3
	70	0.6:1	1.6
	60	1:1	2
	50	1.7:1	2.7
	45	2:1	3
	40	3:1	4
	35	5:1	6
	30	8:1	9
	28	10:1	11
	24	25:1	26

*Assuming 20.9% oxygen in air.
†Total flow of mixed air and oxygen can be calculated by multiplying the total ratio parts times the oxygen flow rate (ℓ/min).

Resistance to flow in these devices causes back pressure and a *decrease* in air-entrainment.[69] This results in an *increase* in oxygen concentration entering the mask and a *decrease* in total flow rate, and it may negate the ability for a controlled FI_{O_2}.

Air-entrainment systems have generally been shown to deliver relatively consistent and reliable oxygen concentrations when used properly.[54-57,71] Measurement of the oxygen percent entering the mask for these devices should be routine, and an attempt should be made to provide adequate total flow rates.[73] Monitoring the inspired oxygen in sick patients by sampling from the hypopharynx has been reported as a relatively simple procedure and can provide additional information and security concerning the FI_{O_2} in these and other oxygen devices.[57]

These masks are generally best used for relatively short periods when precise control over inspired oxygen is needed, such as in acute respiratory failure. They are less well tolerated for long-term oxygen use than are nasal cannulas because of their relative size, comfort, and appearance. The masks must also be removed for eating and drinking whereas removing cannulas is not necessary. The high airflow produced by these masks can be quite drying and attempts have been made to humidify the gases.[74,75] While simple humidifiers can be used for the oxygen flow to the jet without changing the FI_{O_2},[74] very little increase in humidification of all the gases occurs because of the relatively large amounts of room air entrained, especially with 40% oxygen or less (see Table 12-9). A better method is to add aerosol to the entrained air, being careful to not affect the size of the entrainment ports inadvertently on some models.[75]

Air-entrainment nebulizers. Heated nebulizers have long been used in respiratory therapy. Most of these have air-entrainment capabilities, and a general description of them is given in Chapter 10. Generally these nebulizers have settings for 40%, 60% or 70%, and 100% oxygen, or a variable entrainment port continuously adjustable from near 30% to 100%. As mentioned in Chapter 10, these nebulizers have a relatively limited flow available because of the size of both the jet and the air-entrainment port. When the nebulizer is set in its 40% (or lowest) position, maximum total flow is usually available. Studies and clinical experience reveal that with typical tubing set-ups of 4 to 6 feet in length, 40% is often not obtained.[76] Rather, 45% to 50% is measured, because of the slight resistance provided by the tubing. This is more pronounced when the tubing has water in it from condensation of water vapor,[76] although about 70% of the tubing's lumen can be occluded before changes in oxygen percent occur.[77]

The maximum flow to the jet of common entrainment nebulizers is often 12 to 15 ℓ/min from a 50 psig oxygen source. With minimum oxygen concentrations available of about 45% to 50%, the total flows resulting will be about 32 to 48 ℓ/min. This may be barely adequate for some patients and inadequate for patients with dyspnea and increased peak inspiratory flow rates.

Studies have shown that these units do not provide adequate total flows for controlled oxygen delivery unless they are used on the 40% setting, and some variance may still occur.[56-58] When set for a 60%, 70%, or 100% setting the total flow decreases, and room air is inspired at the mask with little gain in actual F_{IO_2}.

Air-entrainment nebulizers can provide a low oxygen percent by using compressed air to drive the jet and add oxygen after the entrainment site.[5,78,79] Again the unit must be set to provide its greatest air-entrainment. Oxygen is titrated into the system until the desired percent is *measured*.

The most significant advantages these systems provide are their humidification and heat control capabilities, especially for intubated patients (Chapter 10). The oxygen and aerosol can be delivered by an aerosol mask, tracheostomy mask, or an aerosol T connector,[5] often called a Briggs adapter.[52]

Oxygen blender systems. Oxygen blenders are devices that use 50-psig sources of oxygen and compressed air and mix the two gases by way of a proportioning valve.[5] Concentrations from 21% to 100% are available, usually at any flow of about 2 to 100 ℓ/min, depending on the model. Blenders can be used to provide a fixed concentration by using an open mask or connector with high flow rates (above the patients peak inspiratory flow rate). They can also be used with a well-fitted nonrebreathing mask or connector (as described earlier) at flows exceeding the patient's minute volume.

Hoods for pediatric patients. Oxygen hoods are the most convenient method of providing therapy to infants.[38] They cover only the head, leaving the patient's body available for nursing care. Controlled oxygen therapy can be given when blenders are used. Depending on the size of hood, flows of 10 to 15 ℓ may be needed to keep the oxygen concentration from fluctuating. It is especially important for a premature infant to receive the oxygen warmed and humidified since cool air over the baby's face can cause an increase in oxygen consumption.[38] The temperature of the gases in the hood should be similar to that of premature infants' ambient environment.[40]

Hoods or "head tents" for adults have been used for decades,[50] but the other methods of oxygen delivery just described have nearly eliminated their use.

Tents. Oxygen tents were once very popular for use in both adults and children. Their use today is rare in adults, but they are still used in pediatric patients. In general, tents are air-conditioned or cooled by ice to provide a relatively comfortable temperature within a plastic sheet enclosure. Oxygen concentrations are quite difficult to control and are usually limited to 50% at flows of 12 to 15 ℓ/min of oxygen for larger tents and 8 to 10 ℓ for some smaller pediatric tents. Frequent opening and closing of the plastic canopy causes great fluctuations in oxygen. A more common use for tents today is to provide an enclosed environment for high-humidity and aerosol therapy for children with croup, epiglottitis, or cystic fibrosis. Oxygen therapy is sometimes also given, but it is more difficult to control with the tent.

Any enclosure such as a tent with an oxygen-enriched atmosphere can provide an increase risk of fire. All electrical appliances with the potential for sparks, such as nurse-call devices and electric toys, should be kept out of an oxygen tent.

A few comments must be made concerning the fire hazard of oxygen, a question that the therapist may expect to encounter occasionally. A frequent source of worry is the presence of static electrical sparks often generated by the friction of movements of the patient in bed or by uniforms of personnel rubbing against bed clothing. This subject has been studied in some detail, and the respiratory therapist should be aware of the following data.

To start any fire three conditions must be met: Flammable material must be present; oxygen must be present; and the flammable material must be heated above its flash or igniting temperature and kept there by some external heat or the heat of its own combustion. Thus for any spark to ignite flammable material, the spark must be able to generate enough heat energy to start the process. In relation to the patient in bed, it was determined that the maximum energy capacity was to be found in the ungrounded bed itself (estimated to be less than 100 micromicrofarads); and it was further estimated that the electrical potential of a hospital bed is about 20,000 volts. Theoretically, such a combination could produce a spark some $^{7}/_{10}$ inch long with a maximum energy of 0.02 joule. The likelihood of a casual, random static spark of this magnitude was thought to be very remote. Under conditions of oxygen concentrations varying from 21% to 100%, sparks exceeding this potential were applied to such fabrics as vinyl plastic canopy material, tissue paper, nylon, wool, cotton, muslin, and dacron-cotton. With a barrage of sparks at a frequency of 60 per minute, ignition was achieved with elevated oxygen concentrations, but under no circumstances was a single spark able to produce fire.

Further experiments were conducted with fabrics impregnated with petroleum jelly or lanolin, simulating conditions that might be expected in the presence of surgical dressings. Again, even with high concentrations and frequent sparking, few ignitions occurred. The conservative conclusions were drawn that the overall hazard from static sparks with the fabrics in common use, even in high oxygen concentrations, is very low but not nonexistent. The static sparks just do not have sufficient heat energy to raise the material to their flash points. The minimal risk that may be present can be further reduced by maintaining a relative humidity in the tent of 60% or greater.

It should be strongly emphasized that the above refers only to static sparking, *not* sparks from electrical equipment such as meters or exposed switches, which are very dangerous. All appliances that transmit house current should be kept out of oxygen tents. The energy of battery-operated current, such as might be found in the many appliances being developed for cardiac support, probably is of too small a magnitude to constitute a risk, especially if well grounded, but the specifications of these appliances should include this information. Recording equipment, such as cardiac monitors, are not hazards, since they pick up only minute physiologic currents and amplify them for inspection outside the high-oxygen environment. It is expected that the therapist is fully aware of the precautions to take against the presence of open flames about a tent and the prohibition of smoking in the room with an operating tent.

One last note of caution should be made, more for completeness than for anything else. With an attached appliance an oxygen cylinder should be opened slowly to avoid a rush of gas downstream into the appliance. The heat of compression of rapidly flowing oxygen carries the potential risk of elevating to their ignition points such materials as valve seat packing and contaminants in the system. Gradual dissipation of this heat by slow opening of the valve will avoid this hazard.

Incubators. Especially useful for premature infants are incubators, not for their oxygen therapy potential per se but for their controlled temperature and humidity environment. Because of the relatively large air space of most incubators it is difficult to provide controlled oxygen therapy, so hoods are often used while infants are in incubators.

Heat loss is critical for premature infants, and cold stress (excessive heat loss) can cause increased oxygen consumption, apnea, and other problems. Newer incubators are incorporating a double-wall construction to help slow radiant heat loss from infants and help decrease oxygen consumption by significant amounts.[80,81] The role of incubators, oxygen therapy, and heat and humidity control and their physiologic consequences in premature infants are beyond the scope of this section. Those readers especially interested are encouraged to read other sources.[38-40]

Some incubators have systems for limiting oxygen levels to 40% by using an entrainment system. Because hoods provide greater overall oxygen control, they are more often used in intensive care nurseries.

Oxygen analyzers. Whenever possible, oxygen therapy systems should be analyzed to monitor the concentrations given. This is especially true for fixed-performance devices and for hoods, tents, and incubators. Monitoring can be continuous or intermittent, such as every 1 to 2 hours or after any change in settings. Common commercially available analyzers for routine bedside use are of three basic types: physical, electrical, and electrochemical.

The *physical analyzer* uses a small glass dumbbell suspended on a taut quartz fiber in the field of a permanent magnet. In the absence of oxygen, the forces of the torque of the quartz fiber and the magnetic field are equal and in balance. If oxygen is introduced into the system, because of its unique capability among all the gases of being magnetized, it is drawn into and augments the magnetic field. This upsets the balance, as the torque of the quartz fiber is overcome, and the glass dumbbell rotates in response to the new magnetic force. A small mirror attached to the fiber reflects a beam of battery-powered light onto a translucent scale calibrated to translate motion into oxygen percent. A major advantage of this oximeter is its ability to detect and measure concentrations of oxygen in any mixture of gases, and the instrument can safely be used with flammable and explosive gases. It is most affected by the partial pressure of oxygen present, since the P_{O_2} will determine the number

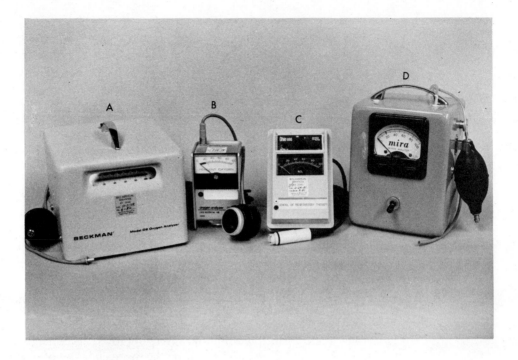

Fig. 12-19   Example of oxygen analyzers. **A,** Physical analyzer; **B,** galvanic fuel cell electrochemical analyzer, **C,** polaragraphic electrochemical analyzer; **D,** electrical analyzer.

of oxygen molecules that will occupy a given space such as in the measuring chamber.

The *electric analyzer* consists of a battery-powered Wheatstone bridge of platinum wires, two arms of which are subjected to the test gas, the other two exposed to air, functioning as references. The instrument is designed only to measure differences in concentrations in a mixture of oxygen and nitrogen and is not to be used with any other gas or gas mixture. A physical property of oxygen is its ability to remove heat from a warmed object faster than nitrogen can; so the higher the concentration of oxygen, the cooler the object (the platinum wires in this instance). Since the electrical resistance of a wire varies directly with the temperature, the resistance will reflect the oxygen concentration. The instrument is calibrated before use by the drawing of room air into it and balancing the Wheatstone bridge by adjusting the scale to read 21%. The test gas is then entered, and variations in oxygen concentration will upset the balance of the Wheatstone bridge through the effect on electrical conductivity, an event noted by an ammeter whose indicating needle reads out on a scale calibrated in oxygen percent. These units are not as popular as the other types presented here but are still used occasionally.

The *electrochemical analyzers* can be subdivided into two types: polarographic and galvanic fuel cell. Both of these can provide continuous monitoring and display. Each operate on a similar principle. The probes of these units contain an anode and a cathode in electrolytic gel separated from the air by a semipermeable membrane such as Teflon. Oxygen diffuses through the membrane at a rate proportional to its partial pressure and is chemically reduced in the electrolyte gel, producing an electric current proportional to the oxygen present. The polarographic analyzer polarizes the probe by providing a small current from a battery. The galvanic fuel cell uses only the current produced by the oxygen reduction to operate its meter and requires no battery unless accessory alarms are provided.

Common oxygen analyzers are pictured in Fig. 12-19. Further descriptions of these and other gas-analyzing devices can be found in other sources.[5,82,83]

Summary

Because of the wide variety of techniques of administering oxygen, it is obvious that there is no one best method, and although the decision to give oxygen to a patient is a medical one, it is not always easy for the physician to know which procedure will be the most effective in a given instance. Clinical observation of the patient, coupled with experience, will often suffice for the physician to initiate treatment, and in the not too distant past these were the only guides. More recently, however, improved technology in both instrumentation and diagnosis have made the therapeutic use of oxygen much more rational and precise.

In our discussion of oxygen equipment, values of oxygen concentration are suggested for each type. Such data certainly have merit, but only in a very general way, for the delivered concentration of gas from any appliance is subjected to many modifying influences such as condition of the equipment, technique of application, cooperation of the patient, and the ventilatory pattern of the patient. It is probably necessary to know only, for example, that the delivery of high oxygen concentrations can best be accomplished by a well-fitted nonrebreathing mask; intermediate concentrations by a simple mask, tent, or high flows with a cannula or catheter; and low concentrations with cannula, catheter, and entrainment device. It is much more important to recognize that complete relief of hypoxia may be easily achieved by low-flow cannula oxygen in one patient and be impossible by mask therapy in another. Indeed, there may be instances in which, at least for a period of time, full correction of hypoxia may not even be desirable. The point to be grasped here is that the pathology of the disease under treatment is the major determinant of the effectiveness of oxygen administration. Except for short-term therapy such as prophylaxis or for conditions felt to be very transient, safe and rational treatment must depend on the actual measurement of blood oxygenation. At the present time, in view of current techniques, this means the determination of oxygen tension of arterial blood. We consider in this section the major pathologic and physiologic changes that disease can effect in ventilatory and gas exchange functions of the lung, and it is easy to visualize that there may be little correlation between the fractional concentration of inhaled oxygen and the realization of a normal arterial oxygen content. Unless the initial degree of hypoxia is quantitated by direct measurement and such measurements continued through therapy until stability is reached, treatment can be based on little more than guesswork.

The correction of hypoxia as part of the management of patients with acute or chronic ventilatory failure requires special care because of the disturbance in the acid-base balance. Because of the risk of untoward reactions to oxygen in acute failure, many techniques of oxygen administration have been suggested that are based on the use of low concentrations of oxygen or oxygen with supporting mechanical ventilation. Although the latter is usually required in severe circumstances and discussed in detail later, oxygen alone may be indicated. We know the great hazard of hypercapnia if therapeutic oxygen obliterates the hypoxic drive mechanism, and to minimize this risk, the use of cannulas or the air-entrainment mask has had various advocates.* Similarly, continuous low-flow oxygen in the treatment of chronic hypoxia has received much attention.[84-86] However, the criteria for the choice of patients for such therapy, as well as an evaluation of its success, are always dependent on the effective arterial oxygen tensions achieved and the response of the acid-base balance. Thus, after the degree of hypoxia has been determined, the choice of technique may require some trials and errors, guided by blood oxygen levels, with thought given to patient comfort as well as the avoidance of over-oxygenation.

Hyperbaric oxygen therapy

Treatment of disorders using increased barometric pressure, with or without increased oxygen concentration, dates back several centuries. It is presently enjoying a great deal of attention and support after many decades of suspicion, abuse, and condemnation. In the majority of instances in the last 100 years, the suspicion and condemnation were justified. Now, with good scientific research and careful attention to conservative applications, the hyperbaric chamber is being recognized as an important tool in the primary treatment of certain disorders and as an adjuvant treatment modality in other disorders.[87]

Hyperbaric chambers come in two types. The expensive multiplace chamber is a walk-in metal-encased room capable of "diving" to many atmospheres below sea level, with many people inside. Whole operating rooms have been functioned inside these types of chambers. The more commonly used chamber is a clear plastic cylinder on wheels designated as a "monoplace" chamber. These chambers allow only "up to" (or "down to") 3 atmospheres, absolute (3 ata) of pressure, can hold only one person at a time, and use 100% oxygen concentration to achieve the high-oxygen tissue tensions needed to be therapeutic.

*See references 11-14, 18, 27, 67, and 68.

Table 12-10	ata	mm Hg	p.s.i.	Feet below sea level
Relationship between air pressures and pressure of water depths	1	760	14.7	Sea level
	2	1520	29.4	33
	3	2280	44.1	66
	4	3040	58.8	99

The way hyperbaric oxygen works is only partially understood, and this understanding requires a basic knowledge of the gas laws (Henry's, Dalton's, and Boyle's laws). These laws have been well covered in other portions of this text.

Oxygen is delivered to the tissues at increased tensions with hyperbaric oxygen, and if an arterial blood sample is taken the Pa_{O_2} might show 1800 to 1900 mm Hg at 3 ata, breathing 100% oxygen. Physiologic effects of increased oxygen tension include (1) new capillary bed formation (neovascularization), (2) arteriolar constriction, and (3) alteration in the metabolism and growth of both anaerobic and aerobic organisms.

The physiologic effects of the increased barometric pressure include reduction in size of bubbles dissolved within the blood.

Over the last 10 years treatment indications designated as categories I to IV* and treatment protocols have been standardized by the hard work of the Undersea Medical Society and have gained wide acceptance by both government agencies and practicing physicians. The treatment protocols of a given disease entity may require 90-minute "dives" to 2 to 3 ata, two to four times a day, many times lasting for months. Caring for patients in these circumstances may be taxing and requires skill and compassion.

The harmful effects of hyperbaric oxygen fall into two areas: central nervous system toxicity and pulmonary toxicity. The CNS toxicity is most commonly manifested by convulsions. Early signs of impending CNS complications include twitching, sweating, pallor, and restlessness. Pulmonary toxicity is not noted early in the treatment because the effects are cumulative. Certain drugs are considered helpful in retarding oxygen toxicity to lung tissue; vitamin E is the most commonly used. Many other drugs, if taken at the same time as the hyperbaric oxygen is being used, can cause acceleration of oxygen toxicity.

Some of the important clinical problems for application of the hyperbaric oxygen unit include carbon monoxide, cyanide poisoning, decompression sickness, gas embolism, gas gangrene, skin grafts, smoke inhalation, actinomycoses, acute peripheral arterial insufficiency, crush injury, intestinal obstruc-

*Category I: Disorders in this category are best treated by hyperbaric oxygen.
Category II: Hyperbaric oxygen is used as adjuvant to other established modes of therapy.
Category III: Some data exist that hyperbaric oxygen may be helpful, but this has not been proved.
Category IV: Theoretic data suggest some benefit might be realized by hyperbaric chamber, but no definitive work has been done to establish this.

tion, refractory osteomyelitis, radionecrosis of soft tissue, osteoradionecrosis, and thermal burns, to name but a few.[87]

The safety aspects of running a hyperbaric chamber are unique and offer added challenges. The safety aspects center around avoiding fires and sudden decompression (blow-outs). Only 100%-cotton material can be used so that fire from static electricity is avoided. No products with an alcohol or petroleum base can be used, and the patient must not wear sprays, makeup, or deodorant.

Helium therapy	In an earlier chapter, reference is made to the use of helium in the treatment of obstructive disease, and we now discuss this technique in more detail. Helium is second only to the highly inflammable hydrogen as the lightest of all gases, with an atomic weight of 4.003 and a density of only 0.1785 g/ℓ. Limited in supply, the source of most commercial helium is deep mines in the Southwest, produced under control of the federal government. Chemically, it is an inert element, and thus physiologically it neither participates in nor interferes with any biochemical process in the body. It is odorless, tasteless. noncombustible, nonexplosive, poorly soluble, and a good conductor of heat, sound, and electricity.

It is the low-density property of helium that makes the gas a valuable therapeutic tool, and its only medical indication is the management of airway obstruction. We know from previous discussions that turbulence characterizes the gas flow pattern through an obstruction and that in such a circumstance the most influential property of a moving gas is its density. With no technical background, we should be able to perceive that the less dense a gas is, the easier it can negotiate an obstruction, but for clarity let us look at the process from two slightly different viewpoints.

First, it should be noted that as a flow of gas passes from a relatively wide passage into one that is realtively narrow, if the driving force is constant, the gas velocity must increase to maintain the same volume leaving as entering the restriction. As Bernoulli's principle demonstrates a decrease in pressure with an increase in gas velocity, there is thus a pressure drop across an obstruction. However, since less driving pressure is required to move a light (low-density) gas than a heavy one, at the same velocity there would be less of a pressure drop. In ventilation this would mean greater efficiency and less work expended in breathing.

Second, the movement of a gas through the narrow aperture of an obstruction subjects it to some of the principles of diffusion, or the passage of a gas across an obstruction in response to a pressure gradient. In Chapter 6 we learn that the rate of diffusion of a gas follows Graham's law and is inversely proportional to the square root of the density of the gas. Obviously, the speed (or ease) of such movement is greater for low- than for high-density gases.

Currently, helium is the only low-density gas acceptable for medical use, and since it is inert and unable to support life, it cannot be used alone but must always be mixed with oxygen. The therapist should keep in mind that helium has no curative properties of its own, in a pharmacologic sense, and that its sole purpose is to lower the total density of any mixture of which it is a part so that such a mixture can ventilate the lungs with minimal effort. All helium-oxygen mixtures must have at least 20% oxygen to supply basic metabolic needs, and a popular combination is the so-called 80-20 mixture, with 80% helium and 20% oxygen. For practical purposes such a mixture is comparable to air, with helium substituted for nitrogen. A patient breathing 80-20 helium is not being provided with any more oxygen than would be provided by air, but because of the low density of the helium mixture, he or she is effectively getting more; the helium more readily reaches the alveoli through obstructed passages and thus more oxygen actually is available for diffusion into the blood.

For a more specific comparison, it should be noted that the density of air is 1.293 g/ℓ, whereas that of 80-20 helium is 0.429 g/ℓ. It may be said that with the same effort three times as much of the helium mixture as of air will ventilate the lungs or that the same volume of helium-oxygen ventilation as of air can be moved with one third the effort. In either case the tremendous advantage of a helium mixture is evident to a patient struggling, often to the point of physical exhaustion, to breathe against severely obstructed airways.

The viscosities of oxygen and helium are almost identical, although both are slightly greater than that of air. The mixing of the two gases therefore does not alter the laminar flow patterns of pure oxygen breathing, and only insignificantly those of air-oxygen mixtures. Table 12-11 lists the densities and relative diffusibilities of air, helium, oxygen, and certain combinations of these and nitrogen, frequently used in therapy.[88]

It is possible to mix pure helium and oxygen at the bedside, but the hazards of error and mechanical failure are so great that it is much safer, as well as more convenient, to use commercially prepared cylinders of premixed gases. In addition to the 80-20 combination, another commonly used mixture is a 70-30. This gives an additional quantity of oxygen, often helpful in correcting severe hypoxia associated with obstruction, and although it does so at a slight cost of low density, as noted in Table 12-11, it is probably the most generally useful mixture.

Barach described the rationale for using helium in 1935[89] for decreasing work of breathing and was still presenting its use for bronchial asthma in 1976.[90] Helium-oxygen therapy has been shown to decrease ventilation, carbon dioxide production, and oxygen consumption in patients with COPD.[91] It has also been shown to decrease resistance to flow in upper airway obstruction.[89,92]

Completely safe to use, helium-oxygen is a most valuable therapeutic tool in the treatment of respiratory disorders and should be available in all hospitals caring for pulmonary patients, even though it may be put to only occasional use. For reasons that are not clear, the use of helium-oxygen has not

Table 12-11
Densities and relative diffusion rates of selected gases (rate of diffusion varies inversely with square root of density)[88]

Gas	Percentage	Density	$\sqrt{\text{Density}}$	Relative diffusibility
Helium	100	0.179	0.423	
Air	100	1.293	1.135	
Oxygen	100	1.429	1.182	
Oxygen-nitrogen	40/60	1.321	1.105	
Helium-oxygen	80/20	0.429	0.655	
Helium-oxygen	70/30	0.554	0.745	
$\dfrac{\text{Oxygen}}{\text{Air}}$	$\dfrac{100}{100}$		$\dfrac{1.135}{1.182}$	0.960
$\dfrac{\text{Oxygen-nitrogen}}{\text{Air}}$	$\dfrac{40\text{-}60}{100}$		$\dfrac{1.135}{1.105}$	1.027
$\dfrac{\text{Helium-oxygen}}{\text{Air}}$	$\dfrac{80\text{-}20}{100}$		$\dfrac{1.135}{0.655}$	1.743
$\dfrac{\text{Helium-oxygen}}{\text{Oxygen}}$	$\dfrac{80\text{-}20}{100}$		$\dfrac{1.182}{0.655}$	1.805
$\dfrac{\text{Helium-oxygen}}{\text{Oxygen}}$	$\dfrac{70\text{-}30}{100}$		$\dfrac{1.182}{0.745}$	1.586

been popular in the past 20 years. Some clinicians have used it frequently, sometimes with dramatic results.[88,89] Helium-oxygen has been used for the patient with diffuse airway obstruction, especially when caused by bronchospasm, as in status asthmaticus, or following instrumentation or other traumatic bronchial irritation. It is also useful in obstruction from extensive secretions, although in this case the major effort should be directed toward airway cleansing. More ordinary therapy is usually employed first, to achieve bronchial patency, and then oxygen administration by conventional techniques next, to combat hypoxia. However, if the obstructive process is unresponsive or the patient is in risk of weakening from fatigue, helium-oxygen should be promptly started before the patient deteriorates to a critical state. There are five points of practical importance to consider in giving helium-oxygen:

1. Helium mixtures must always be given in a tightly closed system because their high diffusibilities will allow them to escape from even small leaks. Tents, catheters, and cannulas are not satisfactory, and the gases should be given by a tightly fitted nonrebreathing mask and bag or through cuffed endotracheal or tracheostomy tubes. They can be administered by inspiratory positive-pressure ventilators.[91]

2. The average hospital gas flow meter is calibrated for oxygen, and since it depends on the kinetic support of a float by the metered gas, gauge readings will not be accurate for the lighter helium-oxygen mixtures. Special meters, calibrated for the helium mixtures, can be used, but they are not necessary because correction can be made for the scales of the

oxygen meters. Table 12-11 shows that an 80-20 helium-oxygen mixture is 1.8 times as diffusible as 100% oxygen, and a 70-30 mixture 1.6 times. This means that for every 10 ℓ/min gas flow recorded on the meter, 18 ℓ/min and 16 ℓ/min, respectively, of the above helium gases would flow. To deliver a desired flow, the flow meter is adjusted to a reading equal to the desired rate divided by either 1.8 or 1.6, depending on the gas mixture being used. Factors for any other combination can be calculated if needed.

3. The low density of the helium mixtures makes them poor vehicles for the transport of pharmacologically active aerosols. Humidifiers, of course, must be used as with any administered gas, but high therapeutic concentrations of water particles cannot be expected.

4. The only side effect directly attributable to helium is a benign one, but one that should be kept in mind. In the low-density gas the spoken word is badly distorted at a pitch so high as to make it almost unintelligible. This is of importance only to the conscious, nonintubated patient, who should be warned of the phenomenon and reassured that it will disappear within a few seconds of discontinuance of therapy.

5. Because of helium's relatively high cost, systems that conserve the gas during therapy should be used. This cost factor and practical problems in administration have probably hampered widespread use of helium-oxygen therapy.

Carbon dioxide therapy

Paradoxic though it may seem, a gas whose removal from the body occupies much of the attention and efforts of the respiratory therapist is sometimes used therapeutically. The therapeutic inhalation of carbon dioxide is not extensive, but the therapist will be called on to administer the gas frequently enough to necessitate becoming very familiar with its characteristics.

At normal atmospheric temperatures and pressure, carbon dioxide is a gas that is colorless, odorless, and about 1.5 times as heavy as air; it will not support combustion or maintain life. Unrefined gas for the commercial production of carbon dioxide may be obtained from the following: combustion of coal, coke, natural gas, oil, and other carbonaceous fuels; by-product gases of ammonia plants, lime kilns, carbide furnaces; fermentation processes; and gases from certain natural springs and wells. From these sources carbon dioxide is refined to a purity of no less than 99.9%.

For safe administration of carbon dioxide the therapist should know its physiologic actions.

Respiratory response. Carbon dioxide is basically a respiratory center stimulant, but maximum stimulation is probably attained with the inhalation of a 10% concentration. Higher concentrations depress the respiratory center after initial stimulation.

Circulatory response. Two major effects are recognized.

Direct stimulation of the cardiovascular brain centers. This leads to an elevation of the systolic and diastolic blood pressures (up to an increase of 40 mm Hg systolic); an increase in the heart rate of up to 20 beats/min; an increase in the force of myocardial contraction; contraction of vascular beds supplied by the sympathetic nervous system, thereby diverting blood flow from general body areas to the brain, whose vessels are not sympathetic-responsive, and increasing the cerebral circulation (conversely, hypocapnia leads to cerebral constriction and a reduced flow).

Local vasodilation. Increased carbon dioxide at the tissue level dilates the vascular bed, as is found in exercising muscle, producing a more active flow for metabolic needs.

Central nervous system response. Generally, high carbon dioxide concentrations produce central nervous system stimulation to the point of convulsions, and low concentrations cause depression. It is vital for the therapist to remember, however, that the administration of 5% carbon dioxide may produce severe mental depression, if given for no longer than 1 hour, and 10% may lead to loss of consciousness within as short a time as 10 minutes.

The clinical indications for carbon dioxide therapy antedate the current techniques of respiratory therapy and in general have been replaced by the latter. Nevertheless, because it is being used, we briefly describe its therapeutic effects. Under *no* circumstance must carbon dioxide be given to a patient unless he or she is definitely known to have a responsive respiratory center. Failure to be assured of this may produce a fatal hypercapnia and respiratory acidosis.

Improve cerebral blood flow. This depends on the physiologic effect described previously and has had long use in attempting to overcome cerebral vascular spasm and to evoke compensatory increased flow following stroke. In general, results have not been spectacular, perhaps largely because many of the patients so treated had associated hardening, or sclerosis, of their vessels, making them impervious to the effect of carbon dioxide. Ophthalmologists sometimes use the gas to dilate vessels in the retina of the eye when thromboses have impaired the circulation.

Overcome hypoventilation. Especially in the aged, or those physically weakened by serious disease, debility results in a low tidal volume of air exchange. Carbon dioxide has been used often to stimulate such patients to deep breathing, effecting a better distribution of inhaled gas. Caution must be employed in such instances to be sure that there is no underlying respiratory dysfunction, since unless the patient can respond to treatment by hyperventilation, not only is the therapy of no value but hypercapnia is a certainty. Modern respiratory therapy equipment and techniques can usually perform this function better and safer than can carbon dioxide.

Prevent postoperative atelectasis. This indication parallels that just described and was often used to stimulate deep breathing in the immediate postoperative state to prevent atelectasis from retained secretions and to overcome the usual postoperative hypoxia following inhalational anesthesia. Better techniques are now generally used.

Assist cough. Oftentimes effective, although tiring, the hyperventilation of carbon dioxide inhalation can aid in the tussive removal of secretions. Again, the available aerosols and other equipment are more effective and safer than carbon dioxide.

Singulation (hiccup, hiccough). Although there are other methods of treating the annoying and sometimes serious condition of singulation, the condition is one of the most specific indications for carbon dioxide therapy. The hiccup is an abnormal spasmodic contraction of the diaphragm against a closed glottis, under the stimulation of an irritated phrenic nerve. Such irritation can come from a host of conditions, including gastric distention or irritation, toxins, and metabolic upsets, and often it plagues patients who are immediately postoperative as well as those who suffer from debilitating diseases.[94] Prolonged hiccupping can produce severe physical fatigue, interfere with eating, and cause emotional distress. We all know some of the traditional maneuvers for stopping hiccups, such as forced inspiratory breath holding, taking long drinks of water, and breathing into a paper bag. The reason these acts have met with variable success is their one common factor: they all withhold carbon dioxide and produce some degree of hypercapnia. This is what stops the hiccups. Subjecting the respiratory center to excessive stimulation of hypercapnia supposedly initiates a rhythmic discharge of impulses to the diaphragm so strong that they override the interposed spasmodic contractions and restore a normal cycle. The administration of low concentrations of carbon dioxide usually accomplishes this more quickly and smoothly and in most instances is effective in stopping the hiccups. Sometimes simple mechanical stimulation of the pharynx, with a catheter, will stop the attack through a reflex mediated by way of the vagus nerve. This technique has been used with success by anesthesiologists on patients suffering from postanesthesia hiccups. For some patients combined therapy, including tranquilization, is necessary to bring relief.

Because carbon dioxide, like helium, does not support life, it must be used in combination with oxygen. In addition to its action as an asphyxiant, carbon dioxide produces toxic effects in excess dosage, and it *must be given with great care*. During its administration the therapist must remain in constant attendance and watch the patient closely because individuals vary in their responses to the gas. It is suggested that each department of respiratory care establish its own rules governing the use of carbon dioxide and that these include such items as the following: (1) unless otherwise specified, all treatments will use a mixture no stronger than 5% carbon dioxide and 95% oxygen, (2) no treatment will exceed a period of 10 minutes, (3) if higher concentrations or longer periods of treatment are ordered, a physician must be present. The carbon dioxide mixture should be given with a well-fitted nonrebreathing mask and bag, and the mask should be held to the patient's face by an attendant, rather than strapped on, so that it can be removed in an instant if necessary.

The potential side effects are many and include headache, dizziness shortly after start of treatment as diastolic blood pressure makes an initial drop, dyspnea, nasal irritation, palpitation, dimming of vision, muscle tremors, paresthesias, sensation of cold, and mental depression. The toxic symptoms indicate serious physiologic injury and should be watched for because they can appear any time after 15 minutes of treatment. Toxicity is manifested by severe dyspnea, nausea and vomiting, disorientation, and a dangerous elevation of blood pressure. When the pressure reaches 200 mm Hg, systolic convulsions and cardiac collapse are apt to occur. It is recommended that carbon dioxide be contraindicated in patients with significant airway obstruction for two reasons. First, it is this type of patient who is most likely to have a less than normally responsive respiratory center and run the risk of hypercapnia. Second, with an active respiratory center the increased work of breathing under carbon dioxide stimulation against obstruction may more than negate any positive value of therapy.

References

1. National Fire Protection Association, 470 Atlantic Ave., Boston, Mass., 02210: Pamphlet nos. 565 and 566.
2. Compressed Gas Association, 500 Fifth Ave., New York, N.Y., 10036: Pamphlet P-2, Characteristics and safe handling of medical gases.
3. Bancroft, M.L., and Steen, J.A.: Health device legislation: an overview of the law and its impact on respiratory care, Resp. Care **23:**1179, 1978.
4. Dorsch, J.A., and Dorsch, S.E.: Understanding anesthesia equipment: construction, care and complications, Baltimore, 1975, The Williams & Wilkins Co.
5. McPherson, S.P.: Respiratory therapy equipment, ed. 2, St. Louis, 1981, The C.V. Mosby Co.
6. Webb, J.M., and Gee, G.N.: In Burton, G.G., Gee, G.N., and Hodgkin, J.E., editors: Respiratory care: a guide to clinical practice, Philadelphia, 1977, J.B. Lippincott Co.
7. Compressed Gas Association: Handbook of compressed gas, New York, 1967, Van Nostrand Reinhold Co.
8. Compressed Gas Association, 500 Fifth Ave., New York, N.Y., 10036: Pamphlet V-1, American Standard Compressed Gas Cylinder Valve Outlet and Inlet Connections.
9. Compressed Gas Association, 500 Fifth Ave., New York, N.Y., 10036: Pamphlet V-5, Diameter Index Safety System.
10. Nunn, J.F.: Applied respiratory physiology, ed. 2, London, 1977, Butterworth & Co., p. 290.
11. O'Donohue, W.J., Jr., and Baker, J.P.: Controlled low-flow oxygen in the management of acute respiratory failure, Chest **63:**818, 1973.
12. Petty, T.L.: Intensive and rehabilitative respiratory care, ed. 2, Philadelphia, 1974, Lea & Febiger.
13. Bone, R.C., Pierce, A.K., and Johnson, R.L.: Controlled oxygen administration in acute respiratory failure in chronic obstructive pulmonary disease: a reappraisal, Am. J. Med. **65:**896, 1978.
14. Sykes, M.K., McNicol, M.W., and Campbell, E.J.M.: Respiratory failure, ed. 2, Oxford, England, 1976, Blackwell Scientific Publications.
15. Clamann, H.G.: Fire hazards, Ann. N.Y. Acad. Sci. **117:**814, 1965.
16. Cullen, J.H., and Kaemmerlen, J.T.: Effect of oxygen administration at low rates of flow in hypercapnic patients, Am. Rev. Respir. Dis. **95:**116, 1967.
17. Massaro, D.J., et al.: Effect of various modes of oxygen administration on the arterial gas values in patients with respiratory acidosis, Br. Med. J. **2:**627, 1962.
18. Mithoefer, J.C.: Indications for oxygen therapy in chronic obstructive pulmonary disease, Amer. Rev. Respir. Dis. **110**(part 2):35, 1974.
19. Hodgkin, J.E., editor: Chronic obstruc-

tive pulmonary disease: current concepts in diagnosis and comprehensive care, Park Ridge, Ill., 1979, American College of Chest Physicians.

20. Hutchison, D.C.S., et al: Controlled oxygen therapy in respiratory failure, Br. Med. J. **2:**1157, 1964.

21. Arnold, W.H., Jr., and Grant, J.L.: Oxygen-induced hypoventilation, Am. Rev. Respir. Dis. **95:**255, 1967.

22. West, J.B.: Pulmonary pathophysiology—the essentials, Baltimore, 1977, The Williams & Wilkins Co.

23. Clark, J.M., and Fisher, A.B.: In Davis, J.C., and Hunt, T.K., editors: Hyperbaric oxygen therapy, Bethesda, Md., 1977, Undersea Medical Society, Inc.

24. Pratt, P.C.: Pathology of oxygen toxicity, Amer. Rev. Respir. Dis. **110**(2):51, 1974.

25. Clark, J.M.: The toxicity of oxygen, Amer. Rev. Resp. Dis. **110**(2):40, 1974.

26. Winter, P.M., and Smith, G.: The toxicity of oxygen, Anesthesiology **37:**210, 1972.

27. Petty, T.L., Stanford, R.E., and Neff, T.A.: Continuous oxygen therapy in chronic airway obstruction: observations on possible oxygen toxicity and survival, Ann. Intern. Med. **75:**361, 1971.

28. Deneke, S.M., and Fanburg, B.L.: Medical progress: normobaric oxygen toxicity of the lung, N. Engl. J. Med. **303:**76, 1980.

29. Mustafa, M.G., and Tierney, D.F.: Biochemical and metabolic changes in the lung with oxygen, ozone and nitrogen dioxide toxicity, state of the art, Am. Rev. Respir. Dis. **118:**1061, 1978.

30. Laurenzi, G.A., et al.: Adverse effect of oxygen on tracheal mucus flow, N. Engl. J. Med. **279:**333, 1968.

31. Caldwell, P.R.B., et al.: Effect of oxygen breathing at one atmosphere on the surface activity of lung extracts in dogs, Ann. N.Y. Acad. Sci. **131:**823, 1965.

32. Hyde, R.W., and Rawson, A.J.: Unintentional iatrogenic oxygen pneumonitis—response to therapy, Ann. Intern. Med. **71:**517, 1969.

33. Northway, W.H., Jr., and Rosan, R.C.: Oxygen therapy hazards in the neonate, Hosp. Pract. **4**(1):59, 1969.

34. Nash, G., et al.: Pulmonary lesions associated with oxygen therapy and artificial ventilation, N. Engl. J. Med. **276:**368, 1967.

35. Pratt, P.C.: Pulmonary capillary proliferation induced by oxygen inhalation, Am. J. Pathol. **34:**1033, 1958.

36. Bruns, P.D., and Shields, L.V.: High oxygen and hyaline-like membranes, Am. J. Obstet. Gynecol. **67:**1224, 1954.

37. Shanklin, D.R., and Wolfson, S.L.: Therapeutic oxygen as a possible cause of pulmonary hemorrhage in premature infants, N. Engl. J. Med. **277:**833, 1967.

38. Klaus, M.H., and Fanaroff, A.A., editors: Care of the high risk neonate, ed. 2, Philadelphia, 1979, W.B. Saunders Co.

39. Thibeault, D.W., and Gregory, G.A., editors: Neonatal pulmonary care, Menlo Park, Calif., 1979, Addison-Wesley Publishing Co., Inc.

40. Korones, S.B.: High-risk newborn infants, ed. 3, St. Louis, 1981, The C.V. Mosby Co.

41. Kensey, V., Jacobus, J., and Hemphill, F.: Retrolental fibroplasia and the use of oxygen, A.M.A. Arch. Ophthalmol. **56:**481, 1956.

42. Kobayashi, T., and Murakami, S.: Blindness of an adult caused by oxygen, J.A.M.A. **219:**741, 1972.

43. Fridovich, I.: Oxygen: boon and bane, Am. Sci. **63:**54, 1975.

44. Crapo, J.D.: Superoxide dismutase and tolerance to pulmonary oxygen toxicity, Chest **67**(suppl.):39s, 1975.

45. McCord, J.M., and Fridovich, I.: Superoxide dismutase, J. Biol. Chem. **244:**6049, 1969.

46. Babior, B.M., et al.: The production by leukocytes of superoxide: a potential bactericidal agent, J. Clin. Invent. **52:**741, 1973.

47. Curvette, J.T., et al.: Defect in pyridine nucleotide dependent superoxide production by a particulate fraction from the granulocytes of patients with chronic granulomatous diseases, N. Engl. J. Med. **293:**628, 1975.

48. Lee, C.J., et al.: Cardiovascular and metabolic responses to spontaneous and positive-pressure breathing of 100% oxygen at one atmosphere, J. Thorac. Cardiovasc. Surg. **53:**770, 1967.

49. Wright, R., et al.: Risk of mortality in in-

terrupted exposure to 100% oxygen: role of air vs. lowered oxygen tension, Am. J. Physiol. **210**:1015, 1966.

50. Leigh, J.M.: The evolution of oxygen therapy apparatus, Anaesthesia **29**:462, 1974.

51. Shapiro, B.A., Harrison, R.A., and Trout, C.A.: Clinical application of respiratory care, ed. 2, Chicago, 1979, Year Book Medical Publishers, Inc.

52. Rarey, K.P., and Youtsey, J.W.: Respiratory patient care, Englewood Cliffs, N.J., 1981, Prentice-Hall, Inc.

53. Rau, J.L., and Rau, M.Y.: Fundamental respiratory therapy equipment: principles of use and operation, Sarosota, Fla., 1977, Glenn Educational Medical Services, Inc.

54. Leigh, J.M.: Variation in performance of oxygen therapy devices, Anaesthesia **25**:100, 1970.

55. Leigh, J.M.: Variation in performance of oxygen therapy devices, Ann. Royal Coll. Surg. **52**:234, 1973.

56. Redding, J.S., McAfee, D.D., and Parham, A.M.: Oxygen concentrations received from commonly used delivery systems, South. Med. J. **71**:169, 1978.

57. Schacter, E.N., et al.: Monitoring of oxygen delivery systems in clinical practice, Crit. Care Med. **8**:405, 1980.

58. Gibson, R.L., et al.: Actual tracheal oxygen concentrations with commonly used oxygen equipment, Anesthesiology **44**:71, 1976.

59. Kory, R.C., et al.: Comparative evaluation of oxygen therapy techniques, J.A.M.A. **179**:767, 1962.

60. Guilfoil, B.A., and Dabe, K.: Nasal catheter oxygen therapy for infants, Respir. Care **26**:35, 1981.

61. Glick, R.V., and Benner, J.N.: Arterial oxygen tension during oxygen breathing, Inhal. Ther. **13**:31, 1968.

62. Poulton, T.J., Comer, P.B., and Gibson, R.L.: Tracheal oxygen concentrations with nasal cannula during oral and nasal breathing, Respir. Care **25**:739, 1980.

63. Collis, J.M., and Bethune, D.W.: Oxygen by face mask and nasal catheter, Lancet **1**:787, 1967.

64. Committee on Public Health: A report: effective administration of inhalational therapy with special reference to ambulatory and emergency oxygen treatment, Bull. N.Y. Acad. Med. **38**:135, 1962.

65. Barach, A.L., and Eckman, M.: A mask apparatus which provides high concentrations with accurate control of the percentage of oxygen in the inspired air and without the accumulation of carbon dioxide, J. Aviation Med. **12**:39, 1941.

66. Barach, A.L., and Eckman, M.: A physiologically controlled oxygen mask apparatus, Anesthesiology **2**:421, 1941.

67. Campbell, E.J.M.: A method of controlled oxygen administration which reduces the risk of carbon dioxide retention, Lancet **1**:12, 1960.

68. Campbell, E.J.M., and Gebbie, T.: Masks and tent for providing controlled oxygen concentrations, Lancet **1**:468, 1966.

69. McPherson, S.P.: Oxygen percentage accuracy of air-entrainment masks, Respir. Care **19**:658, 1974.

70. Scacci, R.: Air entrainment masks: jet mixing is how they work; the Bernoulli and Venturi principles are how they don't, Respir. Care **24**:928, 1979.

71. Friedman, S.A., et al.: Oxygen therapy: evaluation of various air-entrainment masks, J.A.M.A. **228**:474, 1974.

72. Spearman, C.B., et al.: Effects of changing jet flows on oxygen concentrations in adjustable entrainment masks (abstract), Respir. Care **25**:1266, 1980.

73. Woolner, D.F., and Larkin, J.: An analysis of the performance of a variable venturi-type mask, Anesth. Intens. Care **8**:44, 1980.

74. Spier, W.A., et al.: Oxygen concentration delivered by venturi masks with in-line humidification, J.A.M.A. **216**:879, 1971.

75. Cohen, J.L., et al.: Air-entrainment masks: a performance evaluation, Respir. Care **22**:277, 1977.

76. Farney, R.J., et al.: Oxygen therapy: appropriate use of nebulizers, Am. Rev. Respir. Dis. **115**:567, 1977.

77. Klein, E.F., Mon, B.K., and Mon, M.J.: Oxygen accuracy with venturi nebulizer systems, (abstract), Crit. Care Med. **7**:186, 1979.

78. Durham, M., Jr., and Miller, W.F.: Controlled oxygen administration with adequate humidification, Inhal. Ther. **14**:87, 1969.

79. Pierce, A.K.: In Guenter, C.A., and Welch, M.H., editors: Pulmonary medicine, Philadelphia, 1977, J.B. Lippincott Co.

80. Yeh, T.F., et al.: Oxygen consumption and insensible water loss in premature infants in single-versus double walled incubators, J. Pediatr. **97:**967, 1980.

81. Marks, K.H., et al.: Oxygen consumption and temperature control of premature infants in a double-wall incubator, Pediatrics **68:**93, 1981.

82. Wilson, R.S., and Taver, M.B.: Oxygen analysis: advances in methodology, Anesthesiology **37:**112, 1972.

83. Bageant, R.A.: Oxygen analyzers, Respir. Care **21:**410, 1976.

84. Nocturnal Oxygen Therapy Trial Group: Continuous or nocturnal oxygen therapy in hypoxemic chronic obstructive lung disease, Ann. Intern. Med. **93:**391, 1980.

85. Lenfant, F.: Twelve-or 24-hour oxygen therapy: why a clinical trial? J.A.M.A. **243:**551, 1980.

86. Petty, T.L., et al.: Outpatient oxygen therapy in chronic obstructive pulmonary disease: a review of 13 years' experience and an evaluation of modes of therapy, Arch. Intern. Med. **139:**28, 1979.

87. Davis, J.C., and Hunt, T.K.: Hyperbaric oxygen therapy, Bethesda, Md., 1977, Undersea Medical Society, Inc.

88. Egan, D.F.: Therapeutic uses of helium, Conn. Med. **31:**355, 1967.

89. Barach, A.L.: The use of helium in the treatment of asthma and obstructive lesions of the larynx and trachea, Ann. Intern. Med. **9:**739, 1935.

90. Barach, A.L., and Segal, M.S.: In Weiss, E.B., and Segal, M.S.: Bronchial asthma: mechanisms and therapeutics, Boston, 1976, Little, Brown & Co.

91. Ishikawa, S., and Segal, M.S.: Re-appraisal of helium-oxygen therapy on patients with chronic lung disease, Ann. Allergy **31:**536, 1973.

92. Lu, T.S., et al.: Helium-oxygen in the treatment of upper airway obstruction, Anesthesiology **45:**678, 1976.

93. Motley, H.L.: Helium-oxygen therapy, Respir. Care **18:**668, 1973.

94. Souadjian, J., and Cain, J.: Intractable hiccup, Postgrad. Med. **43:**72, 1968.

Chapter 13   Mechanical ventilation

An important part of the respiratory therapist's role relates to patients requiring mechanical ventilatory support of various types. This is true not only because of the technical nature of the apparatus used for such patients but also because it requires the therapist to integrate physiologic, pathophysiologic, and technical knowledge at a rather sophisticated level. Sufficient background information on physiology and pathophysiology has been provided in previous chapters to now present some technical aspects of mechanical ventilation, and we integrate these areas even more in Chapter 14.

Indications

Mechanical ventilatory support is applied in order to provide or maintain adequate ventilation and carbon dioxide removal from the lungs and to provide adequate arterial oxygenation to aid in oxygen delivery to the tissues. Therefore, ventilatory support is indicated whenever gas exchange in the lungs is sufficiently inadequate to warrant mechanical intervention. Conditions causing respiratory failure are discussed in Chapter 14, and these often require that mechanical ventilation be used. However, to help the student fit mechanical ventilation into the total picture of respiratory care, we now take advantage of our increasing experience and look at this subject from the following viewpoint. Reducing the indications for mechanical ventilation to the simplest terms, we can say that it can be used in those conditions that directly cause either or both of the following.

1. *Alveolar hypoventilation,* through interference with neural control of breathing, neuromusculoskeletal ventilatory performance, or expiratory airway conductance. The characteristics defining this category are *ineffective minute alveolar rinsing, hypercapnia, acidemia,* and *hypoxemia.* The last is often a product of the hypoventilation rather than the primary disease, since an air exchange inadequate for carbon dioxide removal will not satisfy oxygen demands. It might broaden the student's thinking to note, although somewhat irrelevantly at this point, that we are discussing indications, and an indication is not a mandate for therapy, since the decision to treat or not is a matter of professional clinical judgment. There is a wide variety of diseases that can cause hypoventilation, and they may roughly be grouped as follows[1]: (a) alveolar hypoventilation associated with normal lungs—respiratory centers damaged by disease, trauma, drugs; paralysis of ventilatory muscles from neurologic diseases; thoracic skeletal deformities as from kyphoscoliosis, trauma, and mutilating surgery; (b) diffuse fibrosis or pulmonary granulomatosis—asbestosis, scleroderma, beryllosis, sarcoidosis, recurrent or chronic infections, and healed destructive tuberculosis; (c) chronic bronchitis–emphysema—combinations of distention, destruction, expiratory obstruction with air trapping, and fibrosis.

2. *Shunt hypoxia,* through decreased ventilation/perfusion ratios (physiologic shunting) not corrected by the unassisted breathing of high concentrations of ambient oxygen. In contrast to the hypoxia secondary to hypoventilation, which reflects a reduced oxygen delivery into the respiratory tract, shunt hypoxia implies a normal, or even an above-normal, air supply and adequate ventilatory mechanics, but with some pathologic process preventing an even intrapulmonary distribution of the inspired air. Consequently, the ventilation/perfusion ratios are reduced in some pulmonary units, producing local areas of physiologic venoarterial shunting. The resulting hypoxia stimulates increased ventilation of unaffected areas, increasing their ventilation/perfusion

ratios. However, the additional oxygen uptake of perfusing pulmonary capillary blood is limited more by the oxygen tension in the ventilated alveoli, which is a function of inspired oxygen tension, than it is by the amount of alveolar hyperventilation. In other words, overventilating one alveolus to make up for another that is underventilated does not necessarily compensate for the oxygen deficiency of the latter, but the increased ventilation will remove from the blood large amounts of easily diffusible carbon dioxide. The characteristics of shunt hypoxia, then, are *hyperventilation, hypoxemia, hypocapnia,* and *alkalemia*. It may be found with small airway obstruction (i.e., bronchiolitis), pneumonia, pulmonary edema or congestion, the adult respiratory distress syndrome, and loss of surfactant, or any other condition that causes increase in alveolar opening pressures in scattered lung areas.

Two points should be emphasized. First, many patients will have both alveolar hypoventilation and shunt hypoxia, and it is thus essential that we watch for elements of each so that we can better judge the need for mechanical ventilation, the time to initiate it, and once started, understand the varying clinical picture that so many of these patients show. Second, although alveolar hypoventilation and shunt hypoxia may present markedly different manifestations, both etiologic and clinical, they have one important common denomi-

Table 13-1
Guidelines for ventilatory support

Data	Normal range	Indication for tracheal intubation and ventilation
Mechanics		
Respiratory rate	12-20	>35
Vital capacity (ml/kg of body weight*)	65-75	<15
FEV_1 (ml/kg of body weight*)	50-60	<10
Inspiratory force (cm H_2O)	75-100	<25
Oxygenation		
Pa_{O_2} (torr)	100-75 (air)	<70 (on mask O_2)
$P(A\text{-}aDO_2)^{1.0}$ (mm Hg)†	25-65	>450
Ventilation		
Pa_{CO_2} (torr)	35-45	>55‡
V_D/V_T	0.25-0.40	>0.60

From Wilson, R.S., and Pontoppidan, H.: Acute respiratory failure; diagnostic and therapeutic criteria, Crit. Care Med. 2:293, 1974. © 1974 The Williams & Wilkins Co., Baltimore.

The trend of values of utmost importance. The numerical guidelines should obviously not be adopted to the exclusion of clinical judgment. For example, a vital capacity below 15 ml/kg may prove sufficient provided the patient can still cough "effectively," if hypoxemia is prevented, and if hypercapnia is not progressive. However, such a patient needs frequent blood gas analyses and close observation in a well-equipped, adequately staffed, recovery room or intensive care unit.

*"Ideal" weight is used if weight appears grossly abnormal.

†After 10 minutes of 100% oxygen.

‡Except in patients with chronic hypercapnia.

nator. In both, the basic functional defect is an impaired ventilation, an inadequate or unbalanced movement of air into and out of the pulmonary lobules. In alveolar hypoventilation this deficit is absolute, with low alveolar minute volumes; in shunt hypoxia it is relative because, while the total alveolar airflow may be normal or above, it still fails to satisfy respiratory needs. Thus, in relation to gas exchange needs, there is respiratory failure in both conditions. In summary, we can simplify terminology by stating that mechanical ventilation is used to support patients suffering from *respiratory failure,* manifested by *alveolar hypoventilation,* or *shunt hypoxia,* or a combination of the two.

There are certain data that are helpful in determining the likelihood of alveolar hypoventilation and hypoxemia caused by increased physiologic shunting. While these are not absolute values, they are helpful guidelines for indicating mechanical ventilatory support for patients with acute respiratory failure. Table 13-1 lists these data under three categories: *mechanics* of ventilation, *oxygenation,* and *ventilation.*

Mechanical ventilatory support aids these problems of respiratory failure by attempting to provide adequate alveolar ventilation and by manipulating airway pressures and lung volumes in an attempt to reduce physiologic shunting. How these goals are achieved for various types of patients and ventilatory modes is discussed in Chapter 14 when management of respiratory failure is considered. The remainder of this chapter deals with general properties of ventilators and types of ventilation and how mechanical ventilation affects physiologic parameters.

It should be noted that there are other terms that are used to indicate that a patient is receiving some sort of ventilatory support; these include *assisted ventilation, artificial ventilation* or *respiration, continuous ventilation, controlled respiration* or *ventilation,* and *resuscitation.*[2-6]

Ventilators: classification and principles

Many available references describe the origin and development of mechanical ventilators, classifying them according to both structural and functional criteria.[3,6-11] Such classifications tend to be based on technical characteristics that are not necessarily clinically oriented. The increasing complexity of ventilators being developed causes an overlapping of principles and makes classification difficult. A rigid classification of equipment is not essential, but some type of grouping allows for an orderly approach to the study of ventilators. We attempt to provide an introduction to concepts used with mechanical ventilators through a systematic approach to their characteristics and available modes. Since there are ample descriptions of individual ventilators in other texts,[3,7,12,13] we use specific ventilators only as examples of principles discussed. However, each person responsible for applying mechanical ventilation must become thoroughly familiar with each ventilator used, and the respiratory therapist should always be the expert on the mechanical ventilator he or she is using, including its principles of operation, capabilities, and limitations.

**Positive- versus
negative-pressure
ventilation**

Moving air into and out of the lungs is basically accomplished by pressure gradients between the alveoli and the upper airways. We learned in Chapter 4 that normal ventilation occurs when the ventilatory muscles contract, enlarging the thorax and dropping the pressure in the alveoli as they expand. This produces a difference between the alveolar pressure and atmospheric, and air moves from the upper to the lower airways. Exhalation is usually passive with the natural recoil of the lungs causing them to become smaller and raising the alveolar pressure to above atmospheric. This reversal in pressure gradient causes the previously inhaled air to now flow out, from the alveoli to the atmosphere.

When a mechanical ventilator is used to provide an inspiration, a pressure gradient from the upper airways to the alveoli can be established either by applying a negative pressure around the chest or by applying a positive pressure to the airways.

Fig. 13-1 schematically illustrates the basic difference in function of these two types of machines during the inspiratory phase of airflow. The negative-pressure ventilator generates a negative pressure (more precisely, a subatmospheric or gauge-negative pressure), or suction, on the external surface of the thorax, as shown by the arrows in Fig. 13-1, A. This negative pressure is transmitted to the interior of the thorax, creating a pressure gradient with the atmosphere, and air flows into the lungs. In contrast, the positive-pressure ventilator, using a power source, forces air into the lungs, developing an intrathoracic positive pressure that expands lungs and chest, as depicted in Fig. 13-1, B. Perhaps the student will observe that the negative-pressure ventilator is more physiologic in its function than is the positive-pressure, since normal ventilation is the product of negative pressure generated in the thorax by the action of the ventilatory muscles.

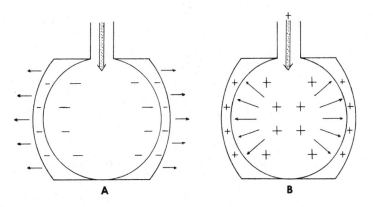

A   B

Fig. 13-1   Diagrammatic illustration of the difference between inspiratory forces of, **A**, negative-pressure and, **B**, positive-pressure ventilators.

Negative-pressure ventilators fall into two basic categories: tank or iron-lung type and cuirass or chest wall type. We reserve a section later in this chapter for a description of these ventilators and their use after we have discussed the more commonly used positive-pressure types.

Let us make two observations here that may help the student avoid later confusion in terminology. First, by custom, unless otherwise specified, the expression *mechanical ventilator* or *mechanical ventilation,* refers to the use of positive-pressure ventilators. Reasons for this will become apparent in the following description of equipment and techniques of their use. Second, regardless of the differences in their operating principles or machine design, positive-pressure ventilators all deliver breathing gas to the patient with positive pressure during inspiration. They thus provide the patient with *inspiratory positive-pressure breathing* (IPPB). For several years IPPB has been the abbreviation of *intermittent* positive-pressure breathing, but many users believe that the adjective "intermittent" is inadequate, since it does not describe the phase of ventilation during which positive pressure is applied, only that it is not continuous. Use of "inspiratory" has recently been recommended as being more realistic, since it specifically separates inspiratory positive pressure from expiratory, a discrimination of considerable importance. Although the new terminology has no official acceptance yet, in this text inspiratory replaces intermittent in the interpretation of IPPB.

Two additional observations are appropriate regarding IPPB. First, and again by custom and habit, IPPB has a definite connotation, referring in respiratory therapy to a short-term treatment procedure by which a patient is subjected to inspiratory positive pressure, often for the purpose of aerosol administration and hyperinflation of the lung. Also, the instrument by which IPPB is given is always a type classified as a pneumatic pressure-cycled assistor, frequently a greatly simplified version. In other words, IPPB therapy is not given by any of the time-cycled or volume-cycled machines listed in the classification below. Second, to differentiate between the uses of the ventilation equipment described next, the term *IPPB* is understood to relate to the treatment defined above using the equipment noted. *IPPV* (ventilation or ventilator) refers to the mechanical support of a patient or the equipment used, regardless of type, as long as it delivers an inspiratory positive pressure. While IPPV admittedly is not an official designation and was not included in the terminology recommendations referred to, it enjoys wide general use and is a helpful term.

Ventilator power and drive mechanisms

Some source of power is required for all ventilators in order to develop a positive pressure at the airway. Modern ventilators are powered either pneumatically or electrically, or they require both power sources.

Pneumatically powered ventilators. Pneumatically powered ventilators require only a pressurized gas source to operate. Often using oxygen at 50 psig, all ventilator functions are pneumatically controlled or can be manually manipulated. These ventilators can vary in complexity from hand-operated units such as the Hand-E-Vent from Ohio Medical Products to the sophisticated model 225/SIMV volume ventilator from Monaghan.[7] In some of these units, such as the Monaghan 225/SIMV, fluidic principles are applied for controlling various functions. Fluidic principles are not covered here, but the reader is encouraged to read the ample descriptions presented in other writings.[3,7,14]

Electrically powered ventilators. Electricity is a common source of power for many of the ventilators in use today.[7] When a ventilator requires only electric current to function, it should be assumed that only room air is being used to ventilate the patient. If oxygen between 21% and 100% is to be used, then a source of compressed oxygen must also be available. However, if the oxygen source were to fail or be depleted, a ventilator that is truly electrically powered would not stop ventilating the patient. In other words, the oxygen source is used to control the inspired oxygen percent but not to drive the ventilator. Often electric motors that drive compressors or pistons are used to produce the positive pressure needed. Examples of ventilators needing only electrical current to operate (using only 21% oxygen) are the Emerson 3-PV, the Bennett MA-1, and the Bourns BEAR 1 models.

Combined power ventilators. Some mechanical ventilators need both a compressed gas source and an electric source in order to function. Often the pneumatic source is used to provide the gas flow needed, while the electric power is used to control various functions of timing and phasing. The Servo ventilators by Siemens are examples of ventilators that must be powered by both compressed gas source and electricity.[3,7] In pediatric ventilators there are several that use electronic systems for the timing controls while utilizing the gas source for flow and pressure controls. Two such devices are the Bourns BP200 and the Sechrist IV-100 ventilators.[3,7,15]

Drive mechanisms. The drive mechanism for a positive-pressure ventilator is the system that produces the *force* needed to ventilate the patient. There are a variety of systems used in modern ventilators to effect a gas flow during inspiration, each type with different capabilities. The drive mechanism a ventilator possesses suggests some of its operational characteristics, and therefore familiarity with drive mechanisms is important to the respiratory therapist. We summarize some of the common types and characteristics here.

Single-circuit and double-circuit systems. Each drive system can be broadly categorized into single- or double-circuit systems. A ventilator with a single circuit is one that provides the gas flow to the patient directly from the driving source. As an example, if a piston is used to provide the necessary driving force and the gases in the piston's cylinder go *directly* to the patient circuit, as in Fig. 13-2, the system is a single circuit.

A double-circuit ventilator is one that uses one circuit to power or drive another. Fig. 13-3 diagrams a piston used again, but instead of the gases from the piston going directly to the patient, they are used to compress a bag, which in turn sends its contents into the patient. In this case, the piston is used as the driving circuit, and the bag and tubing are considered the patient circuit.

Examples of single-circuit ventilators include the Bird Mark 7 and Mark 8,

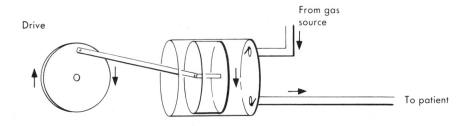

Fig. 13-2   Example of single-circuit ventilator system.

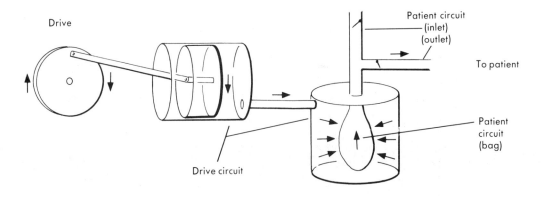

Fig. 13-3   Example of double-circuit ventilator system.

the Bennett PR series, the Emerson 3-PV and 3-MV, and the Servo ventilators 900B and 900C.[3,7] Commonly used ventilators with double circuits are the Engström ER-300 series, the Bennett MA-1 and MA-2, and the Ohio CCV-2, SIMV.[3,7]

During the 1950s and 1960s, the Engström ventilators were common examples of ventilators that had specific flow, pressure, and inspiratory maneuver capabilities because they used a double circuit. Today, however, these same features can be created through the use of electronics on single-circuit ventilators, e.g., Servo 900 models. The functional differences between ventilators are now much less dependent on whether the unit has a single- versus double-circuit design. This feature is included for the sake of completeness.

Rotary-driven piston. Pistons moving back and forth in a cylinder have been used in mechanical ventilators for many years.[3] When powered by an adequate electric motor they provide a convenient mechanism for driving air into a patient's lungs. A *rotary*-drive piston is one that is connected to a motor-driven wheel (Fig. 13-4). If the ventilator is a single-circuit device, then the tidal volume to be delivered can be pulled into the piston during the backward stroke. One-way valves are used to separate the patient's exhaled gases from

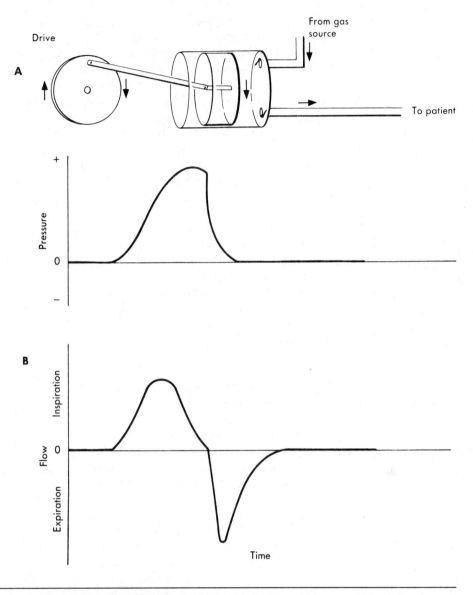

Fig. 13-4   **A,** Example of a rotary-driven piston and **B,** typical pressure and flow wave-forms.

fresh gases during this phase. On the forward stroke of the piston, gases are pushed into the patient's circuit.

A unique flow pattern is established by a ventilator with a rotary-driven piston used as a single-circuit device. Because the piston is connected to a wheel (Fig. 13-4) the piston's movement through the cylinder, and therefore the flow of gas out of the cylinder, occurs in an accelerating, then decelerating, fashion. To illustrate, as the wheel turns, the piston's movements at the beginning of inspiration are slow because much of the movement of the piston's rod is upward and very little is forward. During the middle of the piston's movement through the cylinder, much of the movement is forward, creating an accelerating flow out of the cylinder. The last part of the piston's movement in the cylinder provides a slowing of flow or a deceleration as the piston's movement is less forward again. This type of movement by the piston is termed *sinusoidal,* or producing a sine wave. Thus we often call the inspiratory flow pattern produced by such a device a sine-wave flow pattern, although it is more precisely one half of a sine wave.

Rotary-driven piston ventilators such as the Emerson models 3-PV and 3-MV are powered by electric motors and can provide a very high airway pressure if needed. These devices are very simple and reliable and have proved themselves over the years. The sine-wave flow pattern produced does mimic the typical flow pattern generated by spontaneously breathing healthy people and may offer some advantage over other flow patterns.[16]

Linear-driven piston. If a piston is used for the driving mechanism but it is pushed through its cylinder at the same speed rather than in an accelerating-decelerating fashion, then it is considered to have a *linear* drive. Since the piston's movement is constant throughout its stroke, then the flow of air being pushed into the patient is also constant. This is called a square-wave flow pattern and is discussed further later in this chapter.

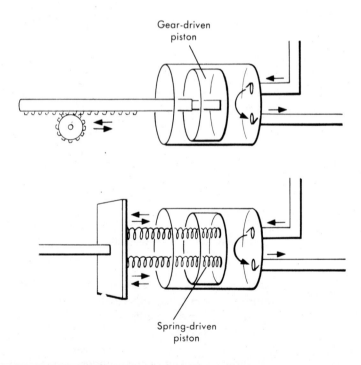

Gear-driven
piston

Spring-driven
piston

Fig. 13-5   Examples of gear- and spring-driven ventilator systems.

Various mechanisms have been used to provide a linear drive system for pistons.[3,7] The Bourns LS104-150 Infant Ventilator uses a gear-driven mechanism, which moves the piston at an adjustable, constant speed. High-tension springs have also been used to push a pistonlike mechanism in the previously produced Searle Volume Ventilator Adult (VVA) ventilator. Fig. 13-5 diagrams these systems.

Compressor-driven bellows. Compressors are convenient devices for producing a positive pressure and are frequently used to power the driving circuit on double-circuit ventilators. In this case, as shown in Fig. 13-6, the compressor supplies pressure to push the bellows upward during inspiration. The bellows contains the gases the patient will receive and is therefore part of the patient circuit. Commonly these compressors are of two general types: those producing relatively low pressures with high flow rates, such as the rotary blower of the Ohio CCV-2, SIMV, or one producing a relatively high pressure but at a low flow rate, such as that used for the Bennett MA-1 and MA-2. In this last system the compressor is used to drive a venturi, which boosts the flow available and limits the driving pressure as compared to the compressor alone.

The flow pattern produced by these systems will generally be square wave or may taper somewhat as pressure increases within the patient circuit.[7]

Pneumatic drive. Some single-circuit ventilators are driven by a blended gas source, often under relatively high pressures of 3 to 50 psig. In these devices

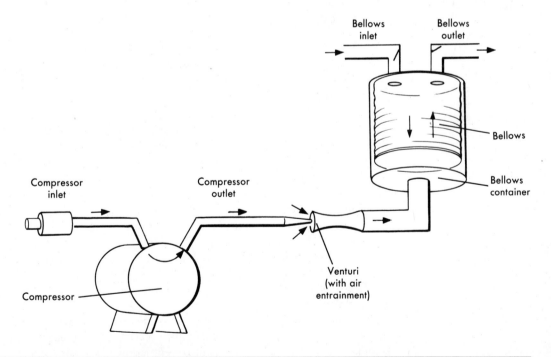

Fig. 13-6   Example of compressor-driven bellows. Venturi serves to increase flow and decrease pressure from the compressor.

a high internal resistance system such as a needlelike valve control is used to control the flow of gas into the patient circuit. Because the driving pressure is relatively high, these units generally produce a constant flow pattern. Examples of ventilators using a single-circuit pneumatic drive are the Bird Mark 7 set on "100%" setting and the Bourns BEAR 1 and BEAR 2.

Venturi drive mechanism. Venturis, also known as "injectors,"[3] are incorporated into some ventilator drive systems. A venturi can boost the flow capabilities of a compressor while decreasing the available pressure. The flow is increased through air entrainment while pressure from the venturi is limited by its maximum forward force. All venturi systems are susceptible to back pressure to some degree and will therefore have a decrease in total flow when significant resistance is applied to them. Ventilators commonly used to administer IPPB, such as the Bird Mark 7 and Bennett PR-1 and PR-2 use venturis for air entrainment.

Weighted drive mechanism. A very simple device used for a driving mechanism in some ventilators is a weight, such as a weighted bellows or piston.[3,7] The weight provides the necessary force to overcome the resistance to airflow during inspiration. This system has also been referred to as "gravity driven." The Chemetron Gill 1 Respirator is an example of a volume ventilator using a weighted piston.[7]

Inspiratory phase

Starting inspiration. There are various ways for a mechanical ventilator to begin a positive-pressure breath, and these provide a convenient way to introduce various modes of ventilatory support.

Assist mode—patient triggered or cycled. When a ventilator has the capability for initiating a positive-pressure breath in response to a very slight effort made by the patient, the ventilator is said to be providing assist mode or assisted ventilation. That is, the patient's very slight effort *triggers* the inspiratory phase of the ventilator. Usually the patient's effort to inhale is sensed by a drop in pressure within the tubing between the patient and the ventilator, although some ventilators use a flow-sensing device. In either case there is usually some mechanism for adjusting the amount of patient effort required before the ventilator cycles on. This adjustable mechanism is usually called the *sensitivity* or *patient-effort* control.

Starting the inspiratory phase is often referred to as *cycling,* but this term is also used to indicate ending inspiration. Basically cycling refers to changing from one phase to another, and we have attempted to indicate which phase change we are referring to when the term is used in the remainder of this text.

Assist mode is commonly used with IPPB therapy, and below we describe its use with prolonged mechanical ventilation (IPPV) when it is combined with controlled ventilation.

Control mode—time triggered or cycled. When some mechanism for timing within the ventilator initiates the inspiratory phase, the ventilator is said to be providing control mode, or controlled ventilation. The rate of pressurized breaths received by the patient is established by the timing mechanism and is independent of the patient's efforts or breathing pattern. In this mode of mechanical support the patient is totally dependent on a functioning ventilator system since many patients receiving controlled ventilation are apneic either from disease or from drugs. More specific considerations for control mode ventilation are presented in Chapter 14.

Specific systems for establishing a controlled breathing rate can vary from one ventilator to another.[3,7] Rate can be set as an individual control that divides each minute in equal time segments, alotting one time segment for each total ventilatory cycle (e.g., Bennett MA-1). With this system, inspiration and expiration are adjusted by using other controls such as flow and volume while the rate remains separate. Separate timers for inspiration and expiration can also set a control rate on some ventilators (e.g., Emerson 3-PV). Changing either or both of these timers can affect the control rate the patient receives.

Assist-control mode. A commonly used ventilatory mode combines patient triggering with a mechanically set rate as a "backup." Generally the patient is allowed to establish an acceptable breathing rate by assisting (triggering the

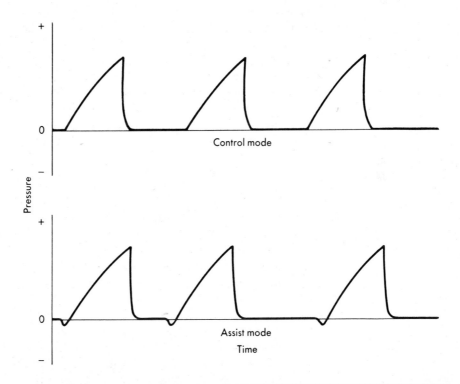

Fig. 13-7 Pressure wave forms for IPPV during control mode (top) and assist mode (bottom). Note regular time intervals for control mode while time intervals for assist mode are more variable. Slight negative pressure "triggers" assist breaths.

ventilator), and a control rate is set somewhat below that of the patient. In this case the control rate is a guarantor in case the patient's breathing pattern slows or stops completely.

Assist-control mode is a convenient mode for mechanically ventilating patients and has been available on modern devices since the 1960s. It is thought that an advantage to assisted ventilation is that it allows patients to establish their own rate and therefore influence their own Pa_{CO_2}. This is not always desirable, and the therapist will encounter some patients who are substantially overventilated by the assist mode because of an abnormal drive to breathe. The hyperventilation and respiratory alkalosis produced causes significant problems, and these are considered in detail in Chapter 14.

Controlled ventilation also has its difficulties, including patients breathing asynchronously with the ventilator, drugs used for respiratory muscle paralysis, and the apneic patient's complete dependence on the ventilator system.

Fig. 13-7 diagrams typical pressure wave forms created during assisted and controlled ventilation. The graph shows units of pressure such as centimeters of water on the vertical axis and time on the horizontal axis. Note that the positive-pressure inspiration begins with a slight *drop* in pressure for assist mode and that the time between breaths in somewhat variable. Control mode shows no such negative pressure starting each breath, and the time between breaths is very regular.

Intermittent mandatory ventilation. IMV is a mode of ventilation that combines a controlled mechanical rate with spontaneous breathing.[6] In this mode, some system is provided for fresh gas from which spontaneous breathing can occur at a rate and volume that is patient determined. This spontaneous breathing occurs *between* the preset mechanical (IMV) breaths (Fig. 13-8). IMV has been used both as a weaning method and as a primary mode of ventilatory support in infants and adults for the past decade.[6]

Not all patients are candidates for IMV, and although it has become a very useful adjunct in ventilatory support, many of its purported advantages are yet to be studied in a controlled fashion.[17,18] IMV allows (or requires) the patient to provide some of the work of breathing during ventilatory support. When the patient is capable of providing more work, the ventilator's control rate is decreased accordingly. This allows for smooth transitions during ventilatory support and may have advantages for decreasing the mean intrathoracic pressure compared to controlled ventilation because of the spontaneous efforts.[6,18] IMV is also useful when it is combined with expiratory pressure maneuvers, which are described subsequently. Some ventilators provide a system for IMV mode,[7] or special circuits can be added.[6]

Synchronized intermittent mandatory ventilation. While IMV is a control rate combined with spontaneous breathing, synchronized intermittent mandatory ventilation (SIMV) is an *assisted* rate combined with spontaneous breathing. With SIMV, each mechanical breath is usually triggered by the patient in the same manner as assist mode. Again a system for providing fresh gas for spontaneous breathing between assisted breaths must be available.

SIMV is really a technical deviation from IMV (see Fig. 13-9), and other-

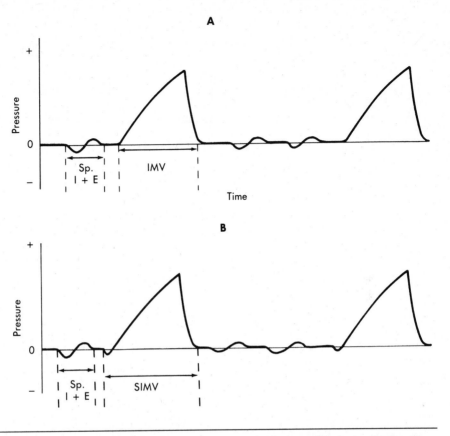

A

B

Fig. 13-8   Pressure wave forms for IMV and SIMV. Spontaneous inspiration and expiration *(Sp. I + E)* are shown combined with pressurized (IMV) breaths. **A,** shows the IMV breaths occurring like control mode breaths while **B** shows IMV breaths triggered by patient (SIMV).

wise they are used in the same manner. Other terms used by manufacturers and authors to describe this same mode are *intermittent demand ventilation* (IDV) and *intermittent assisted ventilation* (IAV).[7,19,20] The real role of SIMV compared to IMV is yet to be determined, although theoretically it should prevent excessive pressures if patients are beginning exhalation when an IMV breath occurs. With SIMV, there is some amount of delay time when a mandatory breath is to occur until the patient begins the next inspiratory effort. One study comparing IMV to SIMV failed to show any significant difference between the two modes when various hemodynamic parameters, blood gases, and pulmonary barotrauma were compared.[21]

Pressure and flow generators. Mushin and associates have proposed a system of classification for ventilators that considers how the positive pressure is applied.[3] Although this system is often more theoretic than specifically applicable, this system is briefly explained and its clinical implications discussed here.

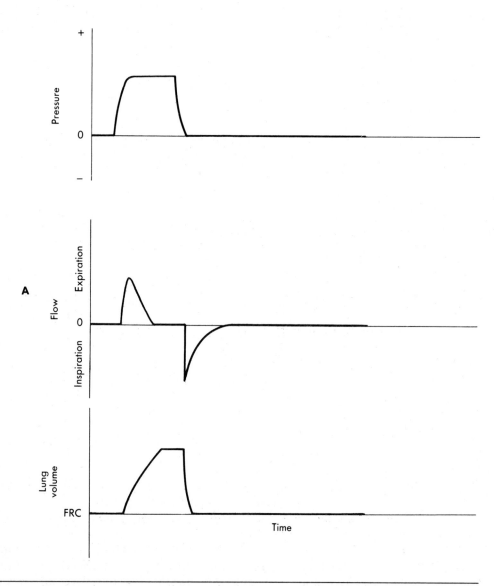

Fig. 13-9   Pressure, flow, and volume wave forms for a constant pressure generator. **A** represents "normal" conditions while **B** illustrates a decrease in compliance and **C** shows an increase in airways resistance. Note the decrease in volume in **B** and the slowly tapering inspiratory flow in **C**.

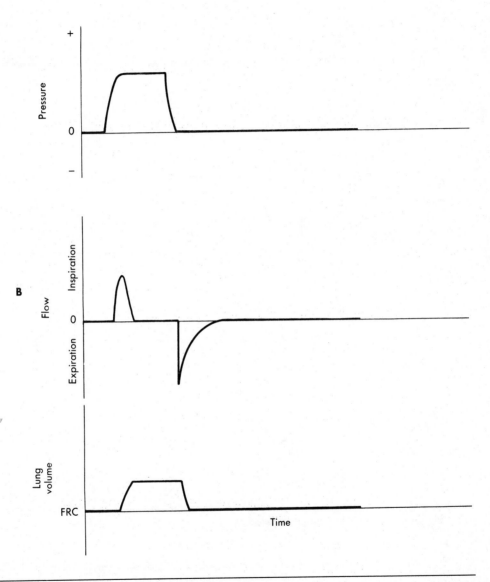

Fig. 13-9, cont'd   For legend see opposite page.   *Continued.*

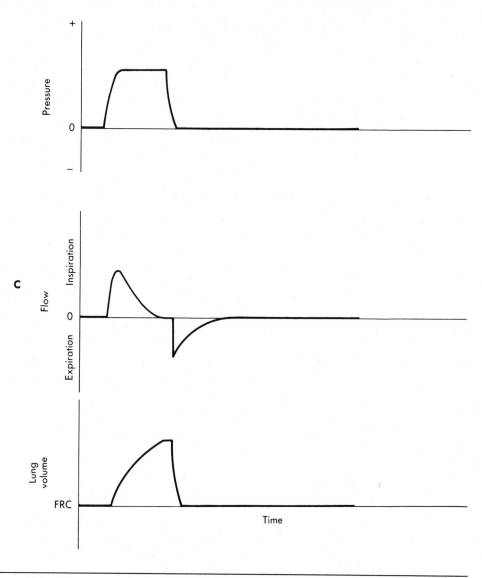

Fig. 13-9, cont'd   For legend see page 506.

A *constant pressure generator* can be defined as a device that produces a relatively consistent pressure throughout inspiration, and this pressure is applied to the airway. Under ideal circumstances this system would produce pressure, flow, and volume patterns seen in Fig. 13-9. Flow into the lungs would start at a high rate because of the initial pressure difference between the airway pressure and the alveolar pressure. As the pressure increased in the alveoli during inspiration, flow would taper in a decelerating fashion because of the decreasing pressure gradient from airway to alveoli. If inspiration were to last long enough, the airway and alveolar pressures would equilibrate, flow would stop, and the volume would be held in the lung until expiration occurred.

The practical application of this principle is not widespread but would include systems with a weighted bellows and some low-pressure generating devices such as a Bennett PR-2. For the PR-2, the pressure generated is not exactly constant under some circumstances, but the differences are relatively minor.

Fig. 13-9 also compares what happens to delivered volume when a pressure generator is used and compliance or resistance changes. Note the volume decreases when the compliance is half normal. Also note that volume can remain constant when resistance is doubled but that more time is required to deliver the same volume. When the resistance to airflow increases, the flow created by the constant pressure is lower initially but will continue until pressure within the alveoli equilibrates with the pressure generated if enough time is given. It is important to notice that in this example of a relatively low-pressure generator, flow and volume can change with changes in the patient's compliance and resistance.

The change in gas flow just described is attributed to the low pressure generated in our example. If the pressure being generated by the ventilator was very high and the pressure allowed in the patient's airways was low, the flow during the breath could remain uninfluenced by the patient pressure. This circumstance produces another parameter of this classification system: the *flow generator.*

A flow generator can be defined as a ventilator that produces the same flow pattern independent of the pressure in the patient system and independent of resistance and compliance changes. Two types of flow generators are *constant flow generators* and *nonconstant flow generators.*

A constant flow generator produces a constant flow throughout inspiration (Fig. 13-10). This produces the characteristic square wave, mentioned previously. With this type of system, the pressure driving the gases is so high that changes in the patient's pressure cannot sufficiently change the pressure gradient, and so flow remains unchanged. For example, Fig. 13-10 illustrates what occurs when the driving force is 50 psig, or about 3500 cm of water. Note that when inspiratory time is held constant, volumes and flow remain unchanged when compliance and resistance worsen, but pressures in the alveoli and airway change instead.

A nonconstant flow generator is one that produces the same *pattern* breath after breath, but that pattern is *not* constant *during* each breath. The most common example is a sine-wave generator, exemplified by the Emerson 3-PV and 3-MV ventilators. Fig. 13-11 illustrates a sine-wave flow generator under changing patient conditions. Again a strong force such as from a rotary-driven piston produces a flow pattern that does not change when resistance and compliance change. Both airway and alveolar pressure can be affected but not the flow pattern. Recently various aspects of ventilation with flow generators were reviewed by Rattenborg.[8]

The primary difference between the pressure generator described and the

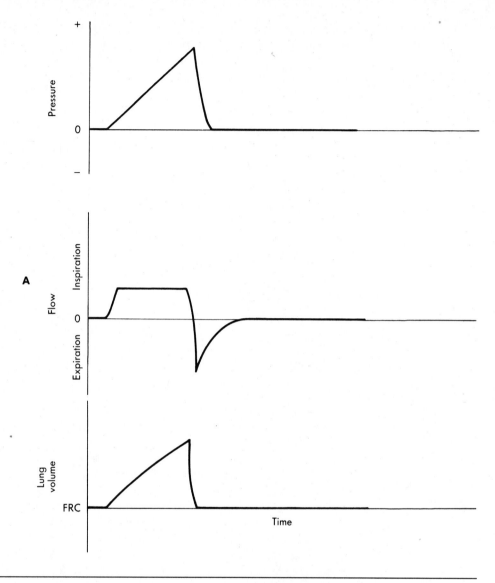

Fig. 13-10   Pressure, flow, and volume wave forms for a constant flow generator under different patient conditions. **A** shows typical wave forms for "normal" conditions. **B** illustrates a worsening of compliance. Note that in **B** the inspiratory flow pattern remains unchanged while inspiratory pressure increases and expiratory flow increases. Lung volume remains about the same for illustration purposes.

flow generators is the amount of driving pressure used. Few ventilators produce very high driving pressures of several psig or more, and so few can be called true flow generators under all patient conditions. From a practical viewpoint however, many ventilators we use maintain nearly the same flow rate or flow pattern until fairly high airway pressures are reached, such as 80 to 100

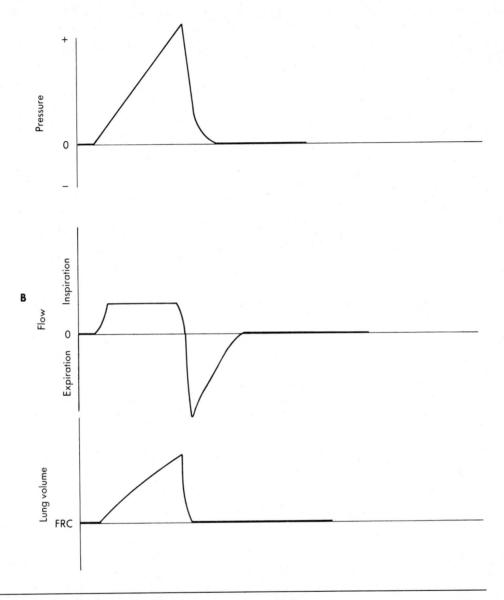

Fig. 13-10, cont'd.   For legend see opposite page.

cm of water. Often, commonly used mechanical ventilators perform like a flow generator for most patients until near maximum pressure is available, at which time flow begins to be influenced by the increasing airway pressure.

Examples of pure flow generators are the Bird Mark 7 and Mark 8 on 100% setting and the Emerson 3-PV and 3-MV ventilators. Examples of ventilators that function as flow generators under *usual* circumstances but not when

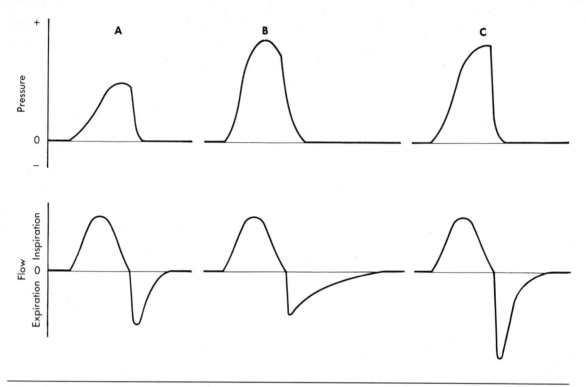

Fig. 13-11   Comparison of pressure and flow wave forms for a nonconstant flow generator (sine-wave type) under various patient conditions. **A** shows patterns for normal conditions while **B** illustrates an increased airways resistance and **C** shows a decreased compliance. Note that the inspiratory flow pattern remains unchanged while generated pressures and expiratory flow patterns vary. **B** shows low expiratory flows due to airways resistance while **C** shows high expiratory flows due to "stiff" lungs.

stressed severely are the Bennett MA-2, the Bourns BEAR 1, the Siemens Servo 900B, and the Ohio CCV-2, SIMV.[7]

Ending inspiration. Various methods are used to stop inspiration and start expiration, and these have important clinical considerations. It is common to see the term *cycle* used to indicate the end of inspiration, but as we mentioned earlier this term may also be used to designate the end of expiration and the beginning of inspiration.[3] *Limit* has also been used to indicate end-inspiration, and the student should be aware of this fact when reading the medical literature. Mushin and associates use the term *cycle* to indicate a change from one phase to the next and *limit* to indicate the maximum amount of some parameter, e.g., pressure or volume, that is available.[3] We use this terminology for the rest of this text. We briefly define common cycling systems first and then later make comparisons of them.

Pressure-cycled ventilators. These ventilators provide a positive-pressure inspiratory phase until an adjustable, preselected pressure has been reached. When the preselected pressure is achieved, inspiration is ended, or "cycled off." These ventilators are most commonly used to administer IPPB therapy but can also be useful for continuous ventilatory support under proper monitoring conditions.

A variety of parameters can affect the ventilation provided by a pressure-cycled ventilator. Depending on the individual unit, changes in the patient's compliance and airway resistance can change the amount of volume, inspiratory time, and flow pattern delivered for a given pressure.

The Bird Mark 7, Mark 7A, Mark 8, Mark 8A, and Mark 14 are all common examples of pressure-cycled ventilators.[7]

Volume-cycled ventilators. A volume-cycled ventilator continues the inspiratory phase until an adjustable, preselected volume has been "delivered" or expelled from the ventilator. Within certain limits, changing compliance and resistance factors cause changes in airway *pressure,* and the volumes remain relatively constant. Inspiratory time and flow pattern remain constant if the ventilator is a flow generator, or they may vary with pressure changes. The preselected *volume* tends to be the consistent parameter regardless of other changes.

Not all of the set volume is delivered to the patient's airways and alveoli from common volume ventilators. Some of this volume is compressed within the ventilator and the connecting tubing circuit between the ventilator and the patient. This is further discussed in a later section when these ventilators are compared with the other types defined in this section.

Common examples of volume-cycled ventilators include the Bennett MA-1 and MA-2, the Bourns BEAR 1 and BEAR 2, the Monaghan 225/SIMV, and the Ohio CCV-2, SIMV models.

Time-cycled ventilators. Time-cycled ventilators end inspiration when a preselected time has elapsed. Delivered volume, pressure, and flow may vary depending on other characteristics of the ventilator and on patient parameters. As the term implies, inspiratory *time* is consistent breath to breath. It should be appreciated that if a time-cycled ventilator is functioning as a flow generator, then both time and flow pattern are constant, and this will also result in a constant volume each breath. If the ventilator is functioning as a pressure generator, then even though inspiratory time is constant, flow and volume delivered can be influenced by changes in the patient's compliance and airway resistance.

Common examples of ventilators that are *primarily* time cycled are the Emerson 3-PV and 3-MV, the Siemens Servo 900, Servo 900B, and Servo 900C, the Bourns BP200, the Sechrist IV-100 and IV-100B, and the Bird Babybird ventilators.

Flow-cycled ventilators. A preselected flow rate could also be used to end the inspiratory phase of a positive-pressure ventilator. In this case, flow might decrease during the breath, and when a specific level was reached the ventilator would cycle off. Volume, pressure, and inspiratory time could be variable and dependent on the patient's lung characteristics.

No ventilator commonly used can provide such ventilation with an *adjustable* flow-cycling level. However, Bennett pressure ventilators such as the PR series, PV-3P, and AP series all cycle inspiration when a very low level of flow is reached.[3,7] Because the special Bennett valve used in these devices closes when a low "terminal" flow rate is passing through it, they are considered to be flow cycled. In these ventilators the terminal or cycling flow is reached because the *pressure* set on the ventilator is nearly reached on both the ventilator and patient sides of the valve. Thus the pressure used to ventilate the patient is also the same each breath, and these ventilators are often considered both pressure- and flow-cycled units.

Manually cycled ventilators. Some ventilators end the inspiratory phase only by a manually operated control. This method is commonly employed with some portable IPPB devices designed to be used in the home. Most often these units function somewhat like pressure generators and limit the amount of pressure being applied. Volumes, flow, and inspiratory time are variable depending on patient conditions and on when the breath is manually released or cycled.

Examples of IPPB units that are manually operated are the Ohio Hand-E-Vent and the Bird Asthmastik ventilators.[7]

Combined cycling. Many ventilators can be cycled off by more than one mechanism. As an example, some volume ventilators also have pressure cycling mechanisms as well. These are usually set so that normally the preset volume cycles the ventilator off, but if excessive pressures are required before volume delivery, the preset pressure is reached first and ends inspiration before the total volume is delivered. In this case the pressure-cycling feature is a safety system on the volume ventilator. This situation is found on the Bennett MA-1 ventilator.

Time cycling is sometimes provided as a backup system to a primarily volume-cycled ventilator. In this case inspiration is ended when some maximum time is reached before volume delivery, should the breath be prolonged for some reason. The Bourns BEAR 1 ventilator provides this feature by its I:E (inspiratory/expiratory) ratio limit system.[7]

The concept of inspiratory limits. As stated previously, the term *limit* has also been used to indicate the end of inspiration. The student should realize that a pressure-cycled or volume-cycled ventilator may be referred to as a *pressure-limited* or *volume-limited* ventilator.[7,22] To make a practical distinction between these terms for our use, we consider *limit* to mean a parameter that has a maximum setting but does not necessarily end or cycle inspiration. As an example, some ventilators use a pressure relief valve, which opens and vents gases when the set pressure is reached and holds that pressure until some cycling mechanism ends inspiration. The pressure is *limited* by the relief valve, but inspiration may *end* by a volume-cycling or time-cycling mechanism. The

Bourns LS104-150 infant ventilator is an example of a volume-cycled ventilator that incorporates a pressure-limiting relief valve. The Sechrist IV-100B and Bird Babybird are time-cycled ventilators using a pressure-limiting relief system.

The Emerson 3-PV and 3-MV ventilators are really time cycled, but inspiration does contain the same volume from their piston breath to breath. Therefore these ventilators are often referred to as being time cycled and volume limited. The Siemens Servo 900 and Engström ER-300 ventilators are also time cycled but normally deliver consistent volumes breath to breath and are therefore also considered to be volume limited. Most ventilators that have adjustments for either tidal or minute volume are considered "volume ventilators" regardless of how inspiration is actually cycled.

Inflation hold. Also called end-inspiratory pause and inspiratory hold, an inflation hold is a maneuver that follows active inspiration and precedes the expiratory phase. Two methods are commonly used to apply inflation hold, and their clinical use is described in Chapter 14. Basically these can be referred to as a *pressure hold* or *peak inflation hold* and a *volume hold* or *plateau inflation hold*.

A pressure or peak inflation hold is a maneuver that maintains the peak pressure against the airway for some time period. Pediatric ventilators are often employed in this manner using their pressure relief valves to set the pressure hold level while their time-cycling mechanisms determine the length of inspiration. This can also be provided by volume-cycled ventilators when a pressure-limiting relief valve is used. In this case the pressure valve holds its set pressure against the airway while the volume-cycling mechanism (e.g., piston or bellows) continues to discharge its volume into the circuit. Both of these systems just described begin to function as a pressure generator once the peak pressure is reached, and therefore both flow and volume delivered to the patient vary with patient compliance and resistance changes.

Volume or plateau inflation hold is commonly found on volume-cycled or volume-limited ventilators. In this system the tidal volume is delivered as usual and then held in the patient's lungs for some preselected time period before exhalation is allowed. During this volume-hold period pressure in the ventilator and tubing system attempts to equilibrate with the patient's lung pressure, and a pressure drop is seen on the ventilator's pressure gauge. The difference between the end-inspiration pressure and the plateau or hold pressure reflects the resistance to flow encountered. The plateau pressure itself indicates the amount of pressure required to hold the delivered volume within the lungs and tubing circuit.

Usually controls for providing plateau inflation hold are calibrated in time increments, often up to 2 seconds or in some percent of total ventilatory cycle time. The Bennett MA-2, the Bourns BEAR 1, and the Siemens Servo 900 series ventilators are examples of volume ventilators with adjustable inflation holds.

Inflation hold maneuvers have been used to increase the distribution of gases in the lung,[16,23] to decrease the V_D/V_T ratio,[23,24] and to aid in monitoring various ventilatory parameters such as resistance and compliance[25,26] (see Chapter 14).

Expiratory phase

During typical IPPB or IPPV, expiration occurs as a function of lung recoil and is considered a passive event, meaning little or no work is involved on the part of the patient. There are certain pressure and flow manipulations that can be therapeutically applied during this phase. Three maneuvers will be defined here: negative end-expiratory pressure (NEEP), expiratory resistance or retard, and positive end-expiratory pressure (PEEP).

Negative end-expiratory pressure. With the NEEP maneuver a subatmospheric pressure is applied to the airway during the expiratory phase (Fig. 13-12). Because the inspiratory positive airway pressure applied during mechanical ventilation can suppress venous return to the right heart, negative pressure during expiration has been used to lower the mean airway pressure and enhance venous return.[3] Problems of airway collapse in both normal and emphysematous patients can offset this potential benefit.[3] NEEP used with mechanical ventilation has also been referred to as "positive/negative pressure ventilation." The use of this maneuver is discussed later in this chapter under Physiologic Effects of Mechanical Ventilation.

Expiratory resistance or retard. Resistance to expiration can be applied during mechanical ventilation to slow the flow from the patient. This maneuver mimics the effect of pursed-lip breathing used by patients with chronic obstructive pulmonary disease and extends the amount of time positive pressure is within the airways. Adding a restricted orifice to the exhalation valve of IPPB systems has been used by individual patients, presumably to replace the pursed-lip effect while receiving IPPB by mouthpiece.

Fig. 13-13 illustrates the effect of adding expiratory resistance following a positive-pressure inspiration. It can be seen that more time is spent with pressure within the lung and therefore the mean airway pressure is increased compared to a positive-pressure inspiration without expiratory resistance. Some mechanical ventilation systems have a significant amount of resistance to expiration because of the sizes of various tubings and ports through which expiratory gases must flow. In general it is best to have a system with the least amount of resistance possible and a mechanism available to add controlled amounts of retard when it seems therapeutically indicated.

Positive end-expiratory pressure. PEEP is a maneuver that applies a positive pressure during expiration. It is commonly applied during assisted or controlled mechanical ventilation and referred to as *IPPV/PEEP, mechanical ventilation with PEEP* (MV/PEEP), or *continuous positive-pressure ventilation* (CPPV).[27-29] PEEP can also be applied during spontaneous breathing with a similar positive pressure also being applied during inspiration such as with continuous positive-pressure breathing (CPPB)[27,30] or continuous positive airway pressure (CPAP).[27,31] When PEEP with spontaneous breathing is combined with inspiration occurring at or near atmospheric pressure, the terms

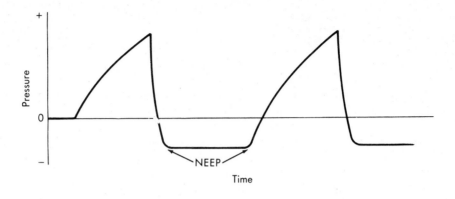

Fig. 13-12   Pressure wave form during IPPV with NEEP added.

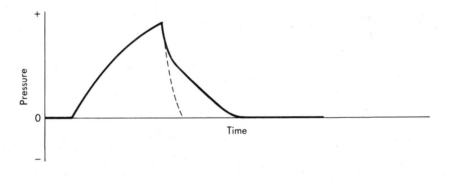

Fig. 13-13   Pressure wave form during IPPV with expiratory resistance (retard) applied. (The dotted line represents the normal slope of the pressure drop from peak to baseline during expiration for comparison.)

spontaneous PEEP (sPEEP) and *expiratory positive airway pressure* (EPAP) have been used.[27,32-35] These spontaneous breathing modes with PEEP can also be added to IMV mode of mechanical ventilation such as IMV/PEEP or IMV/CPAP.[6]

Fig. 13-14 illustrates the pressure wave forms created by these systems. Other terms have also been applied,[27] but we limit our discussion to those just mentioned because they are commonly used or are helpful and descriptive.

PEEP is primarily used to increase functional residual capacity, decrease physiologic shunting, increase oxygenation, and allow for a lower oxygen concentration to be used.[28,29,36-38] Other parameters such as lung compliance and V_D/V_T ratio may also be improved in some patients.[39]

Most currently used volume ventilators have built-in mechanisms to provide PEEP or CPAP.[7] Often these are provided by trapping some pressure in the

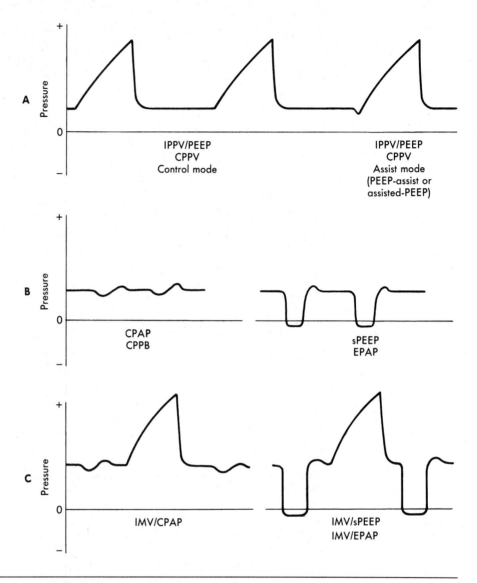

Fig. 13-14 Pressure wave forms for various forms of ventilatory support with end-expiratory pressure at a positive level. See text for description.

exhalation valve of the tubing circuit, which in turn traps a similar pressure in the patient's lungs. A simple column of water can also be used to apply PEEP by directing the exhaled gases under the surface. The distance from the water's surface to the opening of the exhalation tube is equal to the pressure being applied, e.g., 10 cm of distance equals 10 cm of water PEEP. Some systems used to supply PEEP may also offer resistance to flow, and a combined effect of expiratory retard and PEEP is applied.[2] Generally this is less desirable, and ideal PEEP systems offer little or no additional flow resistance.

Up to 15 cm water PEEP is commonly used, although some patients require between 15 and 30 cm water and more than 30 is occasionally needed.[28,37,39,40] When infants are receiving CPAP, usually less than 12 to 14 cm of water is used, though occasionally higher pressures have been used.[41] The clinical application of PEEP for patients in respiratory failure is discussed further in Chapter 14.

Comparison of ventilation methods	Our classification of ventilators suggests several different methods that can be used to ventilate patients. In this section we discuss some of the technical and clinical differences between some ventilators including volume- versus pressure-cycled, time-cycled and pressure-limited, ventilation at high frequencies, and finally negative-pressure ventilation.
Volume- versus pressure-cycled ventilation	**Volume-cycled ventilation.** The most commonly employed ventilator in use today for continuous ventilatory support of critically ill patients is the volume ventilator. Many of the patients treated have a rapidly changing compliance or airways resistance, and it has long been believed that volume ventilators can maintain more adequate ventilation despite these changes, especially when compared to pressure-cycled ventilators.[4,8,10,42-44] Modern volume ventilators generally have substantial pressure available with which to deliver the set volumes, often exceeding 80 cm of water. As compliance decreases, for example, the pressure required to ventilate the set volume *increases*. With a volume ventilator, the airway pressure applied automatically rises, and the volume from the ventilator stays generally the same. If the pressure developed exceeds an established maximum, set as a secondary pressure cycle or limit, inspiration will either end (cycle mechanism) or some of the volume will be vented out of the circuit and lost (limit mechanism, e.g., relief valve).

As mentioned previously, not all the set tidal volume reaches the patient even when the maximum pressure limit is not exceeded. This is because gases under pressure compress and flexible tubing circuits expand. During inspiration pressure rises as gases flow from the ventilator into the patient's tubing circuit and airways. The gases confined in the ventilator and the tubing circuit at the end of inspiration are subjected to the pressure there at that instant. Whatever the volume trapped at that instant in the ventilator and tubing circuit, it will *not* participate in the ventilation of the patient. The next instant when expiration begins, this compressed gas will flow out the exhalation valve and will not have entered the patient's airways. This part of the set tidal volume never reaching the patient is commonly referred to as the *compressible volume*.

The volume of trapped gases during inspiration is a function of (1) the space available, (2) the *compliance* of the system, and (3) the pressure applied.

If all the space available to compress gas is rigid, such as a piston cylinder and stiff, noncompliant tubing, then the amount of gas compressed per each unit of pressure is about 1 ml of gas compressed for each centimeter of water pressure applied for every liter of space available.[7] As an example, a ventilator and tubing system having a 4-ℓ, noncompliant circuit at end-inspiration would compress about 4 ml of gas/cm of water pressure applied. For this example, this system has a *compressibility factor* of 4 ml/cm of water. If the tubing could stretch under pressure, then more volume per unit of pressure could be trapped, such as 5 ml/cm of water. This factor is sometimes referred to as a *compliance factor* and is generally interchangeable with compressibility factor.

Fig. 13-15 illustrates the clinical significance of the compressibility factor for a volume ventilator. In the first example, the tidal volume is set for 800 ml, and the pressure generated at end-inspiration is 30 cm of water. In this example a 4 ml/cm of water compressibility factor is used. To find out how much of the tidal volume is compressed in the system, the airway pressure is multiplied by the factor: 30 × 4 = 120. Thus, only 680 ml out of the set 800 ml reaches the patient's airways, while 120 ml is "trapped" in the system.

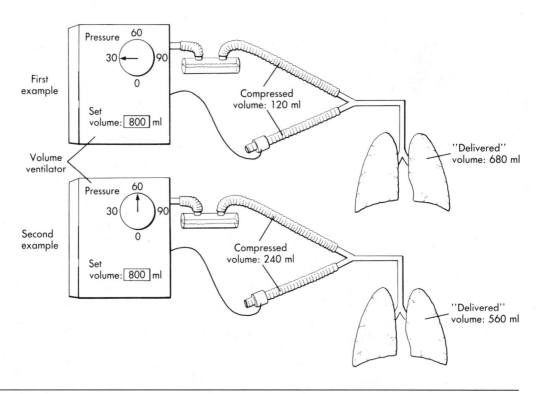

Fig. 13-15   Comparison of volumes delivered to a patient under different end-inspiratory pressures with a volume-cycled ventilator. See text for description of this example.

Let's assume that the patient's compliance decreases, and for our second example of Fig. 13-15 it is now requiring 60 cm of water pressure at end-inspiration. Using the same factor of 4 ml/cm of water we multiply the pressure by the factor again: 60 × 4 = 240. Now only 560 ml of the set 800 reaches the patient, while 240 is compressed in the system. This is a significant drop in patient ventilation although the *majority* of the set volume is still delivered.

It should also be appreciated that if the tidal volume were initially 400 ml, and the factor the same, a similar change in ventilating pressures would have extreme changes in patient ventilation. In general it can be said that *the smaller the tidal volumes desired, the smaller the compressibility factor desired*. This is primarily accomplished by using smaller diameter tubing circuits and by using ventilators that have minimal space internally, which contributes to the compressible volume.

One practical point about compressible volume is that when exhaled volumes are measured from the exhalation valve of a ventilator circuit, the compressed volume of the tubing circuit is also collected. Therefore, an estimation of the patient's exhaled volume can be made only by subtracting the amount of calculated compressed volume from the total collected at the exhalation valve. If the ventilator has a large amount of internal volume besides the volume of the external tubing circuit, there can be a discrepancy between the tidal volume set and the amount collected at the exhalation valve. Fig. 13-16 illustrates this point. In the example shown the internal volume is 2 ℓ, yielding a

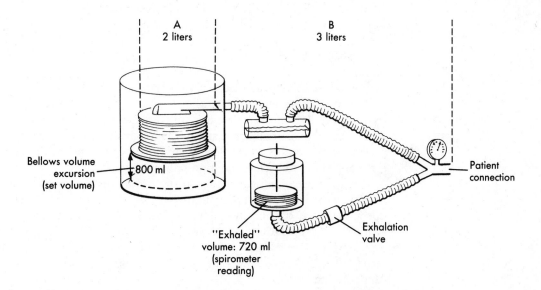

Fig. 13-16   Comparison of internal volume (**A**) and tubing volume (**B**) contributing to compressed volume with a volume-cycled ventilator. See text for description of this example.

factor of 2 ml/cm of water, and the tubing circuit is 3 ℓ with a factor then of 3 ml/cm of water. These two factors together mean 5 ml/cm of water pressure will be compressed and "lost" to the patient each breath. However, only the amount compressed in the external tubing (3 ml/cm of water) will be collected with the patient's exhaled gases because the internal system returns to atmospheric pressure while the bellows falls and refills. The one-way valve shown at the bellows outlet closes, and any compressed gases within simply expand. Thus, if end-inspiratory pressure is 40 cm of water, the set volume is 800 ml; then 80 ml is compressed internally (40 × 2), 120 ml is compressed externally (40 × 3), and the patient receives the remaining 600 ml. Only the patient's 600 ml and the tubing's 120 ml are *collected* during exhalation, while 80 ml remain in the bellows. The set volume of 800 ml differs then from the 720 ml collected because of the internal compressed gas. To determine what the *patient* received in this example from the *exhaled* gases, only the 3 ml/cm of water factor is subtracted from the *collected* amount on the spirometer.

From these examples we can see that a "volume ventilator" may not provide an absolute *constant* volume under all conditions. The physiologic changes that necessitate different pressures may also cause changes in gas exchange parameters such as V_D/V_T ratio and $\dot{V}/\dot{Q}$ matching. Because of these changes, even if our ventilator provided nearly the same overall ventilation against different pressure requirements, the resulting arterial blood gases could still vary. All these factors make it important to monitor exhaled volumes as well as physiologic parameters and to make ventilator adjustments accordingly, even with "volume ventilators."

Because volume ventilators cycle off when a set volume has been expelled from the machine regardless of whether the patient receives all or none of it, they do not compensate for leaks in the system.[8] These are often detected by low exhaled volumes or low inspiratory pressure alarm systems, either built into the ventilator or added to it.[7]

Pressure-cycled ventilation. To contrast volume ventilators, pressure-cycled ventilators terminate inspiration whenever their set pressure is reached, regardless of the volume delivered. This very fact causes these ventilators to be very susceptible to compliance and resistance changes.[8,43,44] Indeed, even if the patient simply begins to exhale actively or to become tense, the pressure will build abruptly and cycle inspiration prematurely.

Pressure-cycled ventilators can be successfully used, however, for selected patients when adequate supervision is provided by a qualified, knowledgeable operator who is continually at the bedside. Patients with normal lungs being ventilated postoperatively for brief periods, patients with stable chronic obstructive lung disease, and patients weaning from controlled ventilation can be managed on pressure-cycled ventilators with appropriate monitoring and other support systems.

Most pressure-cycled ventilators, such as the Bird Mark 7 and Mark 8 and the Bennett PR-1 and PR-2, have both limited pressures (50 to 60 cm of water) and limited flow rates (80 to 100 ℓ/min), and systems for PEEP and

CPAP are not available without special adaptations.[7] Oxygen concentrations with these ventilators can be controlled easily and accurately only with an oxygen blender specially attached. These limitations and the need for adding monitoring devices make pressure-cycled ventilators generally unsuitable for long-term use with patients with severe lung disease.

Bird and Bennett pressure-cycled ventilators generally provide a decelerating (tapering) flow pattern during inspiration.[3,7] This has the potential advantage of providing a decreased turbulence in the airway for the latter part of inspiration, and this may provide an increased distribution of air to airways of varying resistance compared to the square-wave flow pattern common to some volume ventilators. We have observed repeatedly that a specific volume can be delivered at a lesser pressure with these ventilators in postoperative patients than the same volume given with a volume ventilator that produces a square wave.

Under some circumstances pressure-cycled ventilators are better able to compensate for leaks than are volume ventilators,[8] but only if the leak is not so large that it prevents them from cycling off all together. Some models have leak-compensating controls that add gas flow to specifically accommodate the leak (e.g., Bennett PR-2, Bird Mark-14, and the Bird Ventilator).[7]

Because these ventilators are compact and lightweight they are sometimes used with transport systems, both in hospital as well as ground or air transport. They are also used in emergency rooms and as backup units to electrically powered volume ventilators in critical care areas in case of electrical failure. For these reasons it is vital that the therapists responsible for these areas of ventilatory support be thoroughly familiar with the function and application of these ventilators.

Time-cycled, pressure-limited ventilation

Time-cycled ventilation can have either or both volume and pressure change when changes in patient parameters occur, depending on certain features. Flow generators that are time cycled function as the volume ventilators described previously since both flow and time (and therefore volume) are constant. If a pressure relief valve is used as a pressure-limiting device during a timed inspiration, then both flow and volume received by the patient are subject to variables such as compliance and resistance changes. It is this latter type of ventilation system that is currently common in pediatric use, and it is described briefly here as time-cycled, pressure-limited ventilation.[7,15,45]

A common example of this type of ventilation is provided by the continuous flow–type ventilator. That is, a set flow rate continuously moves through the patient's tubing circuit, and spontaneous breathing efforts can be supplied by this fresh gas. Periodically, at preset time intervals, an exhalation valve is closed, and the continuous flow is diverted into the patient's airways. If the pressure limit is reached before inspiration time cycles off, then some or all of the flow begins to vent to atmosphere, and a pressure hold occurs (peak inflation hold).

The volume the patient receives depends *primarily* on two factors if the lung

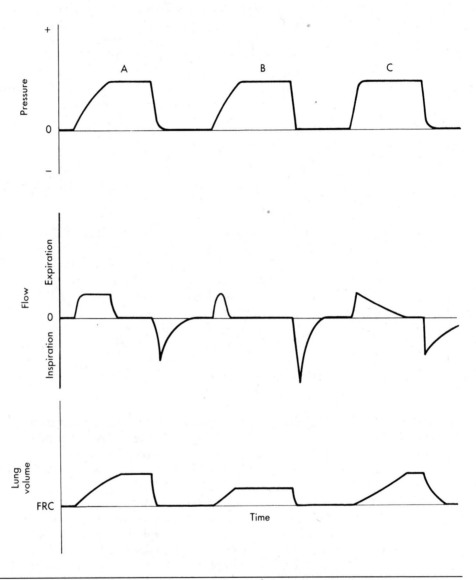

Fig. 13-17   Comparison of pressure, flow, and volume wave forms for time-cycled, pressure-limited ventilation with different patient conditions. **A** shows normal conditions while in **B** there is a decrease in compliance and **C** illustrates an increase in airways resistance. Inspiratory time is equal in **A, B,** and **C.** Note that **B** shows a decrease in volume due to a decrease in compliance. **C** shows the same volume as **A** but more time is required during inspiration to reach that volume in the lung due to the increased airways resistance.

pressure equilibrates with the pressure limit during inspiration: (1) the pressure applied and (2) the patient's lung-thorax compliance. As an example, if an infant has a compliance of 2 ml/cm of water and the pressure limit used is 20 cm of water, then the tidal volume reaching the lung will be 40 ml (2×20) assuming pressure equilibration occurs. If the same infant's compliance drops to 1 ml/cm of water, then the volume received from the same 20 cm of water of lung pressure will be only 20 ml. Because these small volumes are so difficult to measure, especially in a continuous flow system, this change in volume delivered would not be indicated by the ventilator itself. Measurements such as arterial blood gases would have to be used instead.

If the patient using such a system has an increase in airways resistance but the compliance remains unchanged, then volume received may or may not vary. Delivered volume will not change if there is sufficient inspiratory time for the lung pressure to equilibrate with the pressure generated at the airway (pressure limit). The length of time needed before pressure equilibration occurs is longer if airways resistance is increased and shorter if airways resistance is decreased. Fig. 13-17 illustrates these fundamental features of time-cycled, pressure-limited ventilation.

Pressure limits can be increased or decreased to control tidal volumes for patients with stable compliance and resistance parameters. Like pressure-cycled ventilation, monitoring of arterial blood gases and clinical parameters is of utmost importance in this type of ventilation. Details of pediatric ventilation systems can be found in other texts, and the interested student is encouraged to read them.[5,6,15,45]

Ventilation at high frequencies

Recently there has been substantial interest in ventilation systems that use frequencies of from 60 to 900 cycles/min or more.[46-51] Investigations began to appear in the literature with regularity about a decade ago, primarily in Scandinavian journals.[46,51,52] A tremendous interest has developed, exemplified by extensive references cited in two recent review articles[46,51] and by the number of papers presented on the subject at national meetings.[53-55] However, knowledge of these exciting methods of ventilatory support remains limited.[56,57] We introduce the reader to the subject based on some of the literature available and our own limited experience.[46-57]

Although often simply called *high-frequency ventilation* (HFV), there appear to be three general types of ventilation that can be distinguished somewhat from one another based mostly on the rates, volumes, and systems used.[51]

High-frequency positive-pressure ventilation (HFPPV) was introduced by Jonzon and Sjostrand[51,52] and has been used primarily with rates of about 60 to 100/min. Volumes per breath are less than normal tidal volumes, and total minute volume may be nearly the same or twice normal amounts.[51] This system uses a pneumatically controlled valve with a relatively high-pressure gas source to pulse gases down the airway while entraining some gases from a conditioned gas circuit.

High-frequency ventilation or *high-frequency jet ventilation* (HFJV) has been used, primarily with rates of about 100 to 200/min with volumes of from about one to three times predicted anatomic dead space. These systems often encorporate a jetlike system using a 14- to 18-gauge catheter and entrainment of humidified gases.[48,49,58]

High-frequency oscillation (HFO) has been classified as providing rates of over 200/min.[51] Some clinical experience has been reported with rates of 900/min (15 hertz [Hz]: 1 Hz = 60 cycles/min) for adults[49] and from 480 to 1200/min (8 to 20 Hz) for infants.[50] In these studies a sine-wave-producing piston was used to oscillate gases through an endotracheal tube. A source of fresh gas continually flows by the connection, and a resistant tubing is used on the outflow port to create PEEP and aid in creating pressures during oscillation. The volumes used here are somewhat unknown since much of the gas exits through the outflow port during oscillations. However, the volumes reaching the patient per stroke are believed to be less than the predicted anatomic dead space.

It is believed that these high-frequency systems can aid in ventilating patients because of a reduced peak airway pressure, less risk of barotrauma, and decreased or at least similar cardiovascular side effects as compared to conventional mechanical ventilation. There is disagreement about some specific effects of using the high rates, such as how spontaneous breathing efforts are influenced. Some investigators find their systems suppressing spontaneous breathing efforts while others claim there is no interference.[47,49-51,58]

In all these systems, the compressible volume of the system must be kept to a minimum in order to effect proper control of pressure and flow characteristics.[51] The use of conventional mechanical ventilators at an increased breathing rate is *not* the same as the HFPPV, HFJV, and HFO systems described.[51] Although one study of neonates has been published using rates of 80 to 110 with conventional ventilator systems with some success,[59] this should not be confused with these other systems since the mechanisms of ventilatory support may well be different.

Exactly how ventilation at very high frequencies and small volumes maintains adequate gas exchange is not well understood at present.[56,57] It may be that with HFPPV and HFJV systems as currently used, ventilation may occur in a convective manner, similar to conventional ventilation, as well as by an enhancement of gas diffusion within the airways.[51] HFO is thought to primarily enhance gas diffusivity since bulk flow is assumed to be very small.[49,50,60] The differences in the technical apparatus and application of the variety of systems being used experimentally[54,55] make comparisons difficult at best at this time. Still, oxygenation tends to be regulated by PEEP and mean airway pressure while carbon dioxide elimination is affected by the rate and jet pressures (which affect volume), so in this respect at least high-frequency systems are similar to conventional methods.[46-51]

Ventilation at high frequencies appears to hold promise as at least another adjunct in our armamentarium of methods to treat respiratory failure, maintain ventilation under severe circumstances such as bronchopleural fistulas, and decrease the harmful effects of suctioning.[46-58] Much more is left to discover with these systems, and we encourage the reader to follow upcoming reports in the literature and at meetings.

<table>
<tr><td>

Negative-pressure ventilation

</td><td>

The exponent of the negative-pressure ventilation method is the time-honored body tank ventilator, known for so long as the "iron lung."* First described in 1929, the tank ventilator saw widespread, lifesaving use through many poliomyelitis epidemics.[61] The body ventilator is an airtight cylinder that accommodates the patient up to the neck, leaving the head exposed to atmosphere. At the opposite end, or underneath the tank, is a large bellows powered by an electric motor, with a handle for manual operation in the event of electrical failure. Expansion of the bellows creates an intracylinder negative pressure, the magnitude of which is indicated by a pressure gauge calibrated in centimeters of water. Under the influence of the pressure gradient between the interior of the ventilator and the atmosphere, air flows into the patient's lungs, and subatmospheric pressures of up to 15 cm of water are frequently employed.

</td></tr>
</table>

This ventilator has the advantages of ruggedness and durability and relative ease of operation. However, it has many disadvantages and in most institutions has been replaced by equipment of more recent design. The unit is large and cumbersome, requiring considerable space to compensate not only for its physical size but also for its operational noise. From both nursing and medical viewpoints it makes patient care difficult and awkward. Patients ill enough to require ventilator care generally need much personal attention, and yet they are isolated from their surroundings, accessible only through arm ports in the wall of the tank or by being removed from the machine for hurried care. Monitoring of physiologic functions and the administration of intravenous infusions are done under handicaps. Even more important than these inconveniences is the inflexibility of the tank ventilator's function. It is a controller with an adjustable negative pressure that moves the thorax at set, predetermined intervals, with no provisions for patients to use whatever spontaneous ventilation they may possess. There is no way of controlling or regulating flows—a feature that is less important in ventilating patients with normal lungs, such as those with poliomyelitis (with whom the tank had its initial experience), than it is in ventilating the larger number of patients who are disabled with obstructive pulmonary disease. In the latter, flow control may be critical to successful ventilation. As a generalization, a patient in ventilatory failure, but with normal airways and lungs (neuromuscular or central nervous system disease), can usually be ventilated adequately with any of the standard ventilators now available. It is the patient with obstructive or restrictive pulmonary disease who presents the greatest maintenance problems. Finally, the negative pressure by which the tank respirator functions can, itself, be a hazard to the patient. The negative pressure is applied not only to the semirigid

*Drinker-Collins respirator, Warren E. Collins Co., Boston, Mass.

thorax but also to the much more pliant abdomen and is, accordingly, transmitted to the abdominal cavity. Here it tends to cause the venous blood on its return to the right atrium to pool in the large vascular abdominal reservoirs, with a resulting decrease in venous return and cardiac output. The so-called tank shock was not an uncommon complication, as peripheral vascular collapse followed the interference with cardiovascular dynamics. This effect is dealt with in a little more detail, later in this section, in relation to the physiology of positive-pressure breathing.

In an attempt to retain the benefits of negative-pressure ventilation while minimizing the disadvantages of the large tank respirator, the *cuirass*, a shield-like appliance, was developed. Basically, this consists of a rigid shell (available in a number of sizes) with its edges designed to conform to the lateral surfaces of the thorax, base of the neck, and hip-pubic area. From the top of the shell a flexible hose leads to an electric pump. In operation the cuirass functions as does the full body respirator, but the negative pressure is confined mostly to the thorax, avoiding the undesirable effect on the abdomen as described above. At the same time, however, it is less efficient than the tank; and with its own inherent deficiencies, it cannot be relied on to give the support to an apneic patient that is possible with the larger unit. It is frequently difficult to effect the necessary close fit of the shell to the great variety of body contours, and unless it is applied properly, it is undependable. A loose contact between patient and shell not only reduces the available ventilating pressure but can also produce serious chafing of the skin. Like the tank ventilator the cuirass is a controller, and it can "assist" only if its cycling pattern can be adjusted exactly to the patient's spontaneous breathing, although this is not true assisted ventilation by our definition. The main use of the chest respirator, as it is commonly called, is to wean a patient from the body tank. This was especially helpful in the treatment of poliomyelitis, since it allowed access to the patient's extremities for the much needed physical therapy of that disease. Many patients with residual, permanent, partial paralysis of the respiratory muscles who could function adequately during their waking hours have used the chest ventilator regularly on retiring to prevent the occurrence of hypoventilation during sleep.

Although use of the cuirass, along with that of the body ventilator, has declined, an improvement in design has made available a chest ventilator that is an assistor as well as a controller.* Instead of the heavy and rigid chest piece of the original style, the new model uses a lightweight fenestrated plastic shell that sits loosely over the patient's trunk, with no close skin contact. An airtight seal is achieved by a plastic wrapping that encloses the shell and the patient's back and is snugly applied around the legs. A vacuum cleaner–type power unit supplies the negative pressure and can be adjusted for various settings of the control mode. The major feature, however, is a triggering device that permits the patient to initiate the powered inspiratory phase of ven-

*U-Cyclit chest respirator, J.H. Emerson Co., Cambridge, Mass.

tilation at his or her own rate and to support his or her own voluntary breathing. An electronic sensor, attached in front of the patient's nostril, responds with high sensitivity to the slight airflow of the start of the patient's spontaneous inspiration and activates the respirator to assist the rest of inspiration.

We can summarize the status of the negative-pressure ventilators by making a few final comments about the group as a whole. Then in Chapter 14 we discuss details of the use of *intubation* of the airway in mechanical ventilation, which entails passing a tube through the mouth and larynx into the trachea or through a surgical opening beneath the larynx directly into the trachea. This is a procedure usually necessary for the application of positive-pressure ventilators but is not ordinarily required for negative-pressure ventilators. The ability to ventilate a patient without the need for intubation is certainly an advantage in favor of the negative-pressure machines, but it is an advantage that must be viewed with some reservation. First, patients with chronic bronchopulmonary disease in ventilatory failure need frequent aspiration of secretions, done most effectively through an airway. Second, many patients in failure without pulmonary disease, in whom pathologic secretions are not a problem, may have paralyzed or obtunded epiglottal reflexes, and normal oral secretions may pool in the mouth or hypopharynx. In such instances the strong inspiratory suction of a negative-pressure ventilator may draw these fluids into the bronchial tree, with resulting atelectasis or pulmonary infection. Intubation is usually necessary to prevent such complications.

In addition to the problems of size and patient isolation posed by the negative-pressure machines, the much greater versatility of the positive-pressure generators has placed these machines in the foreground of the therapy of ventilatory failure. The original indication for the big tanks was the large number of patients with bulbar, or respiratory paralytic, poliomyelitis, but effective prophylactic medicine has reduced the incidence of this disease to a negligible quantity. At the same time there has been a steady increase in the number of patients with failure caused by airway obstructive disease, and in this group the negative-pressure ventilators are generally less effective than the positive. Nonetheless, because there are some patients who can benefit from the use of negative-pressure support of their ventilation, and especially if the avoidance of intubation is felt to be advisable for some valid reason, ventilators of this group should be available in hospitals with a heavy load of respiratory care patients.

Physiologic effects of mechanical ventilation   Mechanical ventilation cannot be used either safely or effectively until those responsible for it are knowledgeable in its effect on the physiology as well as proficient in its mechanics. When artificially ventilating a patient, we deliberately attempt to change a physiologic condition, hopefully from a poor to an improved status; but we are nonetheless interfering with a level of function, even if that function is pathologic. It is vital that we know what effect our therapy is likely to have on the patient, not only in terms of the objectives we are trying to achieve but also, equally as important, in terms of the effect on organs or systems not directly related to the primary disease and in terms of unwanted adverse sequelae. It is a safe generalization to state that a form of treatment potent enough to alter or correct the progress of a disease is most apt to have some accompanying side effects that may be undesirable. We have already noted with emphasis the caution needed in the administration of oxygen and now consider the physiologic responses, good and bad, to mechanical ventilation. The comments that follow apply primarily to positive-pressure breathing, except where otherwise noted. For convenience, we discuss separately the effects on *ventilation, circulation,* and *metabolism.*

Effects on ventilation

With properly applied assisted mechanical ventilation we can generally expect an improvement in total ventilation, manifested by an increased minute breathing volume, improved alveolar ventilation, an increased distribution of inspired gas resulting from an increased tidal volume, a normalization of blood gases, and a reduction in the patient's work of breathing. It should be apparent to the student that these responses are interrelated and depend on one another but that the degree to which any given one is favorably affected will be determined by the underlying disease and the effectiveness of the ventilator. It is most usual to expect an increase in minute volume and tidal volume, which are dynamic compartments of the total lung volumes, whereas changes in static volumes, the functional residual capacity and the residual volume, are more variable, depending on the bronchopulmonary condition.[62] Theoretically, all five of the functions noted above should be improved or stimulated by mechanical assistance, and if they are not, the cause will be one of the following: (1) The respiratory tract may present a severity of obstruction or a reduction in compliance beyond the ability of the ventilator to surmount. We have described enough of the principles and characteristics of ventilators for the student to accept the fact that such instruments are too severely limited in both scope and flexibility to compensate for all types of failure. (2) Most instances of inadequate mechanical ventilation in daily hospital practice are the result of the wrong choice of instrument for a given circumstance or improper technique in its administration. Both of these responsibilities require in-depth experience in assisted ventilation but are critical to successful therapy. It can be assumed as obvious now that the beneficial effects of mechanical ventilation can be realized only when consideration is given to the establishment of breathing rates and the use of flows consistent with the conducting potential of the airways, coordinated with just the proper delivery pressure. If the student looks into the growth history of positive-pressure breathing, he or she will encounter strong opposing views of its efficacy and safety, especially reported during its early years of use. There is little doubt, in retrospect, that many of the unfavorable opinions originated from failure to achieve satisfactory ventilation because the disease was untreatable with available equipment, the equipment was ill chosen, or especially because the equipment was not effectively used.

The relationship between the distribution of inspired gas in the lung, alveolar ventilation, and the correction of abnormal blood gases and pH is apparent, and in these areas positive-pressure breathing performs some of its most important functions. For the overall stabilization of ventilation, it is not enough merely to increase the gas flow to alveoli already ventilated if there are alveoli persistently nonventilated. A major contribution of PPB is its ability to effect a more normal and uniform distribution of inspired gas to all lung areas by opening up to gas exchange lobules and other pulmonary units that have been nonparticipating. This claim for PPB is made notwithstanding some opinions to the contrary. A study was made of voluntary hyperventilation and IPPB in normal subjects and patients with emphysema.[62] In the normal subjects essentially equal increases in tidal volume were recorded during both hyperventilation and PPB assist, but in the patient group the increase in tidal volume was significantly greater with mechanical aid. In all subjects experiencing an increase in tidal volume, alveolar distribution of air was improved as measured by the nitrogen-washout test, and it is interesting to note that this distribution was improved in patients who could not hyperventilate spontaneously but needed the PPB assistance. In more precise physiologic terms there was an implied improvement in the ventilation/perfusion ratio. On the other hand, another group of patients was reported to show increases in alveolar-arterial oxygen tension differences during positive-pressure breathing.[63] This suggested that the inspired air was not normally distributed among the alveoli in relation to the alveolar perfusion. It was concluded that, since emphysema is characterized by an abnormal $\dot{V}/Q$, PPB might not be expected to improve this relationship in lungs so diseased. However, in comparing divergent results, it is often difficult, if not impossible, to determine how uniform were the techniques employed; unless comparable equipment is used and close attention given to rates, flows, and pressures, comparison is on shaky ground. Many years of clinical observation substantiate the view that an improved $\dot{A}/Q$ ratio incidental to better alveolar distribution of inspired gas is a significant result of properly applied PPB.

Thus improvement in alveolar ventilation, the major objective of the therapy of respiratory failure, coincides with bettering the $\dot{V}/Q$ ratio. More effective alveolar ventilation is evidenced by a decrease in arterial blood carbon dioxide tension and an elevation of arterial blood pH. It must be noted that the effect of PPB on carbon dioxide and pH, well documented and universally accepted, does not necessarily depend on its ability to expand the general distribution of inspired gas, discussed above. Such changes may be accomplished by the hyperventilation of existing functioning alveoli, taking advantage of the easy diffusibility of carbon dioxide. However, it has been aptly demonstrated that not only does PPB decrease the carbon dioxide but it also elevates the arterial blood oxygen tension of hypoxia, even when ambient air is the source gas without added oxygen.[64,65] This was taken as evidence of an increased uniformity of alveolar ventilation and an improved $\dot{V}/Q$ ratio.

Last, but by no means least, an important physiologic service of positive-pressure breathing is a significant reduction in the work energy expended by patients in labored breathing. The respiratory therapist will frequently see the gratifying physical relaxation enjoyed by patients as a mechanical ventilator assumes a major portion of their work. This response to assisted ventilation not rarely is sought to prevent patients, still compensating, from slipping into failure from the cumulative effect of respiratory fatigue. Again, it must be strongly emphasized that merely subjecting patients to mechanical ventilation does not ensure them relief from their struggle to breathe, since unless properly administered, ventilatory "assistance" may seriously handicap them further. Obviously, to aid patients and lessen their work, ventilation must be adequate for their needs. Although this may appear to be so basic as to be redundant, it is an aspect that must be carefully considered to prevent the spontaneously breathing patient from "fighting" the machine. Unless the ventilator can deliver inspired air rapidly enough, the patient will work harder to augment the gas from the instrument, and if flows are too rapid or forceful, the patient may oppose the gas with expiratory efforts. It has been noted that with pressures in excess of 25 cm of water, and with unadjusted flows, alveolar hypoventilation may persist, and the resulting struggle of the patient to get air can increase the work of breathing 250% without benefit.[66] An excellent investigation into the work of breathing explains how effective ventilation helps the patient.[63] It will be recalled that carbon dioxide is metabolically produced by contraction of muscles, including the muscles of ventilation. Indeed, in severe respiratory disability, the energy of all the muscles brought into use to move tidal air may account for a major portion of the carbon dioxide production as well as the oxygen utilization. In short, most of the patient's work may go into driving the machinery that supplies the body's energy fuel, leaving little for other activities. Also relevant to the discussion is the note that the more efficient a muscle is, the less carbon dioxide it produces per unit of work performed compared with a less efficient muscle.

The level of arterial carbon dioxide tension is dependent on both the production of carbon dioxide by the body and the effectiveness of alveolar ventilation and can be expressed in the following proportionality:

$$Pa_{CO_2} \cong \frac{\dot{V}_{CO_2}}{\dot{V}_A}$$

Reduction in the carbon dioxide tension is thus the result of increasing the alveolar ventilation or limiting the carbon dioxide production. In severe airway obstructive disease voluntary hyperventilation is not apt to decrease the arterial carbon dioxide tension significantly because the uneven alveolar ventilation accompanying obstruction prevents the deep breathing from improving the alveolar ventilation. If, by a strenuous effort, the patient is able to effect a better alveolar ventilation, the work involved will increase the carbon dioxide production simultaneously to maintain the same general production in the above equation. It has been determined that the muscles of respiration use one-third less oxygen when passively moved; and thus positive-pressure ventilation increases the alveolar gas exchange, with less patient work, and without raising the carbon dioxide production.

The following list summarizes the potential effects of mechanical ventilation on ventilation:

1. Increased total minute ventilation
2. Increased alveolar ventilation
3. Increased distribution of gases with increased volumes
4. Normalization of blood gases
5. Reduction in work of breathing

Effects on circulation

With the close functional and anatomic relationship between the respiratory and circulatory systems, it is not surprising that interference with the performance of one of them will affect the other. The great potential hazard of circulatory response to mechanical ventilation makes it mandatory for the therapist to understand fully what does and can happen to cardiovascular function when a patient is artificially ventilated.

In our study of the physiology of ventilation, we learned that ventilatory muscle contraction expands the diameters of the thorax, lowering the intrathoracic pressure so that ambient air flows into the lung. The pressure within the thoracic cavity is never above atmospheric with quiet breathing but, rather, is slightly below even at the resting level, and it exceeds atmospheric only during forced exhalation as the expiratory reserve volume is moved. This is illustrated in the ballon-in-box sketches of Fig. 4-6, which depict the fluctuations of intrathoracic pressure from its average resting value of about −5 cm of water, with ventilatory excursions. The cardiovascular system is designed to function with its central power source, the heart, in a subatmospheric pressure, and as noted in Chapter 7, the "thoracic pump" is necessary for venous return to the heart and for an adequate cardiac output. Thus airflow into and out of the lungs and the circulation of blood to and from the heart are both accom-

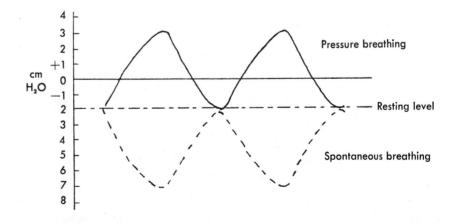

Fig. 13-18   Comparison of *intrathoracic pressure* in positive pressure and spontaneous tidal ventilation with driving pressures of 5 cm of water.

plished most efficiently when the ventilatory cycle starts with a subatmospheric pressure that increases in negativity during inhalation and decreases during exhalation but never exceeds atmospheric except under conditions of stress. Obviously, this normal intrathoracic pressure environment is reversed when positive-pressure ventilation is employed, as inspiratory gas under pressure inflates the lung, raising the intrapulmonary pressure, which is then transmitted through the lung into the pleural "space" to elevate the intrathoracic pressure during inhalation. Passive exhalation returns the pressure to its resting subatmospheric level, as the patient exhales into the ambient atmosphere, and in a functional sense is temporarily disassociated from the machine. Fig. 13-18 is a schematic example of two sets of tidal volume curves, comparing the pressure relationships between normal spontaneous breathing and pressure ventilation. Here the resting level of voluntary ventilation is shown as -2 cm of water, and as air enters the lung, the pressure drops to -7 cm of water, a net pressure change of 5 cm of water; but the pressure at all points is below atmospheric. In contrast, the pressure-ventilated lung starts its cycle from the same resting level of -2 cm of water intrathoracic pressure, but as air is forced into the lung a driving pressure of 5 cm of water is transmitted through the alveoli to the pleural space, raising the intrathoracic pressure to 3 cm of water at end-inspiration. Here several points along the pressure curve are above atmospheric.

For completeness a differentiation should be made here between intraalveolar and intrathoracic pressure fluctuations. As long as the airways are open in unassisted breathing, alveolar pressure immediately equilibrates with atmospheric whenever airflow stops. Thus at the two points of no flow, resting end-expiration (preinspiration) and end-inspiration, intraalveolar pressure is

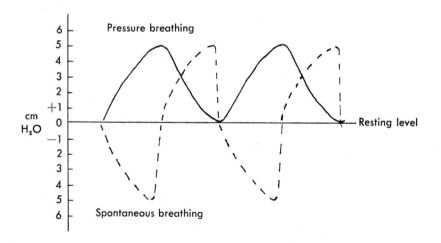

Fig. 13-19   Comparison of *intraalveolar pressure* in positive pressure and spontaneous tidal ventilation with driving pressures of 5 cm of water.

zero gauge. With pressure breathing, positive pressure is maintained in the alveoli from the start of inspiration until the end-expiratory level is again reached. Fig. 13-19 compares alveolar pressures in these two circumstances.

The significance of intrathoracic pressure deviations in their effect on cardiovascular function is one of the most important clinical aspects of mechanical ventilation. During all phases of normal or abnormal pulmonary airflow, those elements of the circulatory system that are located in the thorax, especially the heart and large veins, are subjected to the ambient pressure generated in the thorax, so let us describe details of the circulatory response to both normal and pressure ventilation. The fall in intrathoracic pressure that accompanies a normal spontaneous inspiration enhances the flow of venous blood to the thoracic vessels and hence into the right atrium, increasing the right ventricular output and flow to the lungs. Temporarily, less blood moves from the lungs to the left atrium as the intrathoracic negative pressure fills up the pulmonary vessels, and left ventricular output falls. During passive exhalation, the events are reversed as the increasing (although still subatmospheric) intrathoracic pressure dampens venous return and right atrial filling and output but, at the same time, in a sense, squeezing blood from the pulmonary vessels to increase left atrial filling and left ventricular output. When the lung is ventilated under positive pressure venous return, right atrial filling, and pulmonary blood flow are impaired; but the pressure squeezing the lung, now during inspiration, increases left heart filling and output. However, this lasts for but a few heart strokes, and if the pressure is continued, flow to and from the left heart falls. Exhalation lets the intrathoracic pressure return to normal, encouraging venous return and an increase in pulmonary flow but retarding left ventricular output.

Let us compare these sequences in natural and pressure breathing. During normal spontaneous ventilation, the fluctuations in intrathoracic blood flow are rhythmically synchronized with the breathing pattern, a decrease in one component during inhalation increasing during exhalation, and so on. Thus, whereas venous return accelerates in inhalation and left ventricular output falls, both are reversed in exhalation; the net result, cycle after cycle, is a smooth-flowing circulation. The same description can be given of pressure breathing, with the time sequences of the kinetics turned about, but the efficiency of the net result is markedly modified by one significant factor—supraatmospheric pressure. Several excellent studies have clarified the effect of positive pressure on circulation to explain why such pressure interferes with cardiac function, and we consider the relevant data here.[67-72]

It is necessary to understand the concepts of *mean pressure* and the *pressure-time relationship,* since they are the keys to the problem. Fig. 13-20, *A,* is a biphasic sinelike curve, plotting positive and negative pressures against arbitrary units of time, first traveling from its starting point to a peak pressure of 20 and back to zero pressure in 5 time units, then dropping to -20 units of pressure and back in another 5 time units. For the first 5 time units, positive pressure is being exerted, and for the last 5, negative pressure of the same

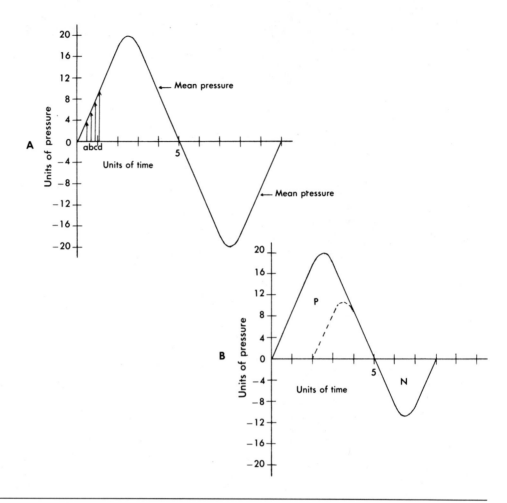

Fig. 13-20 Illustrations of the concept of mean pressure and the relationship between pressure and time: **A,** sketch of a sine curve; **B,** asymmetric biphasic curve. (See text for description.)

magnitude. As we look at the curve, our common sense tells us that the net or final result of these two opposing pressures will be to negate one another, since they will average out to zero. The *mean* pressure of the entire cycle then will be zero, since mean is an arithmetic average. Each half of the curve has its own mean pressure, which is easy to visualize because of the regularity of the curve, but this is not so in curves with changing contours. The mean value of any curve is the average of an infinite number of points along the curve (*a, b, c, d,* etc., in Fig. 13-20, *A*), and although we cannot measure an infinite number of values, the more that are measured, the more accurate will be the calculation. In practice, the calculation of the mean of an irregular curve is done by methods of mathematic calculus or with accurate and rapid electronic calculators, necessary instruments in the modern laboratory. It is obvious in our illustration that the mean pressure of the terminal half of the curve is the same as that of the first but with the opposite sign. If we refer back to Fig. 13-18, we can see that the mean pressure of the upper, positive ventilatory pattern is 0.5 cm of water, whereas that of natural breathing is −4.5 cm of water (the resting level is already at −2 cm of water). The *pressure-time relationship* is the length of time that a pressure is active and refers to the duration of a mean pressure. For example, in the first half of Fig. 13-20, *A,* the pressure continuously changes from time 0 to time 5, but it represents a mean pressure of 10, for 5 time units; and the second half of the curve represents a mean of −10 units of pressure for another 5 units of time. The same interpretations can be derived for the tidal excursions of Fig. 13-18.

It may be evident at this stage that whatever effect pressure will have on circulation will be directly related to the mean pressure to which the circulation is exposed and to the time of this exposure or, in other words, the pressure-time effect. In ventilation the time interval is the duration of the respiratory cycle, or its components, and the pressure is the intrathoracic, which in clinical practice must be measured indirectly. It was noted in the earlier discussion of the lung-thorax relation and compliance that to avoid the risks of a direct measurement of intrathoracic pressure, esophageal pressure is often used, since it reflects changes within the chest, but the student will frequently see reference to *mask pressure* and *mouth pressure* in relation to the kinetics of mechanical ventilation. They refer to the pressure of the ventilating gas as measured at the subject's mouth or administering appliance or the pressure in the trachea of patients who have been intubated. Although the mask pressure is not quantitatively the same as the intrathoracic pressure, the mean values of both are linearly related and thus can be used interchangeably to monitor qualitative changes. When using mask or mouth pressures, the student should remember that the end-expiratory level will be at zero gauge, not subatmospheric.

In Fig. 13-20, *B,* let us consider the positive segment to represent the pressure-time curve of a positive-pressure ventilator generating an arbitrary maximum mask pressure over a 5-unit time period. Regardless of what the mean pressure might be, in a general way the area under the curve *(P)* can be thought of as proportional to the pressure-time effect of the ventilatory pattern, since it represents the total pressure for the total time. The larger the area under a given pressure curve, the greater potential effect it will have on circulation. Let us now imagine a subatmospheric pressure applied to the patient's airway during exhalation that lowers the mask pressure as indicated by the last part of the curve, enclosing pressure-time area *(N).* The net circulatory effect of the pressure over the entire cycle will be proportional to the difference between the areas *P* and *N,* graphically depicted by superimposing *N* on *P,* with the dotted outline. The mean mask pressure for the whole ventilatory cycle has been lowered by the addition of terminal negative pressure, proportionately reducing the effect on circulation that would be expected from the original pressure.

At this point we might pause and summarize our information on the circulatory response to positive intrathoracic pressure. We can say that the determining factor is the relation between the height of the mean intrathoracic (or mask) pressure and the duration of pressure, and we know that the total mean cycle pressure can be kept low by the addition of negative mask pressure during exhalation. In the above description of the circulatory sequences through the natural or pressure-generated ventilatory cycle, we noted the different effects on right and left hearts, depending on the respiratory phase.

However, the picture can be simplified and the "meat" of the matter illustrated in its crudest form as shown in Fig. 13-21, which demonstrates the basic relationship between intrathoracic pressure and the circulation. The thorax is represented by a box with a gas inlet, containing the heart and major vessels. To avoid clutter in the illustration, the lungs are not included, although this does not imply that they play no role. It is assumed, however, that whatever pressure is delivered to the lungs is readily and fully transmitted to the thoracic cavity. Exceptions to this assumption will be noted later. Both

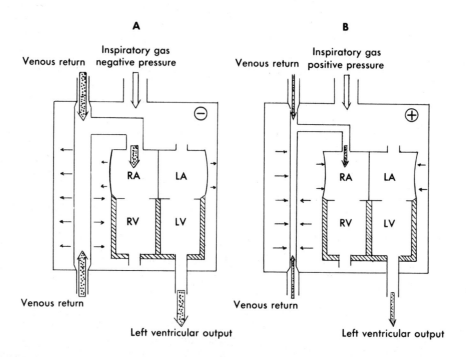

Fig. 13-21   Relationship between intrathoracic pressure and cardiac output in, **A,** negative-pressure and, **B,** positive-pressure breathing. (Details are explained in the text.)

diagrams depict inhalation *(A)* during natural spontaneous breathing and *(B)* during positive-pressure ventilation. Despite the circulatory fluctuations during each ventilatory cycle, the mean intrathoracic pressure of natural breathing is subatmospheric; thus the net pressure effect on blood flow is that of low pressure. This is indicated by the negative sign within the chest cavity and the effect of this *mean negativity* on circulation. Venous return is enhanced, and the negative pressure is shown as dilating the intrathoracic veins and encouraging filling of the atria. In contrast, positive-pressure inhalation produces a higher, or relatively positive, mean intrathoracic pressure, the net circulatory effect of which is just the opposite of natural breathing. The *mean positivity* in the chest depresses venous return by blocking its flow into the thoracic veins. The student is encouraged to consider the conditions demonstrated in Fig. 13-21, *A,* as the normal status, the natural environment in which the heart and supporting vessels developed and grew. In this environment the circulatory dynamics of both inspiration and expiration are such that the body's needs are most efficiently met. It is not so much that the mean negative pressure of spontaneous breathing excessively encourages venous return and a subsequent increase above normal of left ventricular output as it is that *deviations* from the normal mean intrathoracic pressure adversely affect the circulatory efficiency. Therefore, in the positive-pressure breathing of Fig. 13-21, *B,* regardless of whether the left heart filling and output may be temporarily increased by the rising pressure in the thorax, the net effect of subjecting the heart and its tributary veins to an abnormally high mean pressure is to impede venous return and to reduce the arterial blood supplied to the systemic circulation.

When venous blood flows toward the heart from the peripheral areas of the body and encounters an abnormally high pressure as it attempts to enter the thoracic vessels, portions of it will pool in vascular reservoirs, mostly in the huge network of veins and capillaries of the abdominal organs.[73] This can effectively remove from circulation a volume of blood large enough to reduce the left ventricular output, as noted above, and constitute a serious potential danger to the hypoxic patient by reducing cerebral blood flow and further compromising the oxygen supply to the brain. Lesser degrees of the effect of excessively high intrathoracic pressure on cerebral blood flow can be demonstrated in the normal subject by voluntary breath holding at end-inspiration while exerting a strong expiratory effort against the closed glottis. Impaired venous return is manifested by distended neck veins, suffusion of the facial skin, and eventual loss of consciousness or at least faintness. In the mechanically ventilated patient, continued interference with venous return and left ventricular output can lead to a full-blown state of clinical shock, with all the signs and symptoms described for this condition earlier. When precipitated by mechanical ventilation, such vascular collapse is termed *respirator shock.*

So far we have been concerned only with the mechanisms responsible for the physiologic influence of intrathoracic pressure on the circulation, but let us now see how important all of this is in clinical medicine to which the respiratory therapist is exposed. Data from the references cited at the beginning of this discussion, as well as from the observations of those who have managed patients under mechanical ventilation, attest to the reality of this phenomenon. When the mean mask delivery pressure exceeds 7 cm of water, there is a measurable decrease in the left ventricular output, although it need not be clinically evident.[67] In relaxed patients without specific bronchopulmonary disease who were ventilated at a fixed tidal volume and rate, measurement of the mean intrathoracic pressure showed an elevation above normal, ranging from 3.5 to 6 cm of water.[68] The degree to which circulation is impaired and the risk there is in store for the patient are dependent on three modifying factors in addition to the level of pressure.

Cardiac status. The integrity of the heart and circulatory system is an important influence on the effect of an increased intrathoracic pressure. As noted above, even small pressures interfere with cardiac output, and it can be anticipated that anyone subjected to pressure will be so affected. However, the normal healthy heart has a great functional reserve and can tolerate considerable resistance to its action. There is no rule to follow to estimate the risk of circulatory depression from pressure breathing, and the large majority of patients so treated suffer no apparent ill effects. Some have been supported on positive-pressure ventilation for several consecutive weeks without evidence of a compromised circulation. There is no doubt that the patient with overt or potential cardiac disease is a high-risk candidate for trouble. Part of the management of the ventilated patient is a close surveillance of his or her cardiac condition, with appropriate measures taken to support a failing heart so that the needed ventilation can be carried out. Certainly, a circulatory complication might be considered a more likely possibility in an elderly patient than in a young one or in a patient with long-standing pulmonary disease than in one with a new, acute disease. It is this varying response of each individual and the uncertainty of his or her reaction to the pressure of mechanical ventilation that make skillful and intelligent management the keys to successful therapy.

Pulmonary status. Positive pressure generated in a ventilator flows into the alveoli and from there is transmitted across alveolar walls to the thoracic cavity. The ease and the degree to which such transpulmonary transmission of pressure occurs are a function of the physical state of the lung. The more compliant the lung, the more readily will intrapulmonary pressure carry into the thorax, since the flexible lung easily responds to pressure applied to it. The patient with normal bronchi and lungs who needs mechanical ventilation for nonpulmonary hypoventilation is the most likely to demonstrate circulatory interference, a risk greatly enhanced, of course, by concomitant heart disease. In contrast, the patient whose disease has left the lung relatively stiff, with significant loss of compliance, is least likely to transmit intrapulmonary pressure to the thoracic cavity. His or her lungs can tolerate high positive pressures and need such force to move an adequate tidal volume of air. However, such a patient is not free of hazard, since the pressure needed to distend the alveoli also compresses the pulmonary capillaries embedded in alveolar walls, impedes blood flow, and stresses the right ventricle with increased resistance. On the other hand, should the compliance of the chest wall rather than the lung be reduced, there will be a rapid transmission of pressure to the thorax as expansion of the latter is limited. Perhaps the therapist can visualize the difficulty in ventilating a patient with basically normal lungs but whose chest wall is partially immobilized by pain or injury or even extensive postoperative dressings. The compliant lungs and noncompliant rib cage will combine to generate the maximum intrathoracic pressure for any given mask pressure. Finally, allied to the reduced chest wall compliance just described is the resistance to ventilation of the agitated or unrelaxed patient who may have no intrinsic thoracic disability. Patients who "fight" the instrument because poor technique denies them an adequate flow or who are wittingly or otherwise uncooperative will have increased transmission of intrapulmonary pressure. Their muscular activity prevents the necessary chest wall (and diaphragmatic) flexibility for compliant submission to a developing intrathoracic pressure.

Ventilatory pattern. The pattern by which positive-pressured air is delivered to a patient incorporates the concept of the pressure-time effect but applies it to the practical use of mechanical ventilation. Attention was drawn to the importance of pattern when it was observed that a rise in intrathoracic pressure during positive-pressure breathing could be kept minimal if the inspiratory phase was limited to no more than one-third the total cycle time. When we now relate pressure and time to the physiologic process of ventilation, the matter is not as simple as our definition and graphic representation of peak and mean pressures, and it becomes evident that an effective ventilatory pressure-time pattern must be more complex than those used in Fig. 13-20.

The immediate effect of elevated intrathoracic pressure is to interfere with right atrial filling and subsequently to reduce left ventricular output. Thus each atrial diastole is a point of time during which pressure may exert its influence on venous return, and there is another important relationship to consider, that between cardiac rate and the pressure-time curve. Fig. 13-22 is designed to

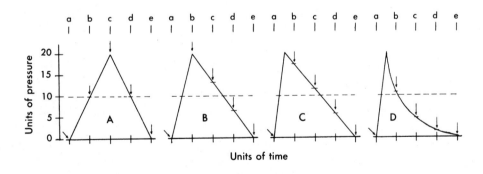

Fig. 13-22   Diagrams illustrating the effect of the relationship between cardiac diastoles and the intrathoracic pressure curve of positive-pressure breathing on the resulting mean pressures affecting cardiac output. (See text for details.)

demonstrate the potential differences in cardiac response to various combinations of the cardiac rhythm and pressure. The vertical bars at the top of the sketches indicate the times of atrial diastole in a heart with a rate of 60 beats/min, the small arrows showing where each atrial diastole falls in the ventilatory cycle. For the sake of comparative uniformity the oblique first arrow represents the last atrial diastole of the previous ventilatory cycle; thus each cycle is correlated with four diastoles. Generation and degeneration of pressure follow linear paths in the three triangular ventilatory patterns of *A*, *B*, and *C*, and the mean pressure of each is necessarily 10 units, since the range is from 0 to 20 units. In curve *A* the final mean pressure affecting the four diastoles is the same as that of the total cycle, that is, 10 units, and even though inspiratory time is reduced in *B*, the pressure mean of the points of diastole is unchanged. Because of the relationship between the heart rhythm and ventilatory time intervals, the student who remembers geometry can see that the diastolic pressure means in both these sketches must be identical. A further, sharp reduction in the inspiratory time of *C*, however, changes the diastole-pressure relation, and the mean of the pressures coinciding with the diastoles has here dropped to 8 units. Careful examination of these illustrations should make it apparent that when diastole occurs with the peak pressure, the mean will be the same as the mean of the cycle. This clear-cut relationship is easy to see in the examples used, the data for which were chosen for simplicity, but with any combination of cardiac rate and ventilatory cycle, it can be demonstrated that the average of diastole-associated pressures will be lower if a diastole does not coincide with peak pressure and if a maximum number of diastoles fall in low-pressure areas of the cycle. This view of the relation of positive intrathoracic pressure and heart action is more of academic interest than anything else, since it is not practical to attempt to correlate the two clinically; but it does give emphasis to the fact that mechanical ventilation has a significant effect on circulation.

The next step in our discussion is of great clinical importance, however. Fortunately, passive exhalation does not follow the simple linear deceleration of the sketches used so far but has a configuration more like that of Fig. 13-22, *D*, somewhat exaggerated.[74] The curved contour of exhalation makes for an early drop in pressure and a reduction of mean pressure during exhalation. Although the mean *inspiratory* pressure of *D* is 10 units, as in the other patterns, more of the *exhalation* curve lies below the 10 units pressure line, showing that mean exhalation pressure is something less than 10 units. It is not necessary mathematically to try to calculate the mean of the curved pressure-drop line, as long as the ventilatory and circulatory advantages of this configuration are appreciated by the student. The projections of diastoles *c* and *d* fall well below the 10 units pressure level so that mean intrathoracic pressure affecting atrial diastolic filling is the least in *D* of the four patterns illustrated. The student should note that the time relationships of *C* and *D* are the same and that the projections of the atrial diastoles of *D* onto the lower pressure levels are entirely a result of the curved shape of the exhalation line. Apart from changing the diastole-pressure relation, the transformation from a straight to curved exhalation line decreases the important pressure-time relation, since the area under sketch *D* is less than the area of the others, and for all practical purposes this is the major contribution of such a ventilation pattern. Modern mechanical ventilators allow the operator great flexibility in determining the most advantageous pressure-time curves for each patient's ventilatory and cardiac status, which is a critical consideration in treating the patient in failure.

The curves in Fig. 13-23 illustrate three clinical points. The patient ventilated by curve *a* experiences a rapid buildup in intrathoracic pressure, which is held as a plateau for a major portion of the cycle before falling precipitiously. The area under this curve is extensive, implying the prolonged exposure of the intrathoracic circulatory system to the steady effects of a high mean pressure. Maximum interference with venous return and consequent left ventricular output can be anticipated from such a pattern. Later we describe a clinical condition for which such a pressure-time curve is highly therapeutic, but for our present purposes we can consider it a serious hazard. Pattern *b* demonstrates a marked modification of pattern *a*. The inspiratory time is slightly prolonged but is still less than one-third the cycle, and it delays somewhat the initial exposure of the circulation to high pressure. The key difference in these two patterns is the immediate drop in pressure as soon as peak has been reached and the rapid falloff to the end of exhalation. The effect on the circulation of curve *b* would be less than that of curve *a* to the same degree that the area

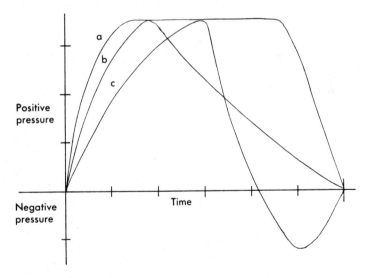

Fig. 13-23   Three pressure-time ventilatory patterns with the same range of positive pressure. Curve *a*, with its sustained peak pressure, has the greatest total pressure effect on circulation. Curve *b* reduces pressure-time by a slower rise and immediate descent. Curve *c* uses terminal negative pressure to offset some of the positive-pressure effect.

under *b* is smaller than the area under *a*. There are occasions when inspiratory needs cannot be fulfilled in the early one third of the cycle because factors of obstruction and low compliance necessitate longer inflationary periods. If possible, duration of exhalation is increased accordingly to maintain a favorable inspiratory/expiratory ratio of 1:1.5 or 1:2 to keep the mean pressure down, but sometimes in assisted ventilation the patient will not tolerate the resulting reduction in ventilatory rate. In such a case, should the prolonged inspiration pose a threat of reduced cardiac output, terminal expiratory negative pressure can be introduced into the system, as in curve *c*. Such a precaution is also applicable to any situation in which, even with a well-balanced ventilatory ratio, cardiac action is embarrassed from other causes. The rapid drop in pressure to below atmospheric increases the venous return during exhalation to make up for a deficit incurred during inspiration. Employing the concept of net pressure referred to earlier, it can be seen that the final effective mean intrathoracic pressure of this type of curve is proportional to the difference between the areas under the curve, above and below the zero line.

Let us summarize the physiologic effect of positive-pressure ventilation on the circulatory system from a clinical viewpoint. Although the primary objective of mechanical ventilation is to ensure an adequate tidal alveolar air exchange, the therapist must always be aware of the side effects of such treatment, especially on cardiac function. When considered over cycle after cycle, the supraatmospheric pressure generated in the patient's chest retards the return of venous blood to the right atrium. The important consequence of this is a drop in the cardiac output, with eventual reduced circulating systemic flow that may develop into a full-blown circulatory collapse or shock. The normal heart can tolerate the restrictive action of high mean intrathoracic pressure for prolonged periods of time, but a heart actually or potentially weakened from disease or one subjected to excessively high pressure may be seriously affected. The degree to which venous return is impeded is proportional to the height of the mean pressure developed in the thorax and the length of time such pressure continues. This gives rise to the concept of the pressure-time relationship, which in a given circumstance with available data on instant-to-instant pressure and time, can be graphically expressed as a curve by plotting pressure against ventilatory cycle time.

The inspiratory-to-expiratory time ratio is an important factor in ensuring adequate ventilation while minimizing the adverse circulatory effects of positive pressure. In general, if an I/E ratio is established so that expiration is longer than inspiration, the mean intrathoracic pressure will be lowered to a level of relative safety. The setting of an I/E ratio requires skill, understanding, and patience of the operator, for the final ventilatory pattern must be able to satisfy inspiratory needs while keeping inspiratory pressure time to a minimum. In our discussion of ventilators, we described the mechanisms for adjusting inspiratory and expiratory times in some of them and found that others had fixed I/E ratios.

Negative pressure during exhalation (NEEP) is available to produce the maximum reduction of mean intrathoracic pressure. Generated by a venturi, 3 to 5 cm of water subatmospheric pressure applied to the airways, when used with a favorable I/E ratio, can reduce the mean pressure in the chest almost to atmospheric. For reasons noted below, negative pressure in exhalation should not be used on a routine basis but reserved for those patients in whom peripheral cardiovascular collapse is an immediate or actual threat. Its use is monitored by close observation of heart rate and blood pressure, and elevation of the first with depression of the second in a patient maintained on positive-pressure ventilation is a most probable indication for instituting negative pressure, regardless of the cause of cardiac dysfunction. Although all other appropriate measures to combat shock are also used, it is not uncommon to observe how easily the stability of the blood pressure can be manipulated by varying the combination of positive and negative pressures.

Artificially induced subatmospheric airway pressure is not without its own inherent hazards, and because it entails a calculated risk its use is restricted to the support of failing circulation only. The two potential dangers of negative expiratory pressure are *air trapping* and *pulmonary edema*. Fig. 8-3 can be used to illustrate the risk of air trapping if we visualize the ventilatory pressures as intraluminal, with positive pressure inflating the alveolus and negative pressure deflating it. The illustrated bronchiolar collapse resulting from extraluminal positive pressure would then be caused by intraluminal negative pressure. This hazard is especially great in patients with chronic bronchopulmonary disease, in whom diseased airways are a major characteristic and many of the smaller passages lack enough connective tissue support to maintain their integrity in the face of subatmospheric pressure. The therapist can understand the seriousness of further restricting the alveolar gas exchange in a patient already in ventilatory failure by cutting short exhalation with airway collapse, retaining air in the lungs and significantly elevating the functional residual capacity. This is why it is necessary to reject the temptation to use negative pressure as a means of aspirating secretions or overcoming airway obstruction, for the suction needed to accomplish these objectives is just as apt to have the opposite effect. The risk of air trapping can be minimized by introducing subatmospheric pressure gradually and limiting it to the least that will achieve the desired purpose.

Negative intrapulmonary pressure also subjects the patient to the danger of pulmonary edema. Like the effect of positive pressure on venous return, the probability of circulatory harm from negative pressure depends on the general health and stability of the pulmonary circulation. Venous return is greatly enhanced during the negative-pressure phase of exhalation as the mean intrathoracic pressure precipitously drops and the pulmonary vasculature fills with blood, creating at least a temporary state of pulmonary congestion. Should some defective function of the left heart make it slow to accept the pulmonary venous outflow, pulmonary vascular hydrostatic pressure will rise and the gradient between the high intravascular pressure and the subatmospheric intraalveolar pressure will force blood water into the alveoli. The same condition can prevail without an undue rise in hydrostatic pressure if there is an abnormal increase in the permeability of the pulmonary capillaries so that the usually well-tolerated capillary to alveolar–pressure gradient is enough to move fluid from circulation to alveoli.

The therapist working in a hospital with a busy pulmonary service will occasionally encounter one of the most difficult patients to ventilate because of a serious physiologic paradox. This is the patient with severe obstruction or impaired compliance who needs relatively high pressure for alveolar ventilation but who has concurrent heart disease, often with myocardial damage from an inadequate coronary artery circulation. Because of the unstable cardiovascular system, not only do high ventilatory pressures easily embarrass venous return and precipitate respirator shock but the corrective measure of expiratory negative pressure induces pulmonary edema. In an extreme example of such a patient, the adjustment of the negative pressure within the range of only a few centimeters of water may find a dropping blood pressure and dry lungs replaced by a rising pressure but accompanied by the wet lungs of edema. The careful and delicate titration of positive and negative pressures against alveolar ventilation and circulatory stability requires the ultimate in physiologic understanding and technical proficiency.

Our discussion of the effects of mechanical ventilation of circulation would not be complete unless we commented on this relationship in *negative-pressure* breathing for comparison. After the above discussion of the action of positive-pressure ventilation, the student may be surprised to be told that the same deleterious effect can be found in the patient treated by a tank respirator. In our description of this instrument, we note that chest expansion and subsequent pulmonary inflation result from the action of subatmospheric pressure on the external surface of the thorax, and the comment is made that this principle is more nearly like that of natural breathing than is positive-pressure breathing. This is a valid observation, since with this technique, intrathoracic pressure never exceeds atmospheric, but there is another factor. If we refer to Fig. 4-16, we will see that in the body respirator negative pressure is applied not only to the thorax but to the rest of the body as well, with the exception of the head and neck. However, because of the relative flexibility of the abdomen compared with the chest, the pressure is readily transmitted into the former, and this is not physiologically similar to natural breathing when inspiration generates positive intraabdominal pressure. The drop in abdominal pressure destroys the normal gradient from abdomen to thorax that aids the return of venous blood to the heart. In consequence there is a dilation of the vast network of abdominal capillaries, as described above in reference to positive-pressure breathing, and pooling of venous blood. Just as with positive-pressure ventilation, the pooled blood is effectively removed from circulation, reducing right atrial filling and ventricular output. Thus the same hazard of circulatory failure is encountered in both types of ventilation. During the years of the poliomyelitis epidemics, when body respirators were extensively used, the circulatory depression caused by distal venous pooling was called "tank shock."

With the large number of patients so treated, this complication undoubtedly would have been more prevalent than it was except that most of the patients were young, with good cardiovascular function. The student can now see an advantage of the chest cuirass other than convenience, since with subatmospheric pressure applied only to the thorax, the circulatory insufficiency produced by both intrapulmonary positive and body surface negative pressures is circumvented.

The following list summarizes the potential effects of mechanical ventilation on circulation.

1. Reduced cardiac output
2. Reduced venous return
3. Decreased ventricular end-diastolic volume
4. Increased pulmonary vascular resistance
5. Reduced shunt, especially with PEEP[76]

Effects on metabolism

In this context, *metabolism* is used to include the function of systems other than the cardiorespiratory system and responses of that system other than those included in the above discussion. An acute and progressively deteriorating state similar to the respiratory distress syndrome in infants has been described in some patients supported by mechanical ventilation and PEEP.[77] Affected patients demonstrate severe dyspnea, tachypnea, hypoxemia refractory to oxygen administration, a large alveolar-arterial oxygen tension gradient, a loss of pulmonary compliance, and a chest x-ray film identical to that seen in acute pulmonary edema. We have considered the damage sustained by the lung after exposure to high oxygen tensions, but in the patients under discussion, unusually high concentrations of oxygen were not used and oxygen toxicity was not considered the cause. With a variety of underlying diseases necessitating mechanical ventilation, it was postulated that damage to pulmonary surface-active material might be responsible for the precipitous loss of lung function. A comprehensive study was made of this condition, reviewing the pulmonary and metabolic status of 100 patients undergoing prolonged mechanical ventilation.[78] In addition to the signs and symptoms noted above, 19 of these patients exhibited a significant retention of body water and either a weight gain or failure to lose weight as anticipated. Also, they showed a drop in concentration of serum sodium (hyponatremia) and a reduction in hematocrit, both consistent with an increase in blood volume (hypervolemia) resulting from retained water (hydremia). This clinical state is called the *adult respiratory distress syndrome* (ARDS) and, being a syndrome, may have a score of causes. We are noting it here because two of its outstanding characteristics, progressive hypoxemia and decreasing compliance, may make a patient who is so affected the most difficult to manage. Mechanical ventilation itself does not cause ARDS, but associated water retention can.

An association between pressure breathing, both positive and negative, and kidney function has long been recognized. A normal subject under continuous positive-pressure breathing may experience a reduction in urinary flow as much as 50%, attributed to a reduced renal blood flow, whereas negative-pressure breathing induces an increase in these functions.[79,80] It was suggested that renal circulation is at least temporarily compromised to compensate for circulatory deficiencies during the stress of positive-pressure ventilation and that one of the mechanisms involved may be an alteration in the so-called *antidiuretic hormone* (ADH). This is a substance secreted by the pituitary gland that is instrumental in regulating body fluid content and concentration by appropriate adjustment of urinary output. By virtue of its name, one can see that the more hormone present, the less excretion of urine and the greater retention of water there will be. The relation of the action of ADH to the patient undergoing mechanical ventilation may lie in the experimental observation that vagal reflexes from the cardiac atria seem to influence ADH activity in response to pressure changes in the atria, and we now know that positive-pressure ventilation markedly alters right heart blood flow and pressure.[81]

Thus, as pointed out in the study noted above,[78] a potentially serious physiologic effect of mechanical ventilation may be the disturbance of the usual body fluid–ADH balance and the selective accumulation of abnormal amounts of water in the lungs, since peripheral edema is not noticeable in the absence of frank cardiac failure. The latter cannot always be ruled out, but the degree of pulmonary fluid appears out of proportion to the sparse indications for heart failure. Certainly the interference with pulmonary function in these patients can reasonably be attributed to pulmonary congestion and edema, an interpretation confirmed by the often rapid and dramatic improvement in the clinical condition and the x-ray picture of the lungs after the administration of a diuretic. It is obvious that management of the ventilated patient must include close attention to maintaining a safe balance between fluid intake and output, since although dehydration must be avoided, so must the risk of overhydration in the event of an increase in ADH activity.

The therapist may feel confused by the apparent paradox of positive-pressure breathing acting to limit the blood volume of the lung as described under its circulatory effects and also precipitating pulmonary edema as just noted. In our first consideration of the physiologic action of positive-pressure breathing, we describe the usual, or expected, effect of pressure, whereas the hazardous metabolic disturbances accompany long-term ventilation, during which many of the body's reserve functions and compensations become depleted. This underscores the lability of physiologic response, especially under the stress of severe disease, and emphasizes the need for intelligent observation of the patient, with an awareness of the possible complications that may develop.

Summarized below are the potential effects of mechanical ventilation on metabolism[82]:

1. Reduced urinary flow caused by increased blood flow to juxtamedullary nephrons and decreased blood flow to cortical nephrons
2. Increased ADH secretion
3. Sodium retention

Methods of intermittent lung hyperinflation

So far, this chapter has dealt with concepts of mechanical ventilators, modes of mechanical ventilation, and physiologic effects of mechanical ventilation. The use of IPPB has been mentioned, and certainly many of the aspects already discussed apply to this intermittently applied therapy. In this section we discuss IPPB as a technique for intermittent hyperinflation of the lungs along with other modes that have more recently been suggested for this purpose.

Two recent symposiums concerning the scientific basis of respiratory therapy have provided summaries of literature reviews on the use and efficacy of IPPB therapy and other mechanical aids to lung expansion.[83,84] We make use of information provided by these conferences, recent editorials, the growing medical literature, and our own experiences in an attempt to provide useful information on this subject.[83-86]

IPPB therapy

We have discussed the use of inspiratory positive pressure in the delivery of assisted or controlled ventilation for the patient with inadequate breathing, and now we consider IPPB as a treatment entity for less acute conditions. IPPB has come rapidly onto the medical scene, enjoying widespread use and acclamation as well as considerable condemnation. As with many innovations, pressure breathing suffered from initial overuse without due regard for proper indications or technique, and when results that were anticipated, but never claimed, for it did not materialize, many users became disenchanted. Much, if not all, of the controversy over the value or harm of IPPB was the result of lack of clear understanding of its capabilities. In addition, the advent of IPPB preceded the development of respiratory therapy as a skilled technical specialty, and pressure breathing was used by many people with little concept of its objectives or knowledge of the mechanics of the instruments or their physiologic effects. It is little wonder that results were less than spectacular and that the treatment was blamed rather than those treating.

Equipment. Most IPPB instruments function according to the principles described for IPPVs, and although the ventilators themselves can be used for intermittent therapy, there are units much simpler in structure designed just for this purpose. Without the need for the many critical controls of ventilators, treatment instruments are generally pressure- or manually cycled, smaller (many are portable), independent of gas cylinders or centrally supplied air, and have their own built-in compressors. Other texts, advertising brochures, and operating manuals from manufacturers will give the student an overview of the specifications of the many competitive units on the market, and we will not pursue the topic further.[7]

Indications for IPPB. In the past, IPPB therapy has been given for a variety of reasons to patients with and without pulmonary disease.[83,84,87-89] Often its use has been linked to the delivery of therapeutic aerosols, prevention or correction of postoperative pulmonary complications, and control of arterial blood gases and as an aid in clearing secretions or to decrease the work of breathing. The actual role, if any, IPPB should play in pulmonary medicine is as yet unresolved.[83-86] We briefly review here what is known currently and what appears to be reasonable use for IPPB.

A distinct feature of IPPB is that it applies a positive pressure to the airways to provide a large volume each breath with or without the patient providing any effort during the breath. For patients in which expansion of the lungs appears indicated but who are unable to produce a large breath, IPPB would seem a rational approach.[90] Patients who cannot breathe deeply or who have difficulty in taking deep breaths include those with neuromuscular disorders, those with pain, and those who are sedated.[91]

While therapeutic aerosols can be given during IPPB therapy there is little evidence that this method has any advantage over simpler methods such as spontaneously breathing mist from a compressor-driven nebulizer as long as the patient can properly use the simpler system.[83,84,88] Some subgroups of patients may benefit from IPPB-administered bronchodilators, such as patients with severe chronic obstructive pulmonary disease with excessive secretions and FEV_1 or MVV of less than 35% of predicted, or patients who cannot properly coordinate their breathing with the nebulizer system.[89,92] Empirical evidence seems to indicate success from aerosol therapy combined with IPPB when used in *selected* patients with pulmonary disease.[93] A multicenter study is currently underway to compare bronchodilator administration by IPPB versus compressor-driven nebulizer for home care of patients with chronic obstructive pulmonary disease. We look forward to the results of this study in hope that it will delineate further the role of IPPB in these patients. Generally, the need for aerosol therapy or for ventilatory assistance by IPPB should be considered separately.

The positive airway pressure applied during inspiration by IPPB can supply all the work necessary for each breath, if properly applied.[94] In order for this to occur the patient must be taught to relax completely during the breath, and the sensitivity and flow-rate controls must be adjusted to minimize patient effort. When IPPB is given in this manner to a patient familiar with or well instructed in the procedure, increased work of breathing can be diminished. Dyspneic states such as those accompanying acute asthma or pulmonary edema can be relieved during IPPB therapy, while bronchodilators and oxygen are also conveniently administered concommittently. However, a high degree of *artful* application must be utilized with these anxious patients for sucessful therapy. While work of breathing can be reduced by properly applied IPPB, so the work can also be increased by *improperly* administered therapy with inadequate control settings.[94]

For some patients an increase in tidal volume may seem more important than an increase in work. For instance, following surgery patients often are thought to benefit from large, deep breaths.[90,95] They are usually capable of increasing the work needed but are often splinting because of pain. One method has been suggested for administering IPPB that encourages the patient to actively inspire *with* the positive pressure rather than relax.[96] This coached maneuver was shown to produce larger volumes than when the patient was not coached during inspiration.[96] While this would certainly increase the work done by the patient, the increase may not be of clinical significance for certain patients. No study has yet been performed to see whether the larger volumes produced by using this technique make any difference to the patient's recovery rate and the technique is not recommended when the work of breathing is already excessive.

IPPB has been used in hope of preventing airway closure and atelectasis, which so often follows repetitive, shallow breathing, such as after surgical procedures. Little evidence exists that IPPB, as currently given, prevents this atelectasis consistently.[90] However, many of the studies reviewed recently were found to be lacking in design or were nonspecific concerning methods of administration of IPPB, and none indicated the tidal volumes used.[90] Many studies have utilized IPPB every 4 hours or three to four times daily, which may not be frequent enough.[86,90] IPPB has also been used to reexpand areas in which atelectasis is already evident, and this use appears more widely accepted by physicians.[88] Again little supportive evidence exists. Using a maximum-*volume*-oriented approach may prove useful in selected patients, especially if other methods have not been successful.[86,97] There does appear to be sound physiologic reasoning for the use of deep breaths to reexpand areas of collapsed lung,[85,95] although it is questionable whether IPPB, instead of other methods, should be used to accomplish this *routinely*.

The effects of the elevated mean intrathoracic pressure during pressure breathing has already been discussed in this chapter. Of special note here is the potential for IPPB to decrease venous return to the heart. The clinical picture of acute pulmonary edema from left ventricular failure is described in Chapter 7, and the student is advised to review it. In this state of impaired pulmonary circulation, regulation of venous return is included as treatment.[98] The use of positive airway pressure in the treatment of acute pulmonary edema has been used with varying degrees of enthusiasm since it was introduced in the 1930s.[30,99-102] Initially the positive pressure was applied throughout the ventilatory cycle such as CPPB or CPAP,[30,99-101] while later IPPB was employed.[98,102]

The use of IPPB in acute pulmonary edema is directed at decreasing the work of breathing, treating hypoxia, and retarding venous return. Reducing the work of breathing requires substantial skill on the part of the therapist to get dyspneic, often panicked, patients to relax. The relief of hypoxia and retardation of venous return are discussed together here because they are managed simultaneously. The treatment of hypoxemia is of the highest priority, and a significant increase in alveolar oxygen tension is necessary to increase diffusion across the fluid barrier of edema. The first move is to give the patient 100% oxygen while readying other measures, preferably by means of a nonrebreathing mask, and oxygen therapy will be continued during the next step of retarding venous return. For many years the reduction of pulmonary blood volume has been recognized as a prime objective in the relief of the acute phase of pulmonary edema, and there are three techniques that will reduce the volume of blood returning to the right atrium.

A phlebotomy is the physical removal of blood from circulation and will certainly reduce the pulmonary blood volume. It was customary in the past to withdraw up to 500 ml rapidly. This can be hazardous, however, since if acute edema has already precipitated circulatory collapse, blood loss will further aggravate shock. This technique has largely been abandoned.

Applied to the extremities, tourniquets will effectively reduce venous return and are much safer than phlebotomy. Rubber straps or blood-pressure cuffs may be used and are applied with a force greater than that of the estimated venous pressure but less than the arterial diastolic pressure. Peripheral pulses must be palpable at all times to avoid the risk of ischemic necrosis. Only three extremities are occluded at a time, and the tourniquets are rotated so that each extremity is free, in sequence, for 20 minutes. When the acute phase is over, the restrictions are released, one at a time of 20-minute intervals, to avoid flooding the pulmonary circulation with a sudden return of flow. This technique is safe and effective and should be used while waiting for and during the next maneuver.

Pressure-controlled inflation of the lungs is more rapid and effective than either phlebotomy or tourniquets, and its administration by IPPB is an important function of the respiratory therapist. As noted earlier, this is an instance in which the usually undesirable generation of high intrathoracic pressures may be lifesaving rather than a hazard. Instead of regulating a ventilator to minimize its circulatory effect, the therapist does just the opposite. He or she uses pressures up to 40 cm of water or higher and flows high enough to reach peak pressure in the shortest possible time. This allows the maintenance of a plateau of high pressure at end-inspiration and blocks the return of venous blood into thoracic vessels. To a considerable degree the volume of blood so retarded can be regulated and controlled in a manner not possible with phlebotomy or tourniquets. In the acutely ill patient, almost a breath-by-breath adjustment of the IPPB unit will be required because of the rapid and difficult breathing; but the great assistance the patient receives from the ventilator gradually eases the work of breathing, reducing frequency and increasing tidal volume. Oxygen (at 100%) is now given through the ventilator so that hypoxia, pulmonary edema, and congestion are effectively treated together. From 20% to 50% ethyl alcohol is sometimes nebulized during treatment, taking advantage of its antifoaming properties to mobilize the edema froth as well as to benefit from the systemic effects after absorption into the circulation. The patient with combined shock and edema is difficult to treat, for positive pressure is a hazard to one, and negative pressure is a hazard to the other. Still, by progressing cautiously, the therapist can provide relief of hypoxia from oxygen administered by gentle pressure breathing and may reverse circulatory collapse and reduce edema. The combined judgment and talents of physician and therapist may determine the outcome.

In summary, it can be stated that acute pulmonary edema may be one of the specific indications for trying IPPB that can provide dramatic results.[98,102]

Frequently, IPPB with an aerosolized bronchodilator is followed by chest physiotherapy, as described in Chapter 15, to facilitate maximum clearance of secretions from the airways. The use of ultrasonically nebulized saline, or saline/propylene glycol may be given before, during, or after the IPPB to water down secretions for later removal by physical therapy. There are many treatment programs that include IPPB, and it is imperative that *IPPB never be used on a dogmatically routine basis*. This is one fault that has exposed the procedure to criticism. There should be a specific objective that IPPB is expected to accomplish in every patient for whom it is prescribed. As yet there are no standard guidelines to judge the efficacy of IPPB therapy, but it is a responsibility of the attending physician to use whatever means are available to evaluate its effects and to indicate its discontinuance. Good clinical observation and examination and judicious use of simple pulmonary laboratory tests will be sufficient in most instances.

There are two cautions in the administration of IPPB that cannot be overstressed, and failure to consider them in the past has contributed to resistance to its use. First, probably most IPPB therapy is poorly done, and many patients would have been just as well, or perhaps better, without it. Unless a trained attendant such as a respiratory therapist or technician can remain with the patient throughout the treatment and actively participate in it, it is doubtful that the therapy will have any beneficial effects. In new patients, IPPB can cause disturbing apprehension, and they must be watched and advised continuously. We often consider that veteran users of IPPB can take care of themselves, and we tend to let such patients treat themselves. *This is a serious error*. Patients cannot be expected to be responsible for the proper performance on themselves of a procedure that requires as much skill as does IPPB. That is our job, as professionals. When left alone for self-treatment, patients almost invariably forget small details of breathing techniques or slouch into positions more comfortable for them but which completely negate the function of the therapy. It is up to the therapist to watch each patient during the entire treatment, instructing and advising, breath by breath if necessary, to help the patient meet the goals set for him or her.

In summary, this means that the minimum criteria for IPPB therapy are that it be given by someone skilled in its use, on a one-to-one therapist-patient relationship during each treatment. Although this is an ideal still a long way from realization, we must recognize that correction of this basic deficiency should be one of our highest priorities.

Second, in our enthusiasm for aggressive action, we sometimes forget that a patient is not a disease but is a person with a disease, and by virtue of illness he or she has less than normal physical stamina. Subjecting patients to a program that may promise to ease their problems, but that pushes them to the edge of exhaustion, will earn them disappointing, diminishing returns. Combining procedures for additive benefit is to be encouraged, as part of a specific therapeutic plan, but it must be done with care and a regard for patients' well-being. To prescribe 15 minutes of IPPB, followed by 30 minutes of ultrasonic aerosol inhalation, then 15 minutes of chest physical therapy, on a 2-hour basis for a 100-pound, 70-year-old woman may stress her to a dangerous point. We frequently must compromise what we would like to do for or to our patient, with concern for the patient's discomfort. Overtreatment is potentially dangerous, but it is preventable by establishing a treatment plan for each patient and prescribing only those procedures that contribute to the plan. Duration of, and intervals between, treatments must be tailored to the specific needs of each patient, progress followed closely, and the program adjusted on a daily basis. This is honest and rational respiratory therapy.

Technique of IPPB administration

Before initiating therapy on a new patient, if meaningful communication is possible, the therapist must be absolutely certain to explain to the patient what is going to be done. Without delivering an academic lecture, the therapist should tell the patient the nature of the treatment and in a general way what is expected of it. Resistance or hostility of patients toward therapy is usually due to one or more of the following: (1) they are irrational from illness or age; (2) they are expressing fright through hostility; and (3) they do not understand what is expected of them. A few moments of reassuring explanation will make the treatment helpful for patients and easy on therapists.

For best results the patient should be seated upright in a relatively straight chair, although this is not always possible for the hospitalized patient. Nevertheless, every effort should be made to avoid a slouched position, which will hamper diaphragmatic mobility. Obesity is a serious hazard to good ventilatory mechanics, and in the supine position, especially if the head of the bed is elevated, abdominal pressure may prevent all but very small diaphragmatic descent. Ventilation can often be greatly helped by IPPB if the patient can be helped to stand by the bed during a treatment. Sitting the obese patient in a chair usually worsens the problem. A mouthpiece is preferred to a mask, and at first a noseclip is best, although this can often be omitted shortly. The edentulous patient presents a problem in achieving necessary airtightness, but a trial of several mouthpieces of different shapes, especially with flanges, will generally locate one that is satisfactory. These appliances should be fitted so that the patient can become acclimated to them before the start of treatment. All initial control settings will be tentative, but sensitivity should be relatively free and pressure started somewhere between 10 and 15 cm of water. The control of flow-adjustable instruments can be set somewhere in the middle of the available range.

As treatment is begun, the patient is instructed to breathe slowly and easily and encouraged to allow the machine to do the work. There is a tendency for respiratory frequency to increase, and the patient often appears to be chased by the respirator so that the therapist may have to urge the patient to maintain a normal or decreased rate. The anxious patient or the patient trying hard to please is especially likely to overbreathe, and this must be prevented because it is easy for him or her to become alkalotic. Not only is alkalosis itself a potential hazard but the hypocapnia reduces central ventilatory drive. On cessation of pressure-assisted breathing there may be a period of hypoventilation until eucarbia returns, during which time blood oxygen levels may drop dangerously low. This consequence of intermittent therapy must be kept in mind.

Pressure and flow may have to be adjusted often during an initial treatment until the patient's pattern stabilizes, but most patients do well quickly, reassured by the therapist's relaxed and confident manner. If overbreathing cannot be corrected by the patient's voluntary efforts, dangerous hypocapnia can be prevented by inserting between the patient and the exhalation valve a piece of breathing tubing, 50 to 150 ml in capacity, for rebreathing of carbon dioxide–rich exhaled air. This should be a temporary expedient, if possible, and efforts continued to help the patient establish a better breathing pattern. It is prudent to inquire after the patient's feelings to determine whether he or she is experiencing dizziness or getting tired. Water, or medication to be aerosolized, must be in the nebulizer at all times, and the treatment must never be given dry; if medication is used, the patient might be instructed to hold his or her breath momentarily at end-inspiration to permit maximum particle distribution.

Tidal volumes being delivered should be monitored, and pressure and flow settings adjusted accordingly. How large the tidal volumes should be is not known, but it has been suggested that either 10% above a spontaneous vital capacity or inspiratory capacity should be generated if large volumes are the primary purpose of therapy.[96,97,103-105] At least, volumes should be measured and a determination of their adequacy evaluated.[85,86,90,106]

Once patients appear at ease with the procedure, if they are obstructed, they should be encouraged to prolong their exhalation within the limits of comfort. If they have difficulty doing this themselves, the therapist can put a *retard cap* over the exhalation port of the instrument. This is a cap that has several holes of different diameters to provide varying degrees of back pressure for slowing down and prolonging exhalation. It is especially useful when air trapping caused by bronchiolar collapse is a problem, since the back pressure developed at the port will help to maintain airway patency to end-expiration. Expiratory retard should not be confused with inspiratory hold, described earlier. Retard does not maintain a pressure plateau but merely delays alveolar-bronchiolar decompression by lengthening exhalation time; in contrast, exhalation following inspiratory hold is usually of normal duration and pattern.

The therapist should also teach obstructed patients to aid exhalation by abdominal contraction. This is often difficult for them to grasp, but it will be easier if the therapist will demonstrate on him- or herself in front of a patient. Then, with a hand on the patient's epigastrium, the therapist can exert gentle but firm pressure during the terminal third of exhalation, pointing out to the patient how this increases the removal of air. Finally, patients are allowed to try epigastric retraction themselves, but they will need close supervision and must not be allowed to tire themselves with this maneuver. For the patient with a severe obstructive problem, there is available an inflatable swathlike belt that can be fitted about the middle and upper abdomen. Coordinated with the ventilator, the belt inflates during exhalation, exerting a forceful squeeze on the abdomen. It does not take the place of active exercise of the abdominal muscles, but sometimes it is helpful in instructing the patient in the purpose of forced terminal expiration and demonstrating what can be accomplished.

Generally, an IPPB treatment of 20 to 30 minutes is sufficient at a frequency of from three to four times daily to hourly, although it is obvious that the schedule must be fitted to each patient's needs. However, the indications for treatment are usually such that an intensity of this degree is necessary, at least at first. Care must be taken not to let IPPB become so routine that all patients are treated alike. On the other hand, both the patient's attending physician and the respiratory therapist need some sort of a working standard procedure to present to a patient for whom therapy is proposed.

Home IPPB therapy may be satisfactory for selected patients if it is subject to certain conditions. First, a series of treatments should be given by a trained therapist in either the inpatient or outpatient service until such time as the therapist is confident that the patient knows the procedure well. There are some patients who never can treat themselves safely or satisfactorily, and the therapist should frankly make this known to the responsible physician. Second, before the hospitalized patient takes his or her instrument home, the therapist should go over it carefully with the patient, reviewing the technique of its use, showing how the components operate, and instructing in its care and cleaning. The outpatient should bring the machine to the ambulatory service for the same purposes, and often arrangements can be made to have the patient's unit delivered to the hospital so that he or she can be instructed when picking it up. It is a responsibility of the patient's physician to follow the progress of home care and, if necessary, to send the patient back to the therapist for an occasional checkup on technique. Experience has shown that many patients on home-care programs are forgotten and tend to become negligent in their treatment. More information on chronic care is found in Chapter 15.

Incentive spirometry— sustained maximal inspiration

Incentive spirometry (IS) is a technique for providing patients with encouragement towards a "maximal" inspiratory volume. As recommended by Bartlett,[106] this maneuver provides for a deep breath with sustained transpulmonary pressure near the end of inspiration and is sometimes referred to as a *sustained maximal inspiration* (SMI). The "incentive" for deep breaths to spontaneously breathing patients is generally provided by a visually evident part of a spirometric device, such as a light or "volume" indicator. A goal is often established for the patient by trials preoperatively or by some arbitrary estimate of achievement. The patient is then encouraged to use the device with or without supervision as often as 10 times per hour.[90,106]

The devices for incentive spirometry generally are activated either by a volume being inhaled from them or by having a flow of gas inhaled through them. Those devices that contain a certain volume from which the patient inhales usually provide a visual estimate of that volume, and the patient may compare this reading to the volume goal established. Some of these volume-oriented incentive spirometers provide a small leak so that some extra volume can be achieved during the sustained maximal effort following the initial inhaled volume. The flow-oriented devices generally use plastic floats in chambers, which are raised during inspiratory flow. The flow rate needed to lift the indicator float and an estimate of how long the float is maintained in an elevated position can provide an estimate of the volume inspired. The amount of flow needed to raise the float is often adjustable so that increasing effort (and hopefully increasing volumes) can be adjusted as goals for the patient as improvement occurs.

The primary goal of this technique of periodic lung hyperinflation is to prevent or reinflate areas of atelectasis.[90,106] Studies of incentive spirometry for this purpose seem to indicate that it is a useful adjunct, but its role compared to other techniques is as yet inconclusive.[90,107] The comparative studies recently reviewed provided conflicting results, probably because of varying control and technique factors.[90] Although SMI is based on sound physiologic principles we do not as yet know what volumes are necessary nor how often the manuever should be done in order to achieve the desired results.[107] It seems reasonable to try this relatively simple method for patients at risk of postoperative pulmonary complications and who are alert and cooperative. If these patients cannot generate the desired inspired volume after suitable trials, then volume-oriented IPPB or some other method could be applied.

It is generally assumed that incentive spirometry techniques are less expensive than IPPB therapy because the equipment involved for IS is less expensive than ventilators used for IPPB. However, the real cost of either of these methods is probably more related to the time involved on the part of the person administering the therapy rather than the equipment per se.[89] If SMI with an incentive spirometer can, in fact, be taught to patients initially and self-administered *reliably* thereafter, then IS can be significantly less expensive than a comparable number of sessions of IPPB with trained personnel in attendance.

Recently some commercially available devices for IS that can be combined with medication nebulizers for concommittent aerosol administration have been introduced. As mentioned previously for IPPB therapy, the *need* for aerosol therapy should generally be considered separately from other maneuvers. If both IS and aerosol therapy are indicated, their simultaneous administration would seem useful to encourage deep breathing during the aerosol delivery. Whether or not a maximal inspiration is needed with *each* breath during 10- to 20-minute periods of aerosol inhalation has certainly not been established and would seem unlikely. These systems may be helpful in training patients in a particular breathing pattern to be used during aerosol therapy, but their combined use for extended periods cannot be recommended at this time.

IS is obviously of no use for patients who are unconscious or who otherwise cannot cooperate in deep breathing techniques.

Other methods   Other methods such as periodic CPAP or PEEP breathing and expiration against resistance, i.e., *blow bottles,* have also been suggested for preventing or reinflating areas of atelectasis.[90] Using PEEP or CPAP to increase the functional residual capacity seems well documented, and these methods have been useful when applied on a continuous basis.[28-40] Little information is available for the periodic or short-term use of these modes for spontaneously breathing patients. One small study recently found that radiographic and blood gas data indicated that patients with CPAP applied briefly on an hourly basis was superior to data for similar patients not receiving CPAP following upper abdominal surgery.[108] All patients in this study also received chest physical therapy procedures. Although this study included only 24 patients, it does suggest that intermittently applied CPAP may be useful in patients postoperatively and that further, larger studies appear warranted.[90]

Blow bottles provide a resistance to expiration as the patient attempts to "blow" water from one bottle to another. There is no evidence that the increased lung pressure provided in this way during exhalation aids in lung expansion.[90] If patients are encouraged to inspire deeply before exhaling against such resistance, then it is likely that improvement in lung volumes would be attributable to the inspiratory rather than the expiratory effort. Further, if patients are encouraged to exhale to below their functional residual capacity, then *closure* of airways would be more likely to occur, defeating the purpose of the maneuver.

Summary

All of the methods of intermittent lung hyperinflation discussed require further study under controlled conditions in order to determine their true efficacy, if any, in respiratory therapy.[83,84,90,107] The use of IPPB, IS, and periodic CPAP or PEEP therapy is more highly recommended for further study than is the use of blow bottles.[107] IPPB therapy may be useful for patients that cannot or will not produce large tidal volumes, such as unconscious patients or those with severely obstructed airways or with neuromuscular disorders.[89-92]

The incidence of complications from each of these methods is not well known.[90] IPPB by mask or mouthpiece can cause gastric insufflation with the possibility of gastric rupture. Both hyperventilation and hypoventilation can occur with IPPB therapy, and patients should be monitored for clinical signs of these conditions.[109] Certainly the potential for adverse circulatory depression by positive pressure is well known, and this should be considered, particularly with patients having known circulatory problems. No such circulatory difficulties are known for IS techniques. Although pneumothorax is highly unlikely as a consequence of IPPB as routinely given, IPPB should *not* be administered to a patient who already has a pneumothorax that is untreated since application of positive pressure can aggravate this problem.

References

1. Fishman, A.P.: The roads to respiratory insufficiency, Ann. N.Y. Acad. Med. **121**:657, 1965.

2. Sykes, M.K., McNicol, M.W., and

Campbell, E.J.M.: Respiratory failure, ed. 2, Oxford, England, 1976, Blackwell Scientific Publications.

3. Mushin, W.W., Rendell-Baker, L.,

Thompson, P.W., and Mapleson, W.W.: Automatic ventilation of the lungs, ed. 3, Oxford, England, 1980, Blackwell Scientific Publications.

4. Safar, P., editor: Respiratory therapy, Philadelphia, 1965, F.A. Davis Co.

5. Klaus, M.H., and Fanaroff, A.A., editors: Care of the high risk neonate, ed. 2, Philadelphia, 1979, W.B. Saunders Co.

6. Kirby, R.R., and Graybar, G.B., editors: Intermittent mandatory ventilation, Int. Anesthesiol. Clin. **18:**1, 1980.

7. McPherson, S.P.: Respiratory therapy equipment, ed. 2, St. Louis, 1981, The C.V. Mosby Co.

8. Rattenborg, C.C., and Via-Reque, E., editors: Clinical use of mechanical ventilation, Chicago, 1981, Year Book Medical Publishers, Inc.

9. Desautels, D.: Ventilator classification: a new look at an old subject, Curr. Rev. Respir. Ther. **1:**82, 1979.

10. Mapleson, W.W.: The effects of changes of lung characteristics on the functioning of automatic ventilators, Anaesthesia **17:**300, 1962.

11. Hunter, A.R.: The classification of respirators, Anaesthesia **16:**231, 1961.

12. Kirby, R.R., et al.: In Burton, G.G., Gee, G.N., and Hodgkin, J.E., editors: Respiratory care: a guide to clinical practice, Philadelphia, 1977, J.B. Lippincott Co.

13. Rarey, K.P., and Youtsey, J.W.: Respiratory patient care, Englewood Cliffs, N.J., 1981, Prentice-Hall, Inc.

14. Smith, R.K.: Respiratory care applications for fluidics, Respir. Ther. **3:**29, 1973.

15. Lough, M.D., Williams, T.J., and Rawson, J.E.: Newborn respiratory care, Chicago, 1979, Year Book Medical Publishers, Inc.

16. Dammann, J.F., McAslan, T.C., and Maffeo, F.J.: Optimal flow pattern for mechanical ventilation of the lungs, part 2, Crit. Care Med. **6:**293, 1978.

17. Fairley, H.B.: In Kirby, R.R., and Graybar, G.B., editors: Intermittent mandatory ventilation, Int. Anesthesiol. Clin. **18:**179, 1980.

18. Luce, J.M., Pierson, D.J., and Hudson, L.D.: Critical reviews: intermittent mandatory ventilation, Chest **79:**678, 1981.

19. Shapiro, B.A., et al.: Intermittent demand ventilation (IDV): a new technique for supporting ventilation in critically ill patients, Respir. Care **21:**521, 1976.

20. Harboe, S.: Weaning from mechanical by means of intermittent assisted ventilation I.A.V: case reports, Acta Anaesth. Scand. **21:**252, 1977.

21. Hasten, R.W., Downs, J.B., and Hesman, T.J.: A comparison of synchronized and nonsynchronized intermittent mandatory ventilation, Respir. Care **25:**554, 1980.

22. Shapiro, B.A., Harrison, R.A., and Trout, C.: Clinical applications of respiratory care, ed. 2, Chicago, 1979, Year Book Medical Publishers, Inc.

23. Lindahl, S.: Influence of an end inspiratory pause of pulmonary ventilation, gas distribution, and lung perfusion during artificial ventilation, Crit. Care Med. **7:**540, 1979.

24. Fulheihan, S.F., et al.: Effect of mechanical ventilation with end-expiratory pause on blood gas exchange, Anesth. Analg. **55:**122, 1976.

25. Bone, R.C.: Monitoring respiratory function in the patient with adult respiratory distress syndrome, Semin. Respir. Med. **2:**140, 1981.

26. Bone, R.C.: Diagnosis of causes for acute respiratory distress by pressure-volume curves, Chest **70:**740, 1976.

27. Eross, B., Powner, D., and Grenvik, A.: In Kirby, R.R., and Graybar, G.B., editors: Intermittent mandatory ventilation, Int. Anesthesiol Clin. **18:**11, 1980.

28. Ashbaugh, D.G., and Petty, T.L.: Positive end-expiratory pressure: physiology, indications and contraindications, J. Thorac. Cardiovasc. Surg. **65:**165, 1973.

29. Kumar, A., et al.: Continuous positive-pressure ventilation in acute respiratory failure, N. Engl. J. Med. **283:**1430, 1970.

30. Barach, A.L., Bickerman, H.A., and Petty, T.L.: Perspective in pressure breathing, Respir. Care **20:**627, 1975.

31. Gregory, G.A., et al.: Treatment of the idiopathic respiratory distress syndrome with continuous positive airway pressure, N. Engl. J. Med. **284:**1333, 1971.

32. Gillick, J.S.: Spontaneous positive end-expiratory pressure (sPEEP), Anesth. Analg. **56**:627, 1977.

33. Sturgeon, C.L., et al.: PEEP and CPAP: cardiopulmonary effects during spontaneous ventilation, Anesth. Analg. **56**:633, 1977.

34. Schmidt, G.B., et al.: EPAP without intubation, Crit. Care Med. **5**:297, 1977.

35. Greenbaum, D.M., et al.: Continuous positive airway pressure without tracheal intubation in spontaneously breathing patients, Chest **69**:615, 1976.

36. Sugerman, H.J., Rogers, R.M., and Miller, L.D.: Positive end-expiratory pressure (PEEP): indications and physiologic considerations, Chest **62**(part 2): 86s, 1972.

37. Gallagher, T.J., and Civetta, J.M.: Goal-directed therapy of acute respiratory failure, Anesth. Analg. **59**:831, 1980.

38. Ralph, D., and Robertson, H.T.: Respiratory gas exchange in adult respiratory distress syndrome, Semin. Respir. Med. **2**:114, 1981.

39. Suter, P.M., Fairley, H.B., and Isenberg, M.D.: Optimal end-expiratory pressure in patients with acute pulmonary failure, N. Engl. J. Med. **292**:284, 1975.

40. Kirby, R.R., et al.: High-level positive end-expiratory pressure (PEEP) in acute respiratory insufficiency, Chest **67**:156, 1975.

41. Gregory, G.A.: In Thibeault, D.W., and Gregory, G.A., editors: Neonatal pulmonary care, Menlo Park, Calif., 1979, Addison-Wesley Publishing Co., Inc.

42. Bendixen, H.H., et al.: Respiratory care, St. Louis, 1965, The C.V. Mosby Co.

43. Elam, J.O., Kerr, J.H., and Janney, C.D.: Performance of ventilators: effects of changes in lung-thorax compliance, Anesthesiology **19**:56, 1958.

44. Fleming, W.H., and Bowen, J.C.: A comparative evaluation of pressure-limited and volume-limited respirators for prolonged post-operative ventilatory support in combat casualties, Ann. Surg. **176**:49, 1972.

45. Reynolds, E.O.R.: In Thibeault, D.W., and Gregory, G.A., editors: Newborn pulmonary care, Menlo Park, Calif., 1979, Addison-Wesley Publishing Co., Inc.

46. Sjostrand, U.: High frequency positive pressure ventilation (HFPPV): a review Crit. Care Med. **8**:345, 1980.

47. Carlon, G.C., et al.: Clinical experience with high frequency jet ventilation, Crit. Care Med. **9**:1, 1981.

48. Carlon, G.C., et al.: Technical aspects and clinical implications of high frequency jet ventilation with a solenoid valve, Crit. Care Med. **9**:47, 1981.

49. Butler, W.J., et al.: Ventilation by high frequency oscillation in humans, Anesth. Analg. **59**:577, 1980.

50. Marchak, B.E., et al.: Treatment of RDS by high-frequency oscillatory ventilation: a preliminary report, J. Pediatr. **99**:287, 1981.

51. Sjostrand, U., and Eriksson, I.A.: High rates and low volumes in mechanical ventilation—not just a matter of ventilatory frequency, Anesth. Analg. **59**:567, 1980.

52. Jonzon, A., et al.: High-frequency positive-pressure ventilation by endotracheal insufflation, Acta Anaesth. Scand. **43** (suppl.), 1971.

53. Heebrink, D.M.: Reports: the high frequency ventilation saga, Respir. Care **26**:991, 1981.

54. Program for the Third World Congress on Intensive and Critical Care Medicine, Tenth Annual Meeting of the Society of Critical Care Medicine, Crit. Care Med. **9**:137, 1981.

55. Abstracts of original papers to be presented at the Ninth Annual Scientific and Educational Symposium of the Society of Critical Care Medicine, Crit. Care Med. **8**:225, 1980.

56. Kirby, R.R.: High-frequency positive-pressure ventilation (HFPPV): what role in ventilatory insufficiency? (editorial), Anesthesiology **52**:109, 1980.

57. Froese, A.B., and Bryan, A.C.: High frequency ventilation (editorial), Am. Rev. Respir. Dis. **123**:249, 1981.

58. Keszler, H., and Klain, M.: Tracheobronchial toilet without cardiorespiratory impairment, Crit. Care Med. **8**:298, 1980.

59. Bland, R.D., et al.: High frequency ventilation in severe hyaline membrane disease: an alternative treatment? Crit. Care Med. **8**:275, 1980.

60. Fredberg, J.J.: Augmented diffusion in

the airways can support pulmonary gas exchange, J. Appl. Physiol. **49:**232, 1980.

61. Drinker, P., and McKhann, C.: The use of a new apparatus for prolonged administration of artificial respiration, J.A.M.A. **92:**1658, 1929.

62. Torres, G.E., et al.: The effects of IPPB on intrapulmonary distribution of inspired air, Am. J. Med. **29:**946, 1960.

63. Ayres, S.M., and Giannelli, S., Jr.: Oxygen consumption and alveolar ventilation during intermittent positive pressure breathing, Dis. Chest **50:**409, 1966.

64. Gray, F.D., Jr., and MacIver, S.: The use of inspiratory positive pressure breathing in cardiopulmonary disease, Br. J. Tuberc. **52:**2, 1958.

65. Motley, H.L.: Intermittent positive pressure breathing therapy, Inhal. Ther. **7:**1, Feb. 1962.

66. Sheldon, G.P.: Pressure breathing in chronic obstructive lung disease, Medicine **42:**197, 1963.

67. Werko, L.: Influence of positive pressure breathing on the circulation in man, Acta Med. Scand., suppl. 193, 1947.

68. Opie, L.H., et al.: Intrathoracic pressure during intermittent positive-pressure respiration, Lancet **1:**911, 1961.

69. Coonse, G.K., and Aufrance, O.E.: The relation of the intrapleural pressure to the mechanics of the circulation, Am. Heart J. **9:**347, 1934.

70. Printzmetal, M., and Kounts, W.B.: Intrapleural pressure in health and disease and its influence on body function, Medicine **14:**457, 1935.

71. Christie, R.V., and McIntosh, C.A.: The measurement of intrapleural pressure in man, and its significance, J. Clin. Invest. **13:**279, 1934.

72. Kilburn, K.H., and Sicker, H.O.: Hemodynamic effects of continuous positive and negative pressure breathing in normal man, Circ. Res. **8:**660, 1960.

73. Bashour, F.A., et al.: Effect of intermittent positive pressure breathing on the cardiac output and the splanchnic blood flow, Inhal. Ther. **13:**47, 1968.

74. Comroe, J.H., et al.: The lung, ed. 2, Chicago, 1962, Year Book Medical Publishers, Inc.

75. Robotham, J.L.: Cardiovascular disturbances in chronic respiratory insufficiency, Am. J. Cardiol. **47:**941, 1981.

76. Dantzker, D.R., Lynch, J.P., and Weg, J.P.: Depression of cardiac output is a mechanism of shunt reduction in the therapy of acute respiratory failure, Chest **77:**636, 1980.

77. Ashbaugh, D.G., et al.: Acute respiratory distress in adults, Lancet **2:**319, 1967.

78. Sladen, A., et al.: Pulmonary complications and water retention in prolonged mechanical ventilation, N. Engl. J. Med. **279:**448, 1968.

79. Murdaugh, H.V., et al.: Effect of altered intrathoracic pressure on renal hemodynamics, electolyte excretion, and water clearance, J. Clin. Invest. **38:**834, 1959.

80. Drury, D.R., et al.: The effects of continuous pressure breathing on kidney function, J. Clin. Invest. **26:**945, 1947.

81. Henry, J.P., and Pierce, J.W.: Possible role of cardiac atrial stretch receptors in induction of changes in urine flow, J. Physiol. **131:**572, 1956.

82. Marquez, J.M., et al.: Renal function and cardiovascular responses during positive airway pressure, Anesthesiology **50:**393, 1979.

83. Pierce, A.K., and Saltzman, H.A., chairmen: Conference on the scientific basis for respiratory therapy, Am. Rev. Respir. Dis. **110**(2):1, 1974.

84. Pierce, A.K.: Scientific basis of in-hospital respiratory therapy, Am. Rev. Respir. Dis. **122**(2):1, 1980.

85. Hughes, R. L.: Points of view: improving post-operative tidal volumes, Respir. Care **26:**985, 1981.

86. O'Donohue, W.J.: Points of view: measures for lung expansion in post-operative patients, Respir. Care **26:**987, 1981.

87. Ziment, I.: Why are they saying bad things about IPPB? Respir. Care **18:**677, 1973.

88. Ziment, I.: In Burton, G.G., Gee, G.N., and Hodgkin, J.E., editors: Respiratory care: a guide to clinical practice, Philadelphia, 1977, J.B. Lippincott Co.

89. George, R.B., Gold, M.I., and Miller, W.F.: Current role of IPPB in pulmonary medicine—a panel discussion from the 1976 AART convention (edited by Kittredge, P.), Respir. Care **22:**610, 1977.

90. Pontoppidan, H.: Mechanical aids to lung expansion in non-intubated surgical patients, Am. Rev. Respir. Dis. **122** (2):109, 1980.

91. Murray, J.F.: Indications for mechanical aids to assist lung inflation in medical patients, Am. Rev. Respir. Dis. **122** (2):121, 1980.

92. Wu, N., Miller, W.F., Cade, R., and Richburg, P.: Intermittent positive pressure breathing in patients with chronic bronchopulmonary disease, Am. Rev. Tuberc. Pul. Dis. **71**:693, 1955.

93. Miller, W.F., Johnston, F.F., and Tarkoff, M.P.: Use of ultrasonic aerosols with ventilatory assistors, J. Asthma Res. **5**:335, 1968.

94. Ayres, S.M., Kozam, R.L., and Lukas, D.S.: The effects of intermittent positive pressure breathing on intrathoracic pressure, pulmonary mechanics and the work of breathing, Am. Rev. Respir. Dis. **87**:370, 1963.

95. Martin, R.J., Rogers, R.M., and Gray, B.A.: The physiologic basis for the use of mechanical aids to lung expansion, Am. Rev. Respir. Dis. **122**(2):105, 1980.

96. Welch, M.A., et al.: Methods of intermittent positive pressure breathing, Chest **78**:463, 1980.

97. O'Donohue, W.J.: Maximum volume IPPB for the management of pulmonary atelectasis, Chest **76**:683, 1979.

98. Egan, D.F.: Management of acute pulmonary edema, Hosp. Med. **2**:20, 1966.

99. Barach, A.L., Martin, S., and Eckman, M.: Positive pressure respiration and its application to the treatment of acute pulmonary edema and respiratory obstruction, Proc. Am. Soc. Clin. Invest. **16**:664, 1937.

100. Barach, A.L., Martin, S., and Eckman, M.: Positive pressure respiration and its application to the treatment of acute pulmonary edema, Ann. Intern. Med. **12**:754, 1938.

101. Poulton, E.P.: Left-sided heart failure with pulmonary edema treated with the pulmonary plus pressure machine, Lancet **2**:983, 1936.

102. Miller, W.F., and Sproule, B.J.: Studies on the role of intermittent inspiratory positive pressure oxygen breathing (IPPB—I-O$_2$) in treatment of pulmonary edema, Dis. Chest **35**:5, 1959.

103. Cheney, F.N., Nelson, E.J., and Horton, W.G.: The function of intermittent positive pressure breathing related to breathing patterns, Am. Rev. Respir. Dis. **110**(part 2):183, 1974.

104. Morrison, D.R., Powers, W.E., and Boocks, R.D.: A proposal for the more rational use of IPPB: volume orientation, Respir. Care **21**:318, 1976.

105. Powers, W.E., and Morrison, D.R.: Evaluation of inspired volumes in postoperative patients receiving volume-oriented IPPB, Respir. Care **23**:39, 1978.

106. Bartlett, R.H.: In Burton, G.G., Gee, G.N., and Hodgkin, J.E., editors: Respiratory care: a guide to clinical practice, Philadelphia, 1977, J.B. Lippincott Co., p. 874.

107. Ingram, R.H., Jr.: Mechanical aids to lung expansion (final report summary), Am. Rev. Respir. Dis. **122**(2):23, 1980.

108. Anderson, J.B., et al.: Periodic continuous positive airway pressure, CPAP, by mask in the treatment of atelectasis: a sequential analysis, Eur. J. Respir. Dis. **61**:20, 1980.

109. Yanda, R.L.: Quality control of IPPB therapy: a baseline study, Respir. Care **18**:33, 1973.

Chapter 14

Respiratory therapy management of respiratory failure

The respiratory therapist will have ample opportunities to apply the skills of respiratory care to a many patients who have a variety of disorders falling under the general heading of *respiratory failure*, either actual or pending. Various terms and definitions have been used to indicate similar clinical entities. The terms *respiratory insufficiency, pulmonary insufficiency* or *failure,* and *ventilatory insufficiency* or *failure* all have been used to describe patients in respiratory failure, and the student should realize that the medical literature on pulmonary diseases is not always uniform in its approach to terminology.

Here we use *respiratory failure* as a general term to describe clinical problems involving or leading to inadequate gas exchange *in the lungs,* usually evidenced by arterial blood gas levels outside the acceptable range. A common definition of respiratory failure by blood gases is a Pa_{CO_2} value of 50 mm Hg or more (not including respiratory compensation for metabolic alkalosis) or a Pa_{O_2} of 60 mm Hg or less, or below that expected for an individual patient's age (not including low Pa_{O_2} caused by *intracardiac* shunt).[1-3] While these numbers are not absolute, they are useful guidelines. Each patient should be evaluated separately for the determination of impending, acute, or chronic respiratory failure.

Generally it is useful to divide respiratory failure into two broad types, realizing that the two may also coexist. The first is respiratory failure causing hypercapnia and is often referred to as "ventilatory" failure since ventilation for clearing carbon dioxide is inadequate.[1] The second type is hypoxemic respiratory failure, in which the primary problem of gas exchange is related to arterial oxygenation.[1] We discuss the causes of hypoxemia in Chapter 8, the worst being the physiologic shunt of nonventilated but perfused areas of the lung. These types of failure can be mixed, and often hypoxemia occurs with the hypoventilation of ventilatory failure. In the early stages of acute respiratory failure causing hypoxemia, the Pa_{CO_2} is often *low* as the patient hyperventilates in response to the low oxygen level. Later, however, fatigue may occur, ventilation may decrease, and Pa_{CO_2} levels return to normal or even elevated values.

Table 14-1 summarizes the various causes of respiratory failure and indicates which are primarily from ventilatory (hypercapnic) failure and which are from hypoxemic respiratory failure.

Patients with respiratory failure often have multisystem derangement, although the primary focus is dramatically on the function of the lungs, and successful management involves several facets of therapy. In patients with inadequate gas exchange, good nursing is a critical factor, nutrition and fluid needs must be met, the control of infection may determine the eventual prognosis, and special care must often be given to cardiac function. Our interest is limited to those aspects of treatment that directly relate to the responsibility of the respiratory therapist. However, the therapist must be aware of and understand the purpose of the efforts and the concern of other medical disciplines involved. Cooperation among members of the medical team is essential, and the rapport among them is as important as that between the team and the patient. In this chapter we discuss such aspects of management of failure as *airway patency, selection of ventilators, ventilatory patterns,* and *monitoring ventilation.* Unavoidably, there is repetition, references to material discussed in other chapters, and cross references among subtopics. We attempt to use this to good advantage to summarize and correlate many principles of physiology and therapy by showing their practical application to patient care.

Table 14-1	Diagnosis	Hypoxemic	Hypercapnic
Causes of acute respiratory failure related to their anatomic reference.*	**Airways**		
	Aspiration of foreign body	1	
	Chronic obstructive pulmonary diseases	1	2
	Near drowning	1	
	Atelectasis	1	
	Lung parenchyma		
	Pneumonia	1	
	Oxygen toxicity	1	
	Toxic gases	1	
	Adult respiratory distress syndrome (ARDS)	1	
	Congestive heart failure	1	
	Fibrosing alveolitis	1	
	Aspiration of gastric contents	1	
	Lung contusion	1	
	Surgical loss of lung tissue	1	
	Blood borne causes		
	Fat embolism	1	
	Venous thromboembolism	1	
	Bacteremia	1	
	Fluid overload	1	
	Chest wall and diaphragm		
	Pneumothorax	1	
	Flail chest	2	1
	Ruptured diaphragm	2	1
	Pleural effusion	1	
	Kyphoscoliosis	2	1
	Spinal arthritis	2	1
	Fibrothorax	2	1
	Rib fractures	1	2
	Obesity	2	1
	Neuromuscular causes		
	Guillain-Barré syndrome	2	1
	Multiple sclerosis	2	1
	Myasthenia gravis	2	1
	Polio	2	1
	Botulism	2	1
	Tetanus	2	1
	Brain and spinal cord infarction	2	1
	Phrenic nerve paralysis	2	1
	Drug overdose	2	1
	Uncontrolled oxygen therapy		1
	Toxic drugs (curare, Colistin, kanamycin, streptomycin, neomycin)	2	1

*For each diagnosis the primary type of blood gas disorder is designated as number 1 and secondary blood gas disorder as number 2 if applicable.

Importance of patent airways

By now we have been well oriented toward the great hazard of airway obstruction and its pathologic origins and can justifiably relate it to the problems of assisting the patient in respiratory failure by the following dictum: *The effectiveness of ventilatory support is directly proportional to the patency of the airways.* The importance of the health of the bronchial tree gives it priority in our discussion. Airway obstruction is a major obstacle to ventilation and an almost constant challenge to the skill of the respiratory therapist—obvious in the patient suffering from chronic bronchopulmonary disease or insidiously developing in a patient otherwise afflicted. Not only is the attempt to administer artificial ventilation against severe obstruction usually futile but the efforts may be demonstrably harmful. Such an attempt may cause a serious increase in dead space ventilation and reduce effective alveolar tidal exchange, since the mechanically driven air rapidly generates back pressure. It may also encourage air trapping, with a subsequent increase in functional residual capacity and an elevation in the resting level, further burdening a lung that may already be abnormally distended.

Before instituting ventilatory support, the therapist should make an estimate of the status of the patient's airways. The therapist should learn something of the patient's background, either from the physician directly or through a study of the clinical chart, to determine whether airway obstruction has been a clinical feature. A significant smoking history may be a valuable warning clue in the patient with no apparent current obstruction; it should caution the therapist to be on the alert for a later complication. At the bedside the experienced therapist can listen for telltale wheezes or rhonchi with a stethoscope for evaluation. Once therapy is under way, indications of obstruction should always be sought. Periodic observation of the assisted patient's ventilation should reveal whether exhalation is unduly prolonged or effortful, whether the pattern is irregular, or whether the rate significantly increases. In the asisted or controlled patient, obstruction may be evidenced by marked shortening of inspiratory time, noted by listening to the cycling of the machine or by observing airway pressure. Air trapping can often be detected by slowing of a tidal volume–metering device to reach its end-expiratory baseline or by an elevation of this baseline.

The pharmacologic agents most frequently used in the treatment of airway obstruction are covered in Chapter 11, and we now consider the mechanical techniques available that may be used before the start of ventilation or introduced into the program at any time needed. The three important procedures with which we must be familiar are *bronchoscopy, intubation,* and *tracheobronchial suctioning.*

Bronchoscopy

Two types of bronchoscopy are now in widespread use—flexible, or fiberoptic, and rigid bronchoscopy. There are similarities and differences in the instruments used, their indications, and techniques. We first describe the older procedure, the introduction of the rigid scope into the airways.

Rigid bronchoscopy. Bronchoscopy is a procedure that is both therapeutic and diagnostic, requiring the services of a skilled and experienced physician, usually a specialist in the fields of either otorhinolaryngology (diseases of the ear, nose, and throat) or thoracic surgery. It is extensively used for direct visual examination of a suspected lesion in the bronchial tree or of one previously noted by x-ray examination. If the lesion is available, the brochoscopist can often remove a small specimen (biopsy) for histologic examination. The instrument is a long, lighted telescopic tube, with a tip that can be rotated through several degrees by remote control, and provided with lenses for looking into bronchial orifices. The procedure is usually performed in a room provided for it, although in extraordinary emergency situations it can be done at the bedside. The pharynx and larynx are locally anesthetized, and with the patient supine and head hyperextended, the operator introduces the tube through the mouth into the airway. Each side is examined in turn, and as the instrument is advanced deep into the main bronchi, the orifices of the branches are visualized. A long metal aspirator is inserted down the tube, and secretions are sucked out; often large plugs that may have obstructed large bronchi are removed.

Major problems with the rigid bronchoscope include its inability to reach all bronchi easily, its potential risk for inflicting patient injury, and the need for a special room for its use. Of the two types of bronchoscopies, however, the rigid procedure is the more useful for removing foreign bodies and for controlling intrabronchial bleeding.

Flexible (fiberoptic) bronchoscopy. Endobronchial examinations and therapy enjoyed giant steps forward with the application of fiberoptic technology to medicine.[4-7] Fiberoptic instruments basically consist of bundles of large numbers of fine glass fibers, each fiber capable of transmitting light. When connected to an electrical light source, but bundles of fibers provide a bright spot of light distally, even though the bundles are twisted on themselves into loops and knots. The importance of such flexibility is immediately evident, permitting the construction of a snakelike cable of light, able to reach into the depths of the respiratory tract. Its great virtue lies in the the wide range of circumstances in which it can be used. Local anesthesia is needed, but bronchoscopy can be performed at the bedside or while the patient is seated in a chair. Many patients can be treated as outpatients, thus eliminating expensive hospitalizations and operating room fees. Whereas the rigid scope is seldom used by any except specialists in otorhinolaryngology and thoracic surgery, the fiberoptic scope is being increasingly used by the internist specializing in pulmonary disease.

The value of bronchoscopy in treating and preventing serious atelectasis is obvious. In many patients suffering acute obstruction from secretions, a single drainage by this technique is often adequate, but if the disease is extensive enough to require repeated suctioning, other methods, described below, are preferred. Certainly, bronchoscopy is the most direct approach to the problem of excessive secretions, but it has little if any value in diffuse bronchospastic obstruction. Indeed, the mechanical irritation of the procedure itself may precipitate or worsen bronchial spasm. There are varying degrees of patient discomfort, both during and after the procedure; many patients complain of soreness of the throat for several hours. The introduction of the instrument into the respiratory tract constitutes an obstruction to breathing, and this can be a serious hazard to the patient already severely hypoxic. Finally, when rapid relief of acute obstruction is needed, the responsible personnel may not be immediately available for the most opportune use of bronchoscopy, and delay may not be justified.

The uses of the flexible bronchoscope extend not only to biopsy of the mucosal wall in the peripheral airways but also to biopsy of lung parenchyma. Some centers use the flexible bronchoscope for lung lavage, recovering the lavage cells for examination to determine the underlying causes of interstitial lung disease. Using special catheters and techniques, sterile samples can be obtained to diagnose pneumonias and the agent causing the inflammation. Without these techniques the sample obtained is contaminated with upper-airway and mouth organisms. Foreign body removal techniques that allow for the retrieval of solid aspirated substances have recently been well developed.

In the future, fluorescent light and lasar light techniques may be used for the diagnosis and treatment of multicentric, lung carcinoma in situ. This will offer a distinct advantage in the early diagnosis and cure of one of the most devastating cancers presently afflicting mankind.

Fiberoptic bronchoscopy can be used in the critically ill patient to help clear secretions as well as to provide diagnostic information.[4,5] More extensive information on uses and complications associated with bronchoscopy are available from other sources.[4-8]

Introduction to intubation

We explore intubation with artificial airways in considerable detail because it is almost a standard procedure in the patient with severe respiratory failure, and the therapist will work extensively with patients so treated. In contrast to bronchoscopy, which is a short-term technique, intubation is the placing of a rigid or semirigid tube in the respiratory tract and leaving it for varying periods of time, from a few hours to permanently, to ensure patency of the upper airway.

The following points should be noted about intubation: First, the tube itself is space occupying in the airway, and its use constitutes somewhat of a compromise in that the tube reduces the caliber of the natural lumen, although it ensures that the narrower passage is clear. Second, intubation is indicated for the access it provides to the bronchial tree for the aspiration of secretions (described in detail below). Third, it is a means of administering mechanical ventilation. Under certain limited circumstances, pressured air may be given to a patient by means of a face mask, but a moment's reflection will bring to mind several practical inadequacies of such a measure.

1. Because of the great variations in contours of the human face, a secure fit between mask and face is difficult to achieve, and if delivered pressure is to be responsible for ventilation, a leak in the system is hazardous.

2. With the best-designed face mask, considerable pressure must be applied to hold it in place to prevent slippage as well as leaks. The dependability of head straps or a harness is highly questionable, and with the force required, the risk of pressure necrosis of the skin is very real. The alternative method of the therapist manually holding the mask in place can be effective sometimes for short periods but is obviously impractical for *prolonged* supportive therapy.

3. There is a great risk of oropharyngeal obstruction by the lax tongue in the unconscious patient, a complication that is often precipitated by the supine position and the pressure of a mask. In such circumstances a mouth airway must always be used to hold the tongue out of the way and to provide a good channel for the delivered air.

4. In the presence of significant airway resistance, the flaccid cheeks may absorb enough of the ventilating pressure that pulmonary ventilation is compromised. Thus, except for short-term emergency treatment, the use of face masks is not suitable for positive-pressure ventilation, and a substantial airway must be provided.

For this last indication the tubes are almost always "cuffed." The cuff is a rubber or plastic, balloonlike item found near the lower end of the airway tube and has a narrow tube extending outside the body by which the cuff can be inflated with air. The simple illustration in Fig. 14-1 shows the general relationships of the parts involved. As the cuff fills with air, it seals the airway to prevent the retrograde flow of gas cephalad under pressure. Thus all gas movement is through the indwelling tube. The outer end of the inflating tube has a small pilot balloon that distends with the cuff and serves as a monitor because should the cuff develop a leak, the pilot balloon will also deflate. The cuff is usually filled with air by a syringe, and a clamp or plug is placed prox-

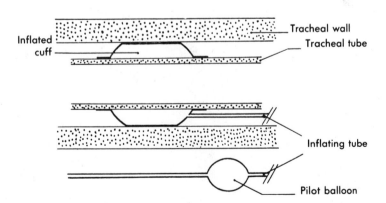

Fig. 14-1   Sketch of intratracheal tube with inflated cuff in place, in longitudinal section of the trachea. Air is introduced into the cuff through an inflating tube, which extends through the surgical incision to the outside. A pilot balloon warns of accidental deflation of the cuff after a clamp is placed distal to it on the inflating tube.

imal to the pilot balloon. More details of cuffs and their management are described later under the subject of tracheostomy.

There are three types of artificial airways for intubation in general clinical use: the *oral endotracheal tube,* the *nasotracheal tube,* and the *tracheostomy tube.* The individual features of each are described here, but characteristics common to all and the general principles of intubation and patient care are discussed with the tracheostomy as the model following a general introduction.

Endotracheal tubes are of plastic or rubber and come in a variety of sizes from 12 cm long with an inside diameter of 2.5 mm to about 38 cm long and an 11-mm inside diameter. They are curved to facilitate introduction into the respiratory tract and are available with attached cuffs, as shown in Fig. 14-2.

Endotracheal intubation, for the most part, is fairly simple, but it carries serious potential risks. At the outset, there is the possibility of an adverse reaction to the local anesthetic, a great hazard to any patient but more so in one with defective ventilation. The larynx is a sensitive organ and often responds to irritation or trauma by becoming spastic, completely occluding the airway, and attempts to force the tube may seriously damage the vocal cords. It is important that every effort be made to pass the cords on the first attempt, since repeated probing will stimulate an almost immediate edema of the cords, greatly hampering the procedure and risking the life of the patient. Intubation should still be considered a medical procedure, not a technical one, and its responsibilities entail legal and ethical considerations such that its use should most often be reserved for the professionally *trained* physician.

There is no doubt that a good therapist can be taught to perform intubation, but the skill with which it is performed is directly proportional to the

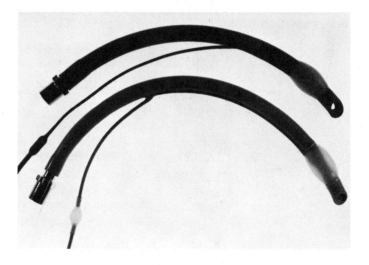

Fig. 14-2   Endotracheal tubes with inflated cuffs and pilot balloons.

frequency of its performance. Even though intubation is widely used in patients receiving respiratory therapy, the actual number of times per week or per month that the average therapist would have occasion to intubate is negligible when compared with its frequency in the daily work of the anesthesiologist. It is recognized that there may be circumstances in which trained professional personnel are not readily available and emergency or routine intubation must depend on the therapist. In this situation then, if competent respiratory therapists are available, they definitely should be given the responsibility. Two recent studies and an editorial support this view.[9-11] In one study 50 consecutive patients were intubated by respiratory therapists specifically trained in the procedure both in the operating room with one-to-one guidance and in emergency situations.[9] All 50 patients were intubed successfully; 35 required one attempt to pass the oral tube, 8 required 2 attempts, 5 needed 3 attempts, and 2 cases needed 4 passes before success was achieved. All procedures were performed under emergency conditions and occurred in the emergency room and various intensive care areas and general wards.

The other study compared respiratory therapist performance in emergency intubations to that of a physician group and a nurse anesthetist group.[10] Again a specific training program was adhered to by the respiratory therapists. Complications during the procedure were compared among groups. Of 47 intubation attempts, therapists had a complication rate of 13 (18%), including 3 unsuccessful attempts, 7 esophageal intubations, and 3 main stream bronchus intubations. This rate was favorable compared to the other groups, which had an *overall* complication rate of 57%.

More studies of larger groups are needed, but these studies do support the practice of training and evaluating respiratory therapists for emergency intubations. However, to maintain their expertise respiratory therapists should practice intubation regularly and frequently in the surgical suite.[11] In summary, each hospital must work out its own solution to providing emergency intubation, but whenever possible, a trained physician, especially an anesthesiologist, should be on first call. It should be remembered that even the most skillful operator is at a serious disadvantage when faced with the task of intubating a larynx already spastic and edematous from a bungled earlier unsuccessful attempt.

Oral endotracheal intubation

Oral endotracheal intubation has long been used to maintain an open airway during surgery, usually instituted after induction of the anesthesia, but with the increasing incidence of pulmonary diseases, it has become an important part of medical management of the conscious or unconscious patient in respiratory failure.

The base of the tongue, the pharynx, and the larynx are rendered insensitive with local anesthetic nebulized or directly applied to the area and sometimes infiltrated into the larynx by injection. With the patient in the supine position, the way is readied for intubation by introducing a laryngoscope into the pharynx. This is an instrument consisting of a handle containing batteries and a small bulb, at approximately right angles to which is a blade that may be straight or curved. Thus, under direct lighted vision, the tip of the laryngoscope blade displaces the epiglottis and exposes the larynx. The endotracheal tube can then be inserted between the vocal cords through the larynx into the trachea just far enough that the cuff clears the larynx. A small oral airway or some other effective "bite block" is fastened between the patient's teeth to prevent accidental compression of the tube by closure of the jaws.

The advantages of oral endotracheal intubation are summarized in a study of this technique.[12] A good airway can be obtained by an expert operator in a short time without the risk and inconvenience of a surgical procedure, as is necessary for tracheotomy. There is no tissue destruction or scarring and no anatomic distortion so that a repeat intubation can be done whenever necessary. Extubation (removal of the tube) time was found to be shorter than with a tracheostomy because there seemed to be less patient and physician dependence on nonsurgical than on surgical intubation. Of great significance was the observation that the return of an effective cough was almost immediate after extubation, whereas there is always some delay after surgical violation of the trachea. Finally, the prior oral intubation of the trachea makes much safer and easier a subsequent tracheotomy, a point that is emphasized below in the discussion of the latter procedure.

In comparison, the disadvantages of oral intubation are of less significance. The most important is some degree of patient intolerance to the awkwardness and inconvenience of the large tube through the mouth. Frequently, much continuous assurance must be given the patient, supported by sedation to allay apprehension and reduce discomfort, obviously not a problem in the unconscious or mentally obtunded patient. Occasionally an agitated patient may pull out the tube, but after replacement, proper restraint will prevent recurrence. Laryngeal edema may be troublesome in the postintubation period, but this has not proved to be a serious hazard, and reintubation can always be done if needed. Until fairly recently it was almost a dictum that oral endotracheal intubation be terminated at 48 hours and that if further therapy were necessary, tracheotomy be done. With increasing experience in its use, the duration of intubation has been greatly expanded, and in the study referred to above, tubes were left in place for periods ranging from 21 to 171 hours with no ill effects.

Other studies have also attempted to evaluate how long endotracheal intubation can be provided before a tracheotomy should be done. A recent study that included both oral and nasotracheal tubes (more than 80% were oral tubes) compared the complications that occurred with these tubes with complications that occurred with tracheostomy tubes.[13] Fifty patients in the endotracheal intubation group had their tubes in place for more than 10 days (up to 22 days). In general, the tracheotomy group had a higher incidence of problems although on the average, they also had the tubes in place longer.

A group of six patients who were intubated from 55 to 155 days (mean 85 days) are the subject of a recent brief report.[14] The authors reported that all six patients had some hoarseness following extubation, three remained hoarse, and three improved. None had any major complications of the airway. Based on the conclusions of other studies[15,16] 1 week to 10 days is probably a more commonly used limit for intubation through the larynx.[14]

Nasotracheal intubation

The objectives of nasotracheal intubation, as well as the tube employed, are similar to those of oral intubation. In this case, however, the tube is introduced first through the nose rather than the mouth and then into the trachea. Although "blind" passage of the tube through the larynx can be attempted, it is much safer to use the same direct visual approach as with oral intubation once the tube has passed the nasal cavity. Nasotracheal intubation has been most extensively used in children but is now finding increasing favor in the treatment of adults, and a study compares its effectiveness with that of tracheostomy in the latter group.[17] With a variety of underlying conditions necessitating intubation, nasotracheal tubes were used for periods ranging from 12 hours to 14 days. The advantages of this procedure are the same as those described for oral intubation with the additional feature of better patient tolerance, better oral hygiene, and less discomfort, since the mouth is free of the large tube. Similarly, the disadvantages are basically those noted previously, with the possible additional risk of some kinking of the tube as it navigates the tortuous nasal passages.

The opinion is frequently heard that a nasotracheal tube must be smaller than an oral or tracheostomy tube and that resistance to airflow will be accordingly increased. The report cited above disputes this, implying that there need be no difference between the oral and nasal tubes, although it would seem reasonable that unfavorable nasal conditions might limit the size of tube that could be effectively used.[17] It further states that despite its greater length, the nasotracheal tube may be less resistant than a loosely fitted tracheostomy tube. It is interesting to note that the survey of the oral endotracheal technique referred to earlier[12] found the use of nasotracheal tubes in adults much less satisfactory than the use of oral tubes and was accompanied by a sharp difference in patient survival. In all probability the differences in opinion reflect the results of personal experiences and interest in one technique over the other rather than any significant inherent difference in these two similar procedures. The therapist will perhaps note that just as we were unable to describe one best mechanical ventilator, endowed with all virtues and no vices, so there is no single intubation technique to satisfy all needs.

A problem that relates to both oral and nasotracheal tubes is one of position in the trachea, and a recent report pointed out the importance of the patient's head in relation to tube position.[18] It was found that for both oral endotracheal and nasotracheal tubes, movement of the head caused a change of position of the tube in the trachea. When the head was tilted with the chin toward the chest (flexation) the tube moved *downward* toward the carina 1.9 cm on the average. Extension of the neck, that is, raising the chin from the chest, caused an average movement of the tube 1.9 cm *upward* in the trachea from the neutral position. This occurred in both types of tubes and regardless of cuff inflation.[18] The report used radiographs to determine this movement, and it points out the need for adequate positioning and securing of the airway once in place.

Tracheostomy intubation

Tracheotomy is a surgical procedure that produces an opening in the trachea (the suffix-*tomy* means "a cutting or incision"), and a *tracheostomy* is the opening so made in the trachea (the suffix-*stomy* coming from the Greek *stoma,* "mouth"). A *tracheostomy tube* is therefore a tube designed to be placed in the trachea through a tracheostomy. This technique has been a lifesaving procedure for some 3 centuries, to and including the present, and is the most precise and definitive way to establish and maintain a free upper airway.

The indications for a tracheostomy can be enumerated as follows: (1) to establish and maintain a patent and accessible airway after endotracheal intubation or when the latter is not considered desirable; (2) with a cuffed tube, to prevent aspiration of regurgitated gastric contents or blood from facial or oral trauma, as in a comatose patient or one with obtunded reflexes; (3) to permit the aspiration of bronchopulmonary secretions, a maneuver easier through a tracheostomy tube than through the longer endotracheal tube; (4) with a cuffed tube, to permit long-term, positive-pressure mechanical ventilation; and (5) to reduce the anatomic dead space and relieve the work of breathing. By short-circuiting the nasal, oral, and pharyngeal passages, the tracheostomy tube affords the spontaneously breathing patient less distance to move air from atmosphere to alveoli. Reference is made to this again later, but it should be observed that the cost of reducing the dead space is a reduction in the lumen of the upper airway, since the tracheostomy tube itself is an obstruction. It has been shown that resistance to breathing does not drop significantly below normal in the adult patient until the internal diameter of the tube exceeds 9.5 mm, and this is larger than the three most commonly used tubes.[19]

Tracheotomy procedure. Tracheotomy itself is not to be taken lightly, since it is a surgical procedure carried out on a patient with a severly compromised major system. Emergency tracheotomies have been performed under a variety of circumstances, and may well be, of necessity, in the future. However, every attempt should be made to see that conditions for it are as ideal as possible, and in the modern hospital the bedside tracheotomy is denounced. Even in the most critical situations, tracheotomy should be an elective procedure, done in the operating room with due regard for preparation and careful technique. With the recognition of airway obstruction severe enough to warrant mechanical interference, the patient should immediately be intubated endotracheally to ensure survival; supportive therapy should be given, and surgery performed, when both the patient's condition and the operating facilities are at their best.

The techniques of tracheotomy may vary, but in general the incision into and through the skin and subcutaneous tissue is made high enough so that the trachea can be entered at the level of either the second or third cartilage. This site is essential so that the tip of the tube will not impinge on the carina. Selection of a tube of proper size and shape is critically important, for the tube must be neither too tight nor too loose if the complications (described later) are to be avoided. Once firmly in place, the tracheostomy tube is secured by a fabric tape around the patient's neck. Tracheotomy carries with it definite surgical risks; the mortality directly attributed to the procedure, as opposed to the underlying disease, is estimated at 3% and serious complications at nearly 50% in some series,[17] and 1.6% mortality and about 16% complication rate in another, large study.[20] The three most important immediate surgical complications can be classifed as follows.

Bleeding. Bleeding is an exceptionally potential hazard, for not only is the involved anatomic area naturally very vascular but congestion in the vessels is often increased as a result of the hemodynamic changes incidental to both pulmonary disease and supportive ventilation. Every bleeding source must be meticulously attended because these patients can ill afford the stress of excessive blood loss.

Tissue emphysema. The great variety of neck contours seriously challenges the surgeons, and the probing and dissection in some patients hold the risk of invading the apices of the lungs with subsequent pneumothorax. Not rarely, air escapes from the opened trachea and works its way through exposed tissues to accumulate under the skin of the face, neck, and thorax, a condition known as *subcutaneous emphysema.* More serious is the movement of air along the paths of the major airways into the mediastinum, *mediastinal emphysema,* where it builds up in response to the negative pressure of the patient's inspiratory efforts and may embarrass the intrathoracic cardiorespiratory mechanics. Fortunately, most of the time such events are correctable or tolerated by the body, but since they can occur even when tracheotomy is done with operating room care, the therapist can understand the risk of operating in haste.

Cardiovascular collapse. There are two types of adverse cardiovascular reactions to the tracheotomy procedure itself, similar in their end results but differing markedly in their mechanisms. First, one of the immediate hazards is acute cardiac arrest, most often encountered during a hurried tracheotomy but fortunately becoming less frequent with adherence to currently accepted practices. At one time believed to be caused by some vagal reflex accompanying the trauma of surgery, arrest is now attributed to a severe and sudden hypoxia superimposed on the hypoxia of the underlying disease, as ventilation is impaired during the manipulations of the procedure. This is the major reason for prior intubation and efforts to improve oxygenation before surgery and for maintaining good mechanical or amnual ventilation until the new airway is adequately functioning. Second, cardiovascular and sometimes respiratory collapse may be the paradoxic result of rapidly achieving a good airway during tracheotomy.[21] Shortly after the airway is secured and secretions cleaned out, the patient may become acutely hypotensive and pulseless and go into complete apnea. This reaction is believed to be caused by the sudden washout of accumulated carbon dioxide from the body as alveolar ventilation is precipitously increased and the respiratory acidosis reversed. Such a rapid swing in acid-base balance is known to produce arrhythmias and hypotension. The accompanying apnea is the sequela of cerebral blood flow reduction from both the circulatory failure and vascular dilation of sudden hypocapnia. Before, during, and immediately after tracheotomy, the patient's blood pressure should be checked frequently and vasopressors kept close at hand to prevent the shock from becoming irreversible.

It might be of interest to note that a secondary, but definitely helpful, benefit of preoperative intubation is the increased ease of locating, mobilizing, and handling a trachea already identified and supported by an indwelling tube. In summary, we can say that the incidence and seriousness of tracheotomy complications are inversely related to the degree that the procedure is performed under elective, controlled conditions.

Tracheostomy tubes. There are many types of tracheostomy tubes now available. For many years only silver tubes were used, but disposable plastic tubes have become popular and for the most part have replaced the metal. We first describe the traditional silver tube (Fig. 14-3) because it is occasionally used, and its parts can be disassembled for descriptive purposes. Then we consider the features of plastic tubes that have given them their position of prominence.

Silver tubes. The tubes are curved to accommodate the anatomy of the trachea and to facilitate introduction and removal, varying from an outside diameter of 3 mm and a length along the outside of the curve of 1.75 inches to an outside diameter of 14 mm and a length of over 4 inches. The tracheostomy tube is basically a cannula within a cannula (Fig. 14-3). The *outer cannula* maintains the patency of the airway, whereas the *inner cannula* is removable for cleaning to prevent secretions from obstructing the tip. If there were but a single tube and it became plugged with secretions, it would have to be removed, thereby disrupting the entire surgical area. This is avoided by the removable inner cannula.

The styluslike accessory is called an *obturator,* and it is used only for the initial introduction of the outer cannula to prevent scraping of the tracheal wall. Once the outer cannula is in place, the obturator is withdrawn and the inner cannula inserted. The two cannulae are held snugly together by a locking mechanism on the metal units or by friction on the plastic. The head of the inner cannula is designed to accept adapters that permit the attachment of ventilators to the system.

Plastic tubes. Plastic tracheostomy tubes generally follow the pattern described for silver tubes, but they have some decided advantages of their own. A major advantage of the plastic tracheostomy tube is its disposability. Each tube is packaged sterile and after use is thrown away, to be replaced by a new one as needed. Additionally, the tubes are lightweight with no sharp edges—features that reduce the risk of tracheal injury during movement of patient or tube. Plastic tends to soften slightly at body temperature, allowing the tube to

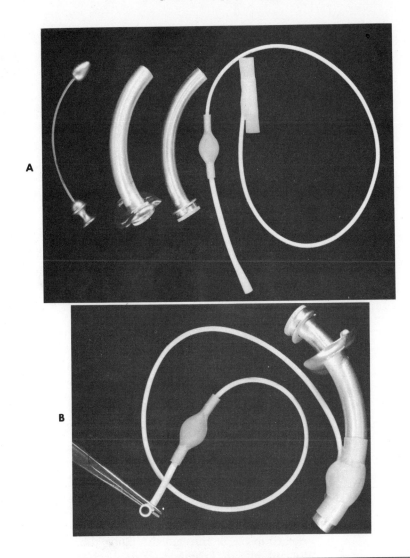

Fig. 14-3   **A,** Components of a disassembled silver tracheostomy tube. On the left is a stylus, or obturator, used only during insertion of the outer cannula, followed by the outer and inner cannulae, and a cuff. **B,** Cuff is in place and inflated, and the inner cannula is seen protruding slightly from the outer tube.

conform to the tracheal contour for a maximum fit. An important asset is the bonded cuff already sealed onto the cannula, eliminating a sometimes difficult task and ensuring that the cuff will not slip off the end of the tube.

Fig. 14-4 shows a common and popular plastic tracheostomy tube. Like many others it has no inner cannula, making frequent suctioning of secretions necessary to prevent obstruction. A variety of tubes are commercially available,

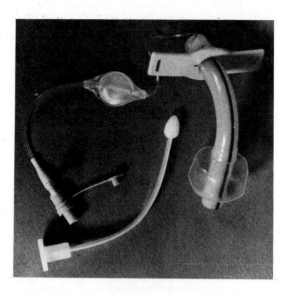

Fig. 14-4   Plastic, low-pressure cuff tracheostomy tube.

and their various features have been presented in other textbooks[22-24] and in journal articles.[25-31] Most of these tubes are made of polyvinyl cloride, silicone, or rubber.[27]

Types of cuffs   We have made frequent references to the cuffs used on intubation tubes, and because of their importance in making effective ventilation available to patients, we describe them here in a bit more detail. A typical cuff for a metal tracheostomy tube is an elastic sleeve whose central segment is thinner walled than its ends and which is slipped over the distal portion of the outer cannula. A small-caliber elastic tube runs from the center of the cuff, along the outer cannula, and through the tracheostomy incision to the outside. A syringe is used to instill air through this filling tube to inflate the distensible center of the cuff, effectively sealing off the trachea around the outer cannula and preventing retrograde air leaks from ventilator positive pressure. The inflating tube is closed by a plug or clamp. Between its outer end and the patient, the tube is equipped with a pilot balloon, which inflates with the distal cuff. This allows the therapist to monitor the integrity of the inflated cuff, for if the cuff should collapse from a leak, the pilot balloon would also deflate. Separate cuffs vary in size from 4 mm to about 13 mm, and success of subsequent ventilation may depend on the proper application of the proper size cuff. As shown in Fig. 14-3, the ends of the cuff are narrower and less elastic than the easily distensible midportion. The tight fit of the ends of the cuff holds it in place on the outer cannula of the tube to prevent both leakage and slippage; a special cement can be used for additional support.

A feature of great value, found with most tubes now used, is the *high-residual volume low-pressure* cuff.[25-30] Designed to occlude the airway with a minimum of intracuff air pressure, thereby reducing the hazard of pressure damage to the tracheal mucosa, low-pressure cuffs are generally of two basic types. The cuff shown in Fig. 14-4 is constructed with a large surface for mucosal contact, thus distributing its pressure over a broad area of mucosa. Lower total pressure is needed for a good seal than if the cuff-tracheal interface were smaller.[32] The second type of low-pressure cuff contains a spongy, air-cell substance, which can be deflated by syringe aspiration for insertion into the airway and which needs no inflation for sealing because of the self-expansion of its air-foam.[30,31]

Both of these types of cuffs differ from the old-style cuffs initially used on tubes. The older style cuffs act more like balloons and must be actively stretched by inflating them with air in order for them to touch the tracheal wall and make a seal. This requires a high pressure within the cuff, and only a relatively small area of contact is made by the cuff against the tracheal wall. In order to create a seal with these cuffs, high pressures are exerted against the trachea.[26-28] At rest these cuffs have little or no volume of air in them and are therefore referred to as *low residual volume, high-pressure* cuffs.

Most low-pressure cuffs can provide an adequate seal of the airway while maintaining pressures of 25 mm Hg or less when used properly.[26] Some tubes have special controlled-pressure devices to help limit the pressure and allow for long-term use with minimal tracheal damage.[22,29,31,33]

We have been emphasizing the primary function of an inflated tracheostomy tube cuff, sealing the trachea between the tube cannula and tracheal wall for use with a positive-pressure ventilator. Often, whenever the patient is not being ventilated, the cuff need not be inflated, but there is an exception. A secondary use of the inflated cuff is prevention of aspiration into the airways of vomitus, secretions pooling in the hypopharynx, or food in patients who are obtunded or with dulled epiglottal reflexes. The length of time a cuff should remain inflated for these reasons alone is a matter of clinical judgement, but in selected patients such protection of the airways may be lifesaving. Always, before the cuff is deflated for any reason, the hypopharynx must be suctioned of any material to prevent its aspiration past the collapsed cuff into the bronchial tree.

Proper cuff inflation requires skill but is somewhat easier if the patient is using a ventilator. In general, the older practice of instilling a fixed volume of air, such as 5 or 10 ml, into the cuff is no longer advised. With the tip of a 10- or 20-ml syringe inserted into the end of the inflating tube, air is slowly introduced while ventilator is attached and operating. Inspiratory air leakage is noted, and cuff inflation is stopped as soon as the leak ceases. Air is then slowly withdrawn from the cuff until a slight leak is once again heard. At this point just enough air can be reintroduced into the cuff to stop the leak, with assurance that occlusion of the cuff is achieved with minimal pressure. As an alternative, the "minimal leak" technique can be used by plugging the filling tube while a slight leak persists. This utilizes the small inspiratory leak to blow cephalad for easier removal of secretions tending to pool around the cuff.

Management of the intubated patient

The management of the tracheotomized patient mechanically ventilated through a cuffed tube constitutes one of the respiratory therapist's greatest responsibilities. There are several factors that the therapist must bear in mind in addition to attention to the efficient functioning of the ventilator. The therapist must remember that the patient is entirely dependent on all medical and nursing attendants. If the patient is alert, he or she will initially be apprehensive and justifiably may be greatly frightened. Reassurance by the therapist through words and action is a *critical* part of therapy, for the patient's emotional status may markedly influence the breathing pattern or acceptance of mechanical ventilation. The therapist must create an atmosphere of calmness and confidence for the patient, aware that the patient watches every move and listens to every word.

It must be remembered that the cuffed patient cannot talk because the vocal cords are bypassed by the tracheostomy tube. With a tracheostomy tube, the patient can speak only after disconnection from the ventilator, deflation of the cuff, and obstruction of the outer opening of the tube so that exhaled air can leak around the tube through the larynx. This may be tiring and should be reserved for those instances when the patient desires to communicate, or when it is necessary to get information from him or her that is essential to therapy.

It was noted previously that adapters are used to attach the ventilator to the end of the inner cannula. For the most part, these are plastic and come in sets to accommodate all sizes of tubes. They are generally held into the inner cannula (a further reduction in the caliber of the airway) by friction, connecting the airway to the machine by a flex tube. It is important to adjust this joint in such a manner that there is a minimum of strain on the connector to reduce the risk of accidental dislodgement, which would completely separate the patient from the major, if not only, source of ventilation. There are various swivel connectors that permit patient mobility without loosening.

The constant potential hazard to the intubated patient, as noted frequently, is obstruction, especially from accumulated secretions. One of the safeguards against this is effective suctioning, the technique of which is described separately below. In addition, if an inner cannula is present, it should be removed and cleaned every 4 hours, or more frequently if needed; for long-term care the entire tube may be removed and changed weekly, even in the absence of malfunction, a responsibility of the physician who did the original surgery or a skilled therapist.[34,35] The final protection against secretion buildup is adequate humidification, and we do not exaggerate when we say that not only will intubation fail to achieve its purpose but it may be positively harmful to the patient if humidity is lacking.

While the patient's dead space has been reduced by tracheotomy, so has the natural humidification mechanism been bypassed, and little can be more detrimental to the respiratory hygiene than a flow of dry air or gas (even room air) directly into the trachea. While the patient is being ventilated, humidification will be provided by the many effective devices available as attachments, especially heated units such as the Cascade humidifier, which delivers water vapor, not aerosolized water, with the latter's capability of carrying bacteria into equipment or the patient's respiratory tract. However, humidification must not be overlooked when the patient is removed from the machine for significant periods of time. A tracheostomy mask or collar that conveniently fits over the opening of the cannula or a T-tube is satisfactory if used with a good humidifier. It is believed by many that secretions will seldom be a serious problem if the patient is supplied with adequate vapor and water aerosol, since most secretions will be wet enough to be easily suctioned. Water in the inspired gas serves another purpose in addition to that of maintaining general health of the respiratory tract. No matter how good is the fit of a tracheostomy tube, there is always some motion of it in response to respiration, patient activity, and handling of the attachments; and a bit of excess water in and about the tube acts as a lubricant to minimize frictional damage to the local mucosa.

Many of the patients who are intubated need supplemental oxygen therapy. Our concern here is not with the indications for or the hazards of oxygen per se, for we have already considered these factors earlier and discuss them again later on; our concern, rather, is with the method of administration. As in the case of humidity mentioned above, during mechanical ventilation oxygen will be provided as needed through the instrument, but a word is in order concerning its use when the patient is not being ventilated. The safest technique is the use of a T or tracheostomy mask, which can combine both oxygen and humidification. Unfortunately, there is an old technique still in use that is to be condemned. This is the insertion of an oxygen catheter directly into the tracheostomy tube. Although arterial oxygen levels can be increased, such a procedure offers a significant resistance to exhalation with a potential danger that outweighs any benefit. This subject was studied with convincing results of the ventilatory burden it imposes. We have already indicated that the tube itself increases the airflow resistance in the respiratory tract, and it is reasonable that the introduction of a catheter, no matter how small, will further increase such resistance. When to this is added the resistance of an oxygen flow directly opposing the passive outflow of air, we can only wonder that such a procedure was ever considered safe. The study logically concluded, but with quantitative proof, that peak expiratory resistance increased as the size of the tracheostomy tube decreased, as the size of the oxygen catheter increased, and as the oxygen flow increased. Should a therapist encounter this procedure in use or being contemplated, it is hoped that he or she will use the greatest diplomacy and tact in suggesting an alternate technique.

Complications of tracheostomy

In addition to the hazards of the surgical procedure of tracheotomy and the clinical precautions to be considered in the management of a tracheotomized patient, there are complications that can be attributed to the presence of the tracheostomy or endotracheal tube itself.[13,25,26,35-39] Although the medical care of such complications is a responsibility of the attending physician, the respiratory therapist should be acquainted with them, for he or she may be the first to note their onset and so stimulate immediate corrective action. Some latitude may be expected in determining what phenomena constitute complications resulting from a tracheostomy, but we include the most important in the following classification.

Obstruction

From secretions. This has already been discussed and is repeated only for emphasis of its importance, but it most certainly is a direct result of the aggravation of preexisting secretions by intubation.

From the cuff. A loosely fitted, single-lumen cuff may partially or completely slip off the end of the cannula, obstructing the airway locally or in either main stem bronchus. This is most apt to occur following rupture of the cuff after it has been in operation, during manipulation of the cannula with the cuff deflated, or during removal of the tube. Clinical and mechanical signs and symptoms of airway obstruction accompanied by inability to inflate the cuff should bring this probability immediately to mind. Because of its better grip on the cannula, a double-lumen cuff is unlikely to become completely dislodged, even when deflated, but it may herniate or hang over the end of the cannula. When it is then inflated, it will occlude both the trachea and the tracheostomy tube as it distends freely across the opening of the cannula. The resulting severe dyspnea in the spontaneously breathing patient will be relieved by deflation of the cuff, and the obstructive response of an attached ventilator will be replaced by evidence of a leak. In such a condition a probing suction catheter will encounter the obstructing inflated cuff but will pass freely when the cuff is emptied of air.

There is also a potential for the large, floppy, low-pressure cuffs to occlude the end of an endotracheal or tracheostomy tube if they are sufficiently *over-inflated*.[40] If the cuffs are inflated just enough to create a seal or with the minimal leak technique, this type of occlusion should not occur. High inflation pressures have also been known to compress plastic or rubber tubes, constricting their lumen and causing obstruction to gas flow.[1,39,41] This is especially likely with low-volume, high-pressure cuffs.[41]

From the cannula. Should the tracheotomy incision be placed too low or too long a tube be installed, the tip of the cannula may impinge on the carina, with resulting severe obstruction. When intubation has been completed and mechanical ventilation started, the attending physician or the responsible therapist should always check to be sure that the cannula is not directed down one or the other main stem bronchi. Should this occur, all the ventilation will go to one lung, whereas the other will become severely atelectatic from complete deprivation of its air supply. Suspicion of this complication should be aroused by the inability to achieve satisfactory ventilation with the respirator (because of the reduced volume of only one functioning lung) and is confirmed by the lack of breath sounds in the bypassed lung as the chest is examined by stethoscope. Immediate correction is mandatory, since this is life threatening.

From abraded mucosa. It has been suggested that many of the instances of obstruction following tracheal intubation may be the result of what has been termed the "snowplow effect" of the tracheal cannula.[42] While the rigid tube remains fairly stable, the respiratory tract moves with the breathing cycle, riding upward during exhalation and downward during inhalation. As a result, if the tube is not centered in the airway and its tip is allowed to rest on the inner tracheal wall, the cephalad expiratory movement scrapes the tracheal mucosa against the unyielding edge of the cannular opening.[40] Debrided epithelium, mixed with secretions, has been demonstrated to form a mass of significant size to obstruct a bronchus and require bronchoscopic removal. Selection of tubes of the proper length and, if necessary, supporting them by packing about the tracheotomy opening will minimize this traumatic risk.

From tracheal stenosis. Obstruction from tracheal stenosis is a serious complication that becomes evident during the weeks following extubation or removal of the tracheostomy tube. As the trachea heals from the double trauma of tracheostomy and intubation, its passage may narrow from fibrous scarring or from the growth of granulation tissue, which is a soft, easy-bleeding mass of proliferating blood vessels, often replacing destroyed tissue. Stenosis usually occurs at the stoma, or incisional opening of the tracheostomy, or at the site of the tracheostomy tube cuff pressure. The stoma probably heals by the joining of severed tracheal cartilage ends, and if the rings are surgically shortened, stenosis results. On the other hand, cuff site tracheal stenosis is often preceded by severe pressure necrosis damage, as the distended cuff impairs local blood supply, causing tissue death and ulceration. Not only is the mucosa injured but the tracheal wall as well, with exposure and destruction of cartilaginous rings. This stage is referred to as *tracheomalacia,* which means a weakness of the tracheal wall usually causing the trachea to dilate. Postmortem studies suggest that some degree of necrosis is probably present in all intubated tracheas.[43] The lesion is circumferential, extending around the trachea, and as destroyed tissue is replaced by granulation and scar, a gradually contracting ring constricts the trachea.[44] Regardless of the cause, if stenosis is symptomatic, interfering with airflow, surgical repair is needed.

There are many informative articles in the pulmonary literature describing stenosis of the trachea after intubation, and the student is advised to make use of them. A recent survey of 40 patients, electively tracheotomized for ventilatory assistance, revealed the following: (1) 10% had complicating bleeding; (2) 17.5% had some problem with tracheostomy management; (3) 16% had asymptomatic narrowing of the stoma site; (4) 16% had asymptomatic defects at the cuff site; and (5) 8% required tracheal resection for stomal stenosis.[35] This study strongly suggests postextubation evaluation of the trachea by fiberoptic bronchoscopy or x-ray examination.[35]

Hemorrhage

From the incisional site. Inadequate hemostasis (control of bleeding) during surgery may allow a recurrence of bleeding from the operative site after therapy has been started. The danger of brisk bleeding is obvious, but even a hidden slow oozing of blood is hazardous, since blood may accumulate about the upper part of the cannula in the trachea and be aspirated into the bronchi when the cuff is deflated during routine care.

From tracheal trauma. Erosion of the tracheal mucosa as described above with "snowplowing" can produce surface bleeding, with subsequent aspiration. Less common, but far more serious, is a frank perforation of the tracheal wall by the indwelling cannula, with damage to a neighboring artery. This may lead to rapid and fatal exsanguination.

Tissue emphysema. The escape of air into body tissues during surgery has already been noted when intrathoracic negative pressure can draw air through the planes of exposed cut tissues, letting it migrate to the mediastinum and subcutaneous areas. During positive-pressure ventilation this is unlikely unless the patient is "fighting" the machine because it is not meeting his or her needs, in which case inspiratory efforts may suck air into the tissues around the incision. However, should there be damage to the airway below the level of the tracheal cuff (as from the end of the cannula), positive-pressure ventilation may force air into the tissues, producing extensive subcutaneous emphysema.

Infection. Some physicians believe that infection is the most troublesome, if not the most significant, of tracheostomy complications.[45,46] It may range from a relatively minor wound sepsis to an overwhelming pneumonia. A frequent major problem is differentiating the infection because of invasion of the respiratory tract through a tracheotomy from that of the underlying pulmonary disease, and at times this is not possible to do with certainty. Many patients have preexisting bronchopulmonary infection at the time of their tracheotomies, and, indeed, such infections may be prominent etiologic factors in the obstructions for which the tracheotomies are performed. There can be little doubt that intubating the trachea increases the possibility of infection, with the deliberate perpetuation of an open wound into the air passages, bypassing the natural filtering mechanism of the upper tract. Handling the tube, frequent introduction of a catheter into the trachea, attaching ventilators to the tube, and serous seepage about the incision all contribute to the risk of infection. However, even positive bacterial cultures of aspirates or wound discharges are not conclusive evidence of a clinical infection; they may be from local contaminants. For the diagnosis of a significant infection, there must be signs and symptoms other than just bacteriologic. Despite the increased chances for sepsis through a tracheostomy, it is not rare to note rapid clearing of a pulmonary infection after the establishment of good bronchial drainage and the aspiration of obstructing secretions.

Especially troublesome is the bacterium *Pseudomonas aeruginosa,* about which the therapist will hear many references. Its frequent culture from tracheotomized patients and their equipment is a constant cause for concern. Because it thrives in dampness, it is a frequent contaminant of equipment and utensils, but an unusual overgrowth of the organism in a patient weakened by disease can be pathogenic in its own right—a serious hazard to the already handicapped patient. Meticulous care is necessary for the tracheotomized patient, and attention to the wound or the tube should be only under conditions of surgically sterile technique. The incision should be treated as any surgical site, with cleaning and asepsis as indicated, and it should be kept dressed as sterile as is consistent with its use. An awareness of the risk of infection in the patient in respiratory failure will help all attending personnel to exercise caution and avoid carelessness.

Summary

The importance of tracheostomy therapy justifies a summation of its place in the management of respiratory failure. If at all avoidable, tracheotomy should never be done as a hurried emergency procedure, since such a circumstance carries with it high mortality and morbidity. Prior intubation should be performed to secure a good airway, for not only does it give technical assistance to the operating surgeon but it also prevents the serious hypoxia that is so likely to damage the patient, even to the point of triggering cardiac arrest. At the same time, overventilation must be avoided or the patient is subjected to the risk of acute alkalosis with cardiovascular collapse and cerebral hypoxia. These two seemingly paradoxic precautions point up the great skill needed to safeguard the patient during the procedure. During follow-up management, medical attendants must watch especially carefully for cuff failure and take all necessary care to prevent tracheal damage. In general, to minimize bleeding and infection the tracheostomy must be treated like the surgical site it is.

Tracheotomy is surgery performed on a physiologically unstable patient in critical condition, and in a real sense it is chosen as the lesser of two evils. The fatality rate among tracheotomized patients has been reported as high as 38% in one group of 300.[47] This is not an indictment against the therapy but, rather, reflects the gravity of the diseases making it necessary. On the other hand, after a careful review it was estimated that a similar 38% of over 400 patients survived their illnesses because they did undergo tracheotomy.[45] In addition to the advantages of airway suctioning and the ability to assist ventilation, tracheotomy carries a physiologic benefit of its own, as shown by a study of the character of spontaneous breathing in a group of emphysematous patients.[48] The subjects experienced a reduction in total ventilation, attributed to a reduction in the volume of the dead space, which was more than enough to offset the increased resistance afforded by the tracheostomy tube, compared with the resistance of mouth breathing. That this was true was indicated in the lowered oxygen consumption, showing a significant reduction in the physical work of breathing. Because less oxygen was needed for ventilatory efforts, arterial oxygen saturation rose, probably aided by a concomitant improvement in the alveolar ventilation-perfusion relationship.

Tracheobronchial suctioning

Suctioning is such an important part of tracheostomy care that it warrants special discussion, for on its effectiveness may rest the success of the tracheotomy and all other associated therapy. Unfortunately, suctioning, or as it is sometimes called, "bronchial toilet," is a facet of patient care that is frequently done ineffectually and harmfully. Except for other specially trained personnel, such as those employed in intensive care units, suctioning of the respiratory tract is best done by experienced respiratory therapists, for they are able to correlate the procedure with the operation of a ventilator or oxygen therapy equipment. Even more significant, their training has impressed on them the importance of maintaining a free airway, on which the successful performance of their work depends. Suctioning is not satisfactorily left to the general ward nursing staff, who, shorthanded and pressed for time, may delegate it to nonprofessional nursing personnel. At best, the instruction and experience in bronchial suctioning vary greatly among nursing school curricula. It is not a difficult task, but it does require understanding of its objectives and hazards and great care. We discuss it in terms of the equipment used, the preparation, and the details of the suctioning technique.

Equipment. A special catheter with a perforated tip through which secretions may be drawn is used to pass into the respiratory tract. It may be of rubber, but many hospitals have found disposable plastic to be more practical and convenient. No matter which type is used, the catheter must be smooth along its length and at its tip; one that has been cut to leave a rough or sharp distal end should never be used. The catheter must be fully sterilized according to standard procedures, and because the ventilated patient will probably need frequent attention, many should be immediately available. For this reason the

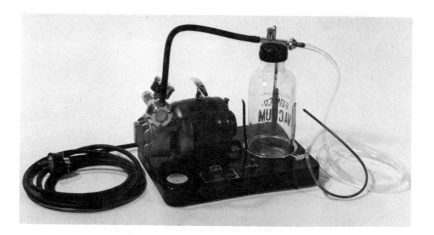

Fig. 14-5   Tracheobronchial aspiration setup using a suction pump. The suction catheter is connected to one arm of a Y-connector, the other arm is left free for thumb-controlled suction. Aspirate is collected in a jar located between the Y-connector and the pump.

individually packed, sterile, disposable units have become popular. For each patient the diameter of the intrabronchial catheter should be no greater than one half the diameter of the tracheostomy tube so that suctioning will not generate dangerous intrapulmonary negative pressure.[49] This is especially important to protect the easily compressed airways of children and the diseased bronchioles of emphysematous patients.

As shown in Fig. 14-5, a collecting bottle for the bronchial secretions is attached to the suction source by suitable tubing and the bottle in turn connected to the stem of a glass Y-tube connector. The cather is attached to one arm of the Y-tube, the other arm left free. After each episode of suctioning the airways, the catheter is discarded, either in the trash if disposable or in a container to be cleaned and sterilized if of rubber. Gone are the days of the single catheter used repeatedly time and again, often left lying on the bedsheet, even dangling to the floor, or futilely immersed in a "germicidal" solution. Examination of such solutions has demonstrated that they very soon become cesspools of bacteria. Once common practice, such mishandling of catheters is inexcusable in the modern hospital.

Preparation. The therapist must carefully open the wrapping of a catheter, making sure not to touch it with the bare hand, letting it set on its sterile covering or some other sterile surface. The therapist must then thoroughly wash his or her hands, preferably scrubbing them with a brush and antiseptic soap, dry them with a sterile towel, and put a sterile glove on the dominant hand. With the unsterile hand the therapist holds the Y-connector and, with the gloved hand, attaches the catheter to one arm of the Y-tube. The ventilator can be disconnected from the tracheostomy tube by an associate, or the therapist, if alone, can do it with his or her uncovered hand. The therapist will take this opportunity to aspirate the mouth and pharynx of secretions, and then deflate the cuff, both to relieve tracheal pressure and to provide the spontaneously breathing patient with some additional airway during the suctioning. If advisable, according to the schedule established for the individual patient, the therapist or a helper can remove the inner cannula for replacement by a fresh sterile one following suctioning. Removal of the ventilator, deflation of the cuff, and removal of the inner cannula can be done by the unaided therapist before scrubbing if the patient is able to tolerate the time off assisted ventilation. Finally, the suction is turned on, and the procedure is ready to begin with a fresh sterile catheter.

We have described the classic aseptic technique, proper performance of which is universally accepted. However, it is time-consuming and awkward without assistance, and often the clinical situation demands faster, more efficient action. An alternative technique that has proved to be safe and effective omits the hand scrubbing and sterile glove. Instead, the operator manipulates the catheter into and out of the airways with a surgical clamp. When not in use, the clamp is kept in a cylindrical container of an effective chemical sterilizer and its tip rinsed in sterile water before the catheter is picked up.

Suctioning. No one without a clear understanding of the anatomic structures of the respiratory tract and a responsible appreciation of the vital role played by the bronchial mucosa in protecting the body from infection should be permitted to suction the airways. All instrumentation of the tract is traumatic to its delicate lining, and the utmost gentleness is required to keep injury to a minimum. During the preparation of the patient and equipment, the patient's airway should be ventilated with 100% oxygen for 1 to 2 minutes. During each interruption in suctioning and at the conclusion of the procedure, ventilation and oxygenation should be repeated. Cardiac arrhythmias have been noted in many patients being suctioned, believed to be a result of accompanying hypoxia.

The operator's sterile hand holds the catheter, and the unsterile hand holds the glass Y-tube connector; with the free end of the Y-tube left open so that *no suction* is applied, the operator gently introduces the catheter into the trachea and one of the main stem bronchi as far as it will easily go. Since both lungs will be suctioned, it generally makes no difference which is treated first, but the catheter may enter either bronchus if the patient's head is turned to the opposite side. As soon as the catheter's progress has stopped, the therapist occludes the open end of the Y-connector and applies suction for 2 to 3 seconds. Suction is stopped by releasing the Y-connector, the catheter is withdrawn a short distance, and suction is again activated. This procedure is repeated in two to four steps until the catheter is in the trachea, at which time it is then withdrawn. While it is stationary and suctioning, the catheter may safely be gently rotated by an easy twirling motion to allow maximum exposure to secretions. An alternate method is to intermittently apply suction while gently rotating the catheter during a steady withdrawal. It must *not* be plunged up and down in the bronchial tree, since it will then ream the respiratory mucosa and denude the airways of much of the all-important cilia. Following vigorous and injurious ramrodding of the bronchi, histologic examination of sediment from the collecting jar has often revealed large sheets of respiratory epithelium with cilia that have been stripped from and sucked out of the airways. Should additional suctioning be needed, the catheter is reintroduced and the sequence repeated, but once withdrawal has started, it should be completed with intermittent suctioning along the way. The opposite lung is then attended, preferably with a new sterile catheter.

The intervals between suctioning sessions will necessarily vary from patient to patient according to need, and evaluation of the need for suctioning should be made every 30 to 60 minutes. The duration of each aspiration will depend on the patient's tolerance but should not be prolonged beyond *15 seconds* even though the patient does not appear adversely affected. Many patients suffer severe apprehension over the procedure, viewing it with great dread and fear, and in some it precipitates distressing coughing and choking. The patient must be closely observed during suctioning because cardiac arrest can occur, especially if the procedure is prolonged. It is felt that arrest is the result of severe hypoxia resulting from the loss of oxygen and lung volume through the catheter.[43] It must be remembered that the therapist is suctioning not only secretions from the lungs but also lung air, reducing the oxygen available to the patient and shrinking the volume of the lungs.

To make the most of bronchial suctioning the therapist should mobilize the secretions as much as possible by humidification. We have adequately emphasized the importance of aerosolized moisture in the breathing gas, but if the secretions are still excessively viscid, they may be rendered more fluid by the installation of 10 to 15 ml of saline directly into the tracheostomy tube before suctioning to increase the aspirate yield. If secretions are predominantly purulent, presuctioning injection into the airways of either acetylcysteine or pancreatic dornase is a helpful preparation for suctioning.

As noted previously, the introduction of a suction catheter may reveal an obstruction above the carina. Difficulty in passing the catheter may be the result of its impingement against the tracheal wall, a dislodged or herniated cuff, or dried secretions occluding the distal end of the cannula. If the cuff is at fault, the entire tube must be removed and completely replaced. The therapist should be alert to these possibilities, for their presence may be noted during routine suctioning before they have had a deleterious effect on the patient.

In some patients requiring mechanical ventilation with PEEP, suctioning can present a special problem. Disconnecting the ventilator to suction removes the therapeutic pressure, and the suctioning process itself removes volumes of air from the lung. While some patients may be protected by preoxygenation with 100% oxygen, clinical experience has shown us that some patients are prone to difficulties when PEEP is removed and suction applied. Special adaptors are available to help with this problem.[50,51] The patient can remain connected while an opening is made in the adaptor, which allows the suction catheter to be introduced. This system helps reduce the problems of disconnection, and the ventilator can ventilate around the catheter while suctioning is applied, minimizing the drop in oxygenation and mean airway pressure.[50,51]

Finally, suctioning through an endotracheal or nasotracheal tube follows the same basic principles described for a tracheotomy. The added distance of the indwelling tube through which the catheter must be passed makes the procedure more awkward and probably a bit less effective. Generally, smaller catheters must be used because of the reduced lumen of the tube and the need to avoid serious additional obstruction by the catheter. For the maintenance of clear airways in the intubated patient whose major problem is not obstructive, suctioning through the tube will usually be satisfactory. If secretions are an important pathologic factor and need frequent attention, the patient should be tracheotomized for the assurance of maximum airway clearance.

Management of the ventilated patient	Because they are among the most critically ill in the hospital, patients being supported for respiratory failure must be treated in an area specifically devoted to intensive care. Attempts to manage such patients on general medical or

surgical floors are inconsistent with good medical practice. Some hospitals have respiratory care units, intensive care areas limited to the acute pulmonary patient. This is theoretically the ideal because it permits maximum concentration of personnel and equipment for each patient. A major drawback is the inevitable duplication of services required to care for patients in the general intensive care unit, or other special care areas, who cannot be moved because of pressing nonpulmonary needs. Probably, in most average general hospitals, mechanically ventilated patients are best managed in the intensive care unit.

The patient on a mechanical ventilator requires constant close attention and observation by both nurses and respiratory therapists who are knowledgeable in the clinical aspects of inaaequate ventilation. As has been pointed out before, the ventilated patient is dependent for every breath on the ventilator and the skill of the attendants. The possibility of mechanical failure and the sudden changes that may develop in the patient's physiology make it mandatory that he or she not be left alone for an instant. It is not enough to have people around; they must be people who know how to respond to the patient's needs and to any emergency that may arise. This obviously leads to the conclusion that the management of the ventilated patient must be delegated only to those with special training in respiratory care at medical nursing and technical levels.

The physician ultimately responsible for the therapeutic details must be experienced in clinical chest medicine and versed in basic cardiopulmonary physiology and pulmonary function evaluation. This extent of preparedness often requires the combined efforts of the patient's attending physician and a specialized consultant. An insight of the interacting physiologic and biochemical forces active in respiratory failure comes only with prolonged exposure, and even the most competent general physician seldom has enough constant experience with this condition to be fully confident in its management, at least during the most acute phases. Certainly, a new house staff should not be given responsibility for the care of respiratory failure without close supervision, for at the present time undergraduate medical education does not give these people adequate preparation. From a teaching point of view the consolidation of respiratory patients in a special care unit provides an unparalleled opportunity to train young physicians in this field and give them the basic knowledge and experience in the minimum time to make them proficient in respiratory care.

General nursing education usually includes pulmonary physiology and respiratory diseases only as segments of overall comprehensive courses, and the nurse who will care for respiratory failure patients must have additional training. In hopsitals with effective respiratory therapy departments, this should be easily accomplished, and it is the responsibility of such departments to make available to all nurses who are interested a course of instruction in the principles and practices of respiratory therapy, with emphasis on acute care.

Let us now consider some of the practical aspects of supporting the patient with a failed respiratory system.

Choice of a ventilator

General factors in selection. We have established that there is no single best ventilator, that there are several machines that are good, with qualifications, yet each has its champions; and we are accustomed to hearing debates extolling the virtues of one over another. The personal preferences among physicians and therapists alike are based on many factors, among which are experience with one type of ventilator, confidence in one over the others, admiration for a particular mechanical principle, and economy. All of these are important considerations but are dependent more on whim than on the specific objectives sought in each individual patient being ventilated. It can be emphasized again that generally the skill and experience of the operating therapist are more important than the specific type of respirator used; but in our discussion of the principles of the various units in common use, we indicated features both favorable and unfavorable. Some of the desirable characteristics that we would like to see in a ventilator would certainly include at least the following:

1. The machine should be able to operate for long periods with a minimum of servicing and maximum freedom from the risk of mechanical breakdown.
2. There should be provisions for operating the instrument on room air, pure oxygen, a variable mixture of both, and any other gas desired.
3. Whether the ventilator is basically pressure, time, or volume cycled, there should be dependable control over, or a safe limit to, the generated pressure.
4. Especially important and strongly emphasized earlier, there should be a variable flow control, either manual or automatic.
5. Desirable, but not always essential, is a combination of both control and assist capabilities or greater versatility in handling the changing patterns of breathing so commonly encountered.
6. There should be some means of monitoring airway pressure.
7. There must be provisions for adequate humidification of inspired gas, a need on which the patient's survival may depend.
8. For the patient under controlled breathing, there should be a means of adjusting the inspiratory-to-expiratory time ratio or at least a provision to ensure that inspiration does not exceed expiration.
9. There should be available some means to monitor the delivered tidal volume.
10. The ventilator should have built-in mechanisms, or attachments, to provide positive end-expiratory pressure and intermittent mandatory ventilation maneuvers.

This is not an exhaustive list, and therapists can probably add several more criteria they would like to see met before they would have full confidence in any machine. In summary, we may state that the choice of a ventilator will often depend on which one of all those available in a given hospital is felt to be the safest and most effective for a given patient with due regard for the number, skill, and experience of the therapists who will be responsible for its operation. This choice will be made from among the groups described in the classification of Chapter 13.

As a recapitulation of some of the features of the major ventilators, Table 14-2 compares their major characteristics.

Clinical guides to selection. Let us now consider the possible clinical indications that might favor one type of ventilator over another, grouping patients according to normal lungs, restrictive disease, and obstruction, with the understanding that in actual practice individual circumstances are often complicated by a combination of these factors.

Patients with normal lungs and thorax. This group usually includes those

Table 14-2
Major characteristics
of ventilators

	Emerson 3-PV, 3-MV IMV	Bourns BEAR 1, BEAR 2	Bennett MA-1, MA-2	Ohio 560	Monaghan 225/SIMV	Siemens Servo 900B, Servo 900C
Small					+	+
Quiet	+	+			+	+
Flexible range of F_{IO_2} (21%-100%)	+	+	+	+	+	+
Flexible range of V_T (0.5-2 ℓ)	+	+	+	+	+	+ System is different ($\dot{V}$ and f)
Frequency range (5-60/min)	+	+	+		+	+
$\dot{V}$ up to 40 ℓ/min	+	+	+	+	+	25-30?
Pressure limits to 100 cm H_2O or more	+	+	MA-1 = 80 MA-2 = 120	+	+	+
PEEP/CPAP to 30-50 cm H_2O	+	+	MA-2 45	(12 cm H_2O)	(20 cm H_2O)	+
Sigh	3-PV can be added	+	+	+		+
IMV down to 1/min or less	3-PV with factory modification, 3-MV	+	+		+	+
Inflation hold (plateau)		+	MA-2 only	+		+
Alarms						
Low pressure		+	MA-2	+		
High pressure		+	+	+	+	+
Apnea		+	MA-2			+
V_T		+	+			
Gas failure		+	+	+		
Failure to cycle		+	+	+		
Selectable flow pattern (square wave, tapered wave, or sine)		Square or some taper				Square or sinelike
SIMV		+	MA-2		+	+

with neurologic or muscular pathologic conditions interfering with ventilation. The generalization may be made that a patient in respiratory failure who has a normal lung-thorax and clear airways can be adequately ventilated with any of the standard ventilators, since the only problem is the simple transportation of air into the alveoli against no abnormal barriers. If the removal of bronchial secretions or the risk of aspiration of oral or regurgitated gastric contents is not a clinical consideration, intubation may be avoided and the patient ventilated by the negative-pressure body ventilator. The elective use of the tank implies the need for minimal medical and nursing attention and the ability to control rather than assist the patient's breathing. It is in this group of patients also that the chest respirator has its greatest application, especially in those being weaned from the large tank or who need support of their own spontaneous breathing, such as during the sleeping hours. However, the cumbersome tank ventilator, and the difficult-to-fit-and-adjust chest ventilator, are being used less and less frequently, since increased skills in the management of the intubated patient almost exclusively employ positive-pressure ventilation. The choice of ventilator in this group is therefore based on convenience and comfort rather than on the need to combat a physiologic limitation to gas exchange. Although the management of ventilation is fairly easy, it is not without its hazard, for the risk of serious overventilation is great.

Patients with restrictive lung disease. Restriction that limits ventilation may be a result of involvement of the thorax, as with trauma, and of the pulmonary parenchyma. The primary ventilatory problem in this case is the markedly reduced lung-thorax compliance, which necessitates high driving pressures to deliver adequate tidal and minute volumes. In this circumstance many physicians and therapists favor the use of a volume positive-pressure ventilator that can deliver the necessary tidal volume at whatever pressure is required. The obvious disadvantage of the pressure-cycled respirator is premature end-inspiratory cycling before delivery of the tidal volume if the pressure needs of air delivery exceed the capability of the machine. The factors that will determine whether a volume or pressure ventilator will be necessary are the degree of restriction and the skill of the respiratory therapist. Pressure-cycled ventilators can be successfully used against a considerable loss of compliance and in many patients with chest injury, but success depends on close attention to the pressure-time relationships of the mechanical adjustments by an experienced therapist in constant attendance.

Two observations may help to clarify this problem for the student. First, regardless of the instrument used, the patient with severe restrictive disease is faced with the hazard of the deleterious effects of high intrathoracic pressures that we have already considered in detail. Because of this and progressive loss of compliance, some patients just cannot be sustained with any equipment or techniques now available. In such patients it is more academic than realistic to debate the virtues of delivering air at almost unlimited pressure if the therapy itself puts the patients under increasing risk. Second, in patients with "pure" restriction, the volume-cycled ventilators can support all but those noted above and are probably preferred, especially when there is anything less than ideal technical supervision. However, except in such diseases as the respiratory distress syndrome of the newborn and adults, and a few fibrotic or granulomatous conditions, restriction is frequently associated with obstructive disease, described next, and in this case the ventilator preference may be reversed.

Patients with obstructive disease. By and large, most patients with obstructive disease present the dual problems of increased airway resistance and reduced compliance and may confront the therapist with the greatest technical challenge. The chief prerequisite of a ventilator to manage the obstructed patient is variable flow control, reasons for which have been adequately covered earlier. There is widespread disagreement on the efficacy of pressure versus volume ventilators, but it is futile to engage in debate. With a mechanically dependable instrument that has flow control, the clinical results obtained depend entirely on the skill and experience of the operator. Theoretically, it makes little difference whether a ventilator is volume cycled or pressure cycled if it possesses flow control, but practically, this reduces the selection to the IPPV type.

We should point out here that for the respiratory therapist who understands basic pulmonary physiology and mechanics as well as the detailed functions of his or her equipment, it makes little difference whether a volume is delivered to a patient at a required pressure or a pressure is delivered to achieve a desired volume, as long as the flow of the gas can be adjusted to ensure its delivery. It is the responsibility of the therapist to determine what variables will respond to changes in adjustable controls for each ventilator he or she is expected to use. The opinion is expressed here that in the face of the unstable and interacting forces of obstruction and loss of compliance, the patient whose ventilation fails because of chronic obstructive disease can best be managed by a ventilator which gives independent control over pressure, flow, and I/E ratio. Both skill and patience are needed, since frequent resetting of controls ensures the maintenance of ventilation through the shifting course of the disease, but maximum flexibility is thereby available to the therapist who is able to give tailor-made treatment to the patient.

Summary. There are no hard-and-fast criteria for ventilator selection, and whatever guidelines one may have are becoming harder to follow because new makes and models of equipment continue to become available. The following personal observations and opinions are offered to help the therapist formulate his or her own views.

1. Respiratory therapy literature of ventilatory care contains few references to economy, as if the grave nature of respiratory failure precludes such a consideration. The student is urged to note the cost differential between most pressure-cycled and volume-cycled ventilators. It is suggested that if properly observed many patients can be successfully supported on flow-adjustable, pressure-cycled machines (Bird Mark 7 or 8, Bennett PR class) and that these are practical for general use because of their portability, adaptability to emergencies, versatility in ventilating normal and obstructed lungs, and economy of cost and space.

2. More skill is required to use the full potential of pressure-cycled ventilators than volume-cycled. Thus availability of personnel trained and experienced in the operation of pressure-cycled units is an important factor in choosing a machine.
3. Rapidly changing compliance is a strong indication for ventilation by volume cycling.
4. Negative pressure ventilators should be limited to the uncommon patient whose ventilatory failure is caused by neuromuscular disease rather than obstruction or loss of compliance and whose physical condition requires little medical or nursing attention and to those instances where the equipment is compatible with available space and the comfort of other patients. There is actually little need for the large tank ventilator and only rare indications for the chest cuirass.
5. Assistor-controllers have always had distinct advantage over assistors, although current techniques in mechanical ventilation, described later in this chapter, have made this difference less important.

Instituting and maintaining ventilation

Most of this section refers to the patient who is apneic or whose breathing is weak and ineffective and who thus needs complete ventilatory control. It is usually obvious where comments also apply to the assisted patient, but where necessary, this is stipulated.

Initiating tidal volume and rate. The first problem to be faced by the respiratory care team is the determination of a suitable tidal volume and rate. For the adult patient with no spontaneous breathing, a rate is generally established somewhere between 10 and 20 breaths/min, although this decision may have to be modified by tidal volume needs. Because of the great variations in body mass among the many patients being mechanically ventilated, the choice of tidal volume can be a difficult one. Obviously, an attempt is made to establish a pattern of breathing that will give the patient the best alveolar gas exchange, and the *only* way this can be determined is to measure arterial oxygen and carbon dioxide tensions and pH. We emphasize a little later the necessity of this technique throughout the entire management period, but it should be stressed here that in many instances ventilation cannot be delayed while waiting for laboratory data. Often the initiation of artificial ventilation must rely on clinical evaluation, and especially on a background of extensive experience in treating respiratory failure. Highly skilled therapists will base their judgment on the size of the patient, the depth and ease of chest movements during ventilation, and the many combinations of pressures and volumes that they have had occasion to use in the past. It is quite remarkable how effective this clinical approach can be when later confirmed by blood gas determinations.

The therapist is not without some assistance in setting combined tidal volumes and rates, since there are available nomograms to use as initial guidelines to get ventilation under way. One device applicable for general use is the Radford nomogram, a reproduction of which can be found in Appendix 13.[52] It should be clearly understood that no nomogram or formula for determining tidal or minute volumes is precise. The nomogram is used only to suggest a reasonable starting point with a minimum of delay, with necessary modifications as indicated by clinical observation or physiologic data. However, the Radford nomogram is useful because of the ease and speed with which it can be used, factors of great importance in the often hurried atmosphere of the failing patient.

The Radford nomogram bases its values on the three parameters of weight, respiratory rate, and sex, but it is vitally important to understand that the data refer to *basal* requirements in *healthy* subjects. This means that the chart is composed of information obtained from large numbers of healthy individuals, of a variety of sizes and ages, of both sexes, at complete rest, with all bodily functions at a minimal level of activity. Obviously, then, the direct information provided by the nomogram does not apply to the patient whose physiologic disturbance may raise metabolic activity far above the basal level. To compensate for such effects of illness, provisions are made to adjust the nomogram values by specific percentages, according to the clinical situation. The effect of a tracheostomy on ventilatory needs is illustrated in the chart of nomogram corrections, permitting the reduction of basal tidal volume by a significant amount. Also, the adjustment referred to as the dead space of "anesthesia apparatus" reflects the anesthesia orientation of the nomogram but can equally be applied to a ventilator. When the nomogram is used for the apneic patient, respiratory frequency must be established that is consistent with the age as well as the tidal volume. If the patient has spontaneous breathing, the tidal volume actually moved by the patient is measured and compared with that predicted by the graph to see whether air movement is adequate or intervention is indicated. If the limitations of this nomogram are kept in mind and the therapist has good clinical understanding and judgment, the chart will be useful. It should not be used by inexperienced personnel as a substitute for a clear understanding of the principles of mechanical ventilation.

On the basis of information from many sources as well as personal experience, the average basal tidal volumes by age, weight, and sex, from birth through adulthood are summarized in Table 14-3.[52-58]

The data from the Radford nomogram and Table 14-3 are often suitable starting values for unconscious patients with normal lungs. However, many patients in acute respiratory failure have an increased V_D/V_T ratio, increased physiologic shunting, and an increased drive to breathe.[59] Many clinicians use a simple formula for establishing tidal volume, usually about 10 to 12 or 10 to 15 ml/kg of body weight for adults without chronic pulmonary disease[3,59-62] and 6 to 10 ml/kg for infants and children.[63-67] These larger volumes are generally used with lower respiratory rates and are sometimes felt to lower shunt[61] (especially with PEEP[60]), make conscious patients more comfortable,[3] and aid in overcoming increased V_D/V_T ratios. Because these volumes are often two to three times predicted values slow rates, use of IMV or added mechanical dead space with controlled ventilation are used to control hypocapnia.[1,3,59]

Table 14-3
Estimated basal tidal
volume by age,
weight, and sex

Age (yr)	Normal frequency	Average weight (lb)	Tidal volume (ml)	
			Male	Female
Newborn	30-40	8	18-22	18-22
1	25-35	22	55-70	55-70
2	±28	27	80	80
3	±25	32	100	100
4-6	20-25	36-44	125-150	125-145
7-9	20-25	50-65	160-180	155-175
10-14	20-25	65-100	200-265	185-245
15-16	16-18	100-115	300-330	280-300
Adult	12-18	120	350	320
		130	370	340
		150	400	360
		175	450	400
		200	500	440
		225	540	460

For patients with chronic obstructive pulmonary disease with carbon dioxide retention in acute ventilatory failure, 8 to 10 ml/kg has been suggested.[68] Higher pressures associated with the larger tidal volumes can have detrimental effects on circulation, which may already be compromised in these patients,[43] particularly those having an increased compliance and tendency toward air trapping.

Establishing tidal volumes and rates for neonatal patients is both difficult and controversial. Small tidal volumes (often 5 to 10 ml) are very difficult to set in most pediatric ventilators, and there are inevitable leaks around the uncuffed endotracheal tubes used for these patients.[69,70,71] There is also a problem of relatively large amounts of the set volume not reaching the patient because of gas compressibility even when using small tubing circuits.[71] Pressure-limited, time-cycled ventilators are quite common for infant ventilation. Discussions detailing choices for settings of both pressures and rates are presented elsewhere in journals and texts, and we suggest the interested student read them.[63,65-67,69,71,72] It might be added that the tidal volumes of premature infants can be as low as 6 ml, making necessary the use of respirator tubing circuits that have as close to no dead space as possible.

Establishing a ventilatory pattern. We are concerned here not with theoretic pressure or flow curves but, rather, with those factors that contribute to establishing a pattern of breathing most helpful to the patient, emphasizing the clinical problems faced by the therapist.

Relation of pressure, rate, and volume. Once the desired frequency and tidal volume have been determined, volume-cycled ventiators are preset and activated and the actual delivered volume measured by a suitable meter.[22] Slight adjustments are often necessary, since the volume controls are not perfectly precise. If a pressure-cycled ventilator is used, a moderate to low starting pressure is chosen to initiate ventilation and is gradually increased to deliver the desired volume. Whatever instrument is used, an attempt is generally made to keep the pressure below 40 cm of water to minimize interference with the circulation, although this may be difficult in the presence of a significant reduction in compliance. To illustrate this with an oversimplified example, let us assume that we wish to deliver a tidal volume of 400 ml at a frequency of 16/min but find that a pressure of 50 cm of water is needed. Because we know from our earlier studies of physiology that compliance tends to vary inversely with respiratory frequency, we will slow down the controlled rate and see whether ventilation can be accomplished with less force. Perhaps we will find that at a rate of 12 breaths/min, the ventilator can deliver 533 ml of air at a pressure of but 40 cm of water, in which case we will provide the same total minute ventilation. Whether this increase in tidal volume is to the patient's advantage will be a matter of medical judgment to determine, but this fictitious example is presented to demonstrate the need for versatility by both therapist and ventilator in accommodating the requirements of respiratory failure.

Frequently patients will have spontaneous breathing but of a character too weak, rapid, or irregular to effect adequate alveolar gas exchange, and it is often possible to "override" such spontaneous breathing with a volume ventilator. If complete control cannot be achieved at once over a rapid rate, the volume ventilator is adjusted to the patient's frequency, and then attempts are made to reduce the rate of the instrument gradually, allowing the patient to accommodate to the slowing pace, which relieves the patient of much of the effort of breathing. The power of the volume-cycled respirators tends to discourage patient competition unless the spontaneous drive is strong, and in such instances safe ventilation may not be possible without modifying the patient's pattern, to be described below, or switching to a different type of ventilator. Semicontrolled ventilation may be achieved with a pressure-cycled machine in a patient with rapid but weak spontaneous breathing. This technique assists the patient's breathing rather than taking complete control over it but at the same time modifies its pattern. The instrument is adjusted for automatic controlled breathing at a rate less than the patient's own, and he or she is allowed to override the ventilator. If the patient is rationally responsive while benefitting from the assist to breathing, he or she sometimes can be encouraged to relax efforts and give in to the control of the respirator, letting the rate subside to a more efficient level. Even when the patient cannot be brought under full control, continued reassuring support by the therapist will often help the rapid breather to slow efforts so that satisfactory, restful, assisted ventilation will ensure good tidal air exchange. No matter what the technique, the object is to relieve the patient of excessive work, to reduce frequency to the normal range for the patient's age and size, and to deliver to the patient an adequate tidal and minute volume.

Inspiratory/expiratory ratio. There are no shortcuts to setting up a safe and effective respirator. Although the pressure-cycled machines are the most versatile and sensitive with the potential for fine control *if properly used,* they require the most skill and experience. It must be repeated here for emphasis that in the hands of the untrained, such ventilators may constitute in themselves a serious hazard to the welfare inspiratory-to-expiratory time ratio, the rationale for which has been sufficiently covered earlier. Inspiratory time should not exceed expiratory time, and in most instances a ratio of 1:1.5 or 1:2 will be safe. The surest way to establish the ratio is to use a graphic display or a stopwatch, but many experienced therapists have so trained their ears that they are remarkably accurate in balancing the respiratory phases merely by listening as they adjust the controls. This important step is not always easily or quickly accomplished, and the manner in which it is done depends on the instrument used. With some, the matter is simply the adjustment of control switches (e.g., Emerson); with others, it depends on regulating the flow control (e.g., Bennett MA-1); and with yet others, the ratio is machine fixed (Engström ER-300).

The Bird respirator, because it is so amenable to custom setting, offers a good example to use for reviewing the intricacies of the I/E ratio. Fundamentally, controlled inspiratory time depends on the flow at a given pressure setting, whereas expiration is regulated by its own mechanism, and the student must remember the interrelationships among flow, pressure, time, and frequency. For convenience, these are summarized in Table 14-4, which does nothing more than compact in columns what already we have described in some detail. The table compares the effects of various combinations of pressure and flow on inspiratory time and frequency. Horizontal arrows mean no change; double arrows imply a greater response than a single arrow. For example, increasing the pressure while decreasing flow increases (prolongs) inspiratory time more than if flow were kept stable. Once the desired combination of airway pressure and tidal volume has been established, the I/E ratio is

Table 14-4
Relationship between P, V̇, inspiratory time, and frequency for pressure-cycled ventilator (e.g., Bird)

	$P\uparrow$			$P\downarrow$			$\dot{V}\uparrow$			$\dot{V}\downarrow$		
P	✕	✕	✕	✕	✕	✕	→	↓	↑	→	↓	↑
V̇	→	↓	↑	→	↓	↑	✕	✕	✕	✕	✕	✕
Inspiratory time	↑	↑↑	→	↓	→	↓↓	↓	↓↓	→	↑	→	↑↑
Frequency	↓	↓↓	→	↑	→	↑↑	↑	↑↑	→	↓	→	↓↓

adjusted by individually timing inspiration and expiration, while still maintaining a constant frequency.

Let us suppose that we have set a Bird-type ventilator so that a delivery pressure of 30 cm of water provides the tidal volume we feel the patient needs and we wish the breathing pattern to be one of 20 breaths/min with an I/E ratio of 1:2. This means that each breath will be of 3 seconds' duration, of which inspiration will comprise 1 second and exhalation 2 seconds. We will first adjust the control that regulates the time interval between inspirations to get our expiratory time. This will remain independent of other controls, since it is activated by end-inspiration, and its duration is determined by the speed of its bleed-off. The 1-second inspiratory phase will be set by appropriately changing the flow, increasing it to reduce inspiration and decreasing to prolong it. In the absence of any variable factors that might change the dynamics of ventilation we should now have set the ventilator to deliver our predetermined tidal volume at a safe pressure, at a frequency consistent with the size and age of the patient, and with a phase ratio that we feel will protect the patient from harmful pressure effects.

However, if our patient has chronic bronchopulmonary obstructive disease, we must be prepared to make frequent readjustments because the compliance-obstruction status of the airways changes frequently. In addition to bronchospasm, which may well be present, the shifting of secretions in the respiratory tract and their periodic removal by therapeutic aspiration will keep the status of the airways in a state of continual flux. This is why the obstructed patient must be kept under constant observation and the controls of the ventilator frequently changed to maintain as constant ventilation as possible in the face of an unstable tract. Such a patient may put the respiratory therapist's skill to a severe test and often requires full-time services.

Let us now imagine that the compliance drops in the patient we attended in the preceding paragraph. We will find that our machine can no longer deliver the required tidal volume at the initial pressure of 30 cm of water; to restore this volume we must increase the system pressure. As soon as we do this, we note that the inspiratory time increases, since more time is required to transmit the higher pressure to the patient's lungs at the original flow. With a prolongation of inspiration, not only is the I/E ratio disturbed, but the total frequency drops because the expiratory time is unaffected and remains unchanged. Obviously, to restore the initial ventilatory pattern, we will have to increase the flow accordingly and bring the inspiratory time back to its original value. If our patient's problem is primarily one of loss of compliance, we can continue to increase both pressure and flow to deliver a constant tidal volume, up to the limits of the ventilator or to the limit of physiologic safety for the patient. On the other hand, if varying degrees of airway obstruction complicate the condition, our task will be much more difficult.

Ventilating obstructed airways. We are well aware of the problems of ventilating an obstructed passage with pressure-driven air and the great need to be able to vary the flow to compensate for such obstruction. If our patient suddenly reduces the effective caliber of his or her bronchi by spasm or an outpouring of secretions, the back pressure so generated will match the system pressure and cycle end-inspiration before delivery of the full tidal volume and, in this instance, inspiratory time will be markedly shortened. We have a choice of two maneuvers to try to restore tidal ventilation. First, we can increase the system pressure as we did with the compliance defect above, which will prolong the inspiratory time; but our knowledge of gas kinetics tells us that overcoming the pressure drop resulting from obstruction by this method will probably elevate the intrathoracic pressure to dangerously high levels. Second, we can make use of the variable flow control of our ventilator and drop the flow, which will significantly reduce the pressure gradient across the obstruction and deliver a larger pressure (and gas volume) distally with a minimum system pressure and prolong inspiratory time. The response of inspiratory time to both these combinations of pressure and flow are indicated in Table 14-4. However, merely slowing the delivered flow will not necessarily be satisfactory, since overcoming the obstruction may require an inspiratory time so long that the reduced minute rate will prevent an adequate minute alveolar ventilation despite the desired pressure and tidal volume. Also, if the inspiratory time is too prolonged, it can seriously upset the optimum I/E ratio. When faced with this problem, therapists must be prepared to spend a considerable period of time trying to achieve a compromise balance among the many factors involved because there is no standard procedural guide to follow. They will probably find that a combination of lowering the flow and elevating the pressure in gradual steps will give the best control over the ventilation. In addition, they may find that they will have to settle for a reduced frequency to accommodate a necessarily prolonged inspiratory time and then will try to increase the tidal volume enough to ensure a safe minute volume. At any rate they will be aware that a change in either pressure or flow will change the entire balance between pressure, flow, inspiratory time, and frequency; and they will soon develop the patience required to reset controls as they find it necessary to keep up with ventilation needs. Their goal will be the lowest system pressure at the lowest flow that will deliver the desired tidal volume at a normal frequency and with a safe I/E ratio.

Periodic hyperinflation. If students will observe their own quiet breathing during a prolonged period of bodily relaxation, as during a reading session, they will note a phenomenon so natural that they are usually unaware of it. Every now and then they will unconsciously sigh, often rather deeply. The significance of this act and its importance to mechanical ventilation became clear with the rapid increase in use of ventilators. During periods of physical inaction, as metabolic needs approach basal levels, depth of ventilation decreases and the distribution of intrapulmonary inspired air becomes irregular. Some pulmonary units are poorly expanded by the low level of ventilation and get less-than-adequate air exchange. This sets up localized areas of decreased ventilation-perfusion ratios, which actually constitute small physiologic shunts. In the normal subject, with active respiratory control mechanisms, this presents no hazard because the natural periodic sigh hyperinflates the lung, expanding and aerating all segments. It had been frequently noted, however, that patients who were maintained on supposedly adequate mechanically ventilated patterns often suffered deterioration of their pulmonary status and became progressively more difficult to ventilate. A detailed study on anesthetized patients demonstrated the cause for this unfavorable response.[73] Ventilatory and physiologic studies showed that prolonged artificial ventilation at an unvarying and small tidal volume levels leads to a gradual and progressive atelectasis. As increasing respiratory units become airless, significant arteriovenous shunting, or venous admixture, develops, and the pulmonary compliance steadily drops. Further, it was found that this phenomenon could be both prevented and corrected by periodic hyperinflation of the lungs, the introduction into the breathing pattern of an artificial sigh.

Part of the management of the ventilated patient on complete control is the use of the periodic sigh, and most volume ventilators have a mechanism to accomplish this automatically. Controls allow one or more deep breaths to be delivered at preset intervals. With other instruments it is advisable to hyperinflate the lungs with two deep breaths at least every half hour. Manual sighing can be done with the Bird respirator by holding open the cycling valve, for which purpose a rod is provided that extends to the outside of the instrument from the ambient end of the valve. The Bennett PR ventilators can be used to sigh the patient by holding open the rotating valve with a finger on its small projecting rod and increasing the terminal flow. Clinical judgment dictates the hyperinflating volume to be so used, but the short duration of the maneuver holds little risk for the patient.

Sustained hyperventilation. In general, hyperventilation is as physiologically unsound as is hypoventilation, and because it is our responsibility to understand the effects of what we do to our patients, we review in some detail the basic hazards of mechanical hyperventilation. We then consider how hyperventilation *may* be used with benefit under close control in selected circumstances.

In earlier chapters we discussed response of the acid-base balance of the body to ventilation and the hazards of respiratory alkalosis accompanying hyperventilation. It should be readily appreciated that the patient in respiratory failure is already severely ill and there is no justification for subjecting him or her to additional physiologic trauma, since the consequences of ventilator-induced alkalosis are potentially grave. The patient may suffer tetany—convulsive spasms resulting from marked increased reactivity of muscles. A warning of this impending condition may be jumpiness of the patient in response to ordinary stimuli or may be elicited by tapping the patient's cheek and noting a spasmodic contraction of the facial muscles of the tested side. Especially hazardous is an interference with cerebral blood flow, which is described in more detail below. A fall in the concentration of serum potassium has been frequently noted in respiratory alkalosis, believed to be caused by movement of potassium ions from the serum into the cells to replace hydrogen ions that are depleted because of the alkalosis. The hypokalemia (low serum potassium concentration) renders the myocardium susceptible to arrhythmias, especially if the heart is already hypoxic or if it is under digitalis treatment. In the latter instance, digitalis toxicity may be precipitated. Finally, alkalosis produces an unfavorable shift in the oxygen dissociation curve, impairing the cellular uptake of oxygen.

The greatest caution must be exercised in ventilating the patient with normal lungs, for this patient is the easiest to ventilate. It was noted that in the absence of obstruction or loss of compliance, almost any standard respiration can be used effectively. With such a patient, however, there is the ever-present risk of overzealous therapy, especially true if the therapist is simultaneously supervising the management of a patient who is hard to ventilate.

Let us consider the patient with chronic bronchopulmonary disease who is in respiratory acidosis with characteristically elevated arterial carbon dioxide tension and low pH. It is natural that all members of the medical team are anxious to restore the blood values to normal as soon as possible, since this gives reassurance of effective treatment subsiding danger; but it is unnecessary to bring down the carbon dioxide level precipitously. This is especially true if the hypercapnia is of significant duration and less important if it is acutely elevated. Thus, if the hypercapnia has suddenly risen, it can be more safely corrected rapidly than if it gradually rose over a long time. There are two physiologic reasons for this differentiation—one somewhat speculative, the other positive. First, with vascular dilation of the cerebral circulation as a major response to high levels of carbon dioxide, any increase in cerebral blood flow caused by sudden hypercapnia in all probability is somewhat "extra," being superimposed on whatever has been the usual perfusion of the brain in the given subject, and the removal of this additional flow by rapid excretion of carbon dioxide returns the cerebral blood flow to its own normal. In contrast, prolonged hypercapnia may condition the cerebral circulation to an increased level of perfusion and, when suddenly reduced, will produce an ischemia of the brain by deprivation of its usual blood supply. This reaction may manifest itself as a period of mental sluggishness or confusion or may produce the signs and symptoms of an acute stroke, with characteristic speech difficulties or muscular weakness, depending on the location of the brain area affected and the severity of the condition. By and large, chronic hypercapnia is more likely to be found in advanced-age patients, since respiratory failure may develop only after many years, whereas sudden, acute uncompensated hypercapnia is more prevalent in the younger patients subject to chest and head trauma, narcosis and anesthesia, and central nervous system infectious diseases. Thus the patient with acute failure superimposed on chronic hypercapnia often has a preexisting compromised cerebral circulation because of degenerative vascular disease, and the brain is more sensitive to alterations in its circulation than is the one with normal circulation.

We are most commonly concerned with the second reason, which is related to the acid-base status of the body. The more acute the hypercapnia, the more uncompensated is the acidosis, simply because there has not been time for the body to meet the challenge by increasing its available supply of buffering bicarbonate. Basically, the problem in this instance is one of a suddenly high carbon dioxide tension and low pH, and if the excess carbon dioxide can be excreted by the ventilatory route, the acid-base balance will readily return to normal. Much more treacherous to manage is the patient with a chronic but low-grade hypercapnia caused by long-standing disease in whom a respiratory infection, for example, has acutely depressed ventilation, pushing the patient into overt failure. This patient may have as high a carbon dioxide tension in the blood as the one cited above, but the pH will not be as low because he or she already has an increased bicarbonate accompanying the chronic hypercapnia and is thereby in partial compensated respiratory acidosis. If the excess carbon dioxide should be rapidly depleted, and it need not even reach a normal level, large quantities of extra bicarbonate will be left circulating, and the pH can easily jump from a severe acidemia to an iatrogenic alkalemia of serious proportions. As an example of the tremendous acid-base swing that can result from overly aggressive treatment, there is the recorded instance of an arterial pH that leaped from 7.10 to 7.80 in 10 minutes.[74] One can only speculate what effect this must have had on the cerebral circulation and the conductivity of the myocardium. The therapist must keep in mind that in many, if not most patients, intensive therapy can lower the carbon dioxide tension fairly readily, but hyperbasemia can be removed only by renal excretion, and it may take a normally functioning kidney 2 to 3 days to rid the body of an excess load of the antacid. Since many patients in respiratory failure have imperfect renal function, the result of either hypoxia or other accompanying disease, it is easy to see how they may be driven from the frying pan into the fire in terms of their acid-base balance if they are not treated prudently.

The use of buffers poses another ventilation problem with which the therapist should be familiar because it may compound the effect of the elevated bicarbonate of metabolic compensation in respiratory acidosis. There has been a great deal of disagreement over the use of buffers in respiratory acidosis, stemming mostly from a failure to appreciate the physiologic differences between respiratory and metabolic acidosis. For years, part of the standard treatment of metabolic acidosis has been the intravenous administration of sodium bicarbonate (or sodium lactate, which is metabolized in the body to produce bicarbonate) to neutralize excess acid according to the following nonspecific reaction:

$$NaHCO_3 + HA \rightleftharpoons NaA + H_2CO_3$$
$$H_2CO_3 \rightleftharpoons H_2O + CO_2 \uparrow$$

Success of this reaction depends on the ability of the body to remove, by blowing off through the lungs, the carbon dioxide formed. The patient with metabolic acidosis, as from the accumulation of organic acids accompanying diabetes or renal failure, can readily remove large volumes of carbon dioxide if he or she has no associated pulmonary disease. Indeed, one of the clinical characteristics of such a patient is severe hyperventilation. However, the student will recall that metabolic acidosis disturbs the Henderson-Hasselbalch equation by decreasing the numerator as the normal body bicarbonate is depleted by the abnormal circulating acids. In such a circumstance it is logical to replace bicarbonate therapeutically and so restore normal balance. The biochemical situation is different in respiratory acidosis, especially if it is chronic. In the first place, if we substitute for acid *HA* in the above reaction the characteristic acid of respiratory failure, H_2CO_3, the added $NaHCO_3$ merely builds up to high levels because the inherent disability of respiratory acidosis is the inability of the body to blow off even normal amounts of carbon dioxide. Second, when we view respiratory acidosis in terms of acid-base balance, we find it is the result of an increase in the denominator of the H-H equation, not fundamentally a deficiency in bicarbonate. In short, we return to the basic principle of therapy of respiratory acidosis: Acid-base balance can be restored only by actively ridding the body of excess carbon dioxide, not by adding increasing amounts of bicarbonate. Suppose a patient has the extreme physiologic values we used earlier in Table 6-6 to illustrate acid-base balance, with a bicarbonate–to–carbon dioxide ratio of 24/2.4 mEq/ℓ and a pH of 7.10. Even if we add enough bicarbonate to the patient's blood to raise its level to 48 mEq/ℓ, restore a 20/1 ratio, and bring the pH up to 7.40, we still will not correct the basic defect. As long as the carbon dioxide level remains elevated, the patient will be in severe failure although temporarily compensated.

Since it is established that mechanically ventilating the patient in ventilatory failure is the fundamental treatment, let us return to our subject of hyperventilation and see just what are its risks. We will use as examples two fictitious treatment situations as shown in Fig. 14-6, making certain assumptions for the sake of clarity.

Let us imagine a patient before respiratory failure with the blood findings of box *A,* the acid-base ratio expressed in millimoles per liter with the equivalent carbon dioxide tension and the pH consistent with the ratio. Let us now assume our patient develops ventilatory failure (box *B*) with no evident compensation at this stage and a subsequent marked drop in pH. At this point we can permit normal renal compensation to do what it can to minimize the acidemia (box *C*), or we can actively assist this function with the parenteral administration of bicarbonate (box *E*). If we follow the first course, we may find that the physiologic conservation of bicarbonate will elevate the numerator of the H-H equation, let us say for example, to 36 mEq/ℓ and partially relieve the acidemia by raising the pH to 7.28. Because the carbon dioxide tension is still high and thus the underlying hypoventilation uncorrected, we place the patient on a mechanical ventilator and, in our enthusiasm to restore the carbon dioxide level to normal, overventilate him or her. After a few hours of therapy we may find that we have completely corrected the hypercapnia, but because renal bicarbonate excretion lags behind carbon dioxide removal, perhaps the patient's bicarbonate has dropped only to 30 mEq/ℓ and we have

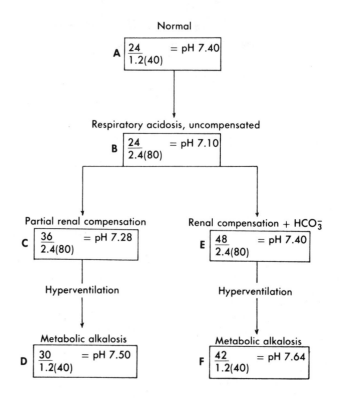

Normal

$$A \quad \frac{24}{1.2(40)} = \text{pH } 7.40$$

Respiratory acidosis, uncompensated

$$B \quad \frac{24}{2.4(80)} = \text{pH } 7.10$$

Partial renal compensation

$$C \quad \frac{36}{2.4(80)} = \text{pH } 7.28$$

Renal compensation + HCO_3^-

$$E \quad \frac{48}{2.4(80)} = \text{pH } 7.40$$

Hyperventilation

Hyperventilation

Metabolic alkalosis

$$D \quad \frac{30}{1.2(40)} = \text{pH } 7.50$$

Metabolic alkalosis

$$F \quad \frac{42}{1.2(40)} = \text{pH } 7.64$$

Fig. 14-6   Schematic outline of the hazard of deliberate hyperventilation in the treatment of respiratory acidosis. The mechanisms by which metabolic alkalosis can be induced are described in detail in the text.

now pushed the patient from a severe respiratory acidemia to a moderate metabolic alkalemia. Although a metabolic swing of this magnitude may not be of any great significance in most patients, it may be in some, and it indicates the ease with which therapy can overcompensate.

Let us now consider the possibilities if we follow the second course and give the patient bicarbonate because it seems reasonable to treat acidity with an antacid. The combination of renal compensation plus administered bicarbonate (box *E*) may effect rapid and complete ratio balance and quickly restore the pH to normal. Assisted ventilation will still be necessary, of course, and the student should realize that starting with a higher bicarbonate level in this instance, with effective ventilation, will make it difficult, if not impossible, to avoid leaving the patient with a significant bicarbonate excess. Box *F* assumes a response similar to that described in the first course, namely a rapid removal of carbon dioxide but with a concomitant reduction in bicarbonate of only 6 mEq/ℓ, giving the patient a severe metabolic alkalemia.

The therapist who thoroughly understands these concepts is now ready to consider exceptions. We often see a patient on a mechanical ventilator who needs a depth of ventilation, to maintain adequate blood oxygenation, in excess of that required for a normal carbon dioxide tension. This is the result of uneven patency of airways to various lung units, preventing uniform distribution of inspired air at tidal volumes judged to be adequate by carbon dioxide blood levels. In other words, easily diffusable carbon dioxide can be sufficiently excreted by ventilation that is unable to correct hypoxemia. In the absence of serious pathology such as surfactant deficiency or massive atelectasis, the problem can frequently be solved by delivering to the patient large tidal volumes, sometimes double or triple that considered normal. Even though the ventilatory rate of a controlled patient can be reduced in an attempt to keep minute ventilation to a minimum, hyperventilation often results, with the rising arterial pH of alkalemia. Unless we can protect the patient from the potential harm of our induced alkalosis, we are not justified in adding another risk to his or her survival.

For the patient on controlled ventilation there are two general procedures that can be used to maintain acid-base balance in the face of deliberate hyperventilation. First, rebreathed volume or dead space (V_D) can be added to the patient tubing, between the patient and the exhalation valve, generally a piece of flexible tubing of known volume. At the beginning of each inhalation the patient breathes this volume of carbon dioxide–rich air trapped in the tubing from the previous exhalation, thus supporting the desired arterial carbon dioxide level despite hyperventilation. It is convenient to have available for this purpose precut lengths of tubing of 50- and 100-ml capacities, measured by water filling. In general, rebreathed volumes of 50 to 300 ml satisfy most needs, but the final determinant is the arterial carbon dioxide tension and pH. Some hospitals routinely include 50 to 100 ml V_D in adult ventilatory circuits and hyperventilate all patients, but it is advisable to use this technique selectively and only when needed. Second, the same objective of elevating inhaled carbon dioxide concentrations can be achieved by adding carbon dioxide to the air-oxygen inspired gas mixture through a special mixing valve, which limits the maximum concentration of carbon dioxide to 3%.* The carbon dioxide mixer is accurate with usual gas flows as long as supply pressure from the oxygen-air mixer to the carbon dioxide mixer is 40 psi, and the carbon dioxide pressure to the carbon dioxide mixer is between 50 and 70 psi. One study found the carbon dioxide mixer more convenient to use than the addition of dead space tubing in controlling Pa_{CO_2}, and demonstrated that carbon dioxide concentrations greater than 3% were neither well tolerated nor necessary.[75]

For the ventilated patient with spontaneous but inadequate breathing, deliberate hyperventilation is probably best and easiest carried out in conjunction with intermittent mandatory ventilation, discussed next.

Perhaps students can see for themselves where the judicious use of bicar-

*CO_2 Ratio Controller, Veriflow Corporation, Richmond, Calif.

bonate may contribute to the overall treatment of ventilatory failure. It is indicated in those patients who have severe acidosis, with a reduction in pH to levels that are a hazard to cellular survival, in whom there has been a negligible metabolic compensatory response. This is exemplified by the patient who does not have chronic hypercapnia caused by long-standing bronchopulmonary disease and in whom there is no chronically elevated bicarbonate but who, for one reason or other, develops sudden carbon dioxide retention. To avoid the damage to this patient's enzyme systems and other cellular functions by subjecting them to a severely acidotic environment, *partial* neutralization of the patient's acidosis by increasing the store of bicarbonate is justifiable. Partial neutralization is further indicated in patients with a combination of metabolic and respiratory acidosis, for in them the ventilator therapy will not correct the underlying metabolic disorder, and the careful use of both modalities will maintain the smoothest acid-base balance. However, such therapy is acceptable only if it is recognized as a stopgap measure to be employed until results can be obtained from definitive assisted ventilation and if the physician is fully aware of the potential risk of overcompensation. As a general rule of thumb, bicarbonate therapy can be recommended, even in obvious respiratory acidemia, when the pH is less than 7.20 if it is discontinued above this level. The patient will be spared the harmful effects of a high hydrogen ion concentration, but the risk of therapeutically induced alkalosis will be minimal. In contrast, the use of supplemental bicarbonate in the patient with an already elevated bicarbonate level from renal compensation is extremely hazardous, and the development of a metabolic alkalosis is almost inevitable. It is a wise precaution for the therapist asked to set up mechanical ventilation to inquire of the medical attendant whether the patient has been given bicarbonate.

We can summarize our comments on the risks of hyperventilation by stating that although the primary need of the patient in ventilatory failure is a mechanically increased alveolar ventilation, such ventilation must be done cautiously and carefully. Especially must judgment be used in treating the patient with chronic hypercapnia and superimposed acute failure, for too great enthusiasm can easily precipitate a potentially harmful metabolic alkalosis to replace acidosis. Supplemental systemic buffers must be used with great reservation, if at all, and every member of the therapeutic team must be aware of the risk involved. The final objective of mechanical ventilation is to return carbon dioxide tension and pH to as close to normal as possible, not to overcompensate. There are times when the so-called normals for a given patient may not be identical with the normals associated with a healthy subject. In some patients with chronic hypercapnia and with adequate compensation before acute failure, it may be satisfactory to return carbon dioxide levels to those with which they have become adjusted. The therapist can be assured that the treatment is safe and effective if he or she first stops the rise in carbon dioxide tension and drop in pH and then notes that both are beginning to return to normal. From then on, as long as the progress is steady, it makes little difference how long the treatment takes, and it is safer to bring down a high carbon dioxide tension over a period of 2 to 3 days than in a matter of hours.

Intermittent mandatory ventilation (IMV). This ventilatory technique has two applications in the management of the mechanically ventilated patient. We describe here the principle of IMV and its role in the support of the patient in ventilatory failure, and later, its use in discontinuing mechanical ventilation. *Intermittent mandatory ventilation* describes a method of operating a ventilator that enables the patient to breathe spontaneously when chosen, bypassing the ventilator, while still delivering to the patient at variable and predetermined volumes and frequencies, machine-powered breaths.[76-78] The adjective *mandatory* refers to the ventilator cycle, over which the patient has little or no control.

The most important concept that the student must grasp at this time is the nature of the patient's spontaneous breathing. All ventilators in common use provide for the patient to cycle the machine spontaneously on demand. The breath so generated is then delivered by the ventilator like any other controlled breath at the preset volume and time. It is an *assisted* rather than a true spontaneous breath, since unless the patient "fights the machine" and prematurely terminates inhalation or otherwise disturbs the inspiratory/expiratory ratio, the patient has no control over the breath. Also, malfunction or inept operation of the ventilator may make its activation by patient effort difficult or impossible. In contrast, a spontaneous breath of the IMV technique is completely *unassisted*, since patient-generated inspiration *does not cycle the ventilator* but bypasses it through a valved circuit, to bring in gas from another source. Not only is initiation of the breath an option of the patient but also full control over its force, duration, and depth.

Fig. 14-7, *A,* is a schematic diagram of a basic volume ventilator setup to which an IMV bypass circuit can be added. Source gas, *A,* supplies ventilator, *B,* and from outflow port, *C,* it passes through humidifier, *D,* patient tubing, *E,* and into exhalation manifold, *F.* During inhalation, pressurized gas from the ventilator inflates balloon-valve, *G,* and gas is directed into intubated patient at *H.* At end-inspiration, the drop in ventilator pressure deflates the balloon-valve and the patient exhales to atmosphere through port *I.*

An IMV system consists of combined ventilator and spontaneous breathing circuits. Fig. 14-7, *B,* demonstrates the relationship of a spontaneous circuit to a ventilator circuit with which it is joined. Source gas, *A,* is carried through the bypass line, *J,* to the wide bore tubing, *K,* of the spontaneous circuit. At the distal end of the circuit, a 3-ℓ anesthesia-type bag, *L,* functions as a reservoir for the continuously flowing breathing gas. The bag bleed-off port may be fitted with an adjustable screw clamp, *M.* The proximal end of the spontaneous circuit is teed or wyed into the ventilator circuit between ventilator and humidifier, where a one-way valve, *N,* permits flow only from the spontaneous circuit into the ventilator circuit. We describe the purpose of the manometer, *O,* tied into the spontaneous breathing circuit when we consider the mechanical ventilatory technique of positive end-expiratory pressure (PEEP) later in this section.

During ventilator delivery, high pressure in the machine circuit closes the one-way valve, preventing gas entering the spontaneous circuit. Breathing gas

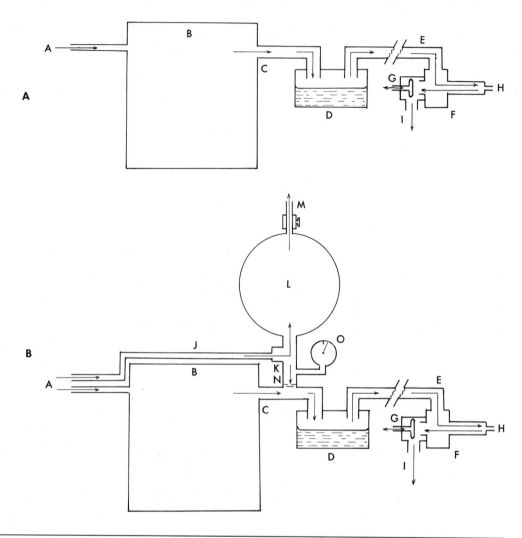

Fig. 14-7   **A,** Simple ventilation setup. **B,** With an added IMV circuit. (See text for description.)

flows steadily into the reservoir bag, and its rate, or the loss of gas through the escape port orifice, should be so adjusted that the reservoir bag does not collapse whenever the patient takes a spontaneous breath. Theoretically, overdistention of the bag by flows greatly in excess of patient needs should not present a serious problem. The increased pressure in the circuit as gas gathers between breaths will allow gas to escape through the one-way valve and vent through the exhalation valve to atmosphere. Only during ventilator delivery, when the balloon-valve blocks egress, will outflow be interrupted. However, in the interests of conservation of gas and maximum precision of technique, seepage of gas through the one-way valve can be prevented by permitting only moderate distention of the reservoir bag. When the patient starts a spontaneous breath, inspiratory subatmospheric pressure in the ventilator circuit opens the one-way valve, and the patient inhales a tidal volume from the reservoir and through the humidifier at a rate and depth of his or her choice. Exhalation pressure closes the valve, and gas flows out to atmosphere.

There is no single routine method of using IMV, and the following general guides may be of help to the inexperienced reader. In some hospitals an IMV system is incorporated in all initial ventilator setups.[76] More experience will be necessary to advise us if it should be immediately available for all patients on ventilators or if it should be used with more selectivity, although there is little doubt that IMV has made mechanical ventilation safer and more effective in many circumstances. It is obviously of no use in the apneic patient but can or should be available when spontaneous breathing returns.

The basic purpose of IMV is to permit mechanically ventilated patients to breathe on their own when they desire so that they may maintain or regain function of their ventilatory system and avoid developing dependence on the machine. In general, the ventilator is initially set to provide fully for a patient's needs, using tidal volumes in the 10 to 15 ml/kg body weight range. Triggering sensitivity of the ventilator must be reduced (resistance to patient triggering increased) so that the patient's inspiratory efforts will open the valve to the IMV bypass circuit rather than initiate a machine cycle. The sensitivity control may be completely inactivated, or as a safety measure only partially so, and thus in the event of gas supply failure to the bypass, a strong patient inspiratory effort will produce a ventilator breath. As spontaneous breathing becomes significant, ventilator breathing (this is the IMV) is gradually reduced in frequency, allowing the patient to assume more responsibility for ventilation. At any given time the IMV rate should be the lowest that is able to maintain normal arterial blood gases and pH, provided the spontaneous rate does not exceed 30 breaths/min. The speed with which IMV is reduced must be highly individualized and based on close observation of the patient. Not uncommonly it is necessary to retreat to higher ventilator rates, allowing the patient more time to adjust to independent breathing. The point at which IMV is discontinued depends entirely on the patient. Ventilator timing mechanisms now provide for IMV rates as low as one breath every 1 to 2 minutes. Thus the transition from controlled, through assisted, to independent breathing can be as gradual as needed.

In the interest of classification and definition, IMV can be designated as a modification of controlled rather than assisted ventilation. Ventilator breaths cannot be initiated by the patient because patient-generated inspiratory efforts open the bypass circuit instead of triggering the machine. Thus, with an IMV circuit in operation, machine assist is not possible. On the other hand, regardless of their frequency, because the ventilator breaths are preset and not influenced by the patient, they are control breaths. IMV therefore is a decreasing mechanically controlled breathing that permits the gradual, simultaneous return of spontaneous, unassisted breathing.

We noted above that IMV provides activity for ventilatory muscles and helps to prevent ventilator dependence. There are two additional physiologic benefits of great significance. *First,* in contrast to machine breathing, the parameters of which are arbitrarily selected to a considerable degree, the true spontaneous breathing of IMV can be the patient's respiratory center response to real gas exchange needs. In other words, as spontaneous breathing gradually becomes a larger segment of total breathing, the patient's own drive can set a ventilatory pattern, and especially a blood carbon dioxide level, more suitable for the patient's needs than we can deliver by machine, based on clinical evaluation and blood gas analysis. A frequently encountered problem is a sequel to ventilator hyperventilation, described a few pages back. Efforts to establish a spontaneous pattern may be frustrated if the dominant ventilator breaths are so large that they produce a hypocapnic alkalosis. The lowered hydrogen ion concentration may be inadequate to stimulate the respiratory center to independent action, and until corrected, will necessitate continuation of machine ventilation. *Second,* under the influence of positive-pressure ventilation, intrathoracic pressure rises abnormally during each tidal volume, elevating the mean pleural pressure, as we have seen. The major risk of such pressure is its retarding effect on venous return and cardiac output. The spontaneous breaths of IMV, on the other hand, are accompanied by subatmospheric intrathoracic pressure, as illustrated in Fig. 13-17. Over a time period, the net intrathoracic pressure is a function of the ratio of machine-to-spontaneous breaths, decreasing as patients take over more of their own breathing. For patients in overt or potential cardiac failure this may be the most important benefit of IMV.

IMV has certainly contributed to patient safety and comfort in many instances, but it must *not* be viewed as an indispensable ingredient in all ventilator management or as a solution to all management problems.[79,80] For example, we must be careful not to burden some patients too early or too frequently with their own breathing. They may have an adequate central drive to breathe spontaneously, but because of their disease, may not possess adequate musculoskeletal power to convert the drive into significant tidal volumes. For such patients, triggered assisted machine breathing may be safer and more effective than IMV until resolution of the underlying disease.[60,80] Thus the timing of introducing IMV may be a critical factor, requiring keen clinical judgment. Again, although many users advise IMV for all ventilated patients, experience continues to show that the tachypneic, shallow spontaneous breather is not always a good subject for it. At times, hyperventilating with the machine will dull the patient's spontaneous drive through alkalosis and slow the rate. Mindful of the hazards of alkalosis, the student can appreciate that such deliberate manipulation of breathing and acid-base balance must be undertaken with great caution. In such circumstances the techniques of spontaneous breathing suppression, described next, may be of considerable short-term use before attempting to institute IMV.

We again consider IMV in conjunction with positive end-expiratory pressure breathing and as part of the process of weaning a patient from a ventilator.[76,78]

Suppressing ventilation. It may be impossible to ventilate adequately a patient with strong spontaneous breathing no matter what instrument is used. Although machine override is often possible, a pattern of breathing that is rapid and shallow or grossly irregular may be forceful enough not to submit to the drive of a preset ventilator. In addition, the patient may "fight the machine," consciously or otherwise, because he or she is severely hypoxic, is fearful or apprehensive, or is mentally unable to cooperate. To continue to assist such a patient is only to perpetuate the pattern, leading to a steady deterioration of respiratory status. Most often the patient will be breathing very rapidly with shallow tidal volumes and is subjected to the following two hazards: First, the tremendous amount of physical work expended in rapid breathing will gradually deplete the patient's energy. Second, rapid shallow breathing is essentially dead space breathing, and although at great energy cost the patient may move large minute air volumes, all that is accomplished is ventilation of the dead space, leaving the alveoli relatively unventilated. If the patient is responsive to metabolic oxygen needs, the resulting hypoxia will continue the ineffective, tiring respiratory pattern. As a general rule, this risk is not great in adults until the frequency exceeds 25, and then, depending on the conductance (opposite of resistance) and compliance of the lung-thorax, rate increases are apt to be accompanied by reduced tidal volumes.

The condition of the patient with strong, ineffective spontaneous respirations who cannot be brought under at least partial control is a grave one, and his or her very survival may depend on the ability of the medical team to correct the deficiency. As soon as it becomes evident that effective assistance or conformance to control is not possible, there is nothing to gain and much to lose by further delay. The decision must be made to abolish the patient's own breathing and place him or her under complete ventilator control. This is a responsibility of the patient's attending physician, although the technical management will fall on the assigned therapist. The responsibility that this technique entails cannot be emphasized too strongly, for when we decide to interfere with natural processes as vital as breathing, thus asserting that we can do better for the patient than the patient can do him- or herself, we are assuming a great burden. The therapist should appreciate that this is not exactly the same as attempting to restore to a patient a function that has been lost completely through injury or disease. Instead, it is the use of our judgment as to the quality and performance of the patient's ability to provide a basic physiologic need, deciding that the patient is inadequate in this function, destroying it, and supplanting it with an artificial substitute of our choosing. This statement is not intended to overdramatize a procedure for which there is no alternative if the patient is to survive, but it is important that the therapist realize the full depth of his or her commitment to the patient who is completely helpless and totally dependent on medical attendants. Respiratory suppression should be undertaken only where facilities are adequate for complete care and in the physical presence of a responsible physician and respiratory therapist. Fortunately, with improved ventilator management techniques the need for going to this extreme measure is becoming less and less. We describe the three common techniques currently used: suppression by oxygen, by morphine, and by neuromuscular blocking agents.

Oxygen suppression of breathing. This procedure is especially effective for the patient with long-standing chronic hypercapnia, whose ventilation has been dependent to a considerable degree on the hypoxic drive that has replaced the damaged function of the patient's respiratory center. It is of interest that in this instance we employ, as therapy, a technique we strongly condemn otherwise. Earlier we discussed in detail the role played by chemoreceptors in the event of respiratory center failure accompanying progressive and chronic pulmonary disease. We stressed the great hazard in administering oxygen promiscuously to such a patient for fear of satisfying hypoxia, thus inactivating the hypoxic chemoreceptor drive and rendering the patient apneic. Now we do exactly that—inactivate the hypoxic chemoreceptor drive—so that we can eliminate the patient's own breathing and ventilate him or her artificially. The patient is given 100% oxygen through the assisting ventilator or by means of a tracheotomy mask, if intubation is required, for a period not to exceed 10 minutes; results should be realized in that length of time if at all. As the patient becomes hypopneic and respiratory energy decreases, he or she is put on ventilator control and the oxygen concentration is reduced to a safe level. Close observation must be maintained to ensure that the patient remains under adequate control and does not return to the previous pattern. If this procedure is unsuccessful, one of the following procedures must be employed.

Morphine suppression of breathing. Morphine sulfate is a potent addicting narcotic with the ability to relieve pain, produce lethargy, and induce a deep-to-stuporous sleep. One of its most specific activities, however, is its depression of respiration by directly suppressing the activity of the medullary respiratory center. Like high concentrations of oxygen, morphine is contraindicated in general medical use in any patient with compromised breathing, and many deaths have been attributed to it in patients with asthma, chronic bronchopulmonary disease, and cerebral injury. The respiratory depressant effect of morphine is directly related to dose and is evident to slight degrees even with small doses given, for example, for pain relief. The respiratory response is a decrease in both frequency and tidal volume.

When used to stop spontaneous breathing, morphine can be best controlled if given by intravenous injection. By this route, maximum respiratory depression for a given dose occurs within 10 minutes, compared with 1 hour or more if given intramuscularly. There are no hard-and-fast rules for its administration, but a good basic program is 5 mg intravenously, repeated every 10 minutes until the desired effect is realized, to a maximum of 20 mg for the series. In most patients, if morphine is to be effective, it will be before this amount of the drug has been used. For maintenance 2 to 3 mg can be given as needed to keep the patient well relaxed. The duration of morphine therapy is usually too short to warrant concern over addiction, but there are occasional side effects that can prove troublesome. Among the most common are nausea and vomiting, which sometimes preclude further use of the drug. Occasionally morphine causes hypotension and must be used cautiously, if at all, in the patient in incipient or overt shock. The automatic movements of the intestine, or peristalsis, are retarded or stopped by morphine, and this can lead to gaseous distention of the bowel severe enough to impair diaphragmatic motion and interfere with ventilation. The face and neck of patients may appear flushed, and the skin or nose may itch as the effects of the drug subside. Generally speaking, the intravenous administration of morphine is a safe and effective method of suppressing unwanted spontaneous ventilation and relaxing patients so that they may be ventilated effectively. It has often been life-saving.

Neuromuscular blocking agents to suppress breathing. A neuromuscular blocking agent is a drug that blocks the transmission of motor nerve impulses to skeletal muscles, effectively paralyzing those muscles. They are widely used in surgery to gain maximum muscular relaxation along with anesthesia, making manipulation of muscular tissues much easier by eliminating their normal tonal contraction. In respiratory therapy there are two indications for neuromuscular blocking—momentary paralysis for ease of endotracheal intubation of a tense or agitated patient, and prolonged action to override unwanted spontaneous breathing in a patient on a mechanical ventilator. In neither instance is total body paralysis desired, but only enough muscular relaxation to achieve the desired results.

These drugs must be used under the closest supervision, and patients under their influence must *never* be left unattended. If patients are alert before the administration of blocking agents, they should first be tranquilized or sedated, since the completely helpless feeling of paralysis to patients aware of their condition can be one of the most frightening of experiences.

We do not take the time to examine pharmacologic differences of the several blocking drugs available to the anesthesiologist, but we note the major characteristics of three of them often used in the control of ventilation—*d*-tubocurarine, succinylcholine, and pancuronium bromide.

d-Tubocurarine. *d*-Tubocurarine is a plant alkaloid whose paralyzing action has been known for centuries and which has been widely used in anesthesiology for many years. When given intravenously, the route of choice, its action is evident in 3 to 5 minutes, lasting about 40 minutes; doses of 15 mg may be used almost as needed until the desired effect is reached. In case of a mishap or overdosage, neostigmine methylsulfate should be available as an antidote. *d*-Tubocurarine has potential side effects. Large doses may precipitate hypotension, already a threat to a mechanically ventilated patient. Perhaps even more relevant to patients in respiratory failure is the severe bronchospasm that may follow curarine's use. The bronchospasm is attributed to the release, by the drug, of histamine from its cellular stores into the plasma, and one of the major physiologic effects of histamine is bronchoconstriction.[81]

Succinylcholine. Although a neuromuscular blocking agent like *d*-tubocurarine, succinylcholine (Anectine) differs chemically and in its mode of action. Also given intravenously, it starts acting in less than 1 minute, reaches its maximum in 2 minutes, and disappears within 5 minutes. It has been used in general surgery to provide rapid relaxation for short procedures such as instrumentation. For respiratory suppression a single dose of 20 mg may be given to test the patient's response or to initiate ventilation and may be repeated as needed until a good ventilatory pattern is established. A smoother response will accompany its prolonged administration in an intravenous infusion, as a 0.1% solution, run at a rate of 2 to 3 mg/min. By this method, because the action is so short, very close control over the depth of paralysis can be maintained merely by adjusting the infusion flow. Acute cardiovascular collapse may follow intravenous succinylcholine administration. It is beleved this is caused by a sudden rise in serum potassium concentration (hyperkalemia) with resulting myocardial depression and ventricular arrhythmias.[82]

Pancuronium bromide. Pancuronium bromide (Pavulon) is one of the newer paralyzing drugs recently made available, and although the total experience with it so far is meager compared with the two just described, it appears to have been well received.[83] Major advantages of pancuronium bromide include its nearly complete freedom from unwanted cardiovascular effects and its failure to stimulate histamine release. Its potency is some five times that of *d*-tubocurarine, and it has no effect on consciousness, pain awareness, or mental activity. Nevertheless, because it is a neuromuscular blocking agent, it is as potentially dangerous as *d*-tubocurarine and succinylcholine. Dosage varies with the duration of effect intended. By intravenous injection 2 to 4 mg are usually adequate for intubation, with effects evident in 2 to 3 minutes and a duration of action of up to 90 minutes. For maintenance of paralysis during control of ventilation, 4 to 5 mg of pancuronium bromide can be given at intervals of 1 to 3 hours, depending on response. Some prefer to use succinylcholine for intubation and pancuronium bromide for long-term control.

Correcting hypoxia. The general subject of oxygen therapy is described in Chapter 12, and we now only attempt to correlate certain aspects of it with mechanical ventilation and some specific needs of respiratory failure. Most of the emphasis in our discussion of ventilators centered about the importance of alveolar ventilation and the removal of carbon dioxide, but we must not forget that the most pressing need of the patient in failure is the correction of hypoxia. Unless ventilation can ensure a viable level of arterial oxygen, our efforts will be of no avail. In all instances of significant ventilatory failure we will have to contend with hypoventilation hypoxia or physiologic shunt hypoxia, along with the management problems already discussed. Correction of these two types of hypoxia is discussed separately.

Hypoventilation hypoxia. We have been almost dogmatic in our insistence that oxygen administration for failure resulting from hypoventilation be accompanied by assisted ventilation to avoid the potential hazard of worsening the patient's ventilatory drive, but now that the fundamental precautions of such therapy are well understood, let us examine the state of failure to see if any modifications are justified. Obviously, we are not concerned with the risk of apnea in all hypoxic patients, and if we feel that a given patient has an adequate alveolar ventilation, we do not hesitate to give oxygen as needed. Perhaps there are patients with some degree of hypoventilation who also can be treated with oxygen unsupported by mechanical ventilation. There are many who feel that a trial of oxygen therapy may safely be given when hypercapnia and acidemia appear to be less a risk to the patient than hypoxemia, thereby hopefully avoiding the need for unnecessary intubation and the additional risks inherent in artificial ventilation.

This has been studied by several investigators, and the following program has proved successful in many patients when combined with vigorous therapy to establish or maintain airway patency.[84-86] Arterial blood gas values are obtained as soon as possible while the patient is breathing room air. If the oxygen tension is less than 60 mm Hg (some use 50 mm Hg as the limit) and the pH is above 7.30, the patient is started on a very low oxygen flow, usually by cannula. Since the method employs trial and error, follow-up blood studies are essential, and if a given level of oxygen flow maintains the blood values within the limits specified above, it is continued. If hypoxia is still not corrected, the oxygen flow is increased by very small increments until an arterial oxygen tension of at least 60 mm Hg is reached, provided the pH does not fall at the same time. Should it not be possible to oxygenate the patient without the development of progressive acidemia, he or she is intubated and given supported mechanical ventilation. This is a conservative approach and, if followed under careful observation, may be expected to be successful in many patients whose ventilatory defects result from readily reversible conditions. If oxygen is given by nasal cannula, 2 to 3 ℓ/min often suffices for moderate hypoxia and is unlikely to cause alarming elevations in arterial carbon dioxide tension unless the ventilation-perfusion balance is seriously disturbed.[87] The entrainment mask lends itself well to this type of therapy, since it will deliver a prefixed and relatively stable oxygen concentration at high enough flows to satisfy almost any ventilatory demand; but of course, it does not guarantee any specific blood oxygen level.[88,89]

There are steps to take to control the delivered oxygen concentration, depending on the type of ventilator used.[22] It is fairly simple in the volume ventilator by adding oxygen to the air that is the basic gas used by the machine. The structure of the volume machine makes available a chamber in which the gases can readily be mixed, and for each instrument there is provided by the manufacturer either a guide table or a mechanical control by which to adjust the oxygen flow to obtain a given concentration under specific operating conditions. It is still necessary to analyze samples of delivered gas to determine the exact concentrations in case of malfunction or maladjustment of the blending mechanism.

The use of helium-oxygen mixtures is noted only in passing because of its detailed coverage in Chapter 12. Helium-oxygen should be considered when oxygenation of a mechanically ventilated patient is unsuccessful because of severe diffuse bronchial obstruction.

Physiologic shunt hypoxia. Most of the discussion so far has centered about patients whose greatest needs are the correction of hypercapnia and acidemia, with oxygen support until spontaneous breathing is again normal. However, there are many whose major problem is a hypoxia that persists in the face of normal total alveolar ventilation, as judged by arterial carbon dioxide tensions and pH, or despite satisfactory support of an associated hypoventilation. We now review the principles of management of this condition, based on several good studies and increasing experience.[90-94]

The basic functional defect in shunt hypoxia is a reduction in ventilation/perfusion ratios in scattered areas of the lung. This may derive from the following: (1) small airway or alveolar inspiratory obstruction, producing so-called microatelectasis, resulting from accumulated secretions, edema, or alveolar exudates; and (2) a lack of surfactant, often replaced by a glassy appearing film described as a hyaline membrane, with its associated increase in alveolar surface tension, and which may be caused by (a) congenital absence as a result of prematurity (respiratory distress syndrome of the newborn) or (b) destruction by systemic shock, oxygen toxicity, infection, and probably other unknown factors (respiratory distress syndrome of the adult). It is important to emphasize again that ventilation/perfusion hypoxia often occurs with hypoventilation failure, complicating its management, but the principle of its therapy is the same no matter what the cause.

Both alveolar inspiratory obstruction and increased alveolar surface tension (reduced lung compliance) elevate the pressure necessary to initiate inflation, and the latter requires yet additional force to maintain alveolar distention adequate for gas exchange. Thus the two basic principles of correction of shunt hypoxia are (1) adjustment of inspiration to permit time for the distribution of gas into the slowly ventilating obstructed lobules; and (2) maintenance of sufficient intraalveolar pressure to resist abnormally high collapsing force and

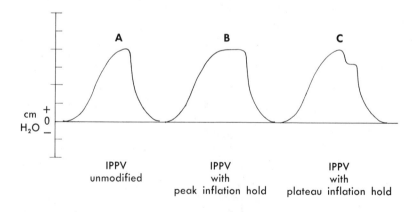

cm H₂O

A IPPV unmodified

B IPPV with peak inflation hold

C IPPV with plateau inflation hold

Fig. 14-8   Inflation hold. Pressure wave forms of two types are compared with unmodified pressure inhalation. (See text for description.)

to limit expiratory alveolar deflation. Two techniques in current use are referred to as *inflation hold* and *positive end-expiratory pressure.*

Inflation hold (Fig. 14-8). A frequent problem in the management of ventilator patients is the ventilation of lung units that are partially blocked by bronchial disease. These areas are referred to as "slow spaces" because of the reduced flow of air into them. Inflation hold is a technique used with IPPV to prolong distention of the lung so that more time is available to ventilate the slow spaces. It is of two general types, depending on the control mechanism provided by the manufacturer: peak inflation hold and plateau inflation hold.

PEAK INFLATION HOLD. Fig. 14-8, *B,* shows the increasing pressure of inhalation reaching its maximum, or *peak pressure,* and holding this pressure until inspiration ends. At this point, either the driving force of the ventilator or a combination of a relief valve and a continuous flow is used to maintain the set pressure until the inspiratory phase is cycled off. Holding inflation gives time for better inspired air distribution than if end-inspiration were only a momentary pause. The peak pressure generated to deliver the desired volume represents so-called mouth or airway pressure and can equilibrate with intraalveolar pressure during the hold period. When the hold is released, exhalation follows the natural passive recoil mechanism to zero gauge resting level. The student should recall that the longer the positive pressure of inspiratory inflation is held the greater will be its possible circulatory effects. This type of hold is common to pediatric ventilators.[22,64,65,70-72]

PLATEAU INFLATION HOLD. Although it is true that peak inflation hold creates an inspiratory plateau, as demonstrated in the sketch, the term *plateau* as we use it here refers to a variation of this pattern. In Fig. 14-8, *C,* inflating pressure is seen to reach the same peak as in *A,* but inspiration cycles off as scheduled. Manual or automatic activation of a control delays the opening of the exhalation valve, and thus for a moment neither gas flow nor pressure moves into or out of the lung. In this brief interval, pressure equalization between airways and alveoli takes place as air that is already in the airways moves further into the harder-to-ventilate alveoli, expanding its volume and dropping its pressure below that at the mouth. The pressure drop is seen in Fig. 14-8, *C,* as a small plateau in the expiratory downslope of the pressure curve, shortly below the peak level. In reality, the plateau causes a hesitation in the descent of the ventilator manometer needle, which may be 1 to 10 cm of water or more below peak pressure, depending on the resistance to airflow during the active phase.

During these moments of no gas flow, between peak and plateau pressures, if we assume that there is complete pressure equilibration throughout the respiratory tract, the mouth pressure as recorded by the ventilator manometer also represents alveolar pressure at the distal end of the tract. The plateau pressure is thus considered to be at least a close approximation of pressure in the alveoli. Measurement of plateau alveolar pressure is both therapeutically and diagnostically useful. Therapeutically, it performs a service similar to that of the peak inflation hold, providing time for ventilation of poorly com-municating lung units. Diagnostically, plateau pressure supplies valuable information about the state of a mechanically ventilated lung.[95-98]

Peak mouth pressure reflects the force required to inflate the lung against the resistance both of the airways and the elastic recoil of the combined lung and chest wall. One of our concerns in the mechanically ventilated patient is evaluating lung-thorax compliance, the amount of lung inflation that can be achieved per unit of ventilating pressure applied. To measure this compliance we must eliminate the factor of airway resistance and consider only the pres-sure relating to the lung-thorax system. This can be done with the plateau hold maneuver, since during the interval between the end of inhalation and the opening of the exhalation valve, once pressure has equilibrated, there is no gas flow in the airways. With cessation of gas flow the contribution of airway resistance to ventilating pressure is removed, and the pressure at the plateau represents the recoil force of the lung-thorax, or conversely, the force needed to inflate the lung-thorax. The therapist can closely estimate what is referred to as the *static compliance* of lung-thorax and tubing circuit by dividing the patient's tidal volume by the plateau pressure minus PEEP (VT ÷ [Plateau pressure − PEEP]), a calculation that should be done frequently during acute stages of mechanical ventilation. It should be emphasized that a true static compliance value depends on an accurate volume measurement, for which ad-equate meters are available, and a static state of no gas flow in the airways, which cannot always be guaranteed with certainty. The time interval for the completion of inspired air distribution among all the lung units depends on the extent of airway patency. In some patients, airway obstruction may be so severe that distribution takes several seconds, and in the presence of severe airway disease, it is possible that a plateau might not be reached before the start of the next ventilator cycle. Thus, to be sure the pressure reading is truly static, expiration should be blocked until it is certain that a real plateau is reached. Although this can be done much more easily with special tools in the laboratory than by the gross method of observing movements of a manometer needle, bedside measurements are fortunately accurate enough for our clinical needs. It would probably be better, however, if we referred to the compliance as *effective static compliance*, because this term acknowledges the possible pres-ence of slight airflow within or between the lungs, even though upper airways may be completely static and because it also represents the compliance of the ventilator tubing system.

Changes in the resistance to airflow as well as changes in compliance can be observed by serial measurements with this inflation plateau hold maneuver when it is used with a volume-cycled ventilator.[95-99] The peak pressure indi-cated during active inspiration reflects the amount of force needed to over-come resistance to airflow from the tubing circuit, artificial airway, and the patient's airways and from the elastic resistances of the lungs. As described above, the plateau or hold pressure indicates an estimate of the elastic recoil of the lungs and tubing circuit. The *difference* between the peak and plateau pressures can indicate the pressure needed to overcome only resistances to airflow such as water in ventilator tubing, bronchospasm, and secretions in the airways.[97,99] This applies only to those ventilators that can produce the same or nearly the same flow pattern each breath regardless of the pressures encountered, i.e., constant flow generators.

As an example, a relaxed patient being ventilated with a constant volume and flow rate has a peak pressure reading of 30 cm of water and a plateau pressure reading of 25 cm of water. One hour later the volumes and flow rate are unchanged, but the peak pressure is now 45 cm of water and plateau hold pressure is still 25 cm of water. This indicates that there is now some obstruction to flow that was not present an hour before. This patient should be further evaluated for signs of bronchospasm, need for suctioning, etc. Since the plateau pressure remained the same, the elastic recoil or compliance has also remained unchanged.

In order to be sure that changes occurring in peak and plateau pressures are only patient or tubing-system related, measurements must only be compared to one another under the same volume and flow settings. If these settings are changed, new *sets* of measurements will need to be made before further comparisons can be done.

Positive end-expiratory pressure (PEEP). One of the most difficult management problems is the patient with persistent hypoxemia, often with hyperventilation, despite the administration of oxygen concentrations of up to 100%. Such a patient may have no significant carbon dioxide retention and may be frankly hypocapnic from hypoxia-induced overbreathing. Obviously, associated airway obstruction further compounds the problem.

The primary functional defect in this situation is widespread physiologic arteriovenous shunting, or venous admixture. Although shunting occurs in a number of diseases, one of its most serious manifestations is as a component of the infant and adult respiratory distress syndromes, where it is the product of accumulated intrabronchial, intraalveolar, and interstitial pulmonary fluid. The fluid interferes with ventilation by (1) physically excluding air; and (2) interfering with action of bronchiolar and alveolar surfactant, causing collapse of bronchioles and alveoli, which in turn (a) decreases pulmonary compliance and (b) reduces functional residual capacity (FRC). The clinical problem therefore is correction of a progressive shunt hypoxia, resulting from airway and alveolar collapse and decreased compliance and FRC.

PEEP is a maneuver that maintains pressure above atmospheric in the patient's lungs at the end of expiration. This combats the collapsing tendency of small airways and alveoli, deprived of effective surfactant, by increasing the FRC. Alveolar inflating force against the resistance of surface tension is inversely proportional to alveolar size. Thus, if more air than normal can be left in the alveoli at end-exhalation (increased FRC), less air pressure will be needed to inflate them (increased compliance). At the same time, because the bronchioles and alveoli are kept in a hyperinflated state at end-exhalation, distribution of inspired gas is greatly enhanced. More effective than inflation hold, the increased FRC improves ventilation of slow spaces and permits air entry into bronchioles and alveoli that otherwise would be partially or completely collapsed. The reversal of severe hypoxemia is sometimes dramatic, but it cannot be stressed too strongly that for this technique to succeed, patency of large and medium airways must be ensured, since significant obstruction at these levels can render PEEP quite useless.

To summarize, PEEP is a procedure that purposely increases FRC when disease has neutralized effective action of pulmonary surfactant. The increased FRC improves compliance, reduces bronchiolar and alveolar occlusion from collapse, improves pulmonary air entry and distribution, and reduces shunting.

The mechanics of increasing FRC by retaining gas pressure in alveoli at end-expiration seem fundamentally simple, but safe clinical application requires sound understanding of the desired objective. Unfortunately, it is not enough that students learn the principles and use of PEEP; they must also cope with the confusion of nonuniform terminology relating to the subject. A problem of definition stems from differences in the use of PEEP on patients who are (1) on controlled or assisted mechanical ventilation or (2) breathing spontaneously without mechanical assistance. These differences will be described, but it can be noted at this time that there is one universal need for effective PEEP: an airtight breathing system. With some exceptions, which will be explained, this means fitting the patient with a cuffed endotracheal or tracheostomy tube.

Terminology of the use of end-expiratory pressure thus depends on whether the patient is on a ventilator or is breathing spontaneously or both. The matter is not this easily settled, however. For example, note the definitions suggested by the ACCP-ATS Joint Committee on Nomenclature, and by an editorial in *Respiratory Care*[100, 101]:

1. ACCP-ATS Joint Committee
   a. Positive end-expiratory pressure (PEEP): a residual pressure above atmospheric maintained at the airway opening at the end of expiration. This may be used *during spontaneous or mechanical ventilation.**
   b. Constant positive pressure breathing (CPPB) (constant positive airway pressure—CPAP): a pressure above atmospheric maintained at the airway opening throughout the respiratory cycle during spontaneous breathing.
2. Editorial, *Respiratory Care*
   a. Positive end-expiratory pressure (PEEP) is *mechanical ventilation** against a threshold resistance.
   b. Continuous positive pressure breathing (CPPB) is nonventilator breathing against a threshold resistance.
   c. CPAP is the same as CPPB.

There is a major difference between the two definitions of PEEP, relating to its application during spontaneous breathing. We will see soon, also, that there is a situation where neither of the definitions limited to spontaneous

*Italics added.

breathing applies. Finally, to add more confusion, there is popular use of the expression, *continuous positive pressure ventilation* (CPPV), as a counterpart to the previously discussed inspiratory positive-pressure ventilation (IPPV) indicating the presence of positive pressure during both phases of ventilation.

Recent uses of combined ventilator breathing and spontaneous breathing at an elevated baseline, that is, IMV with CPAP or PEEP, tend to make the definitions indistinguishable when the use of a ventilator alone attempts to separate the terms.[76] There are also several methods of applying end-expiratory pressure to spontaneous breathing systems, which differ both in pressure wave-forms as well as in potentially important physiologic aspects such as work of breathing and mean intrathoracic pressure. Two terms that recently have emerged in the literature are *spontaneous PEEP* (sPEEP)[102,103] and *expiratory positive airway pressure* (EPAP).[104,105] These are spontaneous breathing systems with end-expiratory pressure but are different from CPAP. These

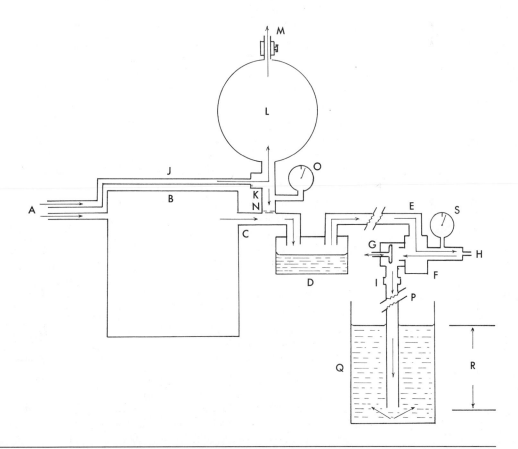

Fig. 14-9 Positive end-expiratory pressure (PEEP) with controlled mechanical ventilation or IMV. (See text for description.)

terms are discussed in more detail later in this chapter. A complete review of terminology, both in current use and proposed, has been presented recently by Eross, Powner, and Grenvik.[106]

We discuss PEEP under the three categories of (1) *PEEP with controlled mechanical ventilation;* (2) *PEEP with assisted mechanical ventilation;* and (3) *PEEP with unassisted spontaneous ventilation.* It is used most frequently on patients with controlled mechanical ventilation, so under this heading we review most of the details of the technique, describing the other two in terms of how they differ.

PEEP with controlled mechanical ventilation. In the interest of conciseness and brevity, we refer to this category as *controlled-PEEP,* understanding that the control status implies the use of a mechanical ventilator.

MECHANICS OF CONTROLLED-PEEP. The reader's attention is drawn to Fig. 14-9, a modification of Fig. 14-7, *B,* illustrating the addition of PEEP capability to IMV circuitry on a volume ventilator system. Breathing gas *A* is delivered by ventilator *B* through humidifier *D* to the patient at *H.* Expired air passes through the ventilator-regulated exhalation valve, *F,* and by tubing of suitable length, *P,* into the resistance of a column of water, *Q.* In the closed, airtight circuit, high-pressure exhaled air bubbles out into the atmosphere, but back pressure of the water column prevents intraalveolar and airway pressures from dropping to atmosphere at the end of exhalation. The amount of pressure, in centimeters of water, remaining in the system at the lung-thorax resting level, keeping alveoli partially inflated and the FRC enlarged, is a function of the distance in centimeters from the end of the exhalation tube to the top of the water column, *R.* When PEEP was first introduced into respiratory therapy, the water-sealed exhalation tube was the usual method of increasing FRC. Now, however, many ventilators have a built-in, manually operated variable control, which produces a plateau of end-expiratory positive pressure by limiting deflation of the exhalation valve diaphragm, *G,* retaining pressurized air in the alveoli.[22] Although water column and mechanical back-pressure devices are often calibrated, tubing resistance to airflow may influence the actual PEEP produced. For accurate monitoring, it is recommended that a manometer, *S,* be integrated into the system as close as possible to the patient.

PEEP and IMV are frequently used together, and special attention must be given to the balance of pressure across one-way valve, *N,* Fig. 14-9. PEEP exerts a continuous positive pressure on the ventilator circuit, holding the valve closed, and since the spontaneous circuit is at atmosphere, the patient must make an inspiratory effort of a force exceeding that of the PEEP to open the valve for a spontaneous breath. Two similar techniques will eliminate the problem. First, adjustment of source gas flow, or of controlled reservoir bag bleed-off, can allow sufficient pressure to develop in the spontaneous circuit to create some gas flow through the one-way valve. The flow may be detected at the exhalation valve port and indicates an erasure of the high to low pressure gradient across the valve from ventilatory circuit to spontaneous circuit.

Second, better flow control can be realized by incorporating a manometer, *O*, into the spontaneous circuit and carefully adjusting gas release from the reservoir bag until the spontaneous circuit manometer approximates the patient circuit manometer, *S*. Slight negative inspiratory pressure by the patient will then open the valve for easy spontaneous breathing.

When only slight drops in pressure (such as 1 to 3 cm of water) occur during spontaneous breathing, then the work of breathing is thought to be reduced compared to systems in which a drop of PEEP to ambient pressure is needed for spontaneous inspiration.[76,102,107-109] However, some patients apparently tolerate this well,[102,105] and there is a potential benefit to this drop in pressure. By having the pressure fall during a spontaneous breath, the mean intrathoracic pressure also falls, and this may be helpful in reducing the circulatory effects of the positive pressure during expiration in some patients[103,108] and not in others.[109] When the pressure is maintained within 1 to 3 cm water of baseline during a spontaneous breath (i.e., CPAP), then work of breathing is probably reduced and mean intrathoracic pressure increased compared to the inspiratory pressure falling significantly or to atmospheric levels (i.e., sPEEP or EPAP). The real benefits of these methods and the question of which patients would be best served by one as opposed to the other need further investigation.[79]

Let us consider intrapulmonary pressure curves *A* and *B* in Fig. 14-10. The

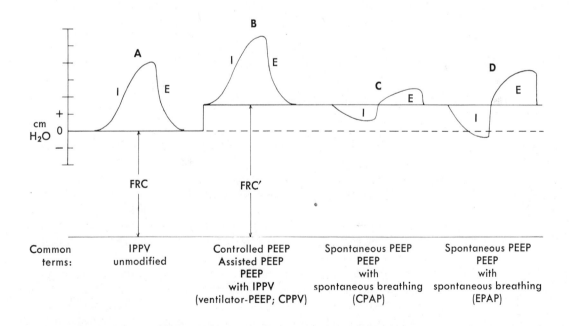

Fig. 14-10   Positive end-expiratory pressure (PEEP). Intrapulmonary pressure curves and lung-thorax resting levels in three applications of PEEP. (See text for description.)

graph is dimensionless and combines pressure with volumes, as the polarity of intrapulmonary pressures is shown with accompanying imaginary FRCs. Curve *A* is a normal curve, for comparison, showing inspiratory and end-expiratory pulmonary pressures of zero gauge and a "normal" FRC volume. Curve *B* uses the same pressure pattern as *A* but differs from *A* in the position of its resting level. The level is elevated because end-expiratory pressure, equal to the difference between the old and new resting levels, has prevented the alveoli from deflating to their volumes in *A,* and consequently FRC has increased to FRC'. The student should note that to maintain a tidal volume after setting a PEEP level, peak inspiratory pressure must also be raised. This occurs automatically with a volume-cycled ventilation. In time, however, as PEEP activates more alveolar units, improved compliance may allow reductions in peak pressure without sacrifice of tidal volumes.

HAZARDS OF PEEP. The use of high pulmonary pressure to hyperinflate the lungs is not without hazards, and some series report complications in as many as 50% of patients so treated, while others report about 10%. The major adverse effects of PEEP are:

1. *High-pressure physical lung damage (barotrauma).* A common manifestation is *subcutaneous emphysema,* the leakage of air from alveoli and its migration along vascular and bronchial paths to the lung roots, expanding out beneath the skin of the upper body. *Pneumothorax,* air leakage into the thorax from alveolar rupture, with varying degrees of lung collapse, while more serious is less frequent and may result from end-expiratory pressures in excess of 20 cm of water.

2. *Reduced cardiovascular function.* If high PEEP can be transmitted to the intrathoracic space, it can retard venous return and reduce cardiac output. Fortunately, in most patients needing the benefits of PEEP, disease has so reduced compliance that the lungs are too "stiff" to carry intrapulmonary pressure to intrathoracic structures, and depressed circulation is avoided. Also, despite high pressure, in some instances myocardial function improves with increased oxygenation.

3. *Reduced urinary output.* We learned earlier that positive pressure ventilation, by elevating intrathoracic pressure, can reduce urinary flow. The addition of PEEP may aggravate this response and require the use of diuretics for correction and control.

Incorporation of intermittent mandatory ventilation in the management plan may help minimize complications.[76,80] Each patient-generated breath will lower the long-term mean effective intrathoracic pressure, potentially relieving strain on other systems.

INDICATIONS FOR, AND CONTRAINDICATIONS OF, PEEP. The general indication for PEEP was described in the opening paragraph of this discussion, but there were no guidelines for its use in specific circumstances. It should be apparent to the reader that there can be no hard-and-fast rules for using PEEP, any more than for starting a patient on mechanical ventilation. The two dangers against which we try to protect these patients are progressive hypoxia and oxygen toxicity as a consequence of treating the hypoxia. When our efforts are inadequate, then we use PEEP. As a rule of thumb, we should at least be prepared to initiate PEEP, when arterial oxygen tension continues to drop below 50 mm Hg, in a patient on IPPV, who is ventilated with an oxygen concentration greater than 50%. Not all patients with hypoxemia are suitable candidates for PEEP. A relative contraindication is, of course, significant hypotension. This is not absolute, because in a given circumstance it may be evident that risk to survival from hypoxia is greater than from hypotension. Also, pharmacologic agents can be used to support circulation, and improved myocardial oxygenation from better gas exchange may protect the cardiovascular system from pressure effects, despite continuation of PEEP.[59,60]

Perhaps more important contraindications to PEEP are known pulmonary hyperinflation before onset of critical hypoxia and a normal or high compliance. The direct effect of PEEP increases both FRC and compliance, and if they are already elevated, little benefit can be expected. In a general way, we can say that PEEP is probably inadvisable for a patient with pulmonary emphysema. Areas of the lung already hyperinflated will be further distended, and excessive intraalveolar pressure may divert pulmonary capillary flow to low-pressurized, poorly ventilated alveoli, increasing venous admixture and worsening hypoxia. The decision to use or withhold PEEP requires careful scrutiny of clinical and laboratory data, establishing priorities of risk to the patient. It should never be employed as a routine procedure, but only when it is judged that the hazards of an increased FRC and elevated intrathoracic pressure are less than the risks of continued hypoxia or oxygen toxicity.

INITIATING AND DISCONTINUING PEEP. So far we have been concerned mostly with the principles of PEEP, and now it is time to consider such practical matters as levels of pressure used and how to start and discontinue it. Although there is no formula available to help us determine what PEEP should be, it is probably safe to say that end-expiratory pressures of 5 to 15 cm of water will accommodate most needs, but often pressures of 20 to 30 cm of water are needed,[59] and rarely pressures more than 50 cm of water.[110] There is no accepted "safe" level of PEEP. For many patients who have maintained fair cardiopulmonary stability, careful clinical observation, with blood gas determinations as needed, can safely guide the use of low PEEP levels. In the very acute patient, when end-expiratory pressures of more than 20 cm of water are needed, more specific cardiovascular monitoring is necessary.

Currently popular for this purpose is the Swan-Ganz catheter, described earlier, which allows the titration of PEEP against cardiac output and degrees of arteriovenous shunt. With this information "optimal PEEP" can be determined as the highest pressure that maximally decreases shunt without impeding cardiac output.[59,78,110] If cardiac output falls before the desired reduction in shunt is achieved, intravascular volumes are treated with appropriate fluid and pharmacologic agents. A modification, described as "best PEEP" has been calculated at the bedside, without using the Swan-Ganz catheter,[111] in normovolemic patients with PEEP up to 15 cm of water. Too much pressure decreases compliance, since overdistention of alveoli exceeds the number of lung units opened up to ventilation. Thus optimum lung function should accompany a level of PEEP that produces maximum compliance. In clinical use the effective static compliance is measured by dividing the tidal volume by the difference between plateau pressure and positive end-expiratory pressure (*not* atmospheric zero gauge). This value is calculated for increasing PEEP levels until additional increments of pressure do not increase compliance. The final end-expiratory pressure (before compliance falls) is considered the "best PEEP." Such a relatively simple maneuver is not intended to replace invasive monitoring techniques, where the latter are indicated, and in patients with crushed chests, for example, where compliance is disrupted, it is inapplicable. This method of "best PEEP" may not work with hypovolemic patients or those receiving more than 15 cm of water. Nevertheless, many patients can be safely managed by the "best PEEP" technique, coupled with knowledgeable clinical observation, and the hazard of intracardiac and intrapulmonary arterial catheterization avoided.

When PEEP is successful, we then have the task of reducing both PEEP and the high concentration of inspired oxygen. Assuming no complications from PEEP, it is advisable to maintain the elevated pressure while dropping inspired oxygen by increments of 10% to 15%, keeping arterial oxygen tension between 60 and 100 mm Hg. When the $F_{I_{O_2}}$ is 40% or less, the PEEP should then be lowered in steps of 5 cm of water until abolished. All patients require tailored schedules, of course, and many can be weaned from PEEP abruptly, whereas others may need a long and gradual withdrawal.

PEEP with assisted mechanical ventilation (assisted-PEEP, PEEP-assist). Enabling a patient to trigger a ventilator, provided with PEEP, into a demand cycle for an assisted breath, requires the same attention to inspiratory effort as does the use of PEEP with IMV discussed a few pages back. Without IMV, spontaneous inspiratory effort should trigger an assisted ventilator breath. Thus machine sensitivity must be increased (as opposed to the use of IMV) so the patient will not have to overcome the PEEP to activate the ventilator. On modern volume ventilators the sensitivity mechanism can be readjusted or it is automatically compensated for PEEP, changing the triggering level from slightly subatmospheric to just below any desired PEEP; then initiating a machine-assisted breath calls for no more patient effort with PEEP than without it.[22,112]

In general, the airway pressure curves of machine-assist, patient-triggered breaths are the same as control breaths under static conditions. Thus curve *B* in Fig. 14-10 represents both controlled-PEEP and assisted-PEEP. It would be more accurate, however, to include a small downward deflection at the start of inspiration of an assist curve, representing patient triggering effort.

Now that assisted-PEEP is technically possible, we should evaluate its role in acute respiratory care.[113] It would appear that the technique of intermittent mandatory ventilation has replaced mechanically assisted ventilation to a considerable degree, but the student must remember that the sudden popularity of a new procedure does not mean that all its predecessors are automatically invalid. Despite the many welcome virtues of IMV, there are still occasional instances when it is advisable to encourage simply an inspiratory effort, even if the patient is unable to effect an adequate follow-up tidal volume. Here, true assisted ventilation is very helpful, and if PEEP is indicated, it can and should be used. It has been suggested that assisted-PEEP might occasionally be useful, in selected patients, when administered by face mask in an attempt to avoid tracheal intubation.[114] Even though perhaps limited in its scope, assisted-PEEP does put at our disposal another valuable tool in the management of ventilatory support.

PEEP with unassisted spontaneous ventilation (CPAP, EPAP). Positive endexpiratory pressure may be indicated in an intubated patient recently weaned from a ventilator or in one whose own breathing has not needed mechanical support but who can be intubated for PEEP. In some circumstances, PEEP can be used for short periods with a tightly fitted face mask.[104,105,115,116] The simplest circuit for *spontaneous-PEEP* or CPAP is shown in Fig. 14-11. Mod-

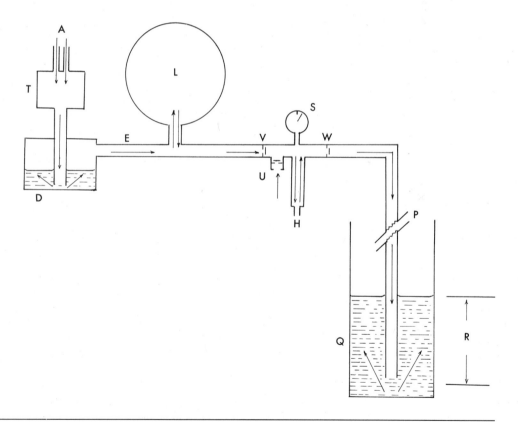

Fig. 14-11   Positive end-expiratory pressure (PEEP) with unassisted spontaneous breathing in an intubated patient. (See text for description.)

ifications can be added to this basic design, but it demonstrates the key elements. Breathing gas mixture from blender, *T,* flows through humidifier, *D,* into patient inspiratory tubing, *E.* Reservoir bag, *L,* makes available adequate gas for any size of tidal volume required by an intubated or tightly masked patient at *H.* As depicted in Fig. 14-9, an extended exhalation tube is immersed in a water column or attached to an adjustable mechanical resistor to create PEEP, the magnitude of which is accurately measured by manometer, *S.* The airways and lungs of a relaxed patient equilibrate with the supraatmospheric pressure in the gas-conducting system, which to the lungs, in a sense, is now "ambient pressure." Spontaneous inhalation and exhalation therefore starts and terminates, respectively, at an elevated lung-thorax resting level, and FRC is enlarged.

Valving in such a system is unnecessary as long as breathing gas supply is adequate and is adjusted to flow steadily through the PEEP generator. It is wise, however, to anticipate the potential disaster of supply failure and include protective safety mechanisms. In the event of a loss gas, atmospheric air is immediately available to the patient through emergency one-way valve *U.* Under the same circumstances, one-way valve *V* prevents exhaled air from taking the retrograde path of least resistance into the inspiratory arm of the patient tubing, creating a large dead space. One-way valve *W* similarly prevents rebreathing of gas in the exhalation tubing, in the absence of the rinsing effect of a steady source gas flow.

The technique just described is commonly referred to as "CPAP" (constant or continuous positive airway pressure) and as "CPPB" (constant or continuous positive pressure breathing) in accord with the two sets of definitions given earlier by the ACCP-ATS Joint Committee and the editorial office of *Respiratory Care.* CPAP (CPPB) implies spontaneous breathing without mechanical assistance against resistance to exhalation for the purpose of increasing FRC. The student's attention is directed to Fig. 14-9, where it can be observed that the circuit through the ventilator is a typical PEEP system, with an end-exhalation resistance to machine-assisted breathing. In contrast, the bypass circuit for spontaneous breathing is essentially the same as the system we have just described for CPAP. In other words, when we add PEEP and IMV capabilities to a ventilator circuit, we are providing both PEEP and CPAP (or CPPB). The battle over terminology and definitions does seem a bit ridiculous in this light because whether the patient is treated with PEEP or CPAP (CPPB) can depend on how he or she breathes—it may be the patient's decision, not ours.[106,117-121]

Early in the description of the PEEP principle, reference was made to exceptions to the need for airtight intubation. The respiratory distress syndrome of infants is an extremely grave condition, most often afflicting the prematurely born. The disease is characterized by progressively falling compliance caused by a surfactant lack of prematurity. Many infants need full ventilator support with intubation, but others with spontaneous breathing may need only assistance in maintaining alveolar patency and can benefit from CPAP.

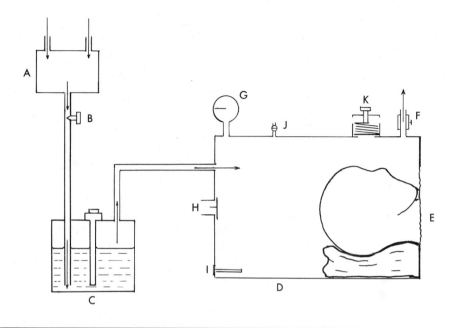

Fig. 14-12   Positive end-expiratory pressure (PEEP) with unassisted spontaneous breathing in a nonintubated infant. (See text for description.)

Intubation in these small patients is difficult, and a CPAP technique has been developed for them that is noninvasive.[93,116]

Fig. 14-12 schematically diagrams the major elements of a spontaneous-PEEP system that is, in reality, a miniature hyperbaric chamber. It surrounds the infant's head with a supraatmospheric pressure, which elevates the lung-thorax resting level and increases the FRC. Air-oxygen mixture from a blender and flow meter, *A,* passes through a flow control valve, *B,* a heated humidifier, *C,* and into a rigid transparent plastic cylinder enclosing the patient's head, *D.* An adjustable soft plastic diaphragm, called an iris, which opens and closes like a camera shutter, forms a partial seal about the infant's neck, *E;* complete airtightness is unnecessary. A balance between entry gas flow and flow out of an adjustable escape port, *F,* maintains desired chamber pressure, which is recorded on an aneroid manometer, *G.* The unit is also supplied with a fitting for emergency manual bag ventilation or sighing, *H,* a thermometer for monitoring chamber temperature, *I,* a sampling port for analysis of chamber gas, *J,* and an adjustable safety pressure relief valve to limit chamber pressure, especially during manual ventilation, *K.* This can also be an underwater seal instead of a mechanical valve. Not shown is a hinged lid on top for easy access to the patient.

Other methods of applying CPAP to infants include the use of nasal prongs and face masks.[116] The nasal prongs are short tubes that fit into the nares much the way a nasal cannula does for oxygen administration. Since neonates are obligate nose breathers, CPAP pressures up to about 10 to 12 cm of water can be applied before an infant's mouth naturally opens and vents further pressures.

CPAP by face mask has been applied to both infants[63,116] and adults.[104,105,115] Problems with administering CPAP by mask include pressure necrosis on the face, increased dead space in the mask, gastric rupture, and eye trauma in infants.[116] Aspiration of gastric contents can occur if the patient vomits when the mask is strapped to the face, but use of a nasogastric tube and careful selection of patients can avoid this problem in adults.[104,105,115] In one recent study, 44 awake, cooperative, spontaneously breathing adult patients with normal or low Pa_{CO_2} and evidence of increased physiologic shunt were treated with CPAP by mask, with all but one avoiding tracheal intubation.[115] In this series no problems with gastric distension or vomiting were reported.

Attention is directed to Fig. 14-10, curve *C*, which has the biphasic intrapulmonary pressure contour of a spontaneous breath. Inspiration generates airflow by lowering intrapulmonary pressure, *I*, and at end-inspiration, as flow stops momentarily, pressure equilibrates with ambient and returns to baseline. Exhalation, *E*, elevates intrapulmonary pressure to force air out, then at end-exhalation pressure again returns to baseline. Two important facts should be noted. First, despite the intrapulmonary pressure oscillations about the baseline during the ventilatory phases, breaths start and stop (end-expiration) at the elevated resting level. Second, and again despite the pressure variation of the breathing curve, all that matters is that end-expiration is at a higher than atmospheric pressure. This is what increases the FRC.

Curve *D* amplifies these points. Assume the patient takes an occasional extra large breath or that his or her regular pattern is large enough that a slight negative pressure is created in the lungs at peak exhalation. The fact that inspiratory pulmonary pressure dips into the negative range in no way interferes with or negates the function or purpose of PEEP. End-expiration still falls at the desired positive pressure of an elevated resting level, and the FRC is correspondingly enlarged. Also, if the patient has the power to create large pressure swings and big tidal volumes, this reflects favorably on his or her functional status. The student is asked to note, however, that in a curve *D* situation, the expressions *constant* or *continuous positive airway pressure* or *positive-pressure breathing* are technically incorrect because of the possibility of inspiratory negative peak pressures. For this reason a term such as *spontaneous-PEEP, EPAP,* or some other that emphasizes the terminal pressure is more appropriate than is *CPAP* or *CPPB,* as defined earlier.

As mentioned earlier, some physiologic differences between these types of curves exist. Several investigators feel that the breathing pattern exemplified by curve *D* may promote venous return because of the lower intrathoracic pressures with this EPAP-type of system.[103,108] This occurs at the expense of apparent greater work of breathing, and some patients may be capable of providing the extra work with no apparent difficulty[102,105] while others become agitated and require a system producing the CPAP-like pattern of curve C.[109] The real cardiovascular effects of the breathing pattern of curve D are not uniform. Although one study showed an improvement in cardiac output in one set of patients,[103] another study did not support these findings.[109] These studies may not be directly comparable in patient groups or control conditions, and further investigation is needed to help deliniate which patients are candidates for which pressure system.

Monitoring mechanical ventilation. The need for close observation of the mechanically ventilated patient has been amply emphasized, as has the value of a respiratory care unit for this purpose.[99] No matter what the physical circumstances are under which treatment is being given, the therapist looks for and checks certain things and follows procedures that experience has shown to be necessary for the patient's safety. We describe three types of monitoring—clinical, physiologic, and mechanical—although there are overlapping areas among them.

Clinical monitoring. Clinical monitoring involves observing the patient and evaluating his or her condition and the effectiveness of ventilation based on signs and symptoms and the therapist's critical knowledge of the physiology of the disease and the expectations of therapy. No sophisticated diagnostic equipment is used. The therapist is interested in the physical and mental comfort of the patient because the patient's attitude is vital to recovery. Since the intubated patient cannot speak, the therapist must be on the watch for signs of pain, restlessness, and apprehension. Often communication can be established through the use of pencil and paper, and although too-frequent annoying questions are to be avoided, the therapist should inquire periodically of the feelings of the patient. The alert and observant therapist soon learns the characteristics of the patient and how best to manage him or her. The patient's color should be watched and both cyanosis and pallor noted. We know that cyanosis is a crude quantitative guage of hypoxemia, but it is a good determinant of changes in oxygenation. Excessive pallor, especially if accompanied by cold moist skin, may indicate developing cardiovascular collapse.

Much valuable information concerning the work of breathing and the effectiveness of therapy can be obtained by noting the muscular components of ventilation. This is especially true before the start of treatment in the patient being assisted rather than controlled in his or her breathing and during breaks in controlled ventilation, as when the patient is being aspirated or equipment is being serviced. Increasing or decreasing use of the accessory ventilatory muscles is noted and is an excellent indication of the energy used by the patient. The therapist should frequently observe the mobility of the upper abdomen, or epigastrium, both when the patient is on and when he or she is off the ventilator. To do this properly the therapist should expose the upper half of the patient's abdomen and kneel by the side of the bed in order to sight across the patient at the abdominal level. Retraction of the epigastrium during the inspiratory phase and protrusion during exhalation constitute paradoxic breathing, described in Chapter 8, and indicate a severe disturbance in the efficiency of ventilation. If present while the patient is being mechanically assisted, they mean that he or she is completely uncoordinated with the instrument and is working against it and that therapy is worsening rather than helping the patient. The degree to which the epigastrium rises during inhalation is a function of the descent of the diaphragm and a rough indication of the tidal volume.

Like the evaluation of cyanosis, the volumetric implication of epigastric movement is valuable as a monitor of changes rather than a quantitative measurement. To appreciate the abdominal motion, the therapist should lay a hand gently on the patient, between the xiphoid cartilage and the umbilicus, and observe as well as feel the movement of the hand. In the obstructed patient with spontaneous breathing, assisted or unassisted, the therapist may be able to feel the expiratory contraction of the abdominal wall as the patient works to express air against heavy resistance.

Finally, in addition to judging the muscular aspect of ventilation, the therapist will be able to ascertain by inspection and palpation of the abdomen whether there is abdominal distention. The accumulation of intestinal gas postoperatively and the swallowing of air by a dyspneic patient given short-term ventilatory assistance through a face mask or mouthpiece can produce serious distention of the abdomen. Not infrequently distention builds up an intraabdominal pressure so great that it seriously interferes with the inspirational descent of the diaphragm. In such an instance the therapist will observe the abdomen to be rounded, its skin stretched smooth, and the wall tense to the touch. A gentle but sharp slap will elicit a tympanic, or drumlike, response. If the therapist notes such distention, he or she should bring it to the attention of the attending physician or nurse, for unless it can be relieved, it may make effective ventilation impossible.

Auscultation of the chest is an examination of the breath sounds through a stethoscope and is a technique with which the therapist should become familiar. It should be clear that the therapist's use of a stethoscope is limted, for diagnostic auscultation is a fine art employed by a physician and takes many years to develop to a point of proficiency. However, the use of a stethoscope will enable the therapist to evaluate the distribution of air in the patient's chest and to evaluate the degree of obstruction. When the ventilator has been set up to the therapist's satisfaction, he or she should listen to the chest with the scope—anteriorly, posteriorly, and in the axillae—comparing the sounds in related areas of both lungs from the apices to the bases. Closing the eyes for maximum concentration, the therapist listens for the intensity of airflow to determine whether there are areas that are not being adequately ventilated.

Since many respiratory patients suffer severe obstruction and have mobile secretions, it is not uncommon to find areas of lung poorly aerated and patterns of air distribution that change from hour to hour. In this regard, special mention should be made of a hazard of intubation referred to earlier in this chapter and illustrated in Fig. 14-13. This is the placement of a tracheal tube too low so that its tip passes the carina into one or the other main bronchus.

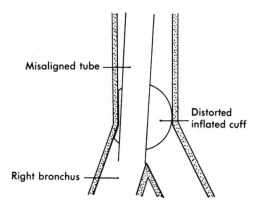

Misaligned tube

Distorted inflated cuff

Right bronchus

Fig. 14-13 Low position of tracheal tube so that its tip enters one main bronchus. The inflated cuff effectively occludes the other air passage, limiting ventilation to only one lung.

This is generally the result of a hasty insertion of an endotracheal or nasotracheal tube, intubation by unskilled personnel, or the use of too long a tracheostomy tube. With most if not all the delivered gas directed into only one lung, the serious disturbance to the ventilation-perfusion balance is obvious. Severe physiologic shunting can increase the venous admixture to the point that hypoxia may be fatal, and in the obstructed patient the resistance to the total airflow's diversion to one lung will prevent compensation for the hypoventilation of the blocked lung, and hypercapnia is probable. Usually the clinical appearance of the patient will warn of this complication, but if the occlusion is not complete, the ineffective ventilation may be attributed to underlying disease and correction attempted by such irrelevant measures as increasing airflow, the use of bronchodilators, etc. Thus, in an intubated patient, signs of sudden disruption of ventilatory pattern, accompanied by auscultatory signs of reduced airflow to one lung, should raise the immediate suspicion of a misplaced or slipped tube or a displaced cuff, and the responsible physician should be alerted at once. With experience the therapist will be able to differentiate the breath sounds encountered in obstructive disease and described in Chapter 8. This will help in evaluating the status of the airways by recognizing obstruction as primarily caused by bronchospasm rather than by secretions; and the better the understanding of the patient, the better will be the therapist's services.

With their knowledge of the effect of mechanical ventilation on circulation, therapists will want to keep themselves informed of their patient's cardiovascular status by frequent checking of heart rate and blood pressure. Although these parameters are traditionally the responsibility of the nursing service, there need be no conflict. Indeed, this is a function whereby cooperation between the nurse and the therapist will be to the advantage of the patient. In a special-care unit, rates and pressures are recorded frequently, and therapists may not need to do the measurements routinely. However, therapists are aware of the speed with which the ventilated patient's condition may change, and they should monitor these values as often as they feel necessary, and especially if they find it necessary to increase inspiratory pressure to a high level in an unstable patient or one receiving prolonged therapy

There is no rule to follow, but in the patient whose cardiac condition is in doubt or who has known cardiac weakness, heart rate and pressure may have to be recorded as often as every 15 minutes until stability is ensured and then at least hourly thereafter. At any time the therapist feels there is a progressive or significant rise in heart rate or a drop in pressure, the attending nurse or physician or the medical director of the respiratory therapy department should be immediately notified. If the responsible physician decides that cardiac output is falling and shock developing, he or she will start corrective measures, and although the therapist knows the role played by expiratory negative pressure in this situation, the physician is the one to order it. However, the tactful therapist may offer his or her services to adjust the ventilator for negative pressure, thus reminding the physician of the availability of this effective measure. If the physician gives approval, it is then the responsibility of the therapist to reevaluate the ventilatory pattern in terms of the I/E ratio and extend the expiratory time as long as possible, while reducing inspiratory pressure as much as is consistent with ventilatory needs. If cardiac rate, dropping blood pressure, and other signs of shock, as described in Chapter 7, are unrelieved, negative pressure during exhalation may be introduced. The physiologic rationale for this maneuver as well as its own risks are detailed in Chapter 13. Let us only repeat here that negative expiratory pressure should never be used indiscriminately and only for correction of reduced cardiac output resulting from positive-pressure ventilation. The hazards of air trapping and pulmonary edema must be watched for closely. Negative pressure should be started gradually, balancing its effect against the blood pressure, and usually 3 to 5 cm of water are adequate. To maintain the same alveolar ventilation as before the introduction of subatmospheric pressure, the therapist may have to increase the tidal volume to make up for additional air removed by expiratory suction at the expense of the functional residual capacity,[122] since in a sense this amounts to increasing the physiologic dead space. Skill is needed to use expiratory pressure safely and effectively, since the procedure entails balancing the negative pressure necessary to protect the cardiac output against a possible increase in positive pressure (if a pressure-cycled machine is being used), to maintain ventilation in the face of the negative-pressure effect on lung volume, and still realize a net drop in intrathoracic pressure.

Physiologic monitoring. In constrast to clinical observation, physiologic monitoring refers to the laboratory measurements of the physiologic responses to disease and treatment. One does not supplant the other, for laboratory findings are of only limited value unless interpreted in the light of what is actually happening to the patient as a whole; but at the same time clinical examinations cannot give us the precise information we need of what is happening inside the patient. The current therapy of respiratory failure is predicated on the availability of facilities to give us this physiologic insight, and the use of modern respirators in controlled treatment is dangerous guesswork without such information. Thus the hospital that is to treat failure must have not only good respiratory therapists but also a pulmonary function laboratory. The organization of such a facility and its relationship to the respiratory therapy service are noted in the final chapter, but let us say here that whatever the structure needed to meet the needs of an individual hospital, the pulmonary function laboratory must work closely with respiratory therapy and its findings made readily available to the therapists. Although the services of such a laboratory may be diverse, in our concern with management of respiratory failure, physiologic monitoring, for the most part, means measurement of arterial oxygen and carbon dioxide tensions and pH, and the calculation of bicarbonate level. By this time the therapist's orientation toward his or her work should be firmly fixed on the importance of these values.

In all probability, before the therapist is called to attend a patient, the diagnostic workup will have included blood gas studies on the basis of which, with clinical findings, the decision to institute therapy was made. Frequently the therapist will see a patient admitted as an emergency, obviously in need of ventilatory assistance, and earlier in this chapter we commented on the therapeutic approach while awaiting physiologic data. Whatever the situation, arterial gas values constitute the basis for definitive therapy and should be obtained as soon as possible. The question is frequently raised concerning the frequency of blood gas examinations during therapy, and for this there can be only one answer—as often as is necessary to ensure the most effective and the safest ventilation. It is not unusual for blood gas determinations to be needed every 15 minutes until the medical team feels confident that management is proper. When the response to therapy is satisfactory, clinical and physiologic signs of stability become evident, and the frequency of blood gas determinations can be gradually reduced. For the sake of safety, once the acute phase has passed and the patient can be considered at a maintenance plateau or recovering, gas tensions and pH determinations should be done at least twice daily. Often this can be modified, however, if hypoxia is felt to be permanently corrected, and monitoring is reduced to carbon dioxide tension and pH measurements. The therapist must keep in mind that despite his or her skill or the sophistication of the equipment, the adequacy of a patient's alveolar ventilation can be ascertained only by these last two values.

The therapist might wonder why venous blood cannot be used for monitoring, since it is considered more readily attainable. The basic objection to venous blood is that, because it is usually drawn from an extremity, it reflects the local metabolic activity of the area drained by the vein chosen and in a sense indicates what is left over after perfusion of local tissues. Arterial blood, on the other hand, shows directly the ability of the lungs to effect gas exchange before any extraction of oxygen or addition of carbon dioxide by the tissues. If venous blood is withdrawn after a needle has been left in the vein without a tourniquet about the extremity for 1 minute, there will be some correlation between venous and arterial carbon dioxide tension and pH but little for oxygen tension.

Arterial blood sampling in infants can be a very difficult procedure, and in some adults repeated "arterial sticks" are hampered by poorly accessible vessels and occasionally threaten vessel integrity. As an alternative to direct arterial sampling, a technique using "arterialized" capillary blood has become popular and practical. Commonly known as a "finger stick" or "heel stick" this procedure consists of puncturing the end of the finger (or toe or heel of an infant) with a sharp blade to obtain a free flow of capillary blood. Before puncture the hand is immersed in hot water for 10 minutes, a technique that has been demonstrated to render blood in the capillaries similar in its characteristics to arterial blood. The blood is collected in a glass capillary or a properly prepared small syringe and analyzed in the same manner as arterial blood. For some time this technique has been considered satisfactory for carbon dioxide tension and pH, but many questioned its reliability for oxygen tension. More comparative experience with it, however, has indicated that all three capillary parameters correlate well enough with arterial blood to be clinically accurate.[123,124] Acceptance of this technique has made physiologic data readily available because this is a procedure that can be done as often as necessary to monitor mechanical ventilation while at the same time sparing the patient repeated arterial punctures. The reliable respiratory therapist may be given freedom to obtain and examine arterialized capillary blood according to his or her own judgment to fulfill the responsibility for maintaining ventilation. The therapist is thus aware of the condition and needs of the patient at all times.

In Chapter 7 and again in the discussion of "optimum PEEP," reference was made to the Swan-Ganz catheter. It and the central venous catheter are primarily tools for cardiac monitoring, but they sometimes are valuable in following patients in respiratory failure, especially if on ventilator support. The data from such intracardiac and intravascular monitoring are described earlier, and we only note here that prevention or rapid correction of cardiovascular complications of mechanical ventilation may be a critical factor in patient survival. Not all patients in respiratory failure need these invasive measures, but their availability is one more option in management.

Of more immediate urgency for the mechanically ventilated patient is an electronic monitor to count cardiac rate, to signal deviations above and below preset ranges, and to display electrical cardiac complexes on a small oscilloscope. There have been unfortunate instances of unnoticed heart stoppage in mechanically ventilated patients. Many efficient commercial models are available, and one of them should be part of all standard ventilator setups.

Mechanical monitoring. For the most part, mechanical monitoring resolves into the use of spirometers to measure tidal and minute volumes. Some ventilators are equipped with such meters, but they often give only an approximation of the amount of air delivered. Extremely useful is a portable meter, the Wright respirometer.*[22] With a face the size of a small clock, the instrument is a flow meter constructed as a small air turbine with one dial calibrated in liters up to 100 ℓ and a second dial calibrated in 10 ml increments up to 1 ℓ. Its minimum flow response is less than 2 ℓ/min, but it should not be subjected to flows exceeding 300 ℓ/min. It is easily adapted to the exhalation port of any ventilator to measure the exhaled air as a gauge of tidal volume, a practical but not always accurate assumption. Obviously, it cannot be so used with expiratory negative pressure. The meter can give rough but usable information about three characteristics of ventilation. First, severe airway obstruction will cause the small needle to "hang up" in response to interference with exhaled flow. Second, in controlled ventilation, if the needle finishes its rotation before the next inspiration begins, it indicates terminal air trapping. Third, if the ventilator pressure and metered tidal volume are noted simultaneously, a working compliance can be calculated. Although not of diagnostic accuracy, this compliance is of importance in monitoring changes in the lung during prolonged ventilation.

Electronic flow sensors are also available for volume monitoring.[22]

Electronic monitors are available that will emit visible and audible signals if preset ranges of rate or phase are not met or are exceeded and if the ventilator fails or disconnects from the patient.[22] Such instruments have a definite value, and with the current interest in instrumentation in so many fields of medicine, there will doubtless be other developments in monitoring respiratory function as there have been for cardiac function. Any assistance that gives support to the patient is desirable, but mechanical or electronic monitors must not be relied on as a substitute for the personal attention of a skilled therapist. A monitor will not correct a deficiency, and its value depends entirely on the capability of the personnel responding to its call.

Also available recently are monitors for measuring mean airway pressure, which can be helpful in determining appropriate ventilator or PEEP therapy.[65,66,72,125]

Weaning from the ventilator

As with all the other aspects of ventilator care, the process of weaning, or gradual removal of the patient from a respirator, must be tailored to the needs of each patient, and only general suggestions can be offered. The therapist must accept the fact that supported ventilation, and especially controlled ventilation, is a harrowing and frightening experience for anyone, accompanied by much psychic trauma. During the course of therapy, the patient develops an understandable dependence on the machine that was responsible for his or her survival. No sooner has the successfully treated patient survived the terror of breathlessness, able to relax with the support of the ventilator, than the patient hears the medical team discussing the possibility of taking it away. The thought may panic the patient, who is far from sure that, since he or she needed mechanical help so recently, he or she is able to do without it now.

*Wright respirometer, Anesthesia Associates, Inc., Hudson, N.Y.

Two dicta of weaning may be stated together. Remove patients from their ventilator as soon as possible, but prepare them for it carefully. There are two general weaning techniques, each with many possible variations—*weaning with unattached ventilator* and *weaning with attached ventilator*. Both systems have advantages, but the student should view them as craftsmen's tools. There are many ways in which they can be used, and they are used according to the need of the work, the work is not fitted to the tool. Despite the aura of scientific precision created by rhythmical ventilators, bedside monitors, and laboratory data slips, separation of a patient from a ventilator is very nearly pure art. The two approaches to weaning are discussed separately and reflect both personal experience and the reported experience of others.[126-130]

Regardless of which method is used—unattached or attached ventilator—certain aspects must be optimized. The patient should be awake and alert, able to follow commands. He or she should be rested—not fatigued and sleep deprived as is commonly seen in the intensive care unit. If life-threatening situations are still present, such as shock or low cardiac output states, weaning is not only futile but dangerous. Nutritionally the patient should be provided with a high-protein diet. The patient should not be receiving a high-carbohydrate load because this allows for increased levels of Pa_{CO_2}, which stimulates unnecessarily high work of breathing levels.[131] If the patient experiences pain with breathing, weaning will not succeed. Other important clinical problems to resolve before weaning include anemia, arrhythmias, fever (infection), and electrolyte imbalance, especially for phosphate (PO_4). Low phosphate levels have been associated with weaning difficulties seen primarily in alcoholic patients, severely diabetic patients, and those receiving total parenteral nutritional support because the supply of both ATP and 2-3 DPG is dependent on adequate phosphate. If these enzymes are not adequate, muscle contraction and oxygen transport are compromised.[132]

The specific respiratory criteria used to suggest that it is safe to start weaning include[130]:

1. Peak inspiratory pressure of at least 20 cm of water.
2. Vital capacity of at least 10 to 15 ml/kg.
3. The ability to double minute ventilation voluntarily.
4. Dead space–to–tidal volume ratio (V_D/V_T) of less than 0.6.
5. Alveolar-arterial Po_2 difference (A-a gradient) while breathing 100% oxygen of less than 350 mm Hg.
6. Shunt fraction of less than 15%.
7. Pa_{O_2} of at least 60 mm Hg breathing 50% oxygen or less.

Whether one, two, a majority, or all of these weaning criteria must be met before weaning can be initiated has not been established, but from experience it is important to note that rarely does only one of these criteria arrive at this range without many of the others rapidly, in concert, arriving at values that fulfill the majority of the parameters listed. Also, it is not feasible to measure all of the them on all patients. It is probably best to select a set, learn to use them well, and build clinical expertise with them.

The timing of the weaning should be regarded as to when, during a 24-hour period, it should be performed. It is unwise to start weaning during a PM or night shift. Laboratory support often is not as good as the first thing in an AM shift. Physicians, allied health personnel, and patients are more rested in the morning. If a patient in the midst of weaning were to "crash," it generally would be better to have it happen during the day than at night.

Weaning with unattached ventilator. Weaning with an unattached ventilator is the older of the two techniques and consists of removal of the ventilator from the patient according to a time schedule. Generally, the longer a patient is ventilated, the more difficult and the longer is the weaning period. In addition, the state of intubation with power-induced ventilation is both unnatural and unphysiologic and carries the risk of secondary infection and injury to the lung the longer it persists. The objective of mechanical ventilation therefore is to support the patient through acute respiratory failure, control or improve the cause of the failure, and restore the patient to spontaneous unassisted breathing as soon as possible.

Conditioning of patients for this move should start well in advance, not by telling them that they will be taken off the ventilator on a given day so that they will anticipate it fearfully, but by giving them encouraging reports of their progress while they are still supported. From the earliest moment in therapy they should be told repeatedly that mechanical ventilation is a temporary measure, designed to give them rest from the stress of breathing until they are better.

It is very helpful to watch carefully the patient's behavior when he or she is removed from the ventilator for the short periods required for suctioning or servicing the tracheostomy tube or ventilator, and if spontaneous breathing is evident at these times, some estimate of its adequacy can be noted. Certainly, such spontaneous breathing must return before weaning can even be considered, and it is often helpful to ask the patient to take an occasional breath while still on control to see if he or she can override the machine. Patients may have to be urged to this effort, since it is so easy for them to conform to the ventilator that they may not exert themselves to see whether they can breathe unless encouraged to do so. For short periods of time patients can be put on assisted ventilation, with take-over control at a lower rate, and the explanation can be given that they must exercise their ventilatory muscles, which have become weak from disuse. Most patients accept as reasonable this need to try breathing on their own, and such periods can be extended to as long as is acceptable to them. The therapist should keep reassuring patients that, should they tire or even fall asleep, the ventilator will automatically start to function.

Once patients' spontaneous breathing has been demonstrated to them, they are ready for the next step. While disconnected from the ventilator for tracheostomy care, patients can be asked if they would like to breathe on their own for a few minutes with the therapist in attendance, and they should be provided with a tracheostomy mask for the delivery of humidified oxygen or air.

Supported ventilation should be resumed before patients tire, but these intervals of spontaneous breathing *with the cuff deflated* are gradually increased until they are breathing on their own most of the time, with occasional periods of restful support.

The therapist should look for certain signs to determine the need for reconnecting the patient to the ventilator. These include signs of hypercapnia, hypoxemia, and acidosis manifested by (1) significant *increases* in respiratory rate, pulse, or blood pressure, (2) a significant *fall* in tidal volume or blood pressure, or (3) development of arrythmias. If these problems occur while the patient is off the ventilator, a blood gas should be drawn to document the level of pH, Pa_{CO_2} and Pa_{O_2} when these problems occurred, and the patient should be reconnected to the ventilator.[133] It may be necessary to provide assisted ventilation during the sleeping hours for a little longer.

The student will find that some authors speak deprecatingly of this "trial-and-error" method of removing patients from ventilator support for periods of time and at intervals that are quite arbitrary. Still, this is a time-tested method that has been successful when supervised by conscientious and knowledgeable medical personnel. It does not take an experienced therapist long to evaluate a patient's ventilatory stamina and to set up a gradual program of ventilator withdrawal that is safe and effective. Some experts advocate removing the patient from the ventilator for a fixed short period of time and gradually shortening the intervals between. As an example, this might mean letting the patient breathe unassisted for 2 minutes of an hour, then 2 minutes each half hour, quarter hour, and so on, until mechanical aid is discontinued. When weaning has started in earnest, oxygenation and humidification in the free-breathing intervals are important. A T-tube blow-by attached to the end of the tracheal tube provides a flow of inspired gas from which the patient breathes. It is advised that inspired oxygen concentration be 10% higher than had been delivered by the ventilator.[130] Humidification should be as close to 100% as possible because the prevention of respiratory mucosal drying is critical at this stage.

Extubation. As mentioned previously, weaning is best started in the morning, so extubation is best done during the AM shift after the night crew has gone home. Some centers have a standardized ritual, which helps to calm everyone's anxieties, the health team's especially. First the patient is allowed to spontaneously breath moist air with an F_{IO_2} at the present level through the T-piece for 30 minutes. A blood gas is then drawn, and the patient is reconnected. When the results of the blood gas return indicating acceptable levels, the patient is now ready for extubation. During this 30-minute period or somewhere close in time some experts like to aerolize a steroid to prevent the possibility of laryngeal edema occurring when the tube comes out. No evidence exists that this is absolutely necessary, but it is part of the "ritual." The patient is then carefully suctioned, and with the *cuff deflated,* the patient is asked to *inhale* deeply and the tube is quickly pulled free. If a cough is needed, the patient's lungs are full of air, and he or she is able to immediately clear the airway. The patient is then given oxygen at 5% to 10% higher then before extubation, and 20 minutes later as blood gas is drawn.

Weaning a person to breathe for several hours through a nasotracheal or orotracheal tube should be considered the ultimate test of whether he or she can be extubated. If the patient can breathe adequately with the increased resistance inherent with these tubes in place, he or she can breathe, cough, sing, talk, and eat, much better with it out.[134]

Removal of a tracheostomy tube is not difficult, but the residual stoma must be covered with one or two gauze pads held loosely with tape. It is treated as any open wound until healed, a matter of a few days in the absence of complications. Many patients are apprehensive about the tracheostomy, but they can be reassured with some simple instructions. Most ventilated patients have excessive sputum production and a cough. A patient newly extubated should be taught to support the tracheal stoma during cough by applying a firm squeezing pressure to the throat over the dressing with the full palm of one hand. With encouragement the patient soon learns to cough past the tracheostomy and bring secretions into the mouth for expectoration. Depending on the flow of secretions, annoying ostial leakage can be expected for 2 to 3 days, and dressings should be changed frequently. Pressurized aerosol therapy can be used with a mouthpiece, shortly after extubation, with little loss of inspired air through the tracheal defect, because the patient uses manual support and is soon able to breathe past it.

Sometimes it is desirable to prevent immediate closure of the stoma, especially when profuse secretions make continued aspiration necessary while a weak patient is regaining his or her own cough power. The use of Kistner tracheostomy tubes or Moore buttons can be very helpful. These are basically short tubes that can be inserted through the tracheostomy and are held in place by flanges on their inner ends. Caps are available for occlusion, some have one-way valves for air intake only, and their small sizes offer little intratracheal airflow resistance.

We now consider two modifications of tracheostomy tube removal that involve special preparation for the actual extubation.

Using a fenestrated tracheostomy tube. For the tracheostomized patient who was difficult to wean, who perhaps is borderline hypoxic, and who may need occasional ventilator support or pressure breathing therapy, the cuffed fenestrated tube can be substituted for the regular style. As illustrated in Fig. 14-14, this tube has an opening (fenestration) cut into its convex surface, and it is supplied with an inner cannula. With the cannula removed and the cuff deflated, the patient can move air through the tube in the usual manner, and by mouth through the fenestration and around the tube. This allows maximum airflow against minimal resistance, supposedly expedites easier coughing and oral removal of secretions, and facilitates phonation, if the tube is plugged. With the cuff inflated and the inner cannula in place occluding the fenestration, pressure-breathing aerosols or assisted mechanical ventilation can be used in a closed system.

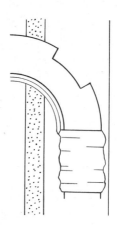

Fig. 14-14   Fenestrated tracheostomy tube. (See text for description.)

Fenestrated tubes are not without danger, and if being used they must be closely watched. The main danger occurs when the tube rocks back so that the opening (fenestration) occludes against the posterior wall of the trachea. These tubes can also migrate forward so that the opening lies within the soft tissue of the neck. If the tube is plugged at its opening when either of these displacements occurs, the patient will suffocate. Also tissue has been known to roll into the fenestration so when the inner cannula is replaced it shears off this tissue, and significant bleeding can occur.

The fenestrated tube therefore is a kind of half-step between ventilator weaning and extubation. It allows the patient a little longer to establish ventilatory and gas-exchange stability before becoming fully independent. At the proper time the fenestrated tube is removed, and the patient is managed as described above.

Plugging the tracheostomy tube. This consists of deflating the cuff, then occluding the tube with a stopper that blocks about half the orifice, and after a variable period of time, replacing it with a fully occluding plug. The purpose is to acclimate patients gradually to breathing through a narrower airway than that provided by the patent tube and to prepare them for the restrictions of their own nasal and laryngeal passages. However, there is an important point here that should be clearly understood. Tracheostomy tube plugging had its origin when tracheostomies were performed mostly for conditions such as laryngeal croup, diphtheria, and the like, or to prevent aspiration of oral secretions in patients with bulbar poliomyelitis who were supported in tank respirators. These patients usually had normal lungs and normal conductance distal to their tracheal tubes. It was reasonable to test their ability to breathe against improving proximal obstruction or to evaluate the degree of return of neuromuscular ventilatory function before extubation. This may still be useful for patients with nonpulmonary ventilatory failure. The many patients we see who are intubated and ventilated for airway obstructive disease present a different problem. Any type of intratracheal tube is space occupying and an impedance to airflow, even when fully patent, and its presence is justified only as long as it is used to support ventilation or remove secretions. There is little rationale in plugging tracheostomy tubes in such patients, adding more obstruction to their already existing difficulties, for which they were intensively treated in the first place. In general, when intubated patients with obstructive disease show signs of improving spontaneous breathing, they will breathe considerably better when the tube is removed.

Weaning with attached ventilator (IMV). This specifically refers to the use of intermittent mandatory ventilation as a means of removing a patient from mechanical ventilation.[135] In our earlier discussion we considered it as a part of general ventilatory management, but of necessity touched on its role in weaning. IMV was originally intended as a weaning device, to be activated in the ventilator circuit as the patient improved. We have already learned, however, that IMV can be available, if felt advantageous, from the beginning of mechanical ventilation.

A recent review of what is presently believed regarding IMV and weaning can be summarized in the following statements.[80] IMV helps prevent asynchronous breathing, may prevent respiratory alkalosis, may shorten weaning time, may allow for weaning with patients who have failed other weaning techniques, helps the psychologic state of some patients, maintains respiratory muscle function, and reduces cardiovascular effects of mechanical ventilation with PEEP. Some suggested, but not well-documented, advantages of IMV include reduced oxygen consumption at a high IMV rate, fewer ventilator complications, and reduced amount of equipment and thus less monitoring of that equipment while weaning.[80]

The disadvantages are that IMV more generally cannot respond to changes in patient status and thus requires more monitoring, increases oxygen consumption at a low IMV rate, prolongs weaning and thus cost if not used properly, and may increase barotrauma risk if the system does not have synchronous IMV mode.

In regard to weaning, IMV is helpful in patients who have failed T-piece weaning, but it is no better than intermittent positive-pressure ventilation unless the patient has asynchronous breathing or hemodynamic compromise or only needs a ventilator for oxygenation and not ventilation.

IMV is less desirable than intermittent positive-pressure ventilation if the patient is unstable and cannot be monitored closely, is depressed immunologically either by disease or by drugs, has an impaired respiratory drive, or is in cardiogenic shock.[80]

No technique if foolproof, and IMV is not an exception. Some patients still require trials off the ventilator, on a T-piece, even though they have been on an IMV system. This does not negate the value of IMV, since perhaps

Table 14-5
Complications of
mechanical ventilation

	Complication	How to spot it	Clinical response
	Zone 1, the patient		
	1. Subcutaneous emphysema	1. Bloating of face and neck, which may extend down to sternum. Skin makes crackling sound when pressed	1. Not a serious complication
	2. Nasal necrosis	2. Skin at nasal opening turns black where nasotracheal tube touches	2. Call attending physician. Retape tube. Potentially serious
	3. Gastric distention	3. Seen following difficult intubation. Abdomen is distended and tympanic, with vomiting sometimes occurring	3. Call attending physician, who will place oral gastric tube. High potential for serious problems
	4. Tube in right main stem bronchus	4. X-ray film shows tip in right side; breath sounds are decreased on left side. Pneumothorax on right side and atelectasis on left may be seen. Pressures on volume ventilator high	4. Call attending physician. Pull tube back until breath sounds are heard bilaterally. Do with supervision; may be lethal situation
	5. Pneumonia	5. Fever, deteriorating blood gases, abnormal breath sounds	5. Call attending physician. Perform x-ray examination of patient, and compare previous films. Obtain sputum for culture and gram stains. Start appropriate antibiotics
	6. Hypotension	6. Sweating, pallor, restlessness, fall in urine output, tachycardia	6. Call attending physician. Check blood pressure. May be serious problem
	Zone 2, tubing and external circuit		
	1. Condensed water in tubing. May give unwanted PEEP effect	1. Gurgling sound from hoses with airflow	1. Drain tubing. *Caution:* Do not drain water back into humidifier; avoid spilling water into patient's airway and lungs
	2. Heater on humidifier malfunctions and overheats humidifier gas	2. Tubing is hot to the touch. High-temperature alarm or reading	2. Replace humidifier heater. Potentially serious; can burn airways and increase patient's core temperature
	3. Tubing may become "switched," or connected to wrong port. Is a problem only with certain circuits. Is more common with increased use of "homemade" IMV circuits	3. Increased or no pressures. Patient turns blue. Increased work of breathing. Low-volume or low-pressure alarms or high-pressure alarm	3. Disconnect patient from ventilator and provide manual ventilation with self-inflating or flow-inflating bag. May be lethal

Table 14-5—cont'd Complications of mechanical ventilation	Complication	How to spot it	Clinical response
	4. Leaks	4. Low pressures on volume ventilator and low exhaled volumes. Decreased or loss of PEEP or CPAP. Some pressure ventilators (e.g., Bird Mark 7) may fail to cycle	4. Carefully check circuit and artifical airway. Change circuit if needed. Notify attending physician if airway needs replacing
	Zone 3, the ventilator		
	1. Alarms turned off and left off. Occurs after suctioning procedures or airway care most often	1. Check the control board for alarm settings	1. Specific inservice instruction and discipline to those responsible. Potentially very serious
	2. Low delivered volumes	2. Evidence on arterial blood gas data of hypoventilation; low exhaled volumes monitored	2. Patient is manually ventilated while someone troubleshoots ventilator quickly or obtains new ventilator if problem is not obvious and easily solved
	3. Inadequate flows	3. Prolonged inspiratory times on volume or pressure-cycled ventilators	3. Same as 2 above
	4. Malfunctioning oxygen delivery system	4. Some ventilators will not cycle, such as pneumatic-powered units, Servo 900 models. Oxygen analyzer or alarms indicate improper oxygen level or pressure	4. Same as 2 above

without it, weaning would have been even more difficult. There is no uniform agreement that IMV is the best weaning procedure to follow, and advocates of unattached ventilator weaning strongly support their method. There is little doubt, however, that IMV has given us a tremendous option in our choice of managing the weaning patient. Principles of extubation are the same as those already discussed.

Complications of mechanical ventilation

The mechanical ventilators are not without serious potential dangers,[136] and a few statements in regard to this are in order. The respiratory therapist standing at the patient's bedside would find it helpful to develop a method for rapidly assessing the patient for complications. To organize this technique it would be useful to break the total problem down into three zones of potential danger so the assessment can be compartmentalized. Zone 1 is the patient; zone 2, the tubing and attached circuits between the patient and the ventilator; and zone 3, the ventilator all the way to the wall outlets for oxygen, air, and electricity. Table 14-5 attempts to summarize these zones.

References

1. Sykes, M.K., McNicol, M.W., and Campbell, E.J.M.: Respiratory failure, ed. 2, Oxford, England, 1976, Blackwell Scientific Publications.
2. Hinshaw, H.C., and Murray, J.F.: Diseases of the chest, ed. 4, Philadelphia, 1980, W.B. Saunders Co.
3. Pontoppidan, H., Giffin, B., and Lowenstein, E.: Acute respiratory failure in the adult, Boston, 1973, Little, Brown & Co.
4. Lindholm, C.E., et al.: Flexible fiberoptic bronchoscopy in critical care medicine, Crit. Care Med. 2:250, 1974.
5. Lindholm, C.E., et al.: Cardiorespiratory effects of flexible fiberoptic bronchoscopy in critically ill patients, Chest 74:362, 1978.
6. Sackner, M.A., Wanner, A., and Landa, J.: Applications of bronchofiberoscopy, Chest 62(suppl.):70s, 1972.
7. Sackner, M.A.: Bronchofiberoscopy, state of the art, Am. Rev. Respir. Dis. 111:62, 1975.
8. Suratt, P.M., Smiddy, J.F., and Gruber, B.: Death and complications associated with fiberoptic bronchoscopy, Chest 69:747, 1976.
9. McLaughlin, A.J., and Scott, W.: Training and evaluation of respiratory therapists in emergency intubation, Respir. Care 26:333, 1981.
10. Conley, J.M., and Smith, D.J.: Emergency endotracheal intubation by respiratory care personnel in a community hospital, Respir. Care 26:336, 1981.
11. Downs, J.B.: Who should intubate? (editorial), Respir. Care 26:331, 1981.
12. Weg, J.G.: Prolonged endotracheal intubation in respiratory failure, Arch. Intern. Med. 120:679, 1967.
13. Stauffer, J.L., Olson, D.E., and Petty, T.L.: Complications and consequences of endotracheal intubation and tracheotomy: a prospective study of 150 critically ill patients, Am. J. Med. 70:65, 1981.
14. Via-Reque, E., and Rattenborg, C.C.: In Rattenborg, C.C., and Via-Reque, E., editors: Clinical use of mechanical ventilation, Chicago, 1981, Year Book Medical Publishers, Inc.
15. Dixon, T.C., et al.: Prolonged endotracheal intubation, Med. J. Aust. 2:529, 1968.
16. El-Naggar, M., et al.: Factors influencing choice between tracheostomy and prolonged translaryngeal intubation in acute respiratory failure: a prospective study, Anesth. Analg. 55:195, 1976.
17. Kuner, J., and Goldman, A.: Prolonged nasotracheal intubation in adults versus tracheostomy, Dis. Chest 51:270, 1967.
18. Conardy, P.A., et al.: Alteration of endotracheal tube position: flexation and extention of the neck, Crit. Care Med. 4:8, 1976.
19. Garson, A.A., et al.: Influence of cannula size on resistance to breathing through tracheostomies, Surg. Forum 14:219, 1963.
20. Chew, J.Y., and Cantrell, R.W.: Tracheostomy complications and their management, Arch. Otolaryngol. 96:538, 1972.
21. Greene, N.M.: Fatal cardiovascular and respiratory failure associated with tracheostomy, N. Engl. J. Med. 261:846, 1959.
22. McPherson, S.P.: Respiratory therapy equipment, ed. 2, St. Louis, 1981, The C.V. Mosby Co.
23. Dorsch, J.A., and Dorsch, S.E.: Understanding anesthesia equipment, construction, care, and complications, Baltimore, 1975, The Williams & Wilkins Co.
24. Caldwell, S.L., and Sullivan, K.N.: In Burton, G.G., Gee, G.N., and Hodgkin, J.E., editors: Respiratory care, a guide to clinical practice, Philadelphia, 1977, J.B. Lippincott Co.
25. Lewis, F.R., Schlobohm, R.M., and Thomas, A.N.: Prevention of complications from prolonged tracheal intubation, Am. J. Surg. 135:452, 1978.
26. Ching, N.P.H., and Nealon, T.F.: Clinical experience with new low-pressure high volume tracheostomy cuffs, N.Y. State J. Med. 74:2379, 1974.
27. Evaluation: Artificial airways, Health Devices 7:67, 1978.
28. Wen-Hsien Wu, et al.: Pressure dynamics of endotracheal and tracheostomy cuffs, Crit. Care Med. 1:197, 1973.
29. Magovern, G.J., et al.: The clinical and

experimental evaluation of a controlled-pressure intratracheal cuff, J. Thorac. Cardiovas. Surg. **64**:747, 1972.

30. Lederman, I.S., et al.: A comparison of foam and air-filled endotracheal cuffs, Anesth. Analg. **53**:521, 1974.

31. Kamen, J.M., and Wilkinson, C.J.: A new low-pressure cuff for endotracheal tubes, Anesthesiology **34**:482, 1971.

32. Carroll, R.G.: Evaluation of tracheal tube cuff designs, Crit. Care. Med. **1**:45, 1973.

33. Bekoe, S., Magovern, G.J., and Shively, J.G.: Prolonged cuff intubation without tracheal injury, CVP **3**(4), 1975.

34. Meyer, J.A.: Tracheostomy care, Int. Anesthesiol. Clin. **4**:675, 1966.

35. Dane, T.E.B., and King, E.G.: A prospective study of complications after tracheostomy for assisted ventilation, Chest **67**:398, 1975.

36. Dobrin, P, and Canfield, T.: Cuffed endotracheal tubes: mucosal pressures and tracheal wall blood flow, Am. J. Surg. **133**:562, 1977.

37. Paegle, R.D., and Bernard, W.M.: Squamous metaplasia of tracheal epithelium associated with high-volume, low-pressure airway cuffs, Anesth. Analg. **54**:340, 1975.

38. Sunderrajan, E.V., et al.: Potentially lethal complications of artificial airways: case reports, Missouri Med. **77**:299, 1980.

39. Blanc, V.F., and Tremblay, N.A.: The complications of tracheal intubation: a new classification and review of the literature, Anesth. Analg. **53**:2, 1974.

40. Galoob, H.D., and Toledo, P.S.: Comparison of five types of tracheostomy tubes in the intubated trachea, Ann. Otol. Rhinol. Laryngol. **87**:99, 1978.

41. Herbert, R.C., and De Sessa, P.C.: Compression of an endotracheal tube lumen by its cuff: a case report, Respir. Care **26**:653, 1981.

42. Dencancq, H.G., Jr.: Tissue "snowplowing": a post-tracheostomy complication, Am. J. Dis. Child. **108**:94, 1964.

43. Bendixen, H.H., et al.: Respiratory care, St. Louis, 1965, The C.V. Mosby Co.

44. Cooper, J.D., and Grillo, H.C.: The evolution of tracheal injury due to ventilatory assistance through a cuffed tube, Ann. Surg. **169**:334, 1969.

45. Head, J.M.: Tracheostomy in the management of respiratory problems, N. Engl. J. Med. **264**:587, 1961.

46. Taylor, H., Mhoon, E., and Matz, G.J.: In Rattenborg, C.C., and Via-Reque, F., editors: Clinical use of mechanical ventilation, Chicago, 1981, Year Book Medical Publishers, Inc.

47. Nelson, T.G., and Bowers, W.T.: Tracheostomy—indications, advantages, techniques, complications, and results. J.A.M.A. **164**:1530, 1957.

48. Cullen, J.H.: An evaluation of tracheostomy in pulmonary emphysema, Ann. Intern. Med. **58**:953, 1963.

49. Feldman, S.A., editor: Tracheostomy and artificial ventilation, London, 1967, Edward Arnold (Publishers), Ltd.

50. Cabal, L., et al.: New endotracheal tube adaptor reducing cardiopulmonary effects of suctioning, Crit. Care Med. **7**:552, 1979.

51. Zmora, E., and Merritt, T.A.: Use of side-hole endotracheal tube adaptor for tracheal aspiration: a controlled study, Am. J. Dis. Child. **134**:250, 1980.

52. Radford, E.P., Jr.: Ventilation standards for use in artificial respiration, J. Appl. Physiol. **7**:451, 1955.

53. Merck manual of therapeutics and materia medica, Rahway, N.J., 1940, Merck and Co., Inc.

54. Dittmer, D.S., and Grebe, R.M., editors: Handbook of respiration, Philadelphia, 1958, W.B. Saunders Co.

55. Growth charts used by Children's Hospital Medical Center, Boston, Mass. Courtesy H.C. Stuart, Department of Maternal and Child Health, Harvard School of Public Health, Boston, Mass.

56. Avery, M.E.: The lung and its disorders in the newborn infant, Philadelphia, 1964, W.B. Saunders Co.

57. Holt, L.E., Jr., and McIntosh, R.: Diseases of infancy and children, New York, 1940, D. Appleton-Century Co.

58. Cooke, R.J.: The biologic basis of pediatric practice, New York, 1968, McGraw-Hill Book Co.

59. Gallagher, T.J., and Civetta, J.M.: Goal-

directed therapy of acute respiratory failure, Anesth. Analg. **59**:831, 1980.

60. Hudson, L.D.: Ventilatory management of patients with adult respiratory distress syndrome, Seminars Respir. Med. **2**:128, 1981.

61. Hedley-White, J., et al.: Applied physiology of respiratory care, Boston, 1976, Little, Brown & Co.

62. Petty, T.L., and Ashbaugh, D.G.: In Petty, T.L., editor: Intensive and rehabilitative respiratory care, ed. 2, Philadelphia, 1974, Lea & Febiger.

63. Brady, J.P., and Gregory, G.A.: In Klaus, M.H., and Fanaroff, A.A., editors: Care of the high-risk neonate, ed. 2, Philadelphia, 1979, W.B. Saunders Co.

64. Williams, T.J.: In Lough, M.D., Williams, T.J., and Rawson, J.E. editors: Newborn respiratory care, Chicago, 1979, Year Book Medical Publishers, Inc.

65. Boros, S.J.: In Lough, M.D., Williams, T.J., and Rawson, J.E., editors: Newborn respiratory care, Chicago, 1979, Year Book Medical Publishers, Inc.

66. Boros, S.J., and Campbell, K.: A comparison of the effects of high frequency–low tidal volume and low frequency–high tidal volume mechanical ventilation, J. Pediatr. **97**:108, 1980.

67. Bland, R.D., et al.: High frequency mechanical ventilation in severe hyaline membrane disease: an alternative treatment? Crit. Care. Med. **8**:275, 1980.

68. Bone, R.C.: Treatment of respiratory failure due to advanced chronic obstructive lung disease, Arch. Intern. Med. **140**:1018, 1980.

69. Kirby, R.R.: Intermittent mandatory ventilation in the neonate, Crit. Care Med. **5**:18, 1977.

70. Mushin, W.W., Rendell-Baker, L., Thompson, P.W., and Mapleson, W.W.: Automatic ventilation of the lungs, ed. 3, Oxford, England, 1980, Blackwell Scientific Publications.

71. Kirby, R.R.: In Thibeault, D.W., and Gregory, G.A., editors: Neonatal pulmonary care, Menlo Park, Calif., 1979, Addison-Wesley Publishing Co.

72. Reynolds, O.: In Thibeault, D.W., and Gregory, G.A., editors: Neonatal pulmonary care, Menlo Park, Calif., 1979, Addison-Wesley Publishing Co.

73. Bendixen H.H., et al.: Impaired oxygenation in surgical patients during general anesthesia with controlled ventilation, N. Engl. J. Med. **269**:991, 1963.

74. Egan, D.F.: Personal experience.

75. Breivik, H., et al.: Normalizing low arterial CO_2 tension during mechanical ventilation, Chest **63**:525, 1973.

76. Kirby, R.R., and Graybar, G.B., editors: Intermittent mandatory ventilation, Int. Anesthesiol. Clin. **18**:1-189, 1980.

77. DeSautels, D.A., and Bartlett, J.L.: Methods of administering intermittent mandatory ventilation, Respir. Care **19**:187, 1974.

78. Civetta, J.M., et al.: "Optimal PEEP" and intermittent mandatory ventilation in the treatment of acute respiratory failure, Respir. Care **20**:551, 1975.

79. Fairley, H.B.: In Kirby, R.R., and Graybar, G.B., editors: Intermittent mandatory ventilation, Int. Anesthesiol. Clin. **18**:179, 1980.

80. Luce, J.M., Pierson, D.J., and Hudson, L.D.: Critical reviews: Intermittent mandatory ventilation, Chest **79**:678, 1981.

81. Greenhouse, B.B.: Muscle relaxants and some problems with their use, Conn. Med. **34**:723, 1970.

82. Thomas, E.T.: Circulatory collapse following succinylcholine, Anesth. Analg. **48**:333, 1969.

83. Smith, J.P., et al.: Acute respiratory failure in chronic lung disease, Am. Rev. Respir. Dis. **97**:791, 1968.

84. Eldridge, F., and Gherman, C.: Studies of oxygen administration in respiratory failure, Ann. Intern. Med. **68**:569, 1968.

85. Kettel, L.J., et al.: Treatment of acute respiratory acidosis in chronic obstructive lung disease, J.A.M.A. **217**:1503, 1971.

86. Anderson, E.F., and Rosenthal, M.H.: Pancuronium bromide and tachyarrhythmias, Crit. Care Med. **3**:13, 1975.

87. Cherniack, R.M., and Hakimpour, K.: The rational use of oxygen in respiratory insufficiency, J.A.M.A. **199**:178, 1967.

88. Mithoeter, J.C., et al.: Oxygen therapy in respiratory failure, N. Engl. J. Med. **277**:947, 1967.

89. Bone R.C., Pierce, A.K., and Johnson,

R.F.: Controlled oxygen administration in acute respiratory failure in chronic obstructive pulmonary disease: a reappraisal, Am. J. Med. **65:**896, 1978.

90. Cheney, F.W.: The effect of respiratory resistance on the blood gas tensions of anesthetized patients, Anesthesiology **28:**670, 1967.

91. Ashbaugh, D.G., et al.: Continuous positive pressure breathing (CPPB) in adult respiratory distress syndrome, J. Thorac. Cardiovasc. Surg. **57:**31, 1969.

92. Kumar, A., et al.: Continuous positive-pressure ventilation in acute respiratory failure, N. Engl. J. Med. **283:**1430, 1970.

93. Gregory, G.A., et al.: Treatment of the idiopathic respiratory-distress syndrome with continuous positive airway pressure, N. Engl. J. Med. **284:**1333, 1971.

94. Trinkle, J.K.: a simple modification of existing respirators to provide constant positive-pressure breathing, J. Thorac. Cardiovasc. Surg. **61:**617, 1971.

95. Bone, R.C.: Thoracic pressure-volume curves in acute respiratory failure, Crit. Care Med. **4:**148, 1976.

96. Bone, R.C.: Compliance and dynamic characteristics curves in acute respiratory failure, Crit. Care Med. **4:**173, 1976.

97. Bone, R.C.: Pressure-volume measurements in detection of bronchospasm and mucous plugging in acute respiratory failure, Respir. Care **21:**620, 1976.

98. Bone, R.C.: Diagnosis of causes for acute respiratory distress by pressure-volume curves, Chest **70:**740, 1976.

99. Bone, R.C.: Monitoring respiratory function in the patient with adult respiratory distress syndrome, Semin. Respir. Med. **2:**140, 1981.

100. ACCP-ATS Joint Committee on Pulmonary Nomenclature: Pulmonary terms and symbols, Chest **67:**583, 1975.

101. Kittredge, P.: The difference between PEEP, CPPB, and CPAP (editorial), Respir. Care **19:**14, 1974.

102. Gillick, J.S.: Spontaneous positive end-expiratory pressure (sPEEP), Anesth. Analg. **56:**627, 1977.

103. Sturgeon, C.L., et al.: PEEP and CPAP: cardiopulmonary effects during spontaneous ventilation, Anesth. Analg. **56:**633, 1977.

104. Greenbaum, D.M., et al.: Continuous positive airway pressure without tracheal intubation in spontaneously breathing patients, Chest **69:**615, 1976.

105. Schmidt, G.B., et al.: EPAP without intubation, Crit. Care Med. **5:**207, 1977.

106. Eross, B., Powner, D., and Grenvik, A.: In Kirby, R.R., and Graybar, G.B., editors: Intermittent mandatory ventilation, Int. Anesthesiol. Clin. **18:**11, 1980.

107. Graybar, G.B. and Smith, R.A.: In Kirby, R.R., and Graybar, G.B., editors: Intermittent mandatory ventilation, Int. Anesthesiol. Clin., **18:**53, 1980.

108. Douglas, M.E., and Downs, J.B.: In Kirby, R.R., and Graybar, G.B., editors: Intermittent mandatory ventilation, Int. Anesthesiol. Clin. **18:**97, 1980.

109. Weinstein, M.E., et al.: Hemodynamic and respiratory response to varying gradients between end-expiratory and end-inspiratory pressure in patients breathing on continuous positive airway pressure, J. Trauma **18:**231, 1978.

110. Kirby, R.R., et al.: High-level positive end-expiratory pressure (PEEP) in acute respiratory insufficiency, Chest **67:**156, 1975.

111. Suter, P.M., et al.: Optimum end-expiratory airway pressure in patients with acute pulmonary failure, N. Engl. J. Med. **292:**284, 1975.

112. Demers, R.R., and Saklad, M.: "Assisted PEEP"—assisted mechanical ventilation with positive end-expiratory pressure, Respir. Care **19:**435, 1974.

113. Gjerde, G.E.: IMV with PEEP versus MV with PEEP, Respir. Care **20:**894, 1975.

114. Ayres, S.M.: Assisted PEEP: helpful or disastrous? Respir. Care **19:**410, 1974.

115. Smith, R.A., et al.: Continuous positive airway pressure (CPAP) by face mask, Crit. Care Med. **8:**483, 1980.

116. Gregory, G.A.: In Thibeault, D.W., and Gregory, G.A., editors: Neonatal pulmonary care, Menlo Park, Calif., 1977, Addison-Wesley Publishing Co.

117. Civetta, J.M., et al.: A simple and effective method of employing spontaneous

positive pressure ventilation, J. Thorac. Cardiovasc. Surg. **63**:312, 1972.

118. Hamilton, F.N., and Singer, M.M.: A breathing circuit for continuous positive airway pressure (CPAP), Crit. Care. Med. **2**:86, 1974.

119. Gjerde, G.E.: A method for spontaneous breathing with expiratory positive pressure, Respir. Care **20**:839, 1975.

120. Sheely, R.B., and Boudria, C.: More on spontaneous breathing with EPP, Respir. Care **20**:1116, 1975.

121. Kenney, F.: Mechanical ventilation and CPPB with modified Ohio 560 ventilator, Respir. Care **20**:655, 1975.

122. Smith, A.C.: Effect of mechanical ventilation on the circulation, Ann. N.Y. Sci. **121**:742, 1965.

123. Stamm, S.J.: Reliability of capillary blood for the measurement of Po_2 and O_2 saturation, Dis. Chest **52**:191, 1967.

124. Begin, R., et al.: Value of capillary blood gas analysis in the management of acute respiratory distress, Am. Rev. Respir. Dis. **112**:879, 1975.

125. Banner, M.J., Gallegher, T.J., and Bluth, L.I.: A new microprocessor device for mean airway pressure measurement, Crit. Care Med. **9**:51, 1981.

126. Downs, J.B., et al.: Intermittent mandatory ventilation: a new approach to weaning patients from mechanical ventilators, Chest **64**:331, 1973.

127. McPherson, S.P., et al.: A circuit that combines ventilator weaning methods using continuous flow ventilation (CFV), Respir. Care **20**:261, 1975.

128. Modell, J.H.: Weaning patients from mechanical ventilation, Respir. Care **20**:373, 1975.

129. Feeley, T.W., and Hedley-White, J.: Weaning from controlled ventilation and supplemental oxygen, N. Engl. J. Med. **292**:903, 1975.

130. Bowser, M.A., et al.: A systematic approach to ventilator weaning, Respir. Care **20**:959, 1975.

131. Bassili, H.R., and Deitel, M.: Effect of nutritional support on weaning patients off mechanical ventilators, J.P.E.N. **5**:161, 1981.

132. Bassili, H.R., and Deitel, M.: Nutritional support in long term intensive care with special reference to ventilator patients: a review, Can. Anaesth. Soc. J. **28**:17, 1981.

133. Gilbert, R., et al.: The first few hours off a respirator, Chest **65**:152, 1974.

134. Petty, T.L., and Nett, L.M.: In Shoemaker, W.C., and Thompson, W.L., editors: Critical care, state of the art, vol. 2, Fullerton, Calif., 1981, The Society of Critical Care Medicine.

135. Downs, J.B., and Douglas, M.E.: In Kirby, R.R., and Graybar, G.B.: Intermittent mandatory ventilation, Int. Anesthesiol. Clin. **18**:81, 1980.

136. Zwillich, C.W., et al.: Complications of assisted ventilation: a prospective study of 354 consecutive episodes, Am. J. Med. **57**:161, 1974.

Chapter 15

Chronic care and rehabilitation of respiratory failure

The steadily improving care of patients with acute respiratory failure is presenting its own problem. As more survive the acute phases of respiratory disease, there is an increasing population of people with chronic pulmonary insufficiency, displaying a wide spectrum of disability. It makes little difference whether they were originally diagnosed as having pulmonary emphysema, fibrotic tuberculosis, chronic asthma, or any of several other conditions, since in their chronic state they have one thing in common—the inability to move to and from their lungs sufficient air for physiologic needs, without being distressingly conscious of the physical effort required. The high incidence of repeated hospitalizations and the progressive disability of these patients make necessary all-out efforts to set up purposeful and supervised chronic-care programs for them, to include not only supportive measures but also vigorous efforts to rehabilitate those with significant cardiopulmonary reserve. This is long-term therapy, for which both trained personnel and physical facilities are in short demand. Many chronically handicapped patients require daily care, some of which can be provided in ambulatory centers, but desperately needed for pulmonary rehabilitation are hospitals primarily intended for the chronic respiratory patient. Only the barest beginning of chronic care can be given in the average general hospital, both the philosophy and cost of which prohibit significant follow-up.

Complete monographs have been written on the subjects of chronic care and rehabilitation, and there are studies in the medical literature.[1-16] We combine information from these sources with our own clinical experience in an attempt to introduce the student to the subject.

Questions are frequently asked regarding the cost-effectiveness of rehabilitation and whether or not it helps survival rates over the long term. What is known is that survival rates of patients with cardiopulmonary disease who are in rehabilitation programs, when compared to matched patients not in rehabilitation programs, show only slight improvement.[2,17] However, the number of hospitalizations is markedly decreased in rehabilitated groups. Patient well-being and activity levels in rehabilitated groups seem to be better.[17] Even though a hospital or clinic does not have a large multidisciplinary team,[1] the important aspects of pulmonary rehabilitation can be made available to the patient by a physician and one or two allied-health persons—a respiratory therapist or a nurse trained in chronic pulmonary care.[17]

The overall objectives of pulmonary rehabilitation are not different from those of other disabling diseases—to increase the patient's physical comfort and performance and help him or her to maintain or regain economic productivity or improved self-care. The following outline gives the needs that should be considered and provided for rehabilitation of chronic bronchopulmonary disease:

A. Medical therapy
1. Control of respiratory infection
2. Maintenance of clear airways
    a. Aerosol therapy
    b. Assisted ventilation
    c. Postural drainage exercises
3. Correction of inefficient ventilation— ventilatory exercises
4. Improvement in ambulation
    a. Graded walking exercises (with or without oxygen)
    b. Physical conditioning exercises
5. Psychosomatic support
    a. Group therapy
    b. Individual therapy as indicated
6. Evaluation of cardiopulmonary function
B. Economic and social adjustment
1. Occupational retraining and placement
    a. Work classification
    b. Employer support
2. Family counseling
    a. Education
    b. Home planning

Although the role of the respiratory therapist may seem more dramatic in the care of the patient in acute respiratory failure, it is no less valuable after passage of the crisis. Many of the same therapeutic and diagnostic techniques apply then as before, but there are some reserved mostly for the convalescent period. We tend to sigh with relief when respiratory compensation is restored to a patient in failure and perhaps congratulate ourselves for normal blood gas values. However, as far as the patient is concerned, this may mark only the start of a long period of disability, threatened with unpredictable relapses and characterized by frustrating physical disability. We are still responsible for the patient, but our aims are somewhat different; and from the convalescent period on we try to accomplish two things simultaneously. First, we attempt to restore as much function as possible to the ventilatory mechanism, and, second, we try to keep the patient out of further episodes of failure. Both are large tasks.

To begin our discussion, let us define the respiratory therapy of chronic pulmonary care as those measures intended to improve respiratory performance rather than to save an acutely threatened life. The chronic state can develop gradually according to its own progression, or it may follow an acute illness, but the management will generally be the same. Chronic care may be started in the hospital as an outgrowth of acute care, or it may be initiated in the ambulatory patient who has never been hospitalized. We discuss here techniques that theoretically and traditionally belong to physiotherapy but that have become not only useful adjuncts to respiratory therapy but an integral part of it. These techniques apply specifically to the treatment of diseases of the chest and, in the United States at least, have been less emphasized by physiotherapists than have other aspects of their field. However, the respiratory therapist found these physically oriented procedures of great interest and use, and in the natural evolution of respiratory therapy, they have been incorporated into the therapist's general function. The encroachment of respiratory care on the domain of physiotherapy therefore was not intentional but developed only as a means to give a full spectrum of care to the respiratory patient.

With the respiratory therapist responsible for administering the basic aids to ventilation and for maintaining the patient during acute illness, it is only reasonable that the therapist also have at his or her disposal any procedures that may further aid the patient's breathing and that will permit the therapist to continue caring for the patient during convalescence and rehabilitation. We will see that some physiotherapy is indicated as part of pressure-breathing treatments, for example, and it is not in the interest of efficiency or good medicine to make the simultaneous services of two technicians necessary when one can do the job or to send the patient back and forth between two departments when only one is needed. The greatest justification for allocating chest physiotherapy to the respiratory therapist, however, is the therapist's specialized knowledge of, as well as interest in, pulmonary physiology and mechanics. It is hoped that the future education of the respiratory therapist will require deeper involvement in the techniques of chronic care, but at this time the training should include the following physical procedures: postural drainage, chest percussion, chest vibration, cough control, acute chest compression, pursed-lip breathing, abdominal breathing, and other ventilatory exercises. These are the subjects we discuss below, but to understand the objectives and techniques of postural drainage, the therapist must know the segmental anatomy of the lung and the spatial relationships of segments and bronchi.

Respiratory therapy of chronic care **Control of infection**	The lung should be a sterile organ even though it is in direct contact with the great outdoors. However, since the patient with chronic lung disease has undergone severe changes to all of the host defense mechanisms designed to maintain this level of sterility, infection is inevitable and is usually continuous. This usually takes the form of chronic bronchitis and frequently full-blown pneumonia.

The common way of looking at these infected states is by referring to them as either *community*-acquired or *hospital*-acquired (nosocomial) infections. Since this is a section on rehabilitation we will assume we are dealing with community-acquired infections and ignore the hospital-acquired infections, which are a completely different group of organisms with a different way of diagnosing and treating.

Patients who continue to smoke in the presence of chronic lung disease, whether it is an obstructive or restrictive disease, are seriously limiting the ability of the treatment program to resolve their infection. Alcohol abuse also has a marked effect on the lung's defense mechanism, damaging especially the macrophages and hindering their ability to combat invading bacteria.[18]

The most commonly acquired colonization of the airways of chronic lung patients is a result of *Hemophilus influenzae* or *Streptococcus pneumoniae*. If the patient's sputum changes in amount, color, or consistency, treatment should be initiated. Usually in well-established lung disease this is done without collecting a sputum for Gram stain or culture. The most commonly used antibiotics are ampicillin (or amoxicillin), tetracycline, erythromycin, or occasionally trimethoprim with sulfamethoxazole. These are all given for approximately 7 to 10 days. Sometimes with patients who have bronchiectasis, it is helpful to give these antibiotics for a set number of days (for example, the first 10 days of each month), regardless of the patient's clinical state.

Medications used in the treatment of cardiopulmonary disease may themselves give infections. An example of this would be a patient receiving an aerosolized steroid who develops moniliasis of the mouth. Frequently this can be prevented by washing the mouth out with water after each treatment. If the infection becomes established, it is relatively easy to control with nystatin (Mycostatin). Potassium permanganate ($KMNO_4$) is also useful but very messy.

Postural drainage	The purpose of postural drainage is to increase the removal of bronchial secretions by so positioning the patient that gravity will aid their cephalad movement. As employed by the respiratory therapist, "tipping," to use the British expression, is often an important part of bronchial hygiene and aerosol therapy. The therapist will have frequent occasion to stop therapy, tip the

patient, percuss and vibrate the chest, and then resume aerosol breathing. In theory, the therapist should have the prior consent of the patient's physician to perform these added services, but in hospitals where the medical staff is properly informed in chest therapy, a reliable therapist may be permitted to use his or her judgment. In the sophisticated respiratory therapy department, such physiotherapy is considered not as "added services" but as much a part of patient treatment as is the use of a respirator. Before initiating drainage, the therapist must consider such factors of the patient's general condition as related diseases, other infirmities, and age, but there are few who cannot benefit from some form of this therapy. This statement does not imply that all patients given bronchial hygiene must have postural drainage, for drainage is specifically reserved for those with significant secretions that cannot be readily removed by other means. It is true, however, that therapies such as inspiratory positive-pressure breathing (IPPB) and aerosol treatment will often fail to achieve their purpose if stubborn secretions are permitted to obstruct the airways, and much time and effort can be wasted on fruitless therapy.

Of the patients the therapist drains, by far the most will have bronchitis-emphysema, and their retained secretions will usually involve the basal segments of the lower lobes. Thus, in a general way, referring to the therapist's average daily work, postural drainage will mean positioning the patient to remove secretions from the lower lobe basal segments, and especially the posterior basal segment, either side or both. The other diseases listed may require

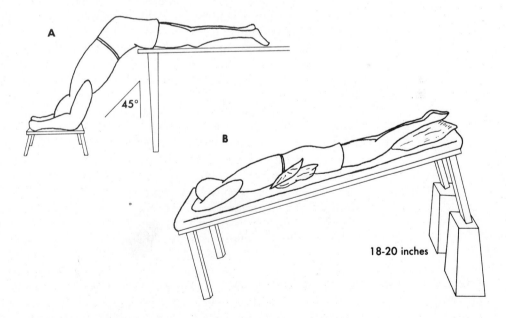

Fig. 15-1   Postural drainage, posterior basal segments. Position **A** is preferred. **B** is reserved for patients for whom the head-down position is not indicated.

treatment of different segments with localization by x-ray examination or bronchography. When a physician specifically orders postural drainage, the area to be treated should be indicated. There are several good manuals on postural drainage describing and illustrating in detail the many available positions and their relationship to the bronchial tree.[19-21] It would be a redundant use of time to reproduce them all on these pages, for the therapist can consult such sources and become familiar with all the techniques. Since our interest is in the common daily use of postural drainage, we confine our discussion to basal segment drainage only but with some recommendations that will apply to all techniques.

Fig. 15-1 illustrates two methods of posterior basal segment drainage. Position *A* is the one preferred if the patient's condition will permit tipping his or her head down. There are three important points to ensure effectiveness with maximum comfort. First, the angle of 45 degrees between the patient's trunk and the horizontal is relatively critical, since this puts the posterior basal segment bronchus in the most favorable position for gravity drainage. Second, the back should be kept as straight as possible, avoiding a tendency to sag, since this impairs effective drainage and strains the back muscles. Third, the patient's arms should be supported or he or she will be unable to maintain the position with any degree of comfort; a footstool, a pile of books, or any other suitable object on which the patient can rest crossed arms may be used. It is not always easy to find a satisfactory surface across which the patient can lie at the desired angle. Many beds are too low or have too much give to them. If a bed is used, it should be adjustable to accommodate the patient's height and its mattress firm enough to be free of sagging. A tilt-table that will allow the entire body to be put at a 45-degree angle is ideal, and this should be part of the equipment of an ambulatory care service of the respiratory therapy department, to which many patients can be brought for therapy. Such a table must have shoulder supports to prevent the patient from sliding off its end.

Position *B* shows an alternate technique for those patients for whom the head-down position is contraindicated. Drainage will be aided if the patient is placed in the prone position with two pillows under the hips and the foot of the bed elevated about 18 to 20 inches. The bed may be raised by blocks of suitable size under the foot legs or by an automobile jack under the foot end to which an extension angle iron has been welded to prevent rocking. Strength of the head legs must be ensured because elevation of the foot places a tremendous strain on the head of the bed. This method is not quite as effective as the head-down position because the body assumes an angle of no more than about 15 degrees, but it has the advantage that it can be maintained for long periods of time. Fig. 15-2, *A,* shows the position that will drain the anterior basal segment, with the foot of the bed raised 18 to 20 inches and a pillow under the knees for comfort. Fig. 15-2, *B,* demonstrates the position for lateral basal drainage, depending on the side on which the patient is placed. A pillow or two is placed under the waist to keep the spine straight.

Judgment will determine whether all three positions should be used in sequence during any one treatment. From a practical point of view, considering the

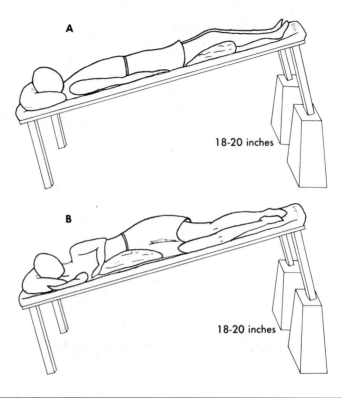

Fig. 15-2   Postural drainage. Position **A** is for anterior basal segments. **B** is for lateral basal segments.

elements of time and patient fatigue, it is probably advisable to use the head-down technique whenever possible and as the first maneuver and, if therapeutic results are satisfactory, to do no more. On the other hand, if the patient presents a particularly difficult secretion problem, it may be necessary to rotate him or her through a series of all three positions. Initially, a patient may be able to tolerate the head-down technique for only a minute, but he or she will soon adjust to it for as long as necessary. When the patient is in position, the therapist should warn him or her not to make a deliberate effort to cough vigorously, since this will markedly raise intracranial pressure. Rather, the patient should be instructed frequently to "clear the throat" with sharp grunting sounds but with only gentle effort. This maneuver will elevate intrathoracic pressure momentarily at intervals, transmitting short bursts of high-velocity air in the bronchi to loosen and move secretions. Both the patient and the therapist should understand that the value of postural drainage is not in the immediate production of a great flow of secretions, since very often the treatment will seemingly accomplish little. Its function is to mobilize secretions intrabronchially for easier removal with a less effortful cough long after the tipping. If the drainage should be effective at once, so much the better, and if it precipitates hard coughing, the patient should sit up until the cough subsides.

Chest percussion   Percussion, also known as tapping or clapping, is a technique of striking the patient's chest to loosen bronchial secretions as an aid to postural drainage. The striking force must be against the bare skin, delivered by the therapist's hand held slightly cupped with fingers and thumb closed so a cushion of air is trapped between the hand and chest wall. The therapist, holding his or her arm with the elbow partially flexed and wrist loose, whips the hand sharply down onto the patient's chest over the area being drained. Best results come from using both hands alternately in rapid sequence for several seconds at a time. It is a noisy procedure, but far from being painful to the patient, it is stimulating and the coarse vibrations set up in the thorax literally shake loose secretions. Naturally, care must be exercised by the therapist to avoid tender areas or sites of trauma or surgery. It is not a difficult technique to master, but skill and experience are needed to determine the force to use for a given chest wall thickness and to maintain a uniform blow throughout the procedure.

Chest vibration   Like percussion, chest vibration is an accompaniment to postural drainage and has the same objective as percussion but through a little different technique. In the classical maneuver the therapist lays one hand on the patient's chest over the involved area and places the other hand on top of the first. Then, while exerting slight to moderate pressure on the chest wall, he or she rapidly produces an even vibratory motion of the hands. In contrast to the more violent percussion, this procedure sets up fine vibrations that are transmitted to the secretions. More effective is the use of an electric hand vibrator. This instrument not only ensures prolonged uniform vibrations to loosen secretions but is also relaxing to the patient.

The combination of aerosol therapy, IPPB, postural drainage, chest percussion, and vibration thus can be considered as a treatment unit, and the physical therapy elements have proved themselves very helpful in increasing the efficiency of pressure breathing and aerosol therapy. In practice, the therapist will often start aerosol or IPPB in the usual manner and then, on noting the apparent presence of resistant secretions that the patient raises with great difficulty, if at all, will stop and position the patient for drainage. The therapist will apply percussion and vibration over the basal areas, giving the patient ample opportunity to cough as needed. Again the therapist will resume aerosol or IPPB and so continue to alternate between pneumatic, aerosol, and physical therapy according to the results obtained. The ability and judgment of the respiratory therapist to use such combined therapy effectively rank equally with his or her skill at maintaining mechanical ventilation.

Cough control   To the patient with a basically normal respiratory tract, a cough is usually a necessary nuisance that gives relief from bronchial irritation. To the patient with chronic pulmonary disease, on the other hand, an effective cough may mean the difference between adequate and inadequate air exchange, and this he or she may not be able to accomplish. In general, patients who need some type of cough assistance are found among those with (1) postoperative or posttraumatic pulmonary restriction (thoracic or abdominal), (2) postventilator weakness, or (3) air trapping. The patient with restriction, usually because of pain, has limited inspiration and is unable to generate enough propulsive power to remove secretions effectively. The therapist can help such a patient by supporting the lower thorax bilaterally with the hands. As the patient inhales, the therapist moves with the expanding chest but still maintains resistance against which the patient must work. At the limit of the patient's inspiration, the pressure exerted by the therapist gives impetus to the start of a cough and continued compression increases the force and velocity of the exhaled air. The therapist can repeat this maneuver several times to mobilize secretions and may be able to teach some patients to do it themselves, although this is usually less effective.

The patient recently weaned from a mechanical ventilator and the patient with air trapping, as from emphysema, may have adequate inspiratory capacities but lack expulsive power for effective removal of secretions. The reasons for their problems differ, however. Prolonged assisted ventilation may allow one patient to lose tone and strength of the ventilatory muscles so that, although he or she can move tidal air satisfactorily, the patient cannot generate cough power. Also, irritation of the throat from intubation or actual laryngeal damage may limit cough. On the other hand, the patient with bronchiolar damage may have commendable vital and inspiratory capacities, but the buildup of intrathoracic pressure during cough compresses the weakened bronchiolar walls to stop the cough before it has had time to be effective. Both these patients can be taught to overcome their problems, a responsibility of the respiratory therapist. The therapist instructs the patients to start their coughs from a midinspiratory position rather than the usual full inspiration, which is more natural. This reduces the volume of air to be removed by the weak patient and lowers the intrathoracic pressure of the air-trapping patient. To compensate for resultant loss of expulsive force, the patients are then told to exhale in a rapid series of "machine gun" bursts of short, sharp coughs, repeated several times always from a midinspiratory position or even the end-expiratory resting level. This technique relieves the weak patient of the strain of a prolonged hard cough, and the staccato rhythm at a relatively low velocity minimizes airway collapse in the air-trapping patient. This technique has a modification called "huffing" whereby the patient is instructed to make the sound of "huff, huff, huff" rapidly with the mouth open, the sound audibly coming from the throat.[2]

Acute chest compression

Acute chest compression is related to the procedure just described for cough control, but it has a specific and often acute indication, especially in the patient with severe emphysema and air trapping. Not only may the mechanism of air trapping interfere with effective cough, as already noted, but it may place the patient's life in jeopardy. The emphysematous patient with chronic bronchial secretions may suddenly be stimulated by the need to cough, take a deep breath, start the cough, and suddenly find airflow shut off before end-expiration. At this point the patient may be unable either to exhale or inhale, and the chest becomes "frozen" and immobile. The patient continues to strain in an attempt to move air, the neck veins distend from the intrathoracic pressure, the face becomes cyanotic, and he or she is suddenly in acute danger of suffocation. Fortunately, most such episodes are self-limiting, as perhaps weakness causes enough relaxation of intrathoracic pressure to permit air to move, but the experience is frightening to patient and family alike, and it severely strains the heart and subjects the brain to acute hypoxia. The respiratory therapist should be prepared to manage this event, since overbreathing from IPPB and breathing exercises may precipitate an attack of acute air trapping. Should this happen or the patient give a history of its occurrence at home, family members should be taught how to treat it. The technique is simple but effective and is applied as soon as the patient's distress is seen because, of course, he or she will be unable to speak. If the patient is relatively slight in stature, the therapist, standing behind the patient, places both hands over the lateral costal margins and lower chest and exerts a series of strong short compressions, releasing completely between each. This develops bursts of enough intrapulmonary pressure to break through airway obstruction and allow completion of exhalation. If the patient is large, with a heavy chest wall, the therapist can exert greater expulsive force by standing to the patient's side and, grasping him or her in a bear hug around the lower thorax, sharply squeezing the patient laterally against his or her own body. The occurrence of acute air trapping whenever an attempt is made to cough indicates the need for intensive therapy to remove offending secretions but at the same time is a warning to use caution in treatment and to try to maintain the patient's ventilation at a level of low velocity. Forceful compression of the costal margins, as described, is not without its hazards, since rib fracture, lung puncture, and injury to liver are possible.

Pursed-lip breathing

Pursed-lip breathing is a simple maneuver that many patients learn for themselves without knowing why, but because it is so useful in breathing exercises and breath control, it should be taught to those unaware of it. Its purpose is to prevent the air trapping caused by bronchiolar collapse, serving the same purpose as the retard cap on the exhalation port of the IPPB respirator, and it is almost exclusively used for emphysema. The patient is instructed to purse the lips as if whistling during exhalation, controlling the velocity of exhaled air to the slowest that is consistent with ventilation. A variation of this, which is not really pursed-lip, consists of placing the tongue on the roof of the mouth and releasing the air slowly as if saying the letter "s." This has no inherent gain over pursing the lips and is certainly noisier. In either case, it is believed that the resistance of the mouth transmits back pressure throughout the bronchial tree, and its gradual release during exhalation prevents intrathoracic pressure from compressing shut those bronchioles weakened by disease.[2] Moreover, it has been shown that pursed-lip breathing slows the respiratory rate.[10] When used with the forceful abdominal-breathing exercises to be described next, the pursed-lip retard of airflow is continued to the end of the prolonged exhalation. At other times, such as during the breath control of quiet breathing or moderate exercise, the pursed-lip retard may be released at midexhalation to allow a normal terminal flow, since the naturally slowing velocity of passive end-expiration carries little risk of air trapping.

Abdominal breathing

Of the many available exercises directed toward improving the mechanics of ventilation, we describe but four, for it is believed that these have the widest application in the general treatment of respiratory deficiencies. Many of the others are designed to improve skeletal muscle performance and posture, but we will let the therapist pursue their uses at his or her leisure. When we discussed the mechanics of ventilation, we learned how such pulmonary pathology as obstruction, destruction of alveoli, and air trapping upset the normal ventilatory pattern, lowering the diaphragm and effectively removing it from useful ventilation and throwing the burden of air movement on the thorax. We learned how inefficient is thoracic breathing, with its need to activate accessory ventilatory muscles, and how the subsequent distortion of a barrel chest aggravates the problem. In this section we are interested in patients with thoracic breathing, especially if paradoxic, for thoracic breathers are expending much more energy moving the chest wall than they would if they had only to move the more flexible abdominal wall. The additional oxygen need for the work of breathing seriously compounds the disability of the underlying disease. Abdominal-breathing exercises are designed to ease ventilatory work by gradually changing the pattern from thoracic to abdominal.

Changing the breathing pattern is a slow and difficult process and requires the utmost patience of the respiratory therapist. The therapist should understand that it is often very difficult for a patient who has developed a thoracic breathing pattern to revert to abdominal, and many never do accomplish it. It is quite remarkable that what was once a natural function, when lost, is so difficult to relearn. There is no set method of teaching effective breathing, but we present suggested techniques on which the therapist can improve with experience and modify according to need.

Before starting a breathing exercise, the therapist should have the patient take two or three inhalations of a bronchodilator aerosol and permit the patient to relax mentally and physically. Before teaching a new exercise, the therapist should demonstrate it plainly to the patient, explaining the purpose of each move and how best the patient can accomplish it.

Forced-exhalation abdominal breathing. The purpose of this exercise is to strengthen the contractile force of the abdominal wall muscles so that they can effectively elevate the diaphragm and empty the lungs. Although it can be done in almost any position, it is best taught in the supine with a pillow under the patient's head and the knees drawn up comfortably to relax the anterior abdominal wall. The principles of technique are illustrated in Fig. 15-3. The patient's hand is placed on the epigastrium, not to exert pressure but only to

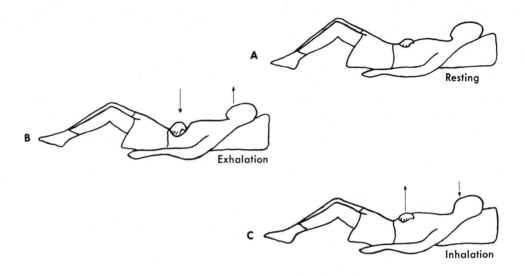

Fig. 15-3 Forced-exhalation abdominal breathing. (See text for description.)

focus attention to this area *(A)*. Much of the success of therapy will depend on the degree to which the therapist can keep the patient's mind on epigastric movement. Exercise is always started in the same manner, by exhaling from the resting level through pursed lips. At the same time the patient is instructed to pull in the upper abdomen gradually, with conscious force, prolonging exhalation as long as possible *(B)*. At end-exhalation the patient is told to inhale easily through the nose, letting the upper abdomen balloon out *(C)*, and the cycle is repeated. From now on, however, exhalation will start from end-inspiration, and the patient is urged to let the air flow out slowly through pursed lips until near the end of normal expiration and then forcibly to contract the upper abdomen to extend expiration to its maximum. The patient is advised to think of all breathing as taking place in the abdomen rather than in the chest; therefore, as the patient fills with air, the abdomen should swell, lifting up the hand, and as he or she expels air, the hand should fall with the receding abdomen.

During the maneuver the therapist must keep reminding the patient to concentrate on all respiratory movement as taking place in the area in contact with the hand and to disregard the chest completely. Many patients, trying hard to cooperate, will suddenly forget the sequence they were taught, contracting the epigastric wall during inhalation and attempting to relax it during exhalation, and may even stop breathing in their confusion. The therapist will find two things of help. The first is the steady repetition over several breathing cycles of "breath in, abdomen out, breath out, abdomen in" to help fix the rhythm in the patient's mind. The second is the placement of a hand over the patient's hand on the abdominal wall to exert gentle but firm pressure, de-

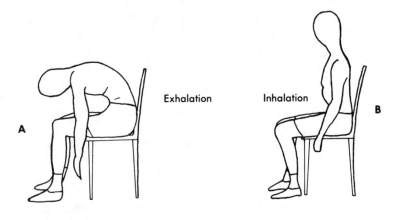

Exhalation   Inhalation

A   B

Fig. 15-4   Forced-exhalation abdominal breathing, seated. (See text for description.)

pressing the epigastrium during the prolongation of exhalation. Much practice may be required for this seemingly simple procedure, but as proficiency is acquired, the patient is encouraged to make a positive effort to keep the chest immobile while ventilating completely with the abdomen.

If the patient has exceptionally poor coordination and is unable to achieve adequate expiratory contraction of the abdomen, the surface on which he or she is lying may be tilted so that the body inclines cephalad about 20 degrees. A pillow may be used under the head, but care is taken that it does not extend beneath the shoulders. In this position the force of gravity shifts the abdominal contents against the diaphragm to assist in elevating it. This technique is useful only to get the procedure under way because success depends on developing sufficient abdominal strength to raise the diaphragm against gravity.

For the breathing exercise to be of value, it must be performed regularly and frequently, not just in the presence of the therapist. A regular schedule of exercise must be set up, perhaps as much as 5 to 10 minutes every hour until clinical results justify reducing it.

To vary the forced exhalation exercise, the patient may be taught to do it in the seated position, employing the added techniques of forward bending as shown in Fig. 15-4. The patient relaxes in a hard, straight-backed chair, sitting upright to commence the maneuver. With the arms hanging loosely by the side to promote relaxation of the thoracic skeletal muscles, he or she slowly exhales through pursed lips while slowly bending forward and retracting the upper abdomen (Fig. 15-4, *A*). When properly timed, flexion of the trunk should be complete at the moment of end-expiration. The body is then raised while the patient inhales through the nose, letting the abdomen distend as the lungs fill. When inhalation is completed, the patient should be back in the upright position. To aid exhalation, the forward bending uses the flexion of the trunk to compress the abdomen and elevate the diaphragm. This exercise is especially helpful to the patient when having trouble with secretions because it enables him or her to hyperventilate slightly and stimulate the mobility of secretions for easier cough removal.

Forced-inhalation abdominal breathing. In contrast to forced exhalation, the physical effort in forced-inhalation abdominal breathing is directed toward inhalation, with exhalation mostly passive. This more closely resembles the normal pattern of breathing. The patient is positioned as for forced exhalation but preferably with a 20-degree head-down tilt, and weight of 10 to 15 pounds is placed over the midabdomen. A set of five fabric bags containing sand or buckshot is helpful, two weighing 5 pounds and three weighing 10 pounds. Since the abdominal weight will make exhalation easy for the patient, attention is directed to strengthening his or her inspiratory effort. After letting air out through pursed lips and terminally contracting the abdominal muscles, the patient is instructed to inhale through the nose, "taking air into the abdomen," with an effort forceful enough to lift the weight visibly. Because of the physical work involved, the initial time tolerated by the patient may be short, but as performance improves, the exercise may be extended to 30 minutes three to four times daily. The abdominal weight is also increased in increments of 5 pounds and over a period of several weeks may reach 30 pounds. This exercise is especially useful for the patient with paradoxic breathing, since it almost forces the patient to accept a normal breathing pattern. At the same time the abdominal muscles are strengthened so that the patient can meet ventilatory needs by this pattern. The therapist must warn the patient not to overdo the exercise, since soreness of the neglected muscles subjected to the strain of exercise is common and, if severe enough, can impede performance.

Forced-exhalation with walking. The primary objective of ventilatory exercise is to increase the patient's tolerance to physical activity, the most important of which is walking. One of the patient's major complaints is the inability to walk comfortably, sometimes even from one room of a home to another, and going out-of-doors may be impossible. Improving walking tolerance will do more to increase the patient's morale than any other therapeutic benefit. The respiratory therapist will observe that many patients who breathe with ease, resting in bed or chair, will revert to severe thoracic or paradoxic ventilation as soon as they start to walk. The purpose of the present exercise is to coordinate walking, and eventually other exertion, to the rhythm of abdominal breathing, using the prolonged phase of exhalation as the period of maximum effort. This implies that the patient has mastered the act of abdominal breathing and fully understands its purpose.

To prepare for walking exercise, the patient must practice abdominal breathing a few times in the standing position. This position, however, should not be rigidly upright but rather slightly bent forward, and although its esthetic effect may be less than desirable, it will make breathing easier. In a straight position the abdominal muscles are under tension, as the string of a bow, but are relaxed by forward flexion and more available for controlled ventilation. The normal subject exerts and adjusts ventilation accordingly to supply body oxygen needs, but the patient who is our concern here has limited ventilation and so must adapt physical activity to it. This makes for an artificial and somewhat awkward relationship between breathing and walking but one that can be mastered profitably with practice. The technique is based on establishing a ratio between a given amount of walking and the phasing of breathing, and experience has shown the following to be practical: The patient is instructed to move and breathe slowly, taking three steps during exhalation and two steps during inhalation. This does two things. It helps the patient to maintain a good ventilatory rhythm whereby exhalation exceeds inhalation, ensuring maximum air clearance of the lung; and it lets the patient perform the most exertion when it is easier, during expiration. Because this exercise is developed so that it can be done smoothly, the patient will find that walking will consume much less energy than when his or her breathing was haphazard.

The rationale of this technique can be explained to the patient in the following way so that he or she will understand the need to persist in what may seem at first to be a silly effort: When the normal subject is faced with a strenuous act, he or she first inhales, closes the glottis to hold the breath, and then contracts the necessary muscles. If the physical action is prolonged, the subject slowly releases the air, often in short bursts, prolonging exhalation while continuing to strain, and then takes a rapid inspiration and repeats until the effort is finished. The point to note is that maximum physical effort is expended during exhalation, not inhalation. With markedly limited ventilation, it is important that our patient with respiratory insufficiency correlate as much of the effort with exhalation as possible. The patient who learns coordinated walking will find the technique applicable to many other activities. It will greatly help in climbing the stairs, ordinarily one of the most difficult chores, if he or she develops the habit of managing two or three steps during exhalation and resting during inhalation. Most emphysematous patients become extremely short of breath when bending to pick up an object. This can be made much easier by exhaling slowly through pursed lips while bending and grasping the object, then inhaling while arising and lifting, much in the manner of doing the forward bending exercise in a chair.

Mobilization of the lower ribs. The final maneuver to be described is not strictly an abdominal exercise, but it is intended to augment abdominal breathing by utilizing a portion of the thorax that does not hinder ventilation. This consists of expanding and contracting the costal margin, which will give maximum mobility to the diaphragm and increase aeration of the lung bases. At first the exercise needs the help of the therapist, but later it can be performed by the patient alone. The patient will best understand the purpose of the exercise if introduced to it in the relaxed supine position; but the maneuver can be as well done seated. The therapist places his or her hands over the costal margins so that they almost cup the lower rib edges, and as the patient exhales through pursed lips, the hands follow the slightly contracting rib margins. Just before the end of exhalation the therapist exerts a forceful crescendo squeeze, holding the pressure firmly. As inhalation begins, the therapist gradually releases the manual pressure but retains some resistance to the expanding ribs. The patient is instructed to "breathe around the waist and push the hands away," to direct attention to this area. The patient is also told to make an effort to squeeze in the costal edge while pulling in the abdomen during exhalation. Finally, the patient is allowed to use his or her own hands to mobilize the lower ribs, and some therapists recommend the use of a swathe or a belt that the patient can use instead of the hands.

Graded exercises   Somewhat as the culmination, or end objective, of the breathing exercises just described, a system of graded exercises is used to condition the patient for prolonged activity, principally walking. As the name implies, the patient's effort is built up gradually against controlled resistance, both to minimize injury and to monitor his or her progress with objective data. A patient is ready for this aspect of rehabilitation only after maximum airway patency has been achieved and after he or she has mastered breath control through abdominal breathing, although it is still frequently necessary to use aerosol therapy, pressure breathing, and postural drainage in conjunction with graded exercise.

Whereas techniques in performing progressive exercises may vary, the general principles are the same. Either a treadmill or an exercising bicycle is used, the resistance of which can be adjusted. Both are satisfactory, but the treadmill has the advantage that it more closely simulates the type of physical activity we are trying to develop—walking—and we use it in our discussion. Supplemental oxygen is usually given to the patient, at least in the early stage of therapy, so that he or she can withstand the stress of activity. A nasal cannula is usually satisfactory, or entrainment masks can be used. Ventilatory function, blood gas determination, cardiac function, and any other evaluation data are obtained before starting the program and are repeated according to the needs of each treatment schedule. The therapist should note that walking on a treadmill is not exactly the same as walking on a stable surface because there is a certain knack to using the legs in a normal manner while the body remains in position and the underfooting moves. This should be explained to the patient and demonstrated by the therapist. The patient should step onto the treadmill mat while it is moving slowly, and although he or she should be allowed to place the hands gently on the safety railing, the patient should be instructed not to let the support bear his or her weight.

The first exposure of the patient to exercise is tentative, to judge response and tolerance and to teach the proper technique. The patient is given oxygen and the treadmill adjusted to 0% grade and a rate not to exceed 1 mph. The therapist must give reassurance and encouragement to many patients who are initially apprehensive, and they may be told that they can step off the moving surface at any time. During the first trial the therapist must see that the patient is using the abdomen to breathe, since it is under such conditions of stress that he or she is likely to revert to thoracic or paradoxic breathing, and this cannot be permitted if the therapy is to be successful.

Whatever program is used, graded exercises are given regularly and daily, sometimes for several weeks. The pitch of the walking surface, its speed, and the duration of exercise are increased in increments tailored to each patient; and these are good criteria for evaluating progress. For example, if a patient walks 10 minutes at 0% grade and 1 mph at one time and later walks 15 minutes at 2% grade and 1.5 mph, this represents significant improvement.

Even more important is the gradual reduction in the need for supplemental oxygen as the intensity of the exercise increases. It may seem paradoxic that increasing exercise of a patient with respiratory insufficiency should lower the oxygen requirement, but the physiologic reason for this is the foundation for this aspect of rehabilitation. We must remember that patients with impaired breathing become sedentary, suffering progressive atrophic weakness of their leg muscles from disuse, and the less efficient the work of a muscle, the greater is the consumption of oxygen for the energy expended by the muscle. To put it another way, more oxygen must be taken in by the body to supply the needs of a poorly conditioned muscle in performing a given amount of work than is required by a well-conditioned muscle.

The clinical improvement from a graded exercise program is attributed to two factors. First, although pulmonary function tests may show little change, ventilatory muscle training improves the patient's pattern of breathing with better pulmonary aeration and an increased ability to satisfy the needs of exertion. Second, the physical conditioning with improved efficiency of ventilatory and leg muscles reduces their oxygen demand. Together, both factors greatly increase the amount of work produced per unit of energy expended. Finally, although strenuous exercise may be contraindicated or must be used with caution in patients with some types of heart disease, cor pulmonale is probably not a contraindication if the heart is not in frank failure. The heart strain is apparently not worsened because of the eventual reduction in metabolic oxygen demand.

The program just described must be carried out in a rehabilitation facility with elaborate equipment under the constant supervision of trained personnel. This is believed to be the most desirable management, but there may be instances in which such supervision is not practical or possible. With proper selection many patients can profit from a well-planned home-care program, and one of the many valuable services of the respiratory therapist is the training and follow-up supervision of patients for such programs. The home-care patient must be carefully taught the postural-drainage and breathing-exercise techniques; it is wise also to teach these techniques to a reliable family member who may have to assist the patient.

Graded exercises with oxygen can be done at home but should be attempted only if both the patient's attending physician and respiratory therapist consider that the patient is responsible and intelligent enough to follow directions accurately. Home exercise can be provided by an exercise cycle, which is space saving, or by level walking, if space permits. Supportive oxygen, gaseous and liquid, is available in small enough containers to be carried by a shoulder sling. Small gaseous cylinders can be refilled from large cylinders, but there is some potential risk in this and it must be advised with caution. According to the patient's capabilities, a graded schedule of walking can be made for him or her, but it must be reviewed frequently for modifications and to assess its results.

Experience has shown that only an exceptional and unusually motivated patient will persist in a graded exercise program at home, away from professional supervision and encouragement, for long enough periods to realize much gain from it as the primary therapy. As a follow-up to a rehabilitation area course of treatment and after the discontinuance of supportive oxygen, home exercises of the postural and kinetic types not only are valuable but for many patients they must be continued indefinitely.

Other aspects of rehabilitation	The rest of our discussion of rehabilitation does not involve the direct technical services of the respiratory therapist, but the therapist should be aware of all the efforts made on the disabled patient's behalf, for each facet of therapy or management has some influence on the others. The more that members of the rehabilitation team know about the patient, the better able they will be to evaluate the patient's progress and their own role in it.
Tracheostomy care	Occasionally patients are discharged to their homes with a tracheostomy tube in place or a permanent stoma constructed. This allows breathing through these appliances for either a full 24 hours or parttime, such as at night while the patient is sleeping. Before discharge the patient must be carefully instructed on how to keep the stoma clear, how to keep the tracheostomy tube clean (often a metal tube is used for permanent tracheostomies), and tricks on how to camouflage with articles of clothing the fact that a tracheostomy tube is in use. This last item will go a long way in improving the patient's self-image and ease in relating to other people.
Long-term oxygen support	Somehow the public has gotten the idea that oxygen is an addicting drug not unlike a narcotic, and if a person is using oxygen outside the hospital he or she is "hooked" and has now started on a rapid slide downhill to death unless higher and higher concentrations of oxygen are used for longer periods of time. Nothing could be further from the truth. A recent study involving 6 medical centers and 203 patients from those centers looked at the mortality of two groups of patients.[22] One group had 102 patients and used nasal oxygen at night only. Their mortality was 1.94 times greater than the group of 101 who used nasal oxygen continuously, 19 to 24 hours each day. The two groups were otherwise well matched for disease severity, etc. These data imply that in fact, oxygen used for longer periods of time each day significantly improves longevity.

Oxygen can be provided in the home by several methods, for instance, with cylinders, liquid systems, or newer devices called *oxygen concentrators*.[4,16,23-26] Briefly, the concentrators are of two types: molecular sieve or membrane. The molecular sieve units can provide about 50% to 90% oxygen at flows of 10 to 2 ℓ/min respectively, while the membrane type produces 40% oxygen at all flows less than 10 ℓ/min. Both types use compressors and separate oxygen from room air, but each functions under different principles, described in the literature.[4,23] Advantages of oxygen concentrators have been related to safety, convenience, and cost, as compared to other systems of home oxygen therapy.[4,24,26,27]

Psychosomatic support

The term *psychosomatic* refers to the relationship between the emotional state or outlook of an individual *(psyche)* and the physical responses of the individual's body *(soma)*. Everyday life is full of such relationships, as, for example, the physical fatigue that follows a period of emotional tension, and many of them are considered part of normal human behavior. Some, however, cause or aggravate an existing physical disability; and it is with this aspect of chronic pulmonary insufficiency that we are concerned. It is important for the respiratory therapist to realize that all his or her skilled technical services, as well as the best pharmacologic therapy, can be negated and a patient driven to a progressively downhill course because of an unfavorable mental attitude. Emotional instability is not unique to patients with respiratory disease alone, of course, for we frequently see severe signs of depression and hostility complicating many acute and chronic diseases. In chronic respiratory disease, however, it may be a double-edged sword, for not only can psychic disturbances affect the general well-being of the patient but they may also directly aggravate the very defects that are responsible for the underlying disability. The ease and frequency with which emotional upsets affect the respiratory function are recognized in such commonly expressed relationships as "holding one's breath in anticipation," or being "choked up with emotion." Thus it is not difficult to imagine that a patient with labored breathing could be made much worse by a psychic stimulus affecting breathing.

The role of emotional and personality problems in the genesis of childhood bronchial asthma is well known and has been extensively recorded in medical literature. It is quite probable that many instances of adult asthma, for which no specific allergic basis can be found, likewise stem from some recent or unresolved emotional conflict. The psychic element in nonasthmatic chronic pulmonary disease is probably of a different nature, although such patients, too, may have preexisting problems. Often the patient with progressive emphysema develops severe anxiety and hostility as a direct consequence of the disability. Because the patient is fearful of economic loss and death, he or she develops hostility toward the disease and often toward those with whom he or she comes into close contact. Patients with chronic respiratory disease are frequently seen to become acutely dyspneic during conversation that touches on subjects arousing fear and hostility.

The therapist should not entertain the impression that all patients chronically ill with pulmonary disability are primarily neurotic or that they imagine their symptoms. From our examinations we know the severe physical impairment of these patients; but we should also recognize that part of their symptomatology may well be a result of psychosomatic influences. Unfortunately, proper attention to this side of their disability has been generally neglected, probably for two basic reasons. First, the great spurt of interest in pulmonary disease of the past two decades has centered mostly on the physiology of diseases and physical therapeutic measures. Second, short as are the facilities for chronic physical care and rehabilitation, those for mental rehabilitation have been even shorter, since psychosomatic therapy demands the services of both psychiatrists and clinical psychologists who are especially interested in the chronically disabled respiratory patient. Such therapy has been used in the management of bronchial asthma, and results justify its wider application to nonasthmatic diseases as well. No suggestions are made here as to how to include adequate psychotherapy into the overall rehabilitation program, but it should be an integral part.[28] It is probable that superficial treatment might be satisfactory in the majority of cases, such as could be provided in group therapy. General observation of patients in a respiratory therapy outpatient service suggests that many derive support and encouragement by association with others, but to be most effective, this association should be professionally guided and directed. On the other hand, some would profit most from private care, in which their personal emotional conflicts should be aired and the relationship of such conflicts to their breathing explained to them. It is hoped that as pulmonary rehabilitation becomes more definitive, some technique of psychotherapy will evolve, directed to the specific needs of the respiratory cripple.

Occupational retraining and placement

Many disabled pulmonary patients are in their economically productive years and are anxious to be self-sufficient. For them, occupational retraining and job placement are necessary ingredients of a purposeful rehabilitation program. Such a program should not be on a hit-or-miss basis but on classifiable data, specific for each patient. Much study is yet needed to categorize occupations in terms of their energy requirements of the respiratory system and to derive simple but informative tests of the work of breathing to enable the rehabilitation team to match patients to those jobs in which they would have the greatest chance of success. Not only must the patient's physical status be considered but education, past experience, and aptitudes as well. Obviously, this is not solely the responsibility of medicine but will require the skills of counselors trained in occupational needs and the cooperation of business and industry in each community. These efforts have already been made in behalf of disability resulting from such conditions as incapacitating trauma and stroke and could be applied readily to pulmonary disability as soon as the specific needs of the last have been classified.

Family counseling   Family counseling is included not merely to round out the program in a general way but because experience has shown its great importance in therapy. Those of us who treat patients with respiratory diseases daily become familiar with the patterns of their diseases, but among the laity there is still a considerable lack of understanding as to the extent of disability that chronic pulmonary disease can produce. Relatives often consider the patient's cough an unnecessary nuisance to them and his or her reluctance to be physically active a manifestation of laziness, an impression supported by a frequently healthy appearance in the resting state. The patient is acutely aware of this attitude and is hurt, discouraged, and anxious. So sensitive are many patients with chronic disability to the discrepancy between how they look and how they feel that they react very irritably to simple greetings by their medical attendants of how well they look. It is essential that members of the patient's family fully understand the nature of the patient's disease and the extent of the disability. It must be stressed to them that there are good reasons why the patient can look comfortable in a chair but may not be able to walk to the next room without assistance. They must also understand the objectives of chronic care and rehabilitation, the duration of treatment, its cost and inconvenience to the family, and the probability of improvement. Because home care is usually an important part of the program, full cooperation of the family is necessary or all efforts will fail.

The first responsibility for educating the family falls to the attending physician, but the follow-up role of the respiratory therapist is equally, if not more, important. The therapist's explanation of technique and procedures to both patient and relatives can do much to ensure understanding of and cooperation with the program. Both the visiting nurse trained in respiratory care and the social worker can offer valuable services by checking on the home progress and helping to correct unfavorable conditions at home that may be detrimental to the patient. In the first category, assistance may be offered to relieve the financial problems so often found with long-term illness and advice given on a more efficient arrangement of home facilities and labor-saving techniques.

One of the most difficult areas for patients with any chronic disease, especially for those with pulmonary disease, to deal with involves maintaining fulfilled sexual relationships. Because of the dyspnea associated with any physical exertion, sexual dysfunction is common among pulmonary patients.[29] It is not within the purview of a respiratory therapist to serve as a counselor to the patient; how to relate to a sexual partner when the patient has pulmonary disease is best left to a trained counselor. However, the respiratory therapist may be the first and only person with whom the patient would dare discuss the problem. An accepting, relaxed attitude toward the patient's problem and reassurance that many have conquered this problem can be very encouraging and set the stage for the patient to agree to follow-up with a person more thoroughly trained in this field.

One way a family can show support for a chronically ill pulmonary patient is in the area of diet. Many times small changes in the way a family eats will have a noticeable effect on the patient, which, if it becomes permanent, may have long-term effects on other family members in improved health for years to come. If the ill patient has to cut out some favored dishes while the rest of the family eats these same foods in front of the patient, compliance by the patient on these dietary changes will be poor. Recent studies suggest that high-carbohydrate diets may cause higher levels of Pa_{CO_2}, thus increasing the work of breathing and acid-base disturbances.[30,31] Low-sodium diets are extremely important in patients with cor pulmonale, and diets high in protein will help maintain weight. Also of importance is care to avoid milk products, since they have been implicated as mucus producers. Potassium replacement, if the patient is receiving diuretics, and calcium, fluoride, and vitamin D replacement, if a patient is receiving steroids, are all very important.

The role of trace elements and vitamins in maintaining health is incompletely understood, but a rounded diet of whole grains, fruit, vegetables, poultry, fish, and lean red meats will help supply these needs. A good diet also improves bowel function. Whereas there are no studies about the effects on heart circulation and lungs of straining down (Valsalva's maneuver) to move a constipated stool followed by the sudden relaxation of intrathoracic pressure, our intuition tells us that this may not be very good for the patient.

Summary

We can summarize the philosophy of chronic and rehabilitative care of the pulmonary disabled patient by emphasizing the following three points: First, in contrast to the treatment of many other chronic illnesses, respiratory therapy depends to a major degree on a well-trained technical specialist who has often followed the patient through an acute illness into the chronic state and is now available to give long-term care based on firsthand knowledge of the patient's present and future needs. The respiratory therapist is a bridge between the acute and chronic phases of the disease and makes possible a valuable continuity of treatment. Second, many of the treatment procedures can be self-administered by the patient, not only relieving the financial burden of care but also putting on the patient some of the responsibility for his or her own welfare and, by such a commitment, helping the patient to become free of complete dependence on others. Third, for maximum rehabilitation of this evergrowing patient population, the team approach is essential. Only through the cooperative efforts of the many whose services can benefit the respiratory patient will we be able to set up a practical program that will permit us to evaluate the patient physiologically, socially, and economically and, on the basis of this evaluation, help him or her to regain optimum well-being and independence.

References

1. Hodgkin, J.E.: Chronic obstructive pulmonary disease: current concepts in diagnosis and comprehensive care, Park Ridge, Ill., 1979, American College of Chest Physicians.
2. Petty, T.L.: Chronic obstructive pulmonary disease, New York, 1978, Marcel Dekker, Inc.
3. Haas, A., et al.: Pulmonary therapy and rehabilitation: principles and practices, Baltimore, 1979, The Williams & Wilkins Co.
4. Brashear, R.E., and Rhodes, M.L.: Chronic obstructive lung disease: clinical treatment and management, St. Louis, 1978, The C.V. Mosby Co.
5. Miller, W.F.: In Backer, T.E., et al., editors: Annual review of rehabilitation, New York, 1980, Springer Publishing Co., Inc.
6. Pierce, A.K., and Saltzman, H.A., chairmen: Conference on the scientific basis of respiratory therapy, Amer. Rev. Respir. Dis. **110**(2):1-204, 1974.
7. Lertzman, M.M., and Cherniack, R.M.: Rehabilitation of patients with chronic obstructive pulmonary disease, Am. Rev. Respir. Dis. **114**:1145, 1976.
8. Miller, W.F.: Rehabilitation of patients with chronic obstructive pulmonary disease, Med. Clin. North Am. **51**:349, 1967.
9. Barach, A.L.: Chronic obstructive lung disease: postural relief of dyspnea, Arch. Phys. Med. Rehabil. **55**:494, 1974.
10. Mueller, R.E., Petty, T.L., and Filley, G.F.: Ventilation and arterial blood gas changes induced by pursed-lip breathing, J. Appl. Physiol. **28**:784, 1970.
11. Pierce, A.K., Paez, P.N., and Miller, W.F.: Exercise therapy with the aid of a portable oxygen supply in patients with emphysema, Am. Rev. Respir. Dis. **91**:653, 1965.
12. Pierce, A.K., et al.: Responses to exercise training in patients with emphysema, Arch. Intern. Med. **113**:28, 1964.
13. Barach, A.L., and Petty, T.L.: Is chronic obstructive lung disease improved by physical exercise? J.A.M.A. **234**:854, 1975.
14. Petty, T.L.: Pulmonary rehabilitation, Respir. Care **22**:199, 1977.
15. Petty, T.L., et al.: A comprehensive program for chronic airways obstruction, Ann. Intern. Med. **70**:1109, 1969.
16. Petty, T.L.: Intensive and rehabilitative respiratory care, ed. 2, Philadelphia, 1974, Lea & Febiger.
17. Petty, T.L.: Pulmonary rehabilitation, Am. Rev. Respir. Dis. **122**(2):159, 1980.
18. Heinman, H.O.: Alcohol and the lung, Am. J. Med. **63**:81, 1977.
19. Gaskell, D.V., and Webber, B.A.: The Brompton Hospital guide to chest physiotherapy, Oxford, England, 1977, Blackwell Scientific Publications.
20. Thacker, E.W.: Postural drainage and respiratory control, ed. 3, Chicago, 1973, Year Book Medical Publishers, Inc.
21. Frownfelter, D.L., editor: Chest physical therapy and pulmonary rehabilitation: an interdiscipliniary approach, Chicago, 1978, Year Book Medical Publishers, Inc.
22. Nocturnal Oxygen Therapy Trial Group: Continuous or nocturnal oxygen therapy in hypoxemic chronic obstructive lung disease, Ann. Intern. Med. **93**:391, 1980.
23. McPherson, S.P.: Respiratory therapy equipment, ed. 2, St. Louis, 1981, The C.V. Mosby Co.
24. Petty, T.L., et al.: Out patient oxygen therapy in chronic obstructive pulmonary disease: a review of 13 years' experience and an evaluation of modes of therapy, Arch. Intern. Med. **139**:28, 1979.
25. Chusid, E.L., et al.: Treatment of hypoxemia with an oxygen enricher, Chest **76**:278, 1979.
26. Brown, H.V., and Ziment, I.: Evaluation of an oxygen concentrator in patients with COPD, Respir. Ther. **5**:55, 1978.
27. Lowson, K.V., Drummond, M.F., and Bishop, J.M.: Costing new series: long-term domiciliary oxygen therapy, Lancet **1**:1146, 1981.
28. Dudley, D.L., et al.: Psychosocial concomitants to rehabilitation in chronic obstructive pulmonary disease: psychosocial treatment, part 2, Chest **77**:544, 1980.
29. Conine, T.A., and Evans, J.H.: Sexual

adjustments in chronic obstructive pulmonary disease, Respir. Care **26:**871, 1981.

30. Saltzman, A., and Salzano, J.V.: Effects of carbohydrate metabolism upon respiratory gas exchange in normal man, J. Appl. Physiol. **30:**228, 1971.

31. Elwyn, D.H.: Nutritional requirements of adult surgical patients, Crit. Care Med. **8:**9, 1980.

Chapter 16

The organization and services of a respiratory therapy department

PATRICK M. McDONALD

The modern respiratory therapy department is a challenging and dynamic place in which to work. Technologic advances in the medical field create an ever-changing environment for therapists nationwide. The one aspect that must remain unchanged, however, is the total commitment to quality—with reference to patient care, to the profession, and to the individual department. Advancements in technology will never replace a dedicated professional.

In attempting to round out our discussion of what a therapist should know of anatomy, physiology, physics, acid-base theory, pulmonary pathophysiology, equipment, and other equally essential elements, it is perhaps most appropriate to discuss the structure and function of the therapist's work unit. While by no means covering respiratory therapy departments in detail, we cover those items that are indeed common and essential to all.

Over the past several years, hospitals have been facing an increasing load of patients with cardiopulmonary diseases. Technologic and educational advances continue to improve the quality of care rendered. The techniques that have evolved for the treatment of these patients require the supervision of highly educated and skilled professionals, whose degree of specialization is beyond the scope of the average attending physician or nurse. In response to this need the technical specialty of respiratory therapy emerged to take its place in the hospital organization. Historically, the predecessor of respiratory therapy was the hospital oxygen service. However, its highly skilled successor bears little resemblance, for during respiratory therapy's evolution, the therapist has undergone intensive medically supervised education and training, enabling him or her to provide skills and service of a very complex and specialized nature. Because of the large number of patients who can benefit from the well-organized services of respiratory therapy, it is the responsibility of every hospital to provide such services. The high use of respiratory therapy services where competent and effective departments operate is ample proof of their acceptance by the medical profession. After observing the growth of this specialty and reviewing the experience of several hospitals with active services, we can make the conservative estimate that a competent and efficient department in a busy hospital will probably provide some form of respiratory therapy to more than half of the patients admitted.

Services of a respiratory therapy department	It is not necessary to describe in detail the services offered by respiratory therapy, as they are covered in previous chapters; the outline below summarizes them. It can be noted that these services may cut across established hospital departmental lines, the administrative implications of which will be mentioned later.

Respiratory therapy services

Therapeutic gases
    Oxygen: mask, catheter, cannula, face tent
    Helium-oxygen mixtures
    Carbon dioxide–oxygen mixtures
Aerosols and humidity
    Bronchodilators, wetting agents, mucolytics, antibiotics, steroids
    High humidity, aerosolized water, high-density aerosols
    Procurement of sputum specimens for cytologic and bacterial examination
Mechanical ventilation
    Inspiratory positive pressure breathing (IPPB)

Administration of aerosols for airway patency
Prevention of postoperative atelectasis
Treatment of acute pulmonary edema
Mechanically assisted volume delivery to those patients unable to take a deep breath
Assisted ventilation for inadequate spontaneous breathing
Continuous ventilation by volume- and/or pressure-regulated ventilators
Monitoring by blood gas analysis, tidal volume, lung compliance
Maintenance of airway patency by tracheobronchial aspiration
Controlled ventilation for apnea
Continuous ventilation by volume-regulated, flow-regulated, pressure-regulated ventilators
Maintenance of adequate volume, flow rate, pressure
Maintenance of cardiopulmonary status
Physical therapy and rehabilitation
Ambulatory service for aerosol and pressure breathing treatments
Postural drainage
Corrective breathing exercises
Oxygen-supported ambulatory services
Pulmonary rehabilitation
Integration of treatments into custom-made progressive program for home care
Patient instruction
Follow-up supervision
Equipment cleaning, sterilization, and storage
Pulmonary function testing
Minimum requirement examinations for routine respiratory care
Spirometry
Lung volume measurements
Nitrogen washout
Helium equilibration
Body plethysmograph
Arterial or arteriolized blood gas analysis
pH
Oxygenation (Pa_{O_2}, oxygen saturation, oxygen content)
Carbon dioxide tension (Pa_{CO_2})
Measurement of metabolic components (base excess, plasma bicarbonate, standard or T_{40} bicarbonate)
Selected examinations
Alveolar ventilation
Dead space volume
Arterial-alveolar carbon dioxide difference
Pulmonary diffusion measurement
Pulmonary compliance measurement
Oxygen uptake measurement
Pulmonary stress tests
Emergency cardiopulmonary resuscitation—endotracheal intubation and airway management
Advanced clinical designations
Patient, staff, physician, and nursing education

Extracorporeal pump operation
Physiologic and hemodynamic monitoring
High-frequency ventilation
Clinical research and cardiopulmonary management and diagnosis
Biomedical and preventive maintenance

This list is by no means complete because the boundaries of respiratory therapy are traditionally flexible. From hospital to hospital there will be variations in the complexities, numbers, and types of services offered. However, respiratory therapy departments in many major centers are already actively involved in most of these pursuits. It is essential that all departments be developed with a philosophy of flexibility and cooperation with other disciplines to allow for future growth.

Departmental structure: administration and personnel	The organization of an effective respiratory therapy department includes some or all of the following personnel: medical director, associate medical directors, technical director (department manager), assistant technical director, shift supervisors, area supervisors, staff respiratory therapists and technicians, pulmonary laboratory technicians, inservice and clinical instructors, equipment technicians, therapists involved in clinical research, pulmonary rehabilitation coordinators, monitoring and surgical technicians, and clerical assistance. Certainly, some departments will not have all of these, and there may be other job specialties, according to individual hospital needs and areas of emphasis.

Fig. 16-1 outlines a suggested departmental organization for a medium to large department, showing the relationship among the components of the department and between the department and the hospital administration. This is presented only as a possible suggestion, flexible enough to lend itself to the needs of any hospital.

The departmental organization should be an independent unit with its own budget and managerial support stemming from the hospital administration. Thus, in administrative and fiscal matters, the director of the department works directly with the hospital administration. The education section applies to those hospitals that include in their structure a respiratory therapy school or that have departments large enough to maintain a continuing inservice educational program. Inservice and continuing education are essential elements of any progressive respiratory therapy department. The medium to small community hospitals will be primarily interested in the service and laboratory functions of their respiratory therapy departments. A small hospital may be adequately served by one medical director supervising a service function and a modest pulmonary function laboratory. In a respiratory therapy department where there is a larger demand, there may be an effective division of labor, with two or more associate directors employed. Here the duties may be divided, with one director responsible for service functions, another for the laboratory, and perhaps yet another for critical care and clinical research projects.

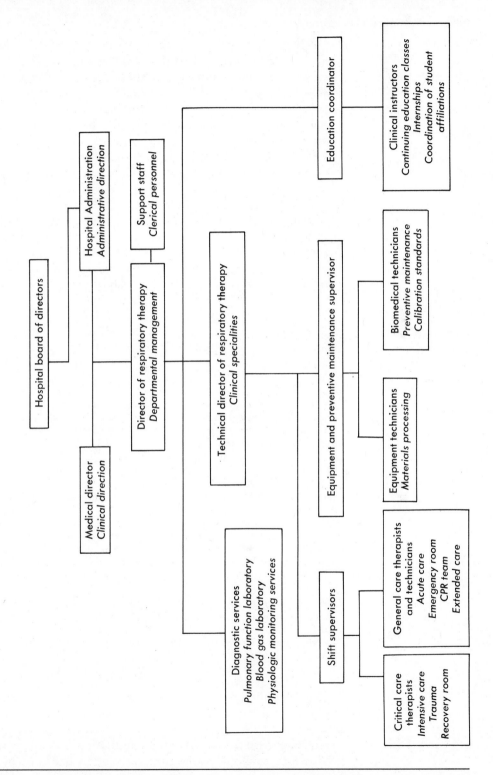

Fig. 16-1 Organizational outline for respiratory therapy service. (Modified from forms used by the Donald N. Sharp Memorial Community Hospital, San Diego, Calif.)

In the largest hospitals, where the work load may be exceptionally heavy, the administrative and professional relationships may be varied again. In some instances, it is practical to consider the service function of the respiratory therapy department, the pulmonary function laboratory, the training and educational facilities in respiratory therapy, and the respiratory rehabilitation program for patients with respiratory diseases all as components of a larger professional unit. Such a facility might have an overall chief, and the various subdivisions of the department might have their own individual directors. Professional cooperation and exchange of ideas with involved physicians ensure the highest degree of patient care.

If a respiratory intensive care unit is available, it should be the direct responsibility of the respiratory therapy department. Its supervision and clinical personnel are taken care of through the regular department personnel and the pulmonary function laboratory. The only nondepartmental services needed are nursing and perhaps physical therapy, and these can be provided through a mutually beneficial agreement with those services.

Classification of personnel

As a result of some significant changes in the field during the past few years, definitions of officially recognized levels in respiratory therapy are as follows:

respiratory therapist A graduate of a school approved by the American Medical Association (AMA) designed to qualify the graduate for the registry examination of the National Board for Respiratory Therapy (NBRT). Usually this means a 2- or 4-year hospital or college affiliation, granting the graduate an associate's degree or bachelor's degree.

registered respiratory therapist (RRT) A respiratory therapist who has successfully completed the registry examination of the NBRT.

respiratory therapy technician A graduate of an AMA-approved school designed to qualify the graduate for the technician certification examination of the NBRT. Usually, this means a 1-year hospital-based program combining a special curriculum of basic sciences with supervised clinical experience.

certified respiratory therapy technician (CRTT) A respiratory therapy technician who has successfully completed the technician certification examination of the NBRT.

respiratory therapy assistant One who has received on-the-job training as part of employment in a respiratory therapy service. For such a program, there are no official guidelines or credentials. On-the-job training is being phased out in favor of one of the two formal therapist or technician programs previously described.

respiratory therapy student One who is enrolled in a program that follows AMA-approved guidelines or essentials of the Joint Review Committee for Respiratory Therapy Education (JRCRTE).

respiratory therapy student trainee One employed in a hospital respiratory therapy service while engaged in a technical or therapist program that follows AMA-approved essentials. For our purposes, the last two categories can jointly be called "students."

Generally, the term *respiratory therapist* often refers to anyone involved in technical respiratory care, but two basic personnel levels exist: the respiratory therapist and the respiratory therapy technician. Their duties and responsibilities often overlap depending on local institutional needs, geographic area, and personnel availability. However, it can be generalized that by virtue of differences of depth and orientation of therapist and technician educational curricula, respiratory therapists often assume responsibilities for managerial or other high-level administrative supervision, clinical supervision in special areas, supervision of teaching programs, development and implementation of special projects and research, the more complex duties of formalized patient assessment, and physiologic monitoring, as well as often assuming the overall responsibility for pulmonary management of patients in critical care. Respiratory therapy technicians, on the other hand, should be responsible for giving most of the general bedside respiratory therapy to patients not critically ill, participating in some clinical instruction, and assisting with special projects.

The functional relationship between therapist and technician is summarized in Table 16-1. Obviously, this format cannot and should not be applied dogmatically, for in real life, the job should and does go to the one who can do it best. Also, education and experience are not the sole indicators of who shall be assigned therapist or technician duties; technical performance, attitude, and commitment to the profession are far more reliable than the label one carries on graduation. In general, however, higher responsibilities, both supervisory and clinical, will fall into the assigned duties of the therapist classification, while the clinical emphasis of the technician's schooling should direct him or her naturally into tasks associated with general patient care. The success of any department will be in direct proportion to the efficiency and skill of its personnel, with emphasis on specific duties.

Table 16-1 Functions of respiratory therapists and respiratory therapy technicians	Therapist	Technician	Therapist	Technician
	Management and supervision		Resuscitation, emergency	X
	Diagnostic procedures		Teaching	
	Arterial blood collection	X	Clinical	X
	Blood gas analysis		Curriculum development	
	Lung volume measurements		Special procedures	
	Compliance studies		Therapy	
	Spirometry, bedside	X	Aerosol/humidity	X
	Spirometry, laboratory		Gas	X
	Equipment		Positive pressure breathing	X
	Evaluation		Ventilation, mechanical	
	Maintenance	X	Initiate	
	Modification		Maintain	X
	Chest physiotherapy		Patient assessment	
	Breathing exercises	X	Therapeutic objectives of care	
	Postural drainage	X	Fiberoptic bronchoscopy assistance	
	Pulmonary rehabilitation		Critical care	
			Clinical research	

Modified from Egan, D.F.: What is inhalation therapy? Clin. Notes Respir. Dis. **11**:3, 1972.

Medical director   The decisions as to whether the departmental directorship should be in the hands of one or more persons or should be fulltime or parttime are matters to be determined by each hospital's needs. Whatever arrangement is made, the hospital can be assured that there will be an increasing amount of time demanded of the medical director as the department grows, and this must be taken into consideration in planning for the future. It almost goes without saying, therefore, that the respiratory therapy department needs a fulltime, *active,* medical director. Such anticipated growth may necessitate the addition of associate directors as time goes on. The medical director must be a physician who is interested in chest diseases and who has had extensive training and clinical experience in this area. Whether the hours are fulltime or parttime, the responsibility as director of the department will be fulltime, and he or she must be reasonably available for consultation and advice for the safe and effective supervision of the department, both to other physicians and to the respiratory therapy staff.

The medical director must be a member of the hospital staff and thus will be affiliated with one of the major hospital departments. From a practical point of view, only two major departments lend themselves well to affiliation with respiratory therapy—pulmonary medicine and anesthesiology. Historically, many departments of respiratory care have been organized under the direction of anesthesiologists for two primary reasons: (1) the common foundation of pulmonary physiology and technical nature of the duties underlying both anesthesiology and respiratory therapy, and (2) the presence of anesthesiologists in the hospital for extended periods of time. Anesthesiologists may be justly credited with much of the early development of respiratory therapy, making it into the specialty it has become. The evolution of respiratory therapy, however, has evoked some subtle changes in its function that affect its relationship to anesthesiology. Whereas the therapist in the early days of the technology performed relatively simple tasks, under the direct guidance of the medical director, the contemporary therapist is permitted a significant degree of independence in judgment and plays an important role in patient care and assessment. Respiratory therapy, as it is now practiced, primarily directs itself to the diagnosis and treatment of diseases and medical complications of surgery or trauma. To realize their full potential, therapists must be well rounded in many aspects of clinical medicine. It is not sufficient for therapists to be skilled merely in specific tasks, but they must understand cardiopulmonary physiology as well as the changes in physiology wrought by disease. Such a view implies a clinical and medical orientation in the teaching and direction of respiratory therapy, most realistically provided by a pulmonary physician trained in the physiologic and clinical aspects of chest diseases. Ideally, the department's medical direction would be provided by a pulmonary physician, with input welcome from the anesthesiology service.

Unfortunately, there is still a shortage of clinicians able or willing to undertake the medical direction of a respiratory therapy department, but there is hope for an improved supply in the future as greater emphasis is placed on postgraduate training in chest disease. It should also be noted that the availability of the anesthesiologist for management of respiratory therapy is often more apparent than real. Since the anesthesiologist's first responsibility is to the operating and recovery rooms, as the work load of respiratory therapy grows, he or she may be increasingly unavailable for its supervision. The choice of the medical director depends on available personnel and the objectives of respiratory therapy in the individual hospital, but a general recommendation can be made. If the treatment of cardiopulmonary disease in a given hospital is to be completely managed by each attending physician, and respiratory therapy is to provide only a skilled technical service of limited scope, supervision and quality, control of such services can be performed by either an anesthesiologist or an internist. If, however, respiratory therapy is to function in state-of-the-art capabilities, integrating diagnostic laboratory facilities, professional consultation, referral services, and outpatient and rehabilitation care, a clinically trained pulmonary physician is preferred as medical director.

The medical director of the respiratory therapy department is professionally responsible for the clinical function of the department. Because of this responsibility, he or she should be afforded considerable authority in establishing the professional policies and practices of respiratory therapy in the hospital, although any major policy involving patient care or relationships between the department and staff physicians should be approved by the hospital executive medical board. This body represents a group of the medical director's peers, and such a move would ensure understanding of policies and procedures as well as guaranteeing maximum cooperation at all levels. The major responsibilities of the medical director include the following: medical supervision of care of patients with respiratory diseases (including consultation and referral), acute respiratory care, intensive care, ambulatory care, and pulmonary function evaluation; development and approval of departmental clinical policies and procedures; medical direction of the respiratory therapy inservice training and education program; education of medical and nursing staffs in pulmonary physiology and pathophysiology; input into the selection and promotion of students, therapists, and technicians; access to personnel records and maintenance of medical records; and input into the preparation of the departmental budget.

The medical director's involvement in personnel and budgetary matters, while by no means extensive, should be welcomed in order to provide integration of medical and administrative thinking into the department's affairs. The normal, continued growth of respiratory care has burdened departmental leadership with problems of major dimensions. A prime challenge to medical and technical directors of respiratory therapy services is to provide increasingly better quality of patient service, but at lower costs. This is the current philosophy of *cost containment* and *cost-effectiveness*. The need for administrative education for medical directors has long been recognized by those active in this work, but only recently has it been given significant exposure. Physicians who contemplate assuming medical directorships of respiratory therapy services must be willing and ready to accept some administrative responsibilities. It is to be hoped that meaningful exposure to relevant aspects of hospital management and medical economics will one day be part of pulmonary education.

As a hospital service, the department provides facilities available on the order of all staff physicians. At the same time, the services so provided are under the responsibility of the medical director of the department. Whereas care must be taken to minimize the risk of interference with the autonomy of the attending physician, close control of the proper use of respiratory therapy services must be ensured by the medical director. These objectives can easily be obtained by stressing cooperation among hospital administration, medical staff, and the respiratory therapy department. Many therapeutic procedures can be classified as "standard," with little ambiguity as to their function and, generally, complete understanding of their clinical application. This group might include such services as oxygen and aerosol therapies. The direct responsibility of the medical director in the application of these services requires little more than ensuring a smoothly running department.

In contrast, the safe and effective use of some respiratory therapy techniques requires much experience as well as specific professional and technical knowledge. This is especially true in the management of the critically ill patient on a ventilator, the techniques of rehabilitation and chronic care, and the interpretation of pulmonary function tests. There are two administrative policies that can be used to handle these sensitive areas, the choice of which will depend on each local hospital situation. First, it can be established that the use of certain specified treatments will require prior official note consultation with the medical director, who will follow the patient's management with the attending physician. Second, the medical director can be given the authority to observe closely all patients receiving the services of his or her department and to interfere with the management at any time the medical director's judgment determines that the best interests of the patient are not being served. The degree of sophistication of the medical staff in the management of cardiopulmonary problems will usually determine the type of medical supervisory program most suitable. It is strongly suggested that the following philosophic observation be accepted: At the present time, respiratory therapy is still a growing field, and the exact legal and moral responsibilities of a respiratory therapy medical director toward other physicians and their patients is not always clear. It must be assumed that the director is responsible for the actions of therapists under his or her jurisdiction and for the safety and efficacy of the procedures of the department. It is only just, therefore, that being asked to assume responsibility, the medical director also be given the authority to control his or her sphere of responsibility. Further experience with the medical staff with which the medical director interacts will be necessary to delineate more precisely the boundaries of the position.

Technical director   The efficiency of departmental operation will depend on the technical director (managing director). This key figure must be well trained in all aspects of respiratory therapy and experienced in its clinical application. He or she must be thoroughly versed in the techniques of therapy and the function of equipment and must possess leadership qualities and management ability. Although the position will probably have more prestige if the director is registered by the National Board for Respiratory Therapy, registration alone is not sufficient, for there are many registered therapists who do not have the other necessary qualities of the technical director. No guideline exists to indicate the depth of experience necessary for this position, but as a generality, to become prepared for the duties of technical director, the average therapist would need a minimum of 3 years of practical experience in the field, following training, and no less than 2 more years in supervisory duties. Whereas the medical director is responsible for the clinical policies and professional functioning of the department, the technical director is responsible for the daily operation and management of this service. The administrative authority of the position must be well understood and completely supported by the medical director, since the technical director is an important link between the medical director and the technical staff. Among the technical director's duties are assignment of staff according to departmental need; the maintenance of payroll data on all personnel; development and enforcement of a system that accurately measures staff productivity; preparation of the departmental budget; development and implementation of special projects; generation of statistical data for reports of departmental activity to justify personnel and new areas of emphasis; advice and assistance to technical personnel; assistance in the training and orientation of new therapists; audits of all phases of patient care with recommendation for their improvement; and major equipment evaluation.

Assistant technical director

One or more assistant technical directors will be needed, according to the size of the department. The assistant should possess technical skills at least equal to those of the technical director but does not need as much administrative experience. He or she has a responsible dual role. In the absence of the technical director, the assistant acts as the director of the department, but in daily operation, he or she is a troubleshooter and may also function as the first shift supervisor. The assistant supervises the service in the respiratory care or intensive care unit and consults with or advises staff therapists in the management of difficult patients, especially when it is necessary to improvise techniques or equipment. The assistant takes an active role in the training and orientation of students and therapists and evaluates all new or recently repaired equipment. He or she is also actively involved in clinical research relevant to respiratory care.

Shift supervisor

The three shift supervisors are responsible for the respiratory therapy service function during their particular segments of the day. Generally, they are directly responsible for the staff therapists and technicians on their shifts, although in large hospitals they may have the assistance of area supervisors or coordinators. Shift supervisors assign duties of subordinates to respond to needs, assist staff personnel with all problems, participate in the work load when necessary, respond to emergency resuscitation calls, assist in clinical training or student supervision, and schedule personnel assigned to their shift. Specific duties of these important people will vary considerably from place to place. The difference in overall hospital activity between shifts also gives different responsibilities to the respective shift supervisors. For example, whereas the first and second shift supervisors might be primarily concerned with fulfilling requests for service, the third shift supervisor might be responsible for overseeing clerical work requiring technical knowledge. These supervisors must be flexible and adaptable, as well as mature, experienced, and totally supportive of the department's philosophy and purpose.

Area supervisor

In areas of the hospital where there is a high concentration of work volume or special services, an area supervisor is needed. Quality of performance can be better achieved in areas of heavy work load by an area supervisor. Perhaps more frequently, there is need for area supervision in specialty areas such as intensive care or respiratory care units, recovery and emergency rooms, and general care, rehabilitation, and outpatient areas. Well-trained area supervisors often serve in these locations, overseeing the performance of staff therapists assigned to them and participating in educational programs to teach new personnel to maintain proficiency of the regular staff. The area supervisor is a specialist with specific technical expertise in a particular area, in contrast with a shift supervisor with wider supervisory skills.

Equipment manager

The equipment manager supervises the overall operation of the equipment area and materials management and preventive maintenance area of the department. He or she coordinates all new product evaluations and solicits input from the medical director, technical director, assistant technical director, and other interested parties. The equipment manager also develops and implements systems to ensure that all equipment is appropriately functioning and that all supply and equipment items essential to the day-to-day operation of the department are always available. Finally, this individual coordinates preventive maintenance of all equipment, which includes calibration and repair. The equipment manager's position is extremely vital to the department, in that it calls for a high degree of communication skill, technical ability, mechanical ability, and the ability to supervise individuals.

Staff respiratory therapist

Staff therapists are expected to know therapeutic modalities of care, including equipment structure, function, indications and contraindications for the use of particular types of equipment, and physiologic hazards associated with use of different types of therapy. They must also know the basic maintenance procedures for equipment in the event of malfunction. Before being allowed to treat patients, therapists must demonstrate an understanding of anatomy and physiology of respiration and circulation, both normal and abnormal, as it applies to respiratory therapy, and have a good working knowledge of the pathophysiology of all diseases that affect the respiratory system. They will be responsible for most, if not all, of the technical functions associated with the respiratory therapy service.

Because respiratory therapists have close and intimate patient contact, it is essential that they be able to establish a good rapport with patients. This requires a stable personality, a strong motivation to work with the sick, a professional appearance, and a strong sense of loyalty to the department and institution in which they will work. They must understand the need for tact and the principles of medical ethics, since patients frequently develop a strong attachment to their therapist and often confide in him or her. The skill of the therapist in managing as well as treating the patient is an important factor in the patient's response to therapy. Extreme care and screening are needed in hiring personnel for this important job.

Pulmonary function and arterial blood gas laboratory personnel

An experienced and well-trained respiratory therapist is especially desirable to operate a pulmonary function laboratory. Background knowledge of cardiopulmonary physiology as well as of clinical chest diseases makes the purposes of pulmonary function testing more meaningful to the therapist than to a technician without this experience. Insight into laboratory procedures makes the therapist a good judge of the reliability of results and better able to recognize inaccuracies or laboratory errors or inconsistencies. Also, a pulmonary function laboratory staffed with respiratory therapists and technicians has close technical rapport with the clinical respiratory therapy personnel.

The technical director of the pulmonary function laboratory must know the details and techniques of all the procedures in the laboratory and be able to train or orient students or new employees. He or she is responsible for supervising the quality of the work done by the therapists, the scheduling of assignments, the maintenance of laboratory records, and the maintenance of an inventory of supplies. The therapist's knowledge of equipment must be sufficient to recognize malfunctions and know what measures are necessary for repair of equipment. He or she also assists the director of the department with special projects.

In many institutions, the pulmonary function laboratory personnel may also perform or be responsible for drawing and analysis of arterial blood gas samples. In small institutions, this may be a duty broadly assigned to the respiratory therapy staff. In larger centers, however, it is not uncommon for both the pulmonary function and blood gas laboratory personnel to be a group of individuals specifically trained in the complexities of many of the tests performed in these areas. Additionally, a select group of pulmonary laboratory personnel is more desirable than "rotating" each staff person through this area, because it ensures quality control and more reproducible results.

The therapists and technicians in the laboratory must be as well versed in the procedures and techniques as the technical director, without the managerial or supervisory experience or authority being a necessity. With careful selection of personnel, it is possible to teach non–respiratory care personnel or those interested in respiratory care (such as students during nonschool hours) to perform such specific duties as blood gas analysis for laboratory coverage.

Education coordinator

Wherever respiratory therapy services are available, there should also be a relevant educational program suitable for the size and sophistication of the hospital and its staff. This may vary from a series of periodic demonstrations of respiratory therapy equipment and techniques to an AMA-approved, structured school of respiratory therapy. For the former, one therapist would be given its responsibility and designated as education coordinator or staff development coordinator, assisted by instructors as needed, drawn from supervision and staff. In the latter, the responsible person is usually referred to as the program director of the school, with an associate as clinical education director. Instructors must be well trained and experienced, able to transmit their knowledge to others. The technical instructors are especially valuable in teaching procedures and equipment function and for supervision of the clinical application of respiratory therapy at the bedside, but other subjects may be delegated to them as their qualifications permit. Capable therapists should be given teaching roles if they are motivated to participate and are truly interested in providing quality educational experiences. An important contribution of the instructor is the evaluation of the student and his or her recommendation of the degree of independent action that a student may be expected to perform. The instructors are accountable under the medical director, correlating their material with the medical director's overall objectives and reporting their findings and recommendations to the director for final action.

In between these two areas, a staff development coordinator in most departments would assume responsibility for regularly scheduled inservices for the respiratory therapy staff, orientation of new personnel, and development of educational programs for new techniques and skills for which the department will assume responsibility. In all cases, nonetheless, a good educational program requires the instructors to be dedicated, knowledgeable, able to present a quality demonstration, and above all, *prepared*.

Equipment personnel

Although not an officially recognized member of respiratory therapy personnel, the equipment aide has been used extensively to great advantage over the years. Many important tasks in an active respiratory therapy service do not require the technical knowledge of a full-fledged therapist or technician. To make the most of valuable labor, nontechnical personnel can be employed to perform these duties. Such functions as cleaning, ordering, restocking, sterilizing, and packaging of equipment, delivery of equipment, repair and maintenance, and some clerical work are better done by those other than patient-care-oriented therapists or technicians. The use of aides where safe and practical is to be encouraged. The best results are to be found in the use of students who are interested in becoming involved in their chosen field and learning as well as enjoying their field during nonschool hours.

Departmental operation: distribution of services

Local hospital needs and available personnel will be the determining factors in time coverage and scope of services. Ideally, respiratory therapy services should be available 24 hours a day, 7 days a week. Every attempt should be made to complete the maximum work volume during the day and afternoon shift, and for this, the full cooperation of the medical and nursing staffs is essential. Physicians should be encouraged to order therapy in advance so that it may be scheduled at the start of each working day. The supervisor should always attempt to leave flexibility in assignments to accommodate emergencies, but this requires careful planning of more routine work.

The provision of services during nights and on weekends always presents a problem. In general, only emergency cases and patients most acutely ill are serviced during those hours. There is no general rule for the classification of patients according to need for respiratory therapy services. However, the following list is offered as a suggested priority scale to help respiratory therapy, medical, and nursing personnel in scheduling priorities of work assignments for respiratory therapy services:

Priorities of patient care
1. Emergency resuscitation
2. Continuous mechanical ventilation
3. Any intensive care area service
4. Emergency room care
5. Postoperative care
6. Oxygen or humidity administration
7. Prescheduled positive-pressure breathing
8. Physical therapy and incentive spirometry
9. Elective diagnostic studies

This grouping represents a common-sense classification of patients from those most in need of attention to those least in need. The objective of such a priority scale is not to restrict the application of respiratory therapy services but rather to enable the department to make maximum use of them. Proper assessment of the needs of patients will determine the acuity of patients, so that the highest quality care can be given by the staff to those patients in the greatest need, and also give justification of the priorities of therapy.

Pulmonary function evaluation facilities should be available wherever respiratory therapy is being used to its maximum potential. At the current stage of respiratory therapy as a clinical specialty, therapeutic modalities frequently need some physiologic evaluation to determine proper therapy. This is especially true wherever patients are being maintained on mechanical ventilation. In such circumstances, it is mandatory that the physiologic status be monitored by frequent examination of blood for pH, carbon dioxide tension, and oxygenation. The experienced therapist will use these data along with other criteria to adjust the ventilators accordingly. Since patients in ventilatory failure are as much in need of close supervision during the night and on weekends as at other times, it is necessary that facilities for blood gas monitoring be available at all hours as well. The ease with which this can be accomplished will be determined by the available laboratory facilities and personnel and is another valuable service the respiratory therapists must perform. It is ideal to have fulltime blood gas laboratory personnel on duty around the clock, 7 days a week.

It is frequently practical to employ the parttime services of personnel who are not respiratory therapists in the blood gas laboratory. Although they may know little cardiopulmonary physiology, if they are receptive and learn thoroughly, they can be taught techniques of blood gas analysis and free the regular staff to perform patient care services during the working day. The success of this approach depends on careful selection, meticulous instruction, and close supervision. As with equipment aides, an individual interested in respiratory therapy as a career will afford the best choice. This can be a prospective student or a current student outside of school hours.

Scheduling of assignments

The assistant director or shift supervisor designates the work areas and assigns patients to the staff therapists or area supervisors at the beginning of the day. A "zone" system is usually the most effective, and with experience, most hospitals can be divided into areas according to the average work load density. One therapist may be designated to circulate, helping in the busy areas, responding to emergencies, and performing such routine duties as monitoring oxygen concentrations, checking oxygen humidifiers, and examining other operating equipment. Arrangements are made to give priority service to intensive care units and the emergency room as needs dictate.

Throughout the day, all calls for services are submitted to the clerical staff in the assistant director's or supervisor's office. A written record should be kept to include date and time, nature of the request, and its disposition. The record is kept on file. The supervisor is responsible for expediting service during the day's operation and shifting personnel on assignments as needed, a critical task that requires skill, judgment, and knowledge of the hospital's day-to-day function and unique logistics.

Records and accounts

Each hospital has its own record and accounting system. Various types of computerized techniques with memory storage and retrieval capabilities allow for great flexibility in statistical work load, billing, and other reporting of data. However, many hospitals must yet rely on manual systems, and every attempt should be made to reduce clerical work to a minimum. The use of a portable or an "in-the-room" charting system enables the therapist or technician to carry around a record card for each patient for whom he or she is responsible. All treatments or services for a given day are entered in this card or chart, and at the end of the day charge tickets are executed for each patient and submitted to the accounting office. From the accumulated patient records, data are obtained for a statistical account of the departmental activities and transferred to a work sheet. The work sheet tabulates such items as the number of patients treated, the number of days the patient has been receiving treatment, the num-

RESPIRATORY THERAPY DEPARTMENT NOTES • GENERAL ACTIVITIES

DATE	TIME	MODE	DESCRIBER	DUR.	VOLUMES SPONT.	AUG.	PULSE PRE	DUR	POST	RESPIRATIONS PRE	DUR	POST	F_1O_2	O_2 LPM	TIMER NO.	METER READING

NOC | DAY | EVE   COMMENTS:

REV | N-REV   NO.   SIGNATURE

A

PULMONARY MEDICINE

JAMES M. SCHIBANOFF, M.D., MEDICAL DIRECTOR

PULMONARY FUNCTION TESTS, RESPIRATORY THERAPY AND BLOOD GAS ANALYSIS

#395.19 3/81

ADDRESSOGRAPH

HOSPITAL NO.

PATIENT NAME _____ AGE ____

PHYSICIAN _____

ROOM NO. OR ADDRESS _____

Continued.

Fig. 16-2 Departmental charting forms, which provide essential patient information and data for billing, statistics, and record-keeping. Copies are routed directly to the department. (Modified from forms used by the Donald N. Sharp Memorial Community Hospital, San Diego, Calif.)

DONALD N. SHARP MEMORIAL COMMUNITY HOSPITAL
7901 FROST STREET, SAN DIEGO, CALIFORNIA 92123

RESPIRATORY THERAPY DEPARTMENT NOTES • CONTINUOUS VENTILATORY SUPPORT RECORD

VENTILATOR	Date
	Time
	Vent
	Mode
	Cycled
	PIP
	Vt Set
	Vt Exhaled
	Static Pressure
	EEP
	Static Comp.
	Dynamic Comp.
	f SET TOTAL
	FIO2 SET Anal
	Flow Rate
	Sighs xf
	Temp Syst
	I:E
	Vdm
	Alarms Y N
	Cuff Press.
BLOOD GASES	pH
	Pco2
	Po2
	HCO3-
	BE
	PT Temp
	Time
	Sample Site
MONITORING	Ve Spont Total
	Spont f
	Vt Spont
	VC
	MIP
	BP
	Pulse
	Therapist

B

395 11

Fig. 6-2, cont'd   For legend see page 693.

RESPIRATORY THERAPY NOTES

SIGNATURE / INITIALS:

PULMONARY MEDICINE

JAMES M. SCHIBANOFF, M.D. — MEDICAL DIRECTOR

PULMONARY FUNCTION TESTS, RESPIRATORY
THERAPY AND BLOOD GAS ANALYSIS

HOSPITAL NO _____

PATIENT'S NAME _____ AGE _____

PHYSICIAN _____

ROOM NO. OR
ADDRESS _____

▲ TYPE, PRINT OR ADDRESSOGRAPH PATIENT IDENTIFICATION ▲

Fig. 6-2, cont'd For legend see page 693.

bers of individual services, and patient charges according to the type of service provided. Each month, the total of the work sheets is recorded in a monthly statistical report, which is submitted to hospital administration, the accounting department, and the director of the department, and these reports form the basis for evaluating departmental progress. Many modifications of this system are possible, especially for recall of group data, and can be achieved by special filing procedures. Because each therapist must keep track of service data on patients scattered all over the hospital, it is essential that the system chosen be as free of potential errors and duplication of effort as possible.

In addition to accounting records, the respiratory care department must maintain a clinical record in each patient's chart. Simplicity is advised in the format of such a record, and a ruled sheet with a place to note date and time, type of therapy, basic physiologic and technical data, comments, and an initial or signature is adequate. Following each treatment, the therapist is expected to note on the sheet a comment concerning the treatment and the patient and any other information considered relevant. This is an invaluable guide for subsequent therapists. If possible, a duplicate record of what is to be entered in the patient's chart should serve as the basis for billing and statistics. This can be a carbon or transfer copy, which ensures as much as possible that whatever is charted is appropriately billed and reported. Also, the same charting form should be able to serve as a genesis for a work load statistical report.

Fig. 16-2, *A,* is a representative example of a patient's general care record. A more detailed record would of course be required in intensive care; Fig. 16-2, *B,* is a representative example of such a form in use in critical care.

Size of respiratory therapy department

Any opinions concerning the number of personnel, size of physical facilities, and type of equipment must be of the most general nature because of the wide variation in individual hospital needs.

Personnel and space

In determining labor requirements, factors such as the *average* work load should be determined. Parttime and "on call" help can supplement increases in the work load, whereas decreases below the average, if predicted or foreseen, will provide time for vacations, special projects, educational endeavors, or opportunities for progressive updating of the entire staff's skills. The most effective way of determining labor needed is to evaluate the work load requirements over a period of several months, with some mechanism derived to convert the amount of work load into actual total hours required to perform that work. Factors such as the number of hours in the time period being monitored, compared to the sum total of all of the hours spent doing actual work, will then, through a series of calculations, yield the number of employees needed to perform the required work.

It is strongly advised that hospitals anticipating physical expansion allow extra space above the immediate needs of the respiratory therapy service, since it can almost be guaranteed that a growing department will find its existing facilities inadequate within 2 to 3 years. The general service area should be large enough to accommodate a generous working space for repair and preventive maintenance of equipment and a convenient area for cleaning and sterilization. Bulk equipment storage space should be near the general departmental area. Provisions should also be made for office space for the medical director, the technical director, and clerical help and a writing area for record-keeping duties of the staff therapists. One of the most important contributions of respiratory therapy will be denied if an adequate outpatient services room is not provided, preferably immediately adjacent to, but separate from, the general service area. Ideally, the space provided for pulmonary function testing should be separate from but near other activities, and this can often be skillfully done by properly placed partitions in the service area or treatment room. The difficulties of incorporating new facilities into existing buildings are well recognized, and makeshift arrangements often must be made. In new construction, however, every attempt should be made to locate the general service room, the laboratory, and the outpatient area as closely as possible, preferably not far from the intensive or respiratory care units.

Equipment

In past years, there was a tremendous increase seen in the use of disposable plastic equipment, presterilized and prepackaged, to save labor costs of cleaning and sterilization. The convenience of an inventory ready to use from dealer to consumer was another asset. Most recently, however, rising costs of disposables, because of increases in the prices of petroleum products and diminishing storage areas, have considerably reduced their advantages. As a result many hospitals are returning for the most part to small inventories of recyclable items, effecting savings in more efficient systems of cleaning, sterilizing, and packaging. The choice of disposables versus nondisposables is made on the basis of cost, a task continuously facing all technical directors of busy departments.

Of nonexpendable therapy equipment, the largest and most expensive pieces are the ventilators. There is no one "best" ventilator obtainable that can perform all functions better than any other, and the decision as to which ventilator to purchase should be left to the technical director and an advisory group of supervisors and therapists. Departmental policy will determine whether it is in the best interest of the hospital to strive for maximum uniformity of procedures through the use of a limited variety of types or for greater flexibility with a wide variety. The *minimum* equipment for the pulmonary function laboratory consists of a spirometer with facilities for measurement of lung volumes, available as a single unit if desired, and a blood gas analyzer, preferably fully automated. Before investing in a large amount of equipment, those involved in the decision to purchase equipment should visit a few established departments of comparable size to determine utilization and techniques employed with that equipment.

Summary

In previous editions of this text, the summary of this section ended with the comment that respiratory therapy was "a new and expanding field seeking its proper place in the health care team." The supposition was made that respiratory therapy, being so closely associated with the treatment of cardiopulmonary disease, would fill the niche and evolve into a field of highly advanced specialization. Since that time, this supposition that respiratory therapy would evolve within the next few years into a clinical cardiopulmonary specialty is becoming more and more an undeniable fact. The outcome of what has popularly become known as the "Sugarloaf Conferences," in which a group of esteemed pulmonary physicians assembled to question the effectiveness of certain respiratory care procedures, has provided the genesis of extensive clinical research in the field of respiratory therapy and pulmonary physiology. The results of this ongoing research, and what is determined to be "appropriate" respiratory care, will produce the future direction of this field. The future of respiratory therapy lies in elements long sought and which, of necessity, have become reality: increased professional responsibility, professional objectivity in determining the value of respiratory therapy procedures, and the professional identity of a mature field.

Bibliography

Burton, G.G., Gee, G.N., and Hodgkin, J.E.: Respiratory care: a guide to clinical practice, Philadelphia, 1977, J.B. Lippincott Co.

Egan, D.F.: The stethoscope and the ledger, Chest **68**:1, 1975.

McLaughlin, A.J.: Organization and management for respiratory therapists, St. Louis, 1979, The C.V. Mosby Co.

Miller, W.F., et. al.: Guidelines for organization and function of hospital respiratory care services: section on respiratory therapy, American College of Chest Physicians, Chest **78**:1, 1980.

Rakich, J.S., Longest, B.B., and O'Donovan, T.R.: Managing health care organizations, Philadelphia, 1977, W.B. Saunders Co.

Yanda, R.L.: The need for leadership in hospital respiratory services, Chest **68**:81, 1975.

Appendix 1 Systems of measurements and equivalents

I. *Scientific notation*
   A. The purpose of scientific notation is to convert a large or small awkward number from its usual form to an integer between 1 and 10, multiplied by the appropriate power of 10 so its value is unchanged.
   B. Tabulation of the powers of 10:

   $10^0 = 1$
   $10^1 = 10$
   $10^2 = 10 \times 10 = 100$
   $10^3 = 10 \times 10 \times 10 = 1000$
   $10^4 = 10 \times 10 \times 10 \times 10 = 10,000$
   $10^5 = 10 \times 10 \times 10 \times 10 \times 10 = 100,000$
   $10^6 = 10 \times 10 \times 10 \times 10 \times 10 \times 10 = 1,000,000$

   $10^0 = 1$
   $10^{-1} = {}^1/_{10} = 0.1$
   $10^{-2} = {}^1/_{10^2} = 0.01$
   $10^{-3} = {}^1/_{10^3} = 0.001$
   $10^{-4} = {}^1/_{10^4} = 0.0001$
   $10^{-5} = {}^1/_{10^5} = 0.00001$
   $10^{-6} = {}^1/_{10^6} = 0.000001$

   C. General rules for writing scientific notation:
      1. For a number larger than 10: Move the decimal to the position to the right of the first integer, and multiply the new number by 10 raised to the power equal to the number of places the decimal was moved. Zeros to the right of the last integer may be dropped. For example:

      $2655 = 2.655 \times 10^3$
      $54,000 = 5.4 \times 10^4$

      $301,010 = 3.0101 \times 10^5$
      $866.67 = 8.6667 \times 10^2$

      2. For a number smaller than 1: Move the decimal to the position to the right of the first integer, and multiply the new number by 10 raised to a *negative* power equal to the number of places the decimal was moved. For example:

      $0.454 = 4.54 \times 10^{-1}$
      $0.00306 = 3.06 \times 10^{-3}$

      $0.00000703 = 7.03 \times 10^{-6}$
      $0.01010 = 1.01 \times 10^{-2}$

II. *Metric system*
   A. There are many excellent descriptions of the history of and justification for the metric system so we shall confine ourselves only to a re-

view of its most salient features.[1] There are three basic units of linear, weight, and volume measurement, respectively the *meter* (m), the *gram* (g), and the *liter* (ℓ), with time calibrated in *seconds* (s). From its scientific use, especially, these parameters have come to be known as the centimeter-gram-second (cgs) metric system. Even though this system has not yet become popular in the United States, there is a move among many European nations to modernize it because it is old to them. Updated metrecation would comprise the so-called *International System of Units* (SI, for Système International).[2,3] The SI consists of the following seven independent measurable quantities and their respective base units: length (meter, m); mass (kilogram, kg); time (second, s); electric current (ampere, A); temperature (Kelvin, K); luminous intensity (candela, cd); and amount of substance (mole, mol). This system is also sometimes known as the meter-kilogram-second (MKS) system.

Other units of measurement are derived from the seven base units described. The SI unit for *force* is the *newton (N)*; $1 \text{ N} = 1 \text{ m} \cdot \text{kg/s}^2$. When applied to a mass of 1 kg, the newton force will cause that mass to an acceleration of 1 m/second during each second.

The SI unit for *pressure* is the *pascal (Pa)*; $1 \text{ Pa} = 1 \text{ N/m}^2$. The pascal is a very small unit of pressure. Because 1 Pa is so small, the *kilopascal* (kPa) is typically used for physiologic measurements when units within the SI system are used. More popular in the United States are centimeters of water (cm H_2O) or millimeters of mercury (mm Hg) pressure, although kPa is gaining ground. Fig. A-1 is a chart for converting from the more traditional units of pressure to SI units and is based on the following relationship:

cm H_2O	kPa	mm Hg
10.197	1	7.501
1.359	0.133	1
1	0.098	0.736

Multiples and divisions of cgs units are related to one another as powers of 10. Multiple prefixes are in Greek, and fractional prefixes in Latin.

deka	da	$= 10^1$	deci	d	$= 10^{-1}$	nano	n	$= 10^{-9}$
hecto	h	$= 10^2$	centi	c	$= 10^{-2}$	pico	p	$= 10^{-12}$
kilo	K	$= 10^3$	milli	m	$= 10^{-3}$	femto	f	$= 10^{-15}$
mega	M	$= 10^6$	micro	μ*	$= 10^{-6}$	atto	a	$= 10^{-18}$
giga	G	$= 10^9$						
tera	T	$= 10^{12}$						

*Micro cannot be abbreviated with a small m because of a conflict with milli, and somewhat paradoxically, the Greek letter *mu*, symbolized μ, was chosen to represent it.

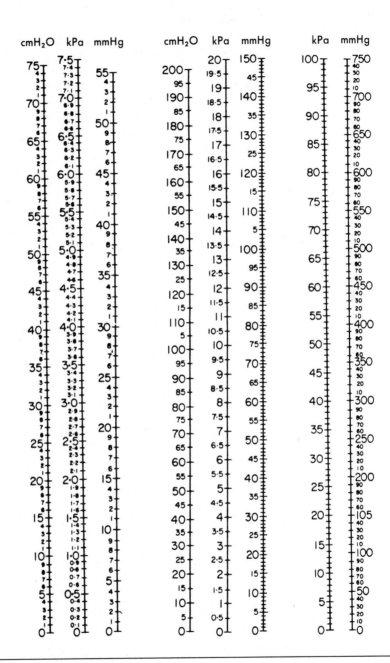

Fig. A-1   Chart for converting the more traditional units of pressure of cm H_2O and mm Hg to SI units: kPa. (From Sykes, M.K., McNichol, M.W., and Campbell, E.J.M.: Respiratory failure, ed. 2, London, 1976, Blackwell Scientific Publications.)

B. Examples of metric measurement terminology

Linear

kilometer (km)	m × 10³
hectometer	m × 10²
decameter	m × 10
meter (m)	
decimeter	m × 10⁻¹
centimeter (cm)	m × 10⁻²
millimeter (mm)	m × 10⁻³
micrometer	m × 10⁻⁶
(μ or μm)	

Weight

kilogram (kg)	g × 10³
hectogram	g × 10²
decagram	g × 10
gram (g)	
decigram	g × 10⁻¹
centigram	g × 10⁻²
milligram (mg)	g × 10⁻³
microgram (μg)	g × 10⁻⁶
nanogram (ng)	g × 10⁻⁹

Volume

kiloliter	1 × 10³
hectoliter	1 × 10²
decaliter	1 × 10
liter (ℓ)	
deciliter (dl)	1 × 10⁻¹
centiliter	1 × 10⁻²
milliliter (ml)	1 × 10⁻³
microliter (μl)	1 × 10⁻⁶
nanoliter (nl)	1 × 10⁻⁹

C. United States customary and metric equivalents

Linear

inch	2.54 cm
foot	3.048×10^{-1} m
mile	1.609 km
micron	3.937×10^{-5} in
centimeter	3.937×10^{-1} in
meter	39.37 in
kilometer	6.214×10^{-1} mi

Weight

ounce (oz)	28.35 g
pound	4.54×10^{-1} kg
gram	3.528×10^{-2} oz
kilogram	2.205 lb

Volume

ounce (fl)	29.57 ml
quart	9.463×10^{-1} ℓ
gallon	3.785 ℓ
cubic inch	16.39 ml
cubic foot	28.32 ℓ
liter	1.057 qt
	61.02 in³
	3.532×10^{-2} ft³

D. Equations to convert between Celsius and Fahrenheit temperatures

$$°C = \frac{5 \ (°F - 32)}{9}$$

$$°F = \left[\frac{9 \times °C}{5} \right] + 32$$

References

1. U.S. Department of Commerce, National Bureaus of Standards: The English and metric systems of measurement, Special Pub. 304A, rev. ed., 1970.
2. Vawter, S.M., and DeForest, R.E.: The international metric system and medicine, J.A.M.A. **218**:723, 1971.
3. Young, D.S.: Standardized reporting of laboratory data, N. Engl. J. Med. **290**:368, 1974.

Appendix 2 — Physiologic and selected physical abbreviations and symbols

Note: A small horizontal line over a symbol signifies a mean, or average value; thus ā equals mean arterial value of whatever measurement is being considered. A prime mark following a symbol indicates an end, or terminal value; thus c′ equals end capillary measurement of some variable.

a	= (1) Arterial blood	
	= (2) Acceleration	
ā	= (1) Mixed arterial blood	
	= (2) Mean acceleration	
ATPD ⎫ APTD ⎬	= Ambient temperature and pressure, dry	
ATPS ⎫ APTS ⎬	= Ambient temperature and pressure, saturated with water vapor	
&	= Alveolar gas	
b	= Blood, generally	
BTPD ⎫ BTPD ⎬	= Body temperature, ambient pressure, dry	
BTPS ⎫ BTPS ⎬	= Body temperature, ambient pressure, saturated with water vapor	
B	= Barometric	
c	= Capillary blood	
C	= (1) Compliance	
	= (2) Concentration of gas in blood	
°C	= Degree of temperature by Celsius scale	
d	= Distance covered by a moving body	
dl	= deciliter (0.1 ℓ)	
D	= (1) Diffusing capacity	
	= (2) Density	
D	= Dead space gas	
ERV	= Expiratory reserve volume	
E	= Exhaled gas	
f	= Respiratory frequency (breaths per minute)	

F	= (1) Fractional concentration of dry gas	
	= (2) Force	
°F	= Degree of temperature by Fahrenheit scale	
FRC	= Functional residual capacity	
g	= (1) Acceleration due to the force of gravity	
	= (2) Gram	
gfw	= Gram formula weight	
s	= Distance covered by a moving body	
S	= Percent saturation of hemoglobin with oxygen or carbon dioxide	
ST	= Surface tension	
STPD ⎫ STPD ⎬	= Standard temperature (0°C), standard pressure (760 mm Hg), dry	
s	= (Subscript to show steady state	
	= (1) Shunt	
t	= (1) Temperature generally	
	= (2) Time	
	= (3) Subscript means total, i.e., Q_t	
T	= Absolute temperature	
TLC	= Total lung capacity	
T	= (1) Tidal gas	
	= (2) Thorax	
v	= (1) Venous blood	
	= (2) Velocity	
gmw	= Gram molecular weight	
H^+	= Ion (hydrogen as an example)	

[H$^+$]   = Molar concentration of ions

IC   = Inspiratory capacity

IRV   = Inspiratory reserve volume

I   = Inhaled gas

K   = Constant of a chemical equilibrium (i.e., dissociation constant of a buffer system)

°K   = Degree of temperature by Kelvin scale

KE   = Kinetic energy

ℓ/min or lpm   = liters per minute

L   = Lung (pulmonary)

mb   = Millibar

mM   = Millimole (M $\times$ 10^{-3})

M   = Mole(s), molar

n   = (1) Number (especially number of molecules)

= (2) nano (10^{-9}, i.e., nM = M $\times$ 10^{-9})

pH   = Negative common logarithm of molar hydrogen ion concentration

pK   = Negative common logarithm of a chemical equilibrium constant (i.e., dissociation constant of a buffer system)

psia   = Pounds per square inch, absolute

psig   = Pounds per square inch, gauge

P   = Gas pressure

Q   = Blood volume

$\dot{Q}$ = Rate of blood flow, volume per time

R   = (1) Resistance

= (2) Respiratory exchange ratio ($\dot{V}CO_2/\dot{V}O_2$)

= (3) Universal gas constant (0.0820561)

°R   = Degree of temperature by Rankine scale

RC   = Respiratory center

RH   = Relative humidity

RV   = Residual volume

$\bar{v}$ = (1) Mixed venous blood

= (2) Mean velocity

V   = Gas volume

VC   = Vital capacity

V$_A$ = Volume of total alveolar space

V$_E$ = Volume of exhaled gas (often used for tidal volume)

V$_D$ = Volume of dead space

VD$_{alv}$ = Volume of alveolar dead space

VD$_{anat}$ = Volume of anatomic dead space

VD$_{phys}$ = Volume of physiologic dead space

V$_{RB}$ = Rebreathed volume

V$_T$ = Tidal volume

$\dot{V}$ = Rate of gas flow, volume per time

$\dot{V}_A$ = Minute alveolar ventilation (ℓ/min)

$\dot{V}_D$ = Minute dead space ventilation (ℓ/min)

$\dot{V}_E$ = Volume of exhaled gas per unit of time (usually ℓ/min, or minute volume)

Appendix 3 Altitude and depth characteristics of atmosphere*

Feet	$t°C$	Atm	psi	mm Hg	Po_2	% O_2 equiv	Density
300,000	-2.2	7.3×10^{-6}	1.1×10^{-4}	0.0055	1.1×10^{-4}	1.4×10^{-5}	8.57×10^{-6}
200,000	33.8	3.2×10^{-4}	4.6×10^{-3}	0.24	5.0×10^{-2}	6.6×10^{-3}	3.28×10^{-4}
100,000	-55.0	0.011	0.155	8.0	1.7	0.22	1.74×10^{-2}
90,000	-55.0	0.017	0.250	12.9	2.7	0.36	2.80×10^{-2}
80,000	-55.0	0.027	0.403	20.8	4.3	0.57	4.52×10^{-2}
70,000	-55.0	0.044	0.649	33.6	7.0	0.92	7.30×10^{-2}
60,000	-55.0	0.071	1.05	54.1	11.3	1.49	1.18×10^{-1}
50,000	-55.0	0.115	1.69	87.4	18.3	2.41	1.90×10^{-1}
40,000	-55.0	0.191	2.72	140.6	29.4	3.87	3.06×10^{-1}
35,000	-54.3	0.236	3.46	178.6	37.4	4.92	3.87×10^{-1}
30,000	-44.4	0.296	4.36	225.7	47.3	6.22	4.67×10^{-1}
25,000	-34.5	0.372	5.46	282.0	59.1	7.78	5.60×10^{-1}
20,000	-24.6	0.460	6.76	348.8	73.1	9.62	6.66×10^{-1}
15,000	-14.7	0.566	8.29	428.6	89.8	11.82	7.86×10^{-1}
10,000	-4.8	0.690	10.11	522.9	109.5	14.41	9.22×10^{-1}
5000	5.1	0.835	12.23	623.3	132.5	17.43	1.08
0	15.0	1.000	14.70	760.0	159.0	20.95	1.25
33		2.000	29.4	1520.0	318.0	41.90	2.50
66		3.000	44.1	2280.0	477.0	62.85	3.75
99		4.000	58.8	3040.0	636.0	83.80	5.00
132		5.000	73.5	3800.0	795.0	104.75	6.25
165		6.000	88.2	4560.0	954.0	125.70	7.50
198		7.000	102.9	5320.0	1113.0	146.65	8.75
231		8.000	117.6	6080.0	1272.0	167.60	10.00
264		9.000	132.3	6840.0	1431.0	188.55	11.25
297		10.000	147.0	7600.0	1590.0	209.50	12.50

*Modified from Dittmer, D.S., and Grebe, R.M., editors: Handbook of respiration, Philadelphia, 1958, W.B. Saunders Co.

Appendix 4 · Factors to convert gas volumes from ATPS to BTPS*

Factor to convert volume to 37°C saturated	When gas temperature (°C) is	With water vapor pressure (mm Hg)† of
1.102	20	17.5
1.096	21	18.7
1.091	22	19.8
1.085	23	21.1
1.080	24	22.4
1.075	25	23.8
1.068	26	25.2
1.063	27	26.7
1.057	28	28.3
1.051	29	30.0
1.045	30	31.8
1.039	31	33.7
1.032	32	35.7
1.026	33	37.7
1.020	34	39.9
1.014	35	42.2
1.007	36	44.6
1.000	37	47.0

Note: These factors have been calculated only for a barometric pressure of 760 mm Hg. Since factors at 22°C, for example, are 1.0904, 1.0910, and 1.0915, respectively, at barometric pressures of 770, 760, and 750 mm Hg, it is unnecessary to correct for small deviations from standard barometric pressure.

$$\text{Factor} = \frac{[760 - P_{H_2O} \text{ at } t_{amb}] \times 0.435}{[t_{amb} + 273]}$$

*Modified from Comroe, J.H., Jr.: Methods in medical research, Chicago, 1950, Year Book Medical Publishers, Inc., vol. 2.
†Water vapor pressures modified from Handbook of chemistry and physics, ed. 28, Cleveland, 1944, Chemical Rubber Publishing Co., p. 1802.

Appendix 5   Temperature correction of barometric reading*

Temperature (°C)	730 mm Hg	740	750	760	770	780
15.0	1.78	1.81	1.83	1.86	1.88	1.91
16.0	1.90	1.93	1.96	1.98	2.01	2.03
17.0	2.02	2.05	2.08	2.10	2.13	2.16
18.0	2.14	2.17	2.20	2.23	2.26	2.29
19.0	2.26	2.29	2.32	2.35	2.38	2.41
20.0	2.38	2.41	2.44	2.47	2.51	2.54
21.0	2.50	2.53	2.56	2.60	2.63	2.67
22.0	2.61	2.65	2.69	2.72	2.76	2.79
23.0	2.73	2.77	2.81	2.84	2.88	2.92
24.0	2.85	2.89	2.93	2.97	3.01	3.05
25.0	2.97	3.01	3.05	3.09	3.13	3.17
26.0	3.09	3.13	3.17	3.21	3.26	3.30
27.0	3.20	3.25	3.29	3.34	3.38	3.42
28.0	3.32	3.37	3.41	3.46	3.51	3.55
29.0	3.44	3.49	3.54	3.58	3.63	3.68
30.0	3.56	3.61	3.66	3.71	3.75	3.80
31.0	3.68	3.73	3.78	3.83	3.88	3.93
32.0	3.79	3.85	3.90	3.95	4.00	4.05
33.0	3.91	3.97	4.02	4.07	4.13	4.18
34.0	4.03	4.09	4.14	4.20	4.25	4.31
35.0	4.15	4.21	4.26	4.32	4.38	4.43

*From U.S. Department of Commerce, Weather Bureau: Barometers and the measurement of atmospheric pressure, Washington, D.C., 1941, U.S. Government Printing Office.

Appendix 6

Factors to convert gas volumes from ATPS to STPD

Observed P_B	15°	16°	17°	18°	19°	20°	21°	22°	23°	24°	25°	26°	27°	28°	29°	30°	31°	32°
700	0.855	851	847	842	838	834	829	825	821	816	812	807	802	797	793	788	783	778
702	857	853	849	845	840	836	832	827	823	818	814	809	805	800	795	790	785	780
704	860	856	852	847	843	839	834	830	825	821	816	812	807	802	797	792	787	783
706	862	858	854	850	845	841	837	832	828	823	819	814	810	804	800	795	790	785
708	865	861	856	852	848	843	839	834	830	825	821	816	812	807	802	797	792	787
710	867	863	859	855	850	846	842	837	833	828	824	819	814	809	804	799	795	790
712	870	866	861	857	853	848	844	839	836	830	826	821	817	812	807	802	797	792
714	872	868	864	859	855	851	846	842	837	833	828	824	819	814	809	804	799	794
716	875	871	866	862	858	853	849	844	840	835	831	826	822	816	812	807	802	797
718	877	873	869	864	860	856	851	847	842	838	833	828	824	819	814	809	804	799
720	880	876	871	867	863	858	854	849	845	840	836	831	826	821	816	812	807	802
722	882	878	874	869	865	861	856	852	847	843	838	833	829	824	819	814	809	804
724	885	880	876	872	867	863	858	854	849	845	840	835	831	826	821	816	811	806
726	887	883	879	874	870	866	861	856	852	847	843	838	833	829	825	818	813	808
728	890	886	881	877	872	868	863	859	854	850	845	840	836	831	826	821	816	811
730	892	888	884	879	875	870	866	861	857	852	847	843	838	833	828	823	818	813
732	895	891	886	882	877	873	868	864	859	854	850	845	840	836	831	825	820	815
734	897	893	889	884	880	875	871	866	862	857	852	847	843	838	833	828	823	818
736	900	895	891	887	882	878	873	869	864	859	855	850	845	840	835	830	825	820
738	902	898	894	889	885	880	876	871	866	862	857	852	848	843	838	833	828	822
740	905	900	896	892	887	883	878	874	869	864	860	855	850	845	840	835	830	825
742	907	903	898	894	890	885	881	876	871	867	862	857	852	847	842	837	832	827
744	910	906	901	897	892	888	883	878	874	869	864	859	855	850	845	840	834	829
746	912	908	903	899	895	890	886	881	876	872	867	862	857	852	847	842	837	832
748	915	910	906	901	897	892	888	883	879	874	869	864	860	854	850	845	839	834
750	917	913	908	904	900	895	890	886	881	876	872	867	862	857	852	847	842	837
752	920	915	911	906	902	897	893	888	883	879	874	869	864	859	854	849	844	839
754	922	918	913	909	904	900	895	891	886	881	876	872	867	862	857	852	846	841
756	925	920	916	911	907	902	898	893	888	883	879	874	869	864	859	854	849	844
758	927	923	918	914	909	905	900	896	891	886	881	876	872	866	861	856	851	846
760	930	925	921	916	912	907	902	898	893	888	883	879	874	869	864	859	854	848

762	932	928	923	919	914	910	905	900	896	891	886	881	876	871	866	861	856	851
764	934	930	926	921	916	912	907	903	898	893	888	884	879	874	869	864	858	853
766	937	933	928	925	919	915	910	905	900	896	891	886	881	876	871	866	861	855
768	940	935	931	926	922	917	912	908	903	898	893	888	883	878	873	868	863	858
770	942	938	933	928	924	919	915	910	905	901	896	891	886	881	876	871	865	860
772	945	940	936	931	926	922	917	912	908	903	898	893	888	883	878	873	868	862
774	947	943	938	933	929	924	920	915	910	905	901	896	891	886	880	875	870	865
776	950	945	941	936	931	927	922	917	912	908	903	898	893	888	883	878	872	867
778	952	948	943	938	934	929	924	920	915	910	905	900	895	890	885	880	875	869
780	955	950	945	941	936	932	927	922	917	912	908	903	898	892	887	882	877	872

$$\text{Factor} = \frac{[P_{B_{abs}} \text{ corrected for } t_{amg} - P_{H_2O} \text{ at } t_{amb}] \times 0.359}{[t_{amb} + 273]}$$

Appendix 7 Factors to convert
gas volumes from
STPD to BTPS at given
barometric pressures

Pressure	Factor	Pressure	Factor
740	1.245	760	1.211
742	1.241	762	1.208
744	1.238	764	1.203
746	1.235	766	1.200
748	1.232	768	1.196
750	1.227	770	1.193
752	1.224	772	1.190
754	1.221	774	1.188
756	1.217	776	1.183
758	1.214	778	1.181

$$\text{Factor} = \frac{863}{[P_{B_{amb}} - 47]}$$

Appendix 8 Low-temperature characteristics of selected gases and water

Substance	Critical temperature °C	Critical temperature °F	Critical pressure atm	Boiling point °C	Boiling point °F	Melting (freezing) point °C	Melting (freezing) point °F
Acetylene	36.0	96.0	62.0	− 88.5	− 119.2	− 81.8	− 114.6
Air	− 140.7	− 221.0	37.2	− 194.4	− 317.9	—	—
Ammonia	132.4	270.3	111.5	− 33.4	− 28.1	− 77.7	− 108.0
Carbon dioxide	31.1	87.9	73.0	− 78.5	− 109.3	− 56.6	− 69.9
Cyclopropane	124.7	256.4	54.2	− 32.9	− 27.2	− 127.5	− 197.7
Freon-12	111.6	233.6	40.6	− 29.8	− 21.6	− 158.0	− 252.4
Freon-14	− 45.4	− 49.9	36.8	− 128.0	− 198.4	− 184.0	− 299.2
Helium	− 267.9	− 450.2	2.3	− 268.9	− 452.1	− 272.2	− 455.8
Hydrogen	− 239.9	− 399.8	12.8	− 252.8	− 423.0	− 259.2	− 434.5
Nitrogen	− 147.1	− 232.6	33.5	− 195.8	− 320.5	− 209.9	− 345.9
Nitrous oxide	36.5	97.7	71.8	− 88.5	− 127.2	− 90.8	− 131.6
Oxygen	− 118.8	− 181.1	49.7	− 183.0	− 297.3	− 218.4	− 361.8
Propane	95.6	206.2	43.0	− 42.2	− 43.7	− 189.9	− 305.8
Water	374.0	705.0	218.0	100.0	212.0	0.0	32.0

Appendix 9

Selected elements and radicals: symbols, approximate atomic weights, valences

Element	Symbol	Atomic weight	Valence
Aluminum	Al	27.0	+3
Argon	A	39.9	0
Arsenic	As	74.9	+3, 5
Barium	Ba	137.4	+2
Bromine	Br	79.9	-1, 3, 5, 7
Calcium	Ca	40.0	+2
Carbon	C	12.0	+2, 4, -4
Chlorine	Cl	35.5	-1, 3, 5, 7
Copper	Cu	63.5	+1, 2
Fluorine	F	19.0	-1
Germanium	Ge	72.6	+4, -4
Helium	He	4.0	0
Hydrogen	H	1.0	±1
Iodine	I	126.9	-1, 3, 5, 7
Iron	Fe	55.9	+2, 3
Krypton	Kr	83.8	0
Lead	Pb	207.2	+2, 4
Magnesium	Mg	24.3	+2
Mercury	Hg	200.6	+1, 2
Neon	Ne	20.2	0
Nitrogen	N	14.0	+3, 5
Oxygen	O	16.0	-2
Phosphorus	P	31.0	+3, 5
Potassium	K	39.1	+1
Silicon	Si	28.1	+4, -4
Silver	Ag	107.9	+1
Sodium	Na	23.0	+1
Tin	Sn	118.7	+2, 4
Sulfur	S	32.0	±2, 4, 6
Xenon	Xe	131.3	0
Zinc	Zn	65.4	+2

Radical	Symbol	Valence
Acetate	CH_3COO	-1
Ammonium	NH_4	-1
Bicarbonate	HCO_3	-1
Borate	BO_3	-3
Carbonate	CO_3	-2
Chlorate	ClO_3	-1
Hydroxyl	OH	-1
Nitrate	NO_3	-1
Nitrite	NO_2	-1
Phosphate	PO_4	-3
Sulfate	SO_4	-2

Appendix 10   Calculation of P_{CO_2} from H-H equation

$$pH = 6.1 + \log \left[\frac{HCO_3}{\text{Dissolved } CO_2} \right]$$

$$\text{antilog } (pH - 6.1) = \frac{\text{Total } CO_2}{0.03 \; P_{CO_2}} - 1$$

$$pH = 6.1 + \log \left[\frac{\text{Total } CO_2 - 0.03 \; P_{CO_2}}{0.03 \; P_{CO_2}} \right]$$

$$\text{antilog } (pH - 6.1) + 1 = \frac{\text{Total } CO_2}{0.03 \; P_{CO_2}}$$

$$pH - 6.1 = \log \left[\frac{\text{Total } CO_2}{0.03 \; P_{CO_2}} - 1 \right]$$

$$P_{CO_2} = \frac{\text{Total } CO_2}{0.03 \times [1 + \text{antilog } (pH - 6.1)]}$$

Appendix 11 Relation of
arterial oxygen
saturation to
capillary unsaturation

With 15 g/dl of hemoglobin and an arterial-venous oxygen content difference of 5.0 vol%, the a-v oxygen saturation difference is 24%. The arterial oxygen saturation required to produce a specific concentration, in grams per deciliter, of unsaturated capillary blood hemoglobin can be computed by the following formula, derived below:

$$Sa_{O_2} = \frac{16.8 - y}{15}$$

(1) Mean capillary unsaturation $= \dfrac{\text{Arterial unsaturation} + \text{Venous unsaturation}}{2}$

(2) $x = Sa_{O_2}$ thus $(1.00 - x) = $ Arterial unsaturation
$(x - 0.24) = Sv_{O_2}$
$(1.00 - [x - 0.24]) = $ Venous unsaturation
$y = $ g/dl unsaturated hemoglobin in capillary blood

(3) Substituting in (1) above:

$$\frac{15 (1.00 - x) + 15 (1.00 - [x - 0.24])}{2} = y$$

(4) $15 - 15x + 15 - 15x + 3.60 = 2y$

(5) $-30x + 33.6 = 2y$

(6) $x = \dfrac{16.8 - y}{15}$

Appendix 12 Alveolar air equation

Accurate measurement of alveolar oxygen tension by direct analysis of alveolar air samples is difficult because of the inability to obtain reliable samples that are representative of all lung areas. The alveolar air equation permits calculation of a close estimation of $P_{A_{O_2}}$ if the $F_{I_{O_2}}$, Pa_{CO_2}, and respiratory exchange ratio ($\dot{V}_{CO_2}/\dot{V}_{O_2}$) are known. Its derivation is well explained by Comroe* and need not be repeated here, but its application will be demonstrated by two examples. The equation is stated as follows:

$$P_{A_{O_2}} = F_{I_{O_2}}(713) - Pa_{CO_2}\left(F_{I_{O_2}} + \frac{1 - F_{I_{O_2}}}{R}\right)$$

Example 1: Calculate $P_{A_{O_2}}$ breathing room air, when $Pa_{CO_2} = 40$ mm Hg, and $R = 0.8$:

$$P_{A_{O_2}} = 0.21(713) - 40\left(0.21 + \frac{1 - 0.21}{0.8}\right)$$
$$= 149.73 - 40(1.198)$$
$$= 149.73 - 47.92$$
$$= 101.8 \text{ mm Hg}$$

Example 2: Calculate $P_{A_{O_2}}$ breathing 40% oxygen, when $Pa_{CO_2} = 55$ mm Hg, and $R = 0.9$:

$$P_{A_{O_2}} = 0.40(713) - 55\left(0.40 + \frac{1 - 0.40}{0.9}\right)$$
$$= 285.2 - 55(1.07)$$
$$= 285.2 - 58.85$$
$$= 226.4 \text{ mm Hg}$$

*Modified from Comroe, J.H., Jr., et al.: The lung, Chicago, 1962, Year Book Medical Publishers, Inc.

Appendix 13 Breathing nomogram*

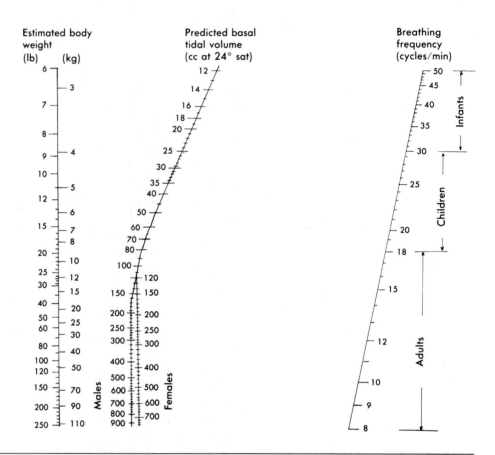

Corrections of predicted basal tidal volumes.
    For patients not in coma: add 10%
    Fever: add 5% for each °F above 99 (rectal)
           add 9% for each °C above 37 (rectal)
    Altitude: add 5% for each 2000 feet above sea level
          add 8% for each 1000 meters above sea level
    Intubation: subtract volume equal to one-half body weight in pounds
          subtract 1 cc/kg of body weight
    Dead space: add equipment dead space

*Modified from Radford, E.P., Jr.: Ventilation standards for use in artificial respiration, J. Appl. Physiol. 7:451, 1955.

Answers
to exercises

Exercise 1-1
- A. 1.161 g/ℓ F. 1.455
- B. 0.759   G. 0.429
- C. 4.65   H. 0.554
- D. 1.250   I. 2.120
- E. 2.857   J. 1.445

Exercise 1-2
- A. 1023.1 g/cm^2
- B. 15.4 lb/in^2
- C. 14.8 lb/in^2
- D. 982.1 g/cm^2
- E. 34.8 ft H$_2$O
- F. 751.2 mm Hg
- G. 30.9 in Hg
- H. 11 mm Hg
- I. 763 mm Hg
- J. 1022 mb

Exercise 1-3
- A. 157.5 mm Hg
- B. 167.7 mm Hg
- C. 668.3 mm Hg
- D. 400.4 mm Hg
- E. 124.5 ft

Exercise 1-4
- A. $P_2 = P_1V_1T_2/V_2T_1$
- B. $T_1 = P_1V_1T_2/P_2V_2$
- C. $V_1 = P_2V_2T_1/P_1T_2$
- D. $T_2 = P_2V_2T_1/P_1V_1$

Exercise 1-5
- A. 137 ml   D. 20.9 ℓ
- B. 2.55 ℓ E. 94.4 ml
- C. 348 ml

Exercise 1-6
- A. 251.6 ml   D. 358.2 ml
- B. 1.896 ℓ E. 2.370 ℓ
- C. 59.72 ml

Exercise 1-7
- A. $V_1 \times 726.4 \times 303/694.6 \times 303$
- B. $V_1 \times 724.7 \times 297/734.6 \times 297$
- C. $V_1 \times 724.1 \times 298/741 \times 293$
- D. $V_1 \times 754.2 \times 295/715.6 \times 288$
- E. $V_1 \times 763 \times 303/734.4 \times 297$

Exercise 2-1
- A. 80.9 g   F. 56.1 g
- B. 32.7 g   G. 49.7 g
- C. 47 g   H. 26 g
- D. 47.3 g   I. 35 g
- E. 17 g   J. 29.15 g

Exercise 2-2
- A. 31.15 g
- B. 55.5 g
- C. 54.7 g
- D. 51.7 g
- E. Al = 32.2 g; OH = 48.3 g; Cl = 96.5 g

Exercise 2-3
- A. 1.99 gEw   D. 0.193 gEw
- B. 0.9 gEw   E. 22.3 gEw
- C. 2.19 gEw

Exercise 2-4
- A. 100 mEq   D. 204.5 mg
- B. 0.1 mEq   E. 1.614 g
- C. 17.8 mEq

Exercise 2-5
- A. 129 mEq/ℓ D. 4.5 mEq/ℓ
- B. 291 mg/dℓ E. 159 mg/dℓ
- C. 5.9 mEq/ℓ

Exercise 2-6
- A. 9 g   F. 500 ml
- B. 1 ml   G. 51.3 g
- C. 25 g:225 g   H. 0.5 N
- D. 249.5 g   I. 100 ml
- E. 2.5 M   J. 114 mg

Exercise 2-7
- A. 22.5 ml
- B. 13 ml
- C. 10.14%
- D. 0.8 ml
- E. 1.5 N

Exercise 2-8
- A. 6.42×10^{-5}
- B. 1.84×10^{-5}

Exercise 2-9
- A. 4.12
- B. 1.52
- C. 11.29
- D. 7.99
- E. 9.06

Exercise 2-10
- A. 6.17×10^{-4}
- B. 1.21×10^{-9}
- C. 9.77×10^{-6}
- D. 5.50×10^{-11}
- E. 2.19×10^{-7}

Exercise 4-1
- A. 13.6 cm H$_2$O
- B. 2.33×10^{-2} cm
  (233 μ)

Exercise 4-2
- C_T = 0.18 ℓ/cm H$_2$O

Exercise 6-1
- 2.01 times as diffusible

Exercise 6-2
- A. 7.49   F. 23.9
- B. 7.32   G. 35.3   33.7
- C. 6.82   H. 31.1   29.9
- D. 53.2   I. 13.1   12.4
- E. 22.6

Index

A